Omega-Z Diet for Weight Loss

Copyright © 2022 by C. Anna Kebles, Ph.D., R. D., CHES

Copyright © 2022 Omega-Z Diet Books

All rights reserved. This publication is protected by copyright. No part of this book may be used or reproduced in any manner whatsoever without written permission. Permission should be obtained by the author prior to any prohibited reproduction, storage in a retrieval system, or transmission in any form or by any means, electronic, mechanical, photocopying, recording or likewise. For information regarding permissions, request forms and the appropriate contacts please visit omegazdietbooks.com

Originally published in paperback and ebook by Amazon.

Paperback: ISBN 978-1-7360024-3-8

ebook ISBN 978-1-7360024-0-7

This book is written as a source of information only. The information contained in this book should by no means be considered a substitute for the advice of qualified medical professionals, who should always be consulted before beginning any diet, exercise or other health program.

All efforts have been made to ensure the accuracy of the information contained in this book as of its date of publication. The authors disclaim responsibility for any adverse effects arising from the use or application of the information contained herin.

Front Cover Credit: Tharin White

Graphic Image Credit: Kayla Follin and Tharin White

Formatting Credit: Kayla Follin

Contents

Acknowledgments

Introduction

Part 1 – Expanding and Clarifying your Nutrition Understanding

Ch 1 – Relationship with Food 1

Ch 2 – Fad Diets 13

Ch 3 – Calories 21

Ch 4 – Micronutrients 29

Ch 5 – Macronutrients 39

Ch 6 – Protein 47

Ch 7 – Fat 55

Ch 8 – Metabolism 65

Ch 9 – Supplements 99

Ch 10 – Exercise 105

References 111

Part 2: Chapter 11 – Rating Popular Diets

The Criteria and Rankings 122

Diets Rated in Alphabetical Order 130

Rating the Diets

02 Diet through Flat Belly Diet 132-199

Flavor Point Diet through Intermittent Fasting Diet 200-224

Jenny Craig Diet through Skinny Vegan Diet 226-292

Slim Fast Diet through Zone Diet 293-323

Acknowledgments

Special thanks go to my friend and colleague, Dr. Mark Hemric, Ph.D., who has been my partner in writing. His knowledge of biochemistry, metabolic pathways and metabolism was essential in accurately relaying the supporting background material for these diets. Mark contributed his expertise to the book's extensive Metabolism chapter, which retains my first-person voice for consistency. Thanks to Mark for his knowledge and insights.

Thanks to my friend and colleague, Lynzi Glasscock, M.P.H., whose organizational, fact checking, and creativity skills were heavily relied upon throughout the creation and execution of this project.

Many thanks to Tharin White and Kayla Follin for their ideas, creativity and skills used in developing many appealing images and icons used to increase the user friendliness of this book.

A special thanks to Kathy Glass for her patience, keen eye and helpful suggestions! She is the best editor ever.

And a special thanks to Kayla Follin who received and adjusted all kinds of documents, images and ideas and pulled them all together to make a beautifully formatted book.

Introduction

I am excited to introduce you to the Omega-Z Diet. It provides you, the Christian Health Care Professional, with the tools needed to evaluate diets that you, your patients, and your clients encounter. Omega (Ω) means the end of something. It can signify a grand closure, or the end of something very long. That is exactly what this book does. It brings closure to the out-of-control chaos many dieters experience while simply trying to understand how to best eat for weight loss. The goal of the Omega-Z Diet is to put an *end* to the dieting chaos and confusion for both dieters and their health care providers. Perhaps this will be the last diet you'll ever try, making it the end of a long search.

A peer-reviewed study published in March 2020 assessed the top 100 best-selling nutritional books for the claims made, along with the credentials and qualifications of the authors making these claims. Some authors have more than one best-selling book. Out of 83 authors, 33 had either an M.D. or Ph.D. Twenty-eight were physicians and only three were dietitians. Many of the authors were personal trainers, bloggers, and even actors. So, you can see, lots of diet information is being dispersed to the public, but not all of it is sound or safe.

The diet industry is a multi-billion-dollar-a-year industry. Yet, diets are like fashion: they come and go. Diets get recycled under different names; minor tweaks are made, then the diets are rebranded. All diets promise wonderful benefits. But because not all diets deliver what they promise, dieters are left wondering where to turn, who to trust, and what is true. In other words, as you already know, many dieters experience mass confusion when it comes to sorting through facts, myths, diet claims, and dieting concepts. And let's be honest, most health care providers didn't have the opportunity to take many courses in nutrition. Yet they often bear the brunt of answering the public's dietary inquiries.

Within these pages are all the tools you need to sort through and evaluate diets, so you can confidently guide your patients and clients who have questions about weight loss. You will find explanations, definitions, and concepts that you can apply to any fad diet that comes your way. This book will equip you with valuable facts so you can help your patients and clients lose weight and keep it off. In this fast-paced, high-tech world, we find that the timeless truths of God's Word apply. Nutrition is important to God. He is the one who created food for our enjoyment and our health. Thus, it should not come as a surprise that the Bible is full of wisdom in all aspects of life, including food, nutrition, and dieting.

In the past 30 years of working with the public I have heard many questions from clients, patients, and students about weight loss. Much of their confusion would not exist if they only understood the key concepts—concepts we will review, explain, and apply to popular fad diets in this book.

How much protein should I eat? Are eggs good for me? Which is the best diet? These are valid questions, and all have one thing in common: the best answer is "It depends." This is because we are all unique individuals created in God's image. We are all in unique situations running the race God has set before us. This uniqueness, combined with the fact that there are so many popular diets, can make sorting through diet books and media hype difficult for your patients and clients. Some diets claim they fuel for peak performance, some diets claim they bring about fast weight loss, some diets claim to reduce the risk of heart disease. Other diets are about cutting out gluten, or cutting carbohydrates, or primarily losing belly fat. As such, there is no one diet that is best for everyone, but the reality is that the diet industry leaves most people confused.

Let's face it: everyone is on a diet. Even if we eat nothing, we are on a diet, the "Starvation Diet." If we eat everything we see, then we are on the "See-Food Diet." This book is specifically designed to help Christian Health Care Professionals assist their otherwise healthy clients and patients lose body fat in a healthy way so they can keep it off. This book is also for people who simply want to make heads or tails of diets out there. Although this book was not designed for people who are on or who need medical nutrition therapy due to having a specific health problem, it addresses many concepts that, if properly applied while under the care of their physician, can help people with excess body fat who may suffer from chronic conditions.

There are many approaches to using *The Omega-Z Diet* book and the systems herein. This book is divided into two parts. Part 1 is a review of basic nutrition concepts and truths related to weight management. It discusses macro- and micronutrients, how the body uses them, and how they impact health. This part provides an in-depth discussion on why so many people struggle with weight loss and how to identify fad diets. Nutrient-dense foods, body composition, phytonutrients, glycemic index/glycemic load, and the dangers of eating too little and too much protein as well as protein's role in weight loss and how much protein is needed are all addressed. This first part also includes information on belly fat, how fat grows, losing belly fat, basal metabolic rate, states of metabolism, metabolic pathways, metabolic hormones, substances that increase satiety, substances that decrease satiety, as well as practical aspects of fasting, proposed benefits of intermittent fasting, ketosis and the ketogenic approach to weight loss, and acid-base balance.

Using colorful, inviting charts, Part 2 rates the most popular weight-loss diets as poor, fair, good, or excellent on 17 different criteria including cost, sustainability, ease of use, and ability to be tailored or to accommodate individual uniqueness of different dieters. This part examines claims made by each diet and discusses scientific truths and myths, as well as positive and negative aspects of each diet. When appropriate, suggestions on how each diet can be improved are also offered, along with practical applications. For dieters who want a deeper understanding of specific concepts, "more information" icons are dispersed throughout this part of the book.

"More information" icons help the reader quickly find relevant information pertaining to a diet(s) of interest. For example, if the metabolic changes that occur while participating in the Ketogenic Diet are of special interest, but time constraints won't allow all of Part 1 to be read, simply read the pages in Part 2 covering the 17 criteria, the claims, truths, myths, and positive and negatives specific to the Ketogenic Diet. Then, following the page numbers identified in the "more information" icons, flip to the pages in Part 1 providing the scientific background and specific concepts involved in the Ketogenic Diet.

This approach allows dieters and health care providers alike to compare and contrast various diets they are considering trying or recommending. It provides dieters with resources to verify claims they hear about diets and different diet approaches to weight loss.

The *Omega-Z Diet for Weight Loss Workbook* is also available for patients or clients wanting to design and execute a personal plan for themselves. The workbook provides templates, recipes, and meal plans along with worksheets to make the plan personal and individualized to meet the dieter's unique needs and lifestyle.

The goal of this book is to put an end to the dieting chaos and confusion. After all, our God is not a God of confusion but of peace.

*Marton RM, Wang X, Barabasi AL, Ioannidis JPA. *Science, advocacy, and quackery in nutritional books: An analysis of conflicting advice and purported claims of nutritional best-sellers.* Palgrave Commun. 2020; 6:43. doi:10.1057/s41599-020-0415-6.

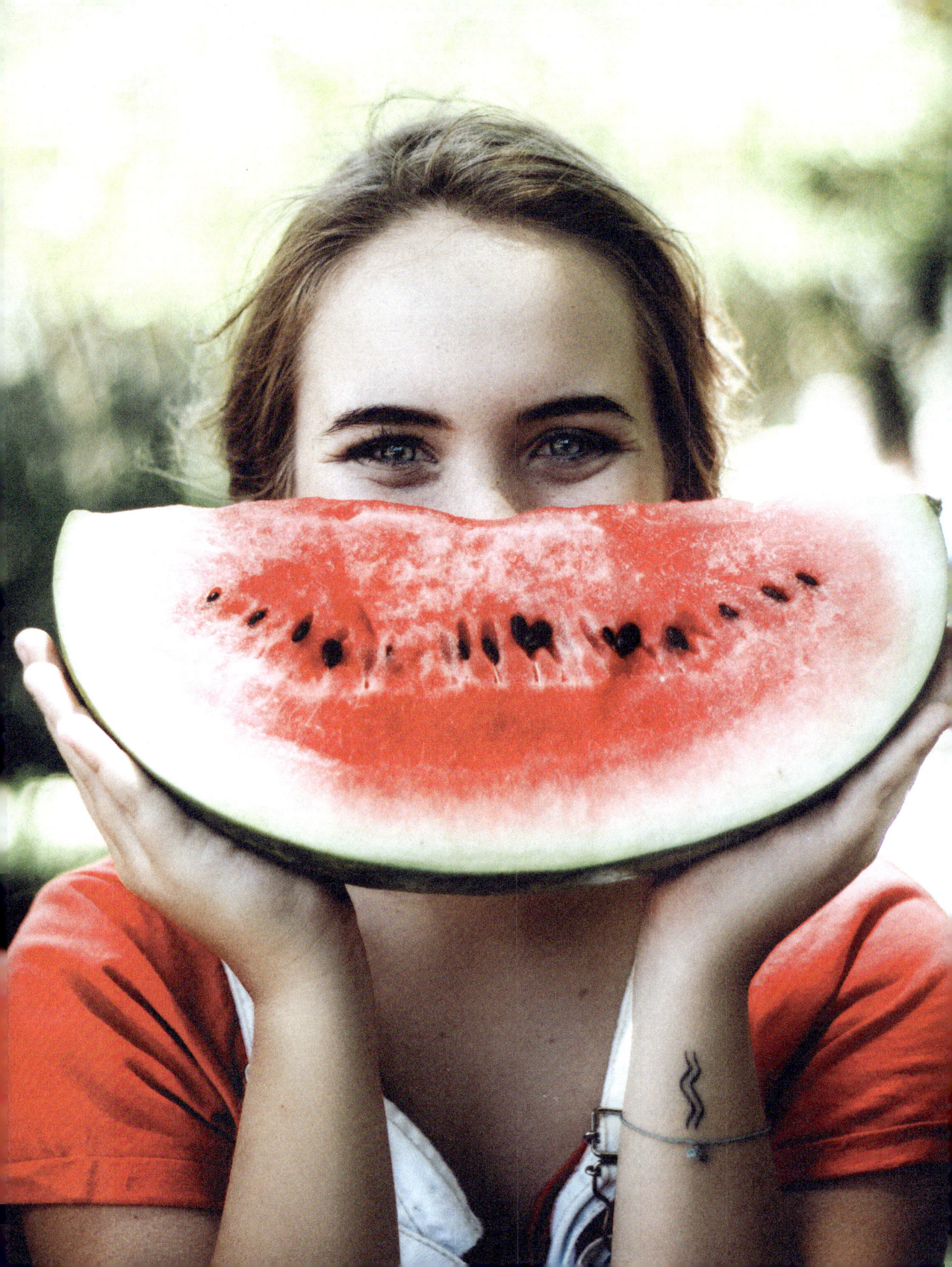

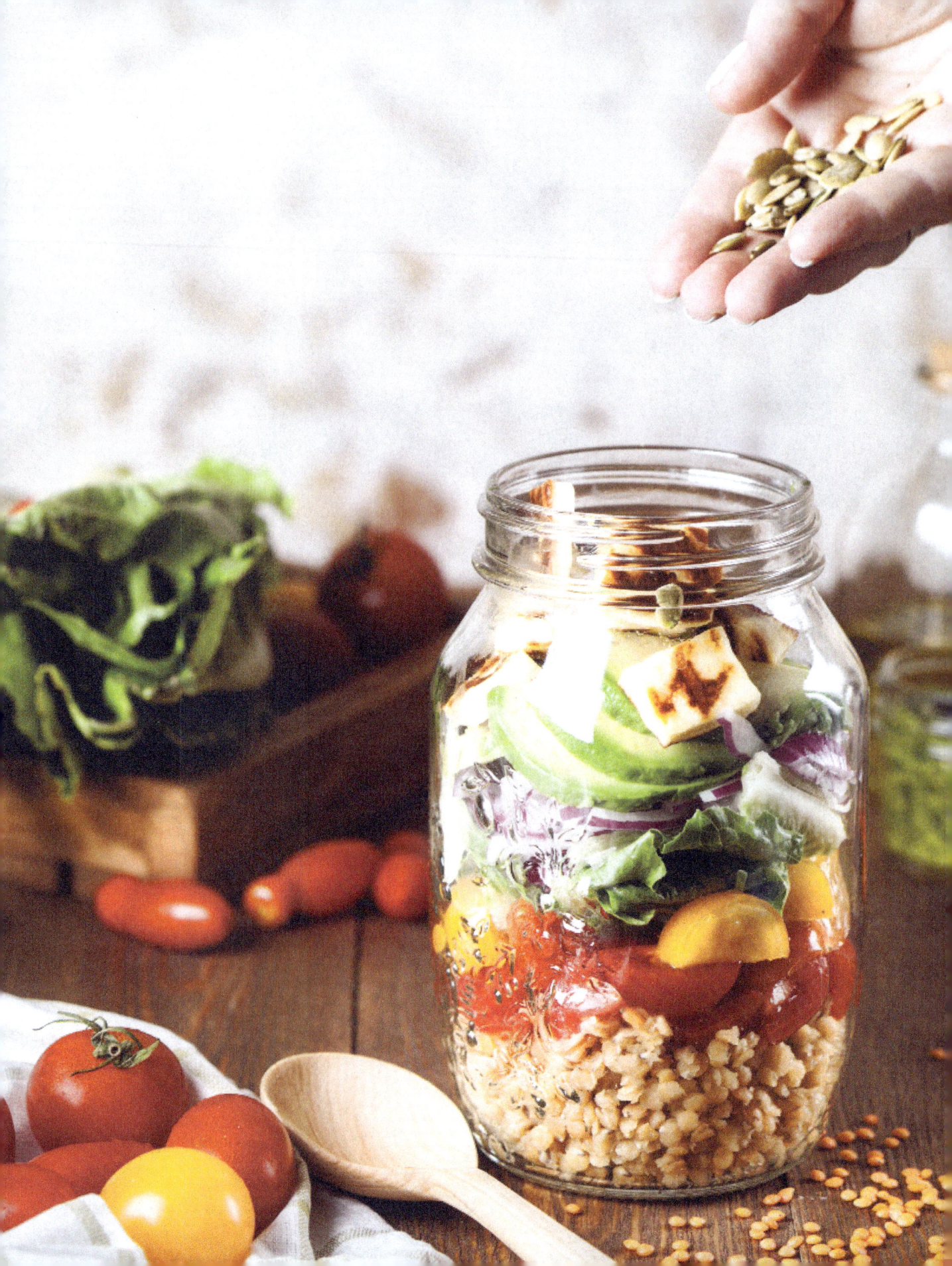

PART 1

Expanding and Clarifying your Nutrition Understanding

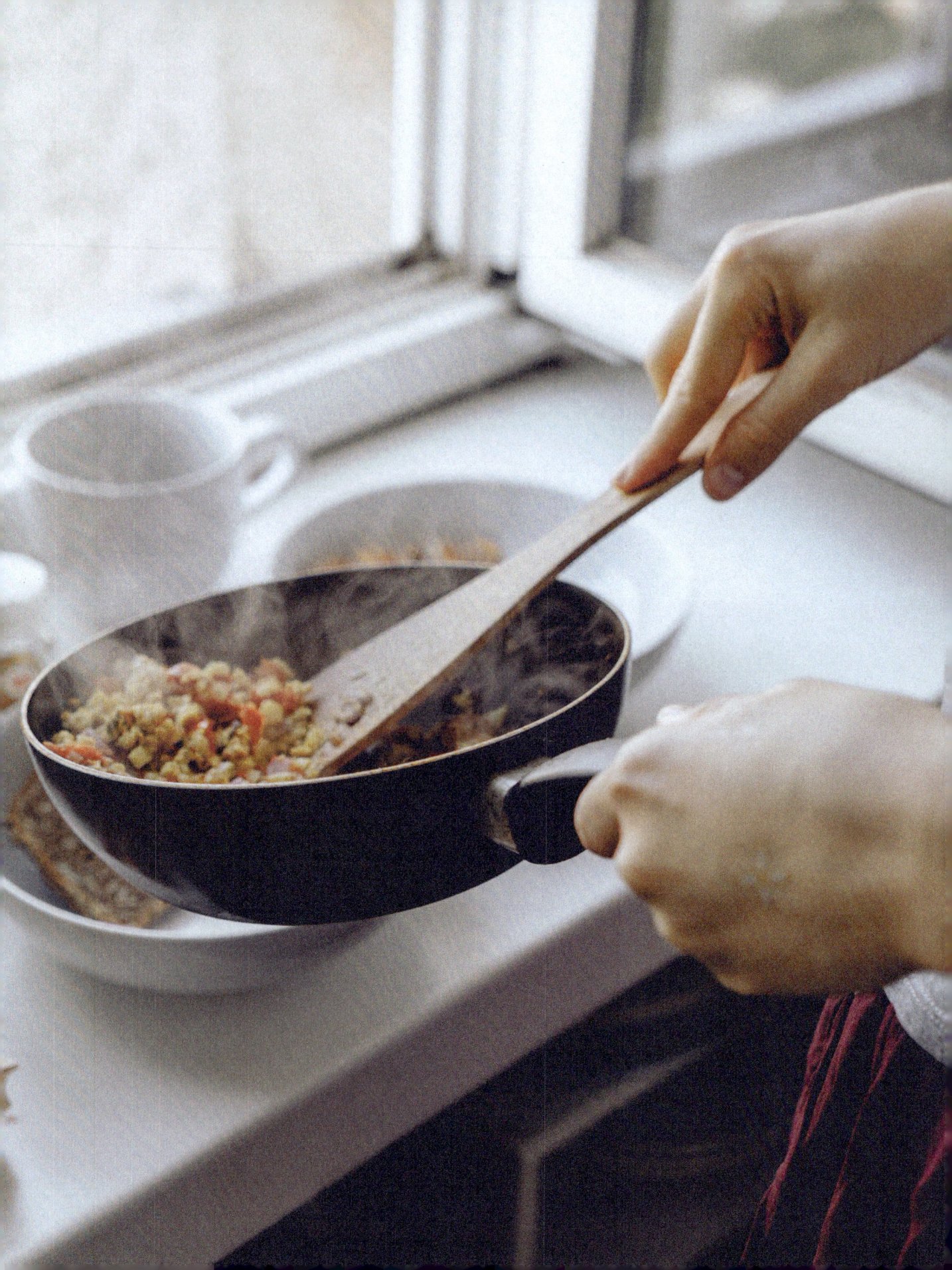

CHAPTER 1
What shapes one's relationship with food?

"Iron sharpens iron, and one man sharpens another." —Proverbs 27:17

It is safe to say that the Lord desires to be glorified through each one of us. Since our bodies are precious gifts from our creator and temples of the Holy Spirit, it is clear that how we care for our bodies affects our relationship with the Lord as well as everything we do. Since eating influences how we fuel our bodies, let's begin by considering what influences eating.

There are many factors that influence food choices and ultimately weight, weight loss, and health. Some influences lead to healthy choices that will enhance and strengthen the body, while other dynamics will lead to unhealthy choices leaving one devoid of energy, disabled, or even closer to premature death. One thing is certain: food choices are personal and complex, and as such, they are often a touchy subject for people. Many people become defensive and feel judged when others ask them about their food choices. And yet, it is a topic into which many people have not put much thought. If your patients or clients have access to many types of foods, why do they choose one food over another? The reality is, everyone has a relationship with food. Some have a healthy relationship with food that brings joy and health, while some have an unhealthy relationship with food that can bring pain and disease.

While genetics may play a part in preferences, life experiences will shape choices and perceptions about food. Let's examine 10 of the top factors that influence food choices. As you review these, think about how they may fit into the lives of your patients and clients.

Consider for a moment your family and how you were raised. Consider what mealtimes were like growing up. Consider not only the foods that were available and how they were prepared, but also who prepared them and how they were presented to you. Consider their impact on your emotions or the emotions of others in the family. If you think about this, it may help you consider and recognize that each patient or client you see has a different set of circumstances that will impact them, and ultimately their health.

> **RECAP:** Every one of us has a unique and personal history and relationship with food. It is important to examine and understand the unique relationship with food that your patients and clients may have.

1. Social Interactions and Celebrations

"Not neglecting to meet together, as is the habit of some, but encouraging one another, and all the more as you see the Day drawing near." —Hebrews 10:25

Many people grow up in homes where food is central to social gatherings. Think for a moment about how your family celebrated important holiday seasons. Are there certain food items that are unique to your family at Thanksgiving celebrations? Perhaps it is sweet potatoes with brown sugar and marshmallows, or maybe it's green bean casserole. For some reason, my family always served red cabbage and creamed onions. Interestingly, Thanksgiving dinner was the only time of the year those two dishes were made in my family. But Thanksgiving wouldn't feel right if those two dishes weren't on the table. They have become a Thanksgiving tradition.

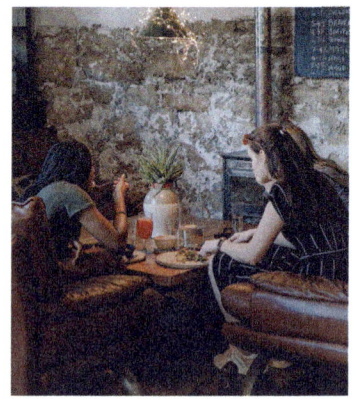

As a child, do you recall having piping hot ramen noodles at a birthday party? Or did you have expectations that cake and ice cream would be served? How would you have felt if there was none? How would you feel if no "goodie bag" was distributed as you left the party? Would that have felt normal? At this point, you have undoubtedly attended several bridal showers, baby showers, and wedding receptions. Do you have expectations that you will be fed at these events? Perhaps you even had expectations that certain kinds of foods would be served at the events. Have you ever been served hot dogs at a wedding reception? Or black licorice as the dessert at a baby shower? While some of you may have answered "yes," most probably answered "no." That is because we have developed certain expectations about food and gatherings. For many people, activities such as watching football bring with them an expectation that certain foods will be enjoyed as part of the event. In the case of football, it is most likely not caviar or orange juice. Gathering and socializing are important. We were created to be part of a family and to commune together. One way people celebrate being together is with food. There are many instances in the Bible of gathering together and sharing a meal:

"Ordering the people to sit down on the grass, He took the five loaves and the two fish, and looking up toward heaven, He blessed the food, and breaking the loaves He gave them to the disciples, and the disciples gave them to the crowds...." —Matthew 14:19

"They began to relate their experiences on the road and how He was recognized by them in the breaking of the bread." —Luke 24:35

"On the first day of the week, when we were gathered together to break bread, Paul began talking to them, intending to leave the next day, and he prolonged his message until midnight." —Acts 20:7

> **RECAP:** Family traditions and social gatherings influence food choices.

2. Taste, Flavor, and Enjoyment

"There is nothing better for a person than that he should eat and drink and find enjoyment in his toil. This also, I saw, is from the hand of God." —Ecclesiastes 2:24

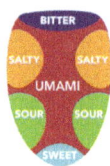

The human tongue has more than 10,000 taste buds that detect and send taste signals to the brain. This unique design allows all parts of the tongue to detect various flavors. Taste buds are certainly a sign that God cares about and loves us. He didn't need to make the tongue this way. He didn't have to create for us the numerous flavors that exist or the ability to enjoy them. From an evolutionary perspective it doesn't make sense that so many different types of taste buds would have evolved. Surely, they all are not necessary for survival! But because the Lord God is creative and loving, I can't help but believe He created these for our enjoyment! Certainly He loves us.

Flavors are often divided into five main types or five common tastes: sweet, sour, bitter, umami (savory), and salty. Of the five, most people enjoy the flavors sweet and salty. But people are unique, and the degree to which each flavor is enjoyed varies. Because food can provide pleasurable sensations and various flavors, it should come as no surprise that taste, more than any other factor, influences food choice. Some people prefer foods that are hot and spicy. They liberally use chili powder and cayenne pepper. Others steer clear of the hot spices in favor of sweet or sour flavors. Preferences for taste or particular textures begin early in life, and when habits and associations are formed early, they can be difficult to change.

> **RECAP:** The number-one influence on our food choices is taste.

3. Time and Convenience

"Be very careful, then, how you live—not as unwise but as wise." —Ephesians 5:15

Life for most people could be defined as a whirlwind. Between children, family, friends, school, and work, it seems they are pulled in 50 different directions. The ever-faster pace of life in Westernized countries today has made convenience an influencing factor in food choices more than ever before. Computers were supposed to make life easier; they were supposed to allow for more leisure time, but this does not seem to be the case. Stress levels have not decreased. Nowadays, people are moving faster and doing more than ever before. It seems the arrival of computers has only increased the demand of the average workload. Many people carry smartphones or tablets with them, and as a result, send and receive email messages and texts from work and friends 24/7. In this fast-paced, high-tech culture, how much time is devoted to meals and fueling our bodies properly?

When it comes to meals, many people want something quick and easy. For reasons related to both time and convenience, more people are eating out and eating on the run than ever before. For example, between 1977 and 1978, foods eaten away from home made up 17% of Americans' calorie intake. In 2011–2012, that figure rose to 34%. In the past twenty years, the frequency of families gathering to share an evening meal declined 33%. In lieu of togetherness, Americans spend 50% of their food budget at restaurants. Sadly, only 3% of those meals at restaurants meet the nutrition standards for children. Foods eaten away from home tend to contain higher amounts of sodium and saturated fat, and less iron, fiber, and calcium. Because, as previously noted, taste is the number-one influencer on food choice, those who frequently eat out tend to not purchase nutrient-dense foods such as fish, vegetables, and nuts, but food heavily laden with salt, fat, and sugar.

When income is considered, folks in higher-income households tend to spend more on foods eaten away from home. They also tend to purchase those meals more frequently. Interestingly, people between the ages of 35 and 44 eat away from home more frequently than other groups, while households with someone over 64 years of age eat out 8% less frequently. In 2010, for the first time, the Americans' budget for foods eaten away from home exceeded their food budget for meals eaten at home. The more frequently someone eats away from home, the less control they have over how that food is prepared and how large a portion they are served. And, let's face it, if we are paying for someone else to prepare our food, it better taste good, and they'd better not skimp on the amount they set in front of us! Nobody wants to feel ripped off. It is no secret that restaurants that do well serve generous portions of food that tastes good. Of course, this has contributed to obesity rates.

While I am all for progress and innovation, I think it is wise to not always plow full steam ahead without periodically glancing back to examine the results made by our waves while we were full throttle. Sometimes, there may be consequences that we did not anticipate. Research shows that participation in family meals has been associated with numerous health-related benefits, as well as positive social development for children. When a family works together to set a table and calls family members to gather around, the environment is set for conversation to ensue. Bonding with one another and sharing thoughts, ideas, and experiences will likely take place. Sharing regular meals together as a family is a natural, wholesome practice with many benefits. This habit has been shown to improve children's diets and eating habits, which can then have promising consequences for children trying to lose weight. Experts in the field have also proposed that family meals can positively contribute to the psychosocial development of children. Gathering around a dinner table for a meal in which we pass bowls of food to one another, look into each other's eyes, and communicate face-to-face is a much more conducive environment for building healthy family relationships, enhancing intimacy among family members, and alleviating negative effects of the day's stress than is passing a bag filled with a hamburger, fries, and a soda to the people in the back seat while the driver speeds away to the next activity.

During a class discussion on the topic, a student once shared her perception of food growing up. She indicated that she grew up eating traditional Czechoslovakian meals, including things like sauerkraut, golumpki, pierogis, pagach, and kielbasa, along with homemade mashed potatoes. She indicated that although these meals were filling and very satisfying, what they imparted most to her was a caring feeling. Those thoughts immediately conjured the awareness that her father's all-day labor in the kitchen over steaming pots and a hot oven containing homemade bread was an indication that he cared about her and her sisters. Tears filled her eyes as she realized that he wanted to work that hard for them. She ended by sharing that she equates a complete, homemade meal with a feeling of being loved. If that is not enough to make you want to slow down and enjoy family dinners together, a longitudinal study that followed children aged 9 to 19 years found that children who ate with their parents had closer relationships and better coping abilities later in life. They were also less likely to smoke or have unhealthy eating attitudes and behaviors. Eating family meals together more often decreases the likelihood of boys engaging in unhealthy weight-control behaviors and girls engaging in unhealthy and extreme weight-control behaviors. Wow! Talk about family values! Unfortunately, despite the nutritional and psychosocial benefits associated with family meals, in the past two decades the frequency of family meals in Westernized countries has declined. Family is central to any society. Family structure matters. Children growing up in healthy, married, two-parent families are more likely to lead happy, healthy, and successful lives than children raised in environments that do not offer the same level of family security and stability. Those in stable families have a higher life expectancy and lower risks of mental illness, alcoholism, and domestic violence. Children are also positively affected in that lower infant mortality rates, lower risk of drug addiction, lower incidences of engaging in criminal activities after puberty, higher academic achievements, lower incidence of many mental illnesses, and fewer unplanned teenage pregnancies are seen. Findings from academic research demonstrate that God's plan for families is best.

> **RECAP:** Modern families pack their schedules with so many activities and obligations that they often leave no time for homecooked family meals, resulting in a sacrifice of familial intimacy and control over food preparation.

4. Nutrition Knowledge

"An intelligent heart acquires knowledge, and the ear of the wise seeks knowledge." —Proverbs 18:15

I once saw a movie about an attorney who was defending a company's actions. Well into representing this company, this defending attorney came across information that proved the company he agreed to represent was, in fact, at fault. Having to share all information with the prosecuting attorney, the defending attorney found himself in a bit of a quandary. But legally, he had to share that information. So, he skillfully shared ALL information. In other words, he bombarded the prosecuting attorney with so many books, reports, and emails that the prosecuting attorney would be hard-pressed to find the needle in the haystack of information. That is kind of how it is with nutrition information. There is so much nutrition information available that the average person feels bombarded and overwhelmed. Most people have a challenging time finding the nuggets of truth in the haystack (or in the sea of internet information).

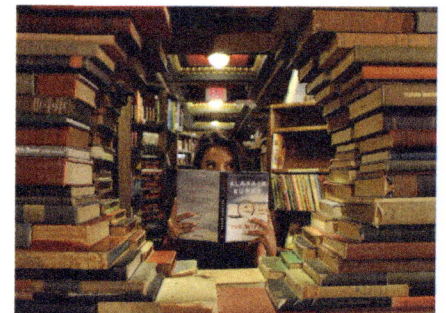

To help sift through all this mostly unnecessary information, we need to be reminded of a few things. Nutrition is a young science. It has not been a field of study for very long. In fact, the first vitamin was not discovered until the early nineteenth century. What this means is that we don't know what we don't even know yet. For example, when I was a dietetic student in the mid 1980s, we never learned 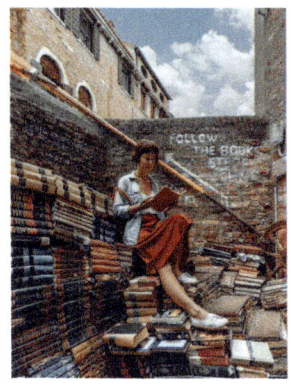 about phytochemicals. That is because they were not well known or understood. There is abundant nutrition information available on the internet today, but the vast majority comes from companies trying to sell products. Our patients and clients need to be careful with where they get their nutrition information, because the reality is that just about any source can be found to justify any position, stance, or diet, and that is not helpful when it comes to locating accurate nutrition information. I tell students in my classes that, whether they recognize it or not, they are truly fortunate to be taking college classes and even more fortunate to be able to sit in on a college nutrition class. I usually tell students they need to go to "peer-reviewed" articles from "scholarly journals" to get accurate nutrition information. But the problem with "peer-reviewed" articles from "scholarly journals" is that they are usually filled with million-dollar words that are difficult to pronounce and even harder for the general public to understand and apply. What that means is only a handful of people can read and interpret them. For example, one of my friends has a degree in aerospace engineering. He is brilliant. During one visit, he asked me about losing weight and eating better. Well, I instantly put on my "professor's" hat and started lecturing him. Almost immediately, he put up his hand and said, "What do you mean, 'resistant starch'?" The truth is, no matter how smart, how educated, or well-read a person is, unless they have a solid foundation in the truths of nutrition, they too can become lost in the vast sea of nutrition myths that plague the internet. So, for the general public, articles found in scholarly journals, although they are excellent resources, don't end up being helpful.

As was indicated earlier, nutrition is a rather young science, and we don't know what we don't even know yet. Because of this, it is important to recall the concept of "The Scientific Method and Procedure." Part of the Scientific Method and Procedure involves repeating studies to see if we get the same results. This is important in science, and it is especially important in the field of nutrition. For example, many studies over the years have been conducted to see if researchers could find vitamin C in oranges. Many researchers have experimented, and each time the same finding emerged. Because studies were duplicated and repeated over time, we can now say with certainty: Oranges contain vitamin C. Nobody disputes this fact. But project this idea forward. With all the new findings in this young field, researchers need time to conduct and duplicate studies. In other words, just because one study has a specific result, it doesn't mean we should begin sharing that finding with clients or patients. That study needs to be repeated and repeated to see how the results vary. This is the reason we must be careful about making diet recommendations to our clients and patients based on the results of a few studies. Furthermore, one sensational study is precisely what the media loves to shine the spotlight on, because the more dramatic and astonishing the results of a study are, the more likely it is to draw attention. While knowledge of food and nutrition is important, knowledge alone does not equal behavior change. If knowledge by itself were the sole necessary ingredient needed for behavior change, there would be no cardiologists who smoke. But knowledge is not enough. In His word, God talks a lot about wisdom. Wisdom involves knowing what to do (and here comes the big one) AND doing it.

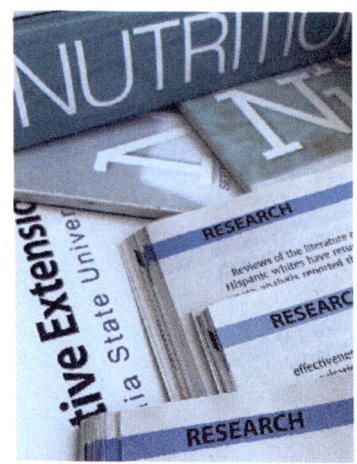

RECAP: We must be careful from where we get our nutrition information because there is a lot of dangerous misinformation available.

5. Cost

"Why spend your money on food that does not give you strength? Why pay for food that does you no good? Listen to me, and you will eat what is good. You will enjoy the finest food." —Isaiah 55:2

Money is an issue for most people in many areas of life, and food costs are no exception. Has a patient or client ever said to you, "I can't afford to eat healthy?" This is a concept that needs challenging. Although the cost of fast food has risen, it is usually still less expensive than most sit-down restaurants. However, the real savings come from shopping for foods in their raw forms and preparing them at home. Not only is this the least expensive way to eat, it is also the healthiest. Look at the chart below.

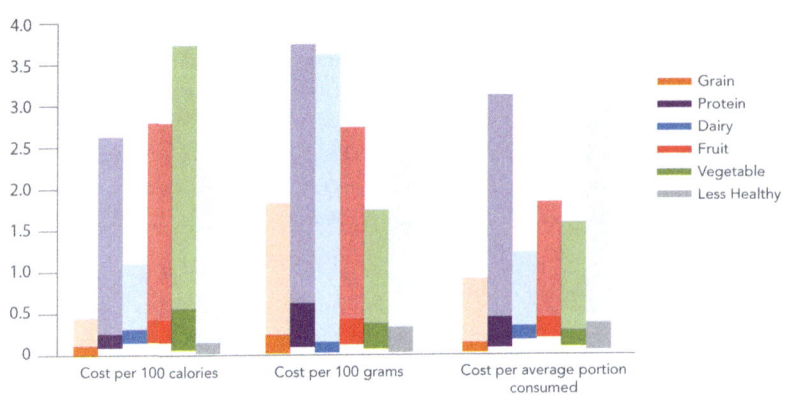

Does it really cost more to eat healthy?

Note: Dark areas of each bar represent the less expensive foods in the category, while the lighter areas represent the higher costing foods. White space at the bottom of the bars represents the start of the price range.

Note: Dark areas of each bar represent the less expensive foods in the category, while the lighter areas represent the higher-cost foods. White space at the bottom of the bars represents the start of the price range.

Adapted from: Carlson A, Frazao E. Are healthy foods really more expensive? It depends on how you measure the price. United States Department of Agriculture. https://www.ers.usda.gov/webdocs/publications/44678/19980_eib96.pdf?v=42321. Published May 2012. Accessed April 7, 2020.

There is a lot going on in this image. The foods are color-coded: the darker areas at the bottom of each bar indicate the less expensive foods in the category, while lighter areas represent higher-cost foods. So, for example, fruit is red. Thus, the dark red could be bananas while the light color red could represent raspberries. White space at the bottom of the bars represents the start of the price range. There are three graphs. The graph to the far left is how food has traditionally always been measured, by cost per 100 calories. And when food is examined like this, yes, fruit, vegetables, and proteins are more expensive. Think about it: cost per 100 calories. Do you know how much broccoli or carrots must be eaten before reaching 100 calories, especially when compared to something like sweets or junk food?

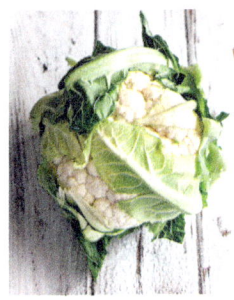

Now look at the graph to the far right; this measures food by how people really consume it, by portion! Here we see that vegetables, grains, fruits, and dairy are less than half the cost of junk food and protein. In other words, price per average portion is the price of the average amount consumed by adults. People don't often sit down and eat an entire head of cauliflower, right? Let's look at cost for a moment. If a head of cauliflower costs $2.99, and a person only eats 1/8 of that head, the portion costs about 37 cents. On the other hand, it is not uncommon for a person to sit down with a family-sized bag of Doritos during a movie and find their fingers scraping the bottom of the bag before the movie ends. In this scenario, their portion costs them the price of the entire bag. (Dare I remind you that the cauliflower is packed with vitamins, minerals, phytochemicals, and fiber, while the bag of Doritos simply contributes to one's calories and sodium intake?) A steady diet of junk food may appear cheaper than a well-balanced diet, but those calculations do not take into account the hospital, doctor's, or prescription fees. Moreover, the true cost, as we have just seen, depends on how we do the math. Let's look at another example. Someone can choose either one apple or one candy bar as a snack. While apples might cost $2.49 a pound (which gets you 2-3 apples), the cost of an apple for a snack would be somewhere around 80 cents to $1.20 per apple. The cost of a candy would be in the same ballpark. As you can see from these two examples, it does not necessarily cost more to eat healthy.

Finishing up this graph, we see that the center graph is price per edible gram. This is the price of food after it has been cooked and the seeds, peels, skins, shells, and bones have been removed. Consistently, we see the protein cost is the highest, but there are several healthy, inexpensive sources of protein to choose from as well. For example, canned tuna (packed in water) and dried beans, peas, and lentils are great sources of protein and other nutrients, and they are pennies per serving.

> **RECAP:** It is possible to eat healthy on a budget. In fact, it is less costly to eat healthy, especially when looking at long-term expenses.

6. Environment, Culture, and Availability

"And I brought you into a plentiful land to enjoy its fruits and its good things…" —Jeremiah 2:7a

One's environment certainly influences what is eaten. Culture, location, climate, soil conditions, and the local geography with its native plants and animals all have an impact. Food availability is a major determinant of what people choose to eat. What is available is often affected by season, geography, economics, living conditions, and even current health status. In many parts of the world, food choices are limited to foods produced locally. Developed countries, on the other hand, have sophisticated shipping techniques that can bring out-of-season items to grocery stores and even to doorsteps. Food availability is a major issue in many inner cities. Many corner stores in inner cities have closed their doors or moved to suburban areas where there is more affluence and crime is lower. This has left many inner-city folks, who do not have a car or who can't afford regular public transportation, in a food desert. It leaves them without access to many essential foods, like fresh produce. On the other hand, there are other locations where fresh fruits and vegetables are available year-round. When caring for patients, it is important to take the time to familiarize yourself with their food availability, as this will greatly influence what they eat.

For many, food plays a significant role in cultural heritage and national identity. Traditions are passed down from one generation to another, and for many people, traditions are a way of preserving not only culture but our memories of loved ones. Not an occasion goes by that I don't think of my grandmother when making our family's traditional "pineapple cookies," and it is a gesture of love when my mother makes homemade cabbage rolls. If cabbage rolls are served, I can be certain someone at the table will start talking about my deceased father, "Pap," as cabbage rolls were his favorite. And if the conversation dies down after the mention of his name, it is certain that while another word may not be spoken, the thoughts of everyone who knew him and his Slovak heritage will spark a smile and a memory before the discussion evaporates. In a world that is ever-changing and becoming increasingly geographically connected, cooking traditional food is a way of preserving culture and family when people move to new places.

> **RECAP:** Culture, environment, and the availability of food can determine what is eaten.

7. Health and Body Image

"So whether you eat or drink or whatever you do, do it all for the glory of God." —1 Corinthians 10:31

As you well know, it is true that most people don't value their health very much…until they begin to lose it. Then, suddenly, it becomes priceless. Perhaps you have had a patient or client who got such a frightening medical report that it motivated them to change their diet. One's desire to be healthy or to get healthier can influence food choices. While working in a hospital outpatient setting, I encountered and counseled many people who were diabetic, on the verge of becoming diabetic, who needed heart transplants, as well as some who simply wanted to feel better and have more energy. All of them were there because they wanted help in learning how to eat to improve their health.

In my experience and interactions with the public, there are several categories into which people fall. One natural method of separation is by their level of motivation. Some people are motivated to change their eating behavior and others are not. It is a difficult situation because, in general, what I have seen is that older people whose bodies have endured years of wear and tear—and in some cases, misuse—are often motivated to change because they either want to feel the way they used to when they were younger or they no longer want to feel sick.

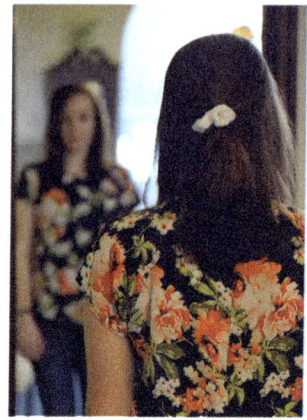

The other group tends to be younger in age, and they often have little motivation to change their eating habits. For them, eating is based on convenience, not fueling their body for health. As a result of feeling fine daily, their eating choices are influenced by factors other than health. Their motivation often stems from "fitting in" with their peer group and having fun socializing. Unfortunately, it is during these developmental years that habits are formed. If unhealthy habits are formed early, they become harder and harder to change as years pass. As these young people grow older, if they don't make dietary changes, they will eventually find themselves in a physician's office just like the first group, receiving bad news that frightens them, and then they become motivated to change. However, at this point, they have decades of entrenched habits that they need to change. It would be much easier and people would be far more successful if the youth would practice healthy eating habits from the beginning. Again, we find God's word to be true: "Train up a child in the way he should go: and when he is old, he will not depart from it." —Proverbs 22:6

Some people make food choices driven by what they think will help them achieve health goals or the body shape they desire. Interestingly, I have encountered many young adults who care little about their health until children come along. I have had many students indicate that it was the addition of children to the family that reinforced healthy habits for them. Many young parents say they want to provide a healthy nutritional foundation for their children because that is what they remember their parents doing for them as children. In fact, many women don't take their health or diet seriously until they become pregnant with their first child because they feel responsible for the little life growing inside them. More and more research in the area of epigenetics is pointing to the notion that a person's diet may influence the health of their grandchildren.

The key word when we talk about health or body image is "intentional." Intentional choices are made with a goal in mind. For example, if someone is told by their physician that their cholesterol is high and they should start paying attention to their diet, they may respond by reading food labels and choosing leaner cuts of meat. Life circumstances often influence when a person begins to take their health and diet seriously and thus make intentional decisions about food choices. Some people refer to this as "mindful" eating.

RECAP: Making intentional and informed choices can help improve health.

8. Habits

"'All things are lawful for me,' but not all things are helpful. 'All things are lawful for me,' but I will not be enslaved by anything." —1 Corinthians 6:12

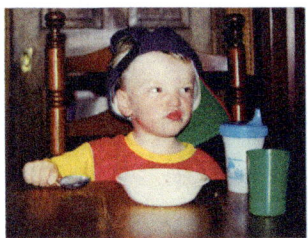

Daily habits and routines affect both what a person eats and when they eat. If someone develops the habit of waking up late as a teenager and not eating breakfast, there is a good chance they will continue that habit into adulthood. On the other hand, if someone develops the habit of waking up early to work out before going to school as a teenager, there is an equally good chance they will continue that habit into adulthood. If someone usually has a vegetable and a salad with their evening meal when young, as they age, they will feel like something is missing if a meal doesn't include a vegetable and a salad. Moreover, if as a youngster someone became accustomed to walking to a nearby park to play after dinner, in their adult years their habits may look different from a peer who became accustomed to plopping down in front of the television with a bowl of ice cream after dinner.

Parents and caregivers play a crucial role in the habit formation of children. As a health professional, I find it is important to encourage parents and caregivers to repeatedly offer initially rejected foods. It is only through this repeated exposure that an unfamiliar food can be transformed into a familiar food that is enjoyed and regularly incorporated into meals. In fact, children may require up to 15 exposures to a new food before trusting it enough to taste it. Furthermore, they may need an additional 10–15 exposures before they actually like the food. Perseverance is important. God speaks about perseverance in Galatians 6:9, "And let us not grow weary of doing good, for in due season we will reap, if we do not give up."

Foods offered are usually linked to the taste preferences of parents. When parents have a narrow or limited diet, many foods are not presented often enough to children to allow sufficient exposure for these foods to become familiar. This also limits opportunities for positive role-modeling to take place. Parental habits can promote the development of either positive or negative behaviors among children.

> **RECAP:** The sooner a person develops healthy habits, the better.

9. Emotions

"Therefore I tell you, do not worry about your life, what you will eat or drink; or about your body, what you will wear. Is not life more than food, and the body more than clothes?" —Matthew 6:24-26

I can still recall being a dietetic student and my professor, Dr. Birdsall, saying, "Some people use food as a source of comfort." With pencil in hand, I wrote the sentence in my notebook, but the statement meant nothing to me. In fact, I didn't really understand it fully until about 25 years later when a friend came to visit with her 3-year-old son. When I opened the front door and invited them in, down the front hallway, through the kitchen, and into the back room, the little 3-year-old spied toys and he took off running toward them. He made it safely down the hallway, but unfortunately for him, the kitchen's bar stools that usually reside under the overhanging countertop of the island had been removed. The poor little guy's head! He was a fraction of an inch too tall. At full "toy-driven steam" he plowed his head straight into the overhanging counter and fell with the distinct slapping sound of tender 3-year-old flesh on polished wooden planks. I remember the moment well, because my friend raced to his rescue and, as if sliding into home plate, she first scooped him up in her arms and then into her quickly formed lap, and with terrified eyes and a voice that could wake the dead bellowed, "Do you have any chocolate?" I was so startled by her fearful reaction that I quickly ran to the pantry and grabbed the remains of an opened bag of chocolate chips and poured several into her hand, then stood back. What took place in front of me, there on my kitchen floor, amazed me. One by one, as my friend fed her boy those chocolate chips, his tears began to subside. It was like a lightbulb went off and I was back in Dr. Birdsall's class. It was all I could do to refrain from saying out loud, "This is what Dr. Birdsall meant when she said, 'Some people use food as a source of comfort'." Now, I ask you, what was that little boy learning? When he hurts, he gets chocolate? When he feels pain, chocolate makes the pain go away? What do you think? No matter how it is worded, it is not a healthy message or habit, but it is one that many people learn.

If you don't mind, to make this point stronger, I'd like to share one more memory; this one is from college. While a dietetic student, I encountered a young man of Polish descent. This man was raised in a small house with both his parents, his sister, and one set of grandparents. As a means of bonding and sharing their day, his grandfather used to steal time away with him from the intrusion of other family members. Their private ritual involved first boiling links of sausage in the kitchen, then sneaking out onto the back porch, where they would savor both the flavor of the sausage and the special time they shared. Now, as a dietetic student, I knew nothing of this young man's background. All I knew was that nearly every time I brought my meal tray to his table, I noticed mounds of sausage links on his plate. Well, being an inexperienced dietetic student and not yet having learned the lesson, "Don't offer advice about what someone is eating unless they ask you for it," I spoke up. "Wow—you sure eat a lot of sausage. You know that's not good for you, right?!" You would have thought I took away birthday cake from a spoiled 4-year-old right before his first bite. This young man exploded with anger! I was totally confused. How could he possibly be so angry over sausage or even a comment about sausage? What I didn't realize was the meaning sausage held for him. Although I never said it, what this young man heard was "You know all those special moments with your grandfather? They were no good! In fact, they were a really bad time, and you should forget them and never revisit them. That stupid, wicked, old man was basically slowly killing you. Very bad!" No wonder he reacted with hurtful anger.

Food can also be used as a punishment, resulting in emotions being aroused by either specific foods or certain situations. For example, a student once told me that whenever he did something wrong, his mother would look at him in anger and say, "Now, just for that, you're going to have broccoli for dinner!" After he told the class that story, I asked that young 21-year-old man, "Do you like broccoli today?" He responded, "I hate it." It has been well established that food-induced emotions contribute to food choices. Emotions such as anger, fear, sadness, and joy have been found to affect eating. Food and emotions are closely linked for many people. It is important for health care providers to encourage patients and clients to identify those foods, as well as the meanings they hold in their lives. In many cases, counseling may help reveal hidden meanings behind foods. This understanding may be necessary before patients and clients can treat foods in a healthy manner.

Research has demonstrated that lower levels of spiritual well-being correlate with higher levels of emotional eating, and that emotional eating contributes to higher caloric intake along with unhealthy eating attitudes and behaviors. With the stressors and responsibilities of modern-day life, it is important to be immersed in God's Word daily. This is a fallen world. It is full of sin, brokenness, instabilities, uncertainty, and struggles. It is a waste of energy and can be overwhelming to try to solve problems in our own strength. But Jesus tells us He will never leave us or forsake us. When fear, anxiety, or depression grabs us, we need to cling with tenacious confidence and childlike trust knowing we can rest in His protective presence. He is our provider and has endless resources. Turning to Him instead of food is undoubtedly precious in His sight and more comforting.

RECAP: It is important to identify foods that hold emotional significance.

10. Advertising

"Keep your life free from love of money, and be content with what you have, for he has said, 'I will never leave you nor forsake you.'" —Hebrews 13:5

Advertising is a multi-billion-dollar-a-year industry. The money is spent simply because advertising works. It is effective in prompting and moving people to make purchases. Yet, when surveyed, most people believe they are immune to the influence of advertising. While they admit looking at ads, they don't believe ads have any influence on them. Generally speaking, most people don't believe that ads affect them because they believe they are above the ad's power. If we were to examine individual ads, indeed, they would seem harmless and insignificant. But when examined in their entirety, we see they create a very powerful environment. There is power in numbers. Advertising is designed to have a cumulative, unconscious effect on people. Environments are difficult to perceive when caught up in them. Interestingly, the fact that advertising is not considered a form of education makes it even more powerful. The function of advertising is to sell products, to get people to buy stuff. One of the roles of advertising is to produce discontent in humans. The message "You are NOT OK" is subtly but repeatedly sent through advertising. The goal is to make people uncomfortable in their personal situation and social standing—in essence, in their lives. Advertising generates endless self-criticism, which works to the advertisers' advantage, because it is in human nature to compare ourselves with others. When this comparison is done with the images that have been carefully and craftily created in the ads that surround all of us, people are left feeling as though something is lacking. This way of thinking is in direct opposition to what God tells us:

"Do not be conformed to this world, but be transformed by the renewal of your mind, that by testing you may discern what is the will of God, what is good and acceptable and perfect." —Romans 12:2

"You shall not covet your neighbor's house; you shall not covet your neighbor's wife, or his male servant, or his female servant, or his ox, or his donkey, or anything that is your neighbor's." —Exodus 20:17

"For where jealousy and selfish ambition exist, there will be disorder and every vile practice." —James 3:16

"For am I now seeking the approval of man, or of God? Or am I trying to please man? If I were still trying to please man, I would not be a servant of Christ." —Galatians 1:10

Because of the magnitude of advertising in today's world, it ends up creating assumptions about the world. It tells us the way the world is. To a large extent, the messages sent through advertising depict who we are and who we should strive to become. The message is: "You must transform yourself, and we can help."

Advertisers know we process images and words differently. While we can argue with words that are stated or written in an advertisement, it is difficult to argue or disagree with images. Thus, advertisers often use images of success, love, and happiness to sell products. Advertisers have studied people's responses to various advertisements. One philosophy involves the concept that we are constantly competing with others around us to be noticed, to be seen, to be admired, or viewed as successful or worthy. Some researchers have suggested that to understand a society, we should examine the advertising of that society. Advertising is everywhere, and as such, it is part of the environment in which we live.

While we may think we are not affected by advertising, it is important to recognize that this advertising world was constructed by someone. It wasn't always here, and it wasn't always like this. Consider today's advertisements for Calvin Klein or Victoria's Secret. Would your grandmother or grandfather respond to those ads the same way someone in their twenties would respond? If the answer is no, think about why not. Part of the explanation would involve the fact that the constructed environments that your grandparents grew up in were different, most likely more conservative, than the environment in which young adults are growing up today.

There are many advertising techniques: "power words" are used to gain attention, "misleading comparisons" can be used to sway the average consumer, "advertising puffery" uses subjective opinions, superlatives, or exaggerations to praise a product, and "weasel words" are modifiers that tend to negate the claim that follows. These include words like "virtually," "reportedly," "looks like," "theoretically," and "as much as." And we can't forget the all-too-famous "testimony" approach, which is a favorite of many advertisers of diets and diet products. These are only a few of the many techniques used to sell diet aids, formulas, and programs.

> **RECAP:** Advertising influences food choices.

As you can see, there are many influences affecting your patients' and clients' eating. It is safe to say, "Education does not equal behavior change." As their health care provider, it is important that you take a broad approach when coming alongside them. While educating them is important, all influences should be considered. This takes time, gentleness, probing questions, conversation, and sometimes referrals to other health professionals.

Before examining other influences on eating such as hormones and biological processes, let's identify fad diets.

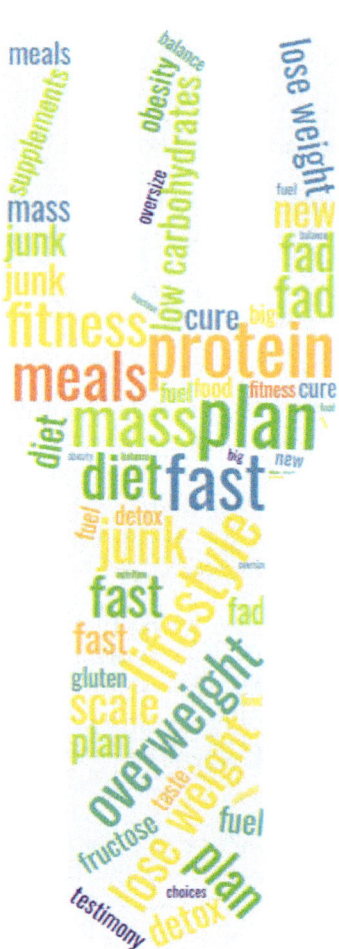

CHAPTER 2
What is a Fad Diet, and how can it be recognized?

"Beware of false prophets, who come to you in sheep's clothing but inwardly are ravenous wolves." —Matthew 7:15

While not on the same level of importance as eternal salvation, it is imperative for health care professionals to be able to identify fad diets if they are going to help their patients and clients. A fad diet is a trendy weight-loss plan or system that frequently claims dramatic results. A fad diet is what people talk about at work around the water cooler. A fad diet is usually what pops up when that four-letter word D-I-E-T is typed into a search engine. A fad diet is the basis of most diet books. Many diets exist and have notoriety because they describe what people want to hear; they are filled with promises of weight loss and happiness.

Undoubtedly, part of the problem is the prevalence of fad diets. Many dieters are impatient and elect to try fad diets that are unhealthy or too low in calories. Research shows that very low-calorie diets (500 calories a day) are associated with a greater loss of fat-free mass. In other words, the weight lost is not fat. To make matters worse, research shows that when a greater percentage of fat-free mass is lost, physical activity is reduced and there is an increased risk the weight will be regained. In other words, when someone loses lean tissue because of being on a fad diet, they tend to exercise less and eat more (especially fat calories) when they go off the diet, and both behaviors lead to regaining the lost weight. A review of the literature reveals 124 determinants influencing the ability to maintain weight loss; 5 were demographic, 59 were behavioral, 51 were psychological/cognitive, and 9 were social or environmental determinants. Demographic determinants were consistently found not predictive of weight-loss maintenance, whereas behavioral and psychological factors were. This means if a diet does not address these issues, the likelihood of keeping weight off over time is low.

Unfortunately, nearly all fad diet approaches are ultimately unsuccessful. Studies show that less than half of overweight people maintain a weight loss of 10% of their maximum weight for a year. So if a dieter starts at 200 pounds, less than 50% of them are able to keep off 20 pounds after a year. Only about one fourth of dieters will be able to maintain that weight loss for five years or more. No wonder so many dieters get frustrated. So, what is successful weight loss?

How do we define success? How long does someone need to keep weight off before they qualify as being successful? How much weight do they need to lose in order to be successful? Researchers continue to look into this area from many angles. There is no set standard definition for the length of time that weight must be kept off in order to be dubbed "successful weight loss," but many researchers consider success as keeping off weight for a year.

What do you think? Is losing weight for one year successful? By definition, that means in 2 or 3 years, your patient could be back at the starting gate. But success was achieved! This is a critical point, because in examining popular diets, many can't claim long-term success. They can't claim it because no long-term studies have been conducted. In other words, when there are no long-term studies, it simply means that during the 6 or 8 or 12 weeks of being on the diet, the subjects lost weight. Well, how impressive is that? If a diet can't claim long-term success, it can't claim the weight was kept off for even a year! This deserves further discussion. Why are there so few studies demonstrating success for one year? One big reason is the diet was too difficult to stay on for a year. Any diet that can't be maintained will end in weight being regained.

Keep in mind, the research shows that the majority of all people who lose weight regain that weight, and most people who lose weight on a fad diet will not only regain that same weight back but will add a few more extra pounds.

RECAP: Keeping weight off for one year defines successful weight loss; many fad diets can't claim "success."

What are your patient's or client's weight-loss goals?

How much weight a person should lose is only one determining factor that may impact success. For example, if someone is carrying around an excess 100 pounds of body fat, while someone else has 20 pounds, those differences will impact research results and therefore our understanding of the findings of weight loss. Weight loss achieved at a slow rate of 1–2 pounds a week is best. In fact, for short, older, frail females the recommended weight loss may be ¼ of a pound a week. The longer someone can maintain a lower weight, the better their chances are for successfully keeping the weight off. Not only that, but people who maintain the weight they lose for a longer time report it becomes easier and easier to maintain that new lower weight. They indicate it is less of an effort to control their weight. That is exciting news!

I realize that the thought of losing just 1 pound a week may be disappointing to many of your patients or clients. We have all been waiting for scientists to find that "magic bullet." We hoped Olestra (1968) might be it, but over time, users found that it caused loose stools and inhibited the absorption of some vitamins. Then, the hope was in obesity drugs like fenfluramine and/or dexfenfluramine, only to find out they were linked to heart valve problems (1997). Artificial sweeteners have been around for a while, which brought glimpses of hope because their sweetness is far more potent than table sugar or high-fructose corn syrup. But research has shown that in and of themselves, they are not enough in the fight against body fat. Moreover, artificial sweeteners are not created equal. Some, like cyclamate, were banned by the Food and Drug Administration (FDA). Additionally, some health care professionals have expressed concern that intense and frequent overstimulation of the taste buds for sweetness may, over time, result in that person avoiding or even rejecting less sweet foods, like vegetables, similar to how an infant is less likely to try peas or green beans if they have already been introduced to bananas and peaches. If continued, the ultimate result of continual use of artificial sweeteners may be rejection of highly nutritious, nutrient-dense foods in favor of consuming more artificially flavored foods that supply less nutritional value. More research is needed in this area.

This brief walk through history shows only a few of the many acclaimed miraculous breakthroughs in the quest for simple, easy weight loss. Alas, to date, there still is no silver bullet. But there are ways of losing weight and keeping it off long term.

Reasons people want to lose weight

People want to lose weight for many reasons. Some fear developing chronic diseases; others want to fit into their bikini by spring break; while others simply want to feel better.

When it comes to weight loss, it is important that your patients and clients lose it in a healthy fashion, using methods that will not land them in the hospital or back at stage one again in a few weeks or months. For your clients and patients who have a lot of excess fat to lose, it is useful to remind them that considerable literature shows losing just 3 to 5% of weight is

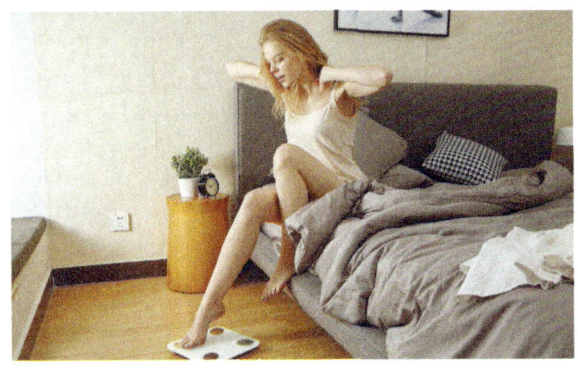

accompanied by a reduction in health risk such as reductions in triglycerides, blood glucose, and the risk of developing type-2 diabetes. It is exciting to know that even a little weight loss provides meaningful health benefits, not to mention feeling better both mentally and physically. Larger weight loss can reduce even more risk factors for cardiovascular disease, such as improving low-density and high-density lipoproteins, cholesterol levels, and blood pressure. This kind of weight loss can even decrease the need for cardiovascular and type-2 diabetes medications. How cool is that! Thus, according to the Academy of Nutrition and Dietetics, a weight loss of 5% to 10% within 6 months is a great goal.

RECAP: Losing no more than 2 pounds a week helps ensure long-term success.

The Illusion of Glycogen as Weight Loss

Another reason fad diets claim rapid weight loss is based on glycogen. The loss of glycogen gives the illusion of fast, easy weight loss. Remember, glycogen is stored carbohydrates in muscles and the liver. While numbers will vary from individual to individual, the average inactive adult stores about 75–100 grams of glycogen in the liver, which equates to about 300–400 calories. Additionally they store between 300–400 grams of glycogen in the muscles which translates into 1,200–1,600 calories. A strenuous two-hour workout can just about deplete both liver and muscle glycogen.

Glycogen is stored along with water. Between 2.7 and 4 grams of water bind with each 1 gram of glycogen. That equates to a lot of weight. On a low-carbohydrate diet, glycogen stores (and its accompanying stored water) are lost. Thus, even small decreases in calories at the start of a low-carbohydrate diet can give the impression of significant fat loss, even if no fat is lost. When the number on the scale drops quickly it gives the illusion of easy weight loss, which can lead to unrealistic expectations of future weight loss. Many fad diets, especially low-carb fad diets, claim fast success, when in fact no fat is even lost.

RECAP: Low-carbohydrate diets cause an impressive initial weight loss. It is glycogen and water loss, not body fat.

Grains of Truth

"You shall not spread a false report. You shall not join hands with a wicked man to be a malicious witness." —Exodus 23:1

Interestingly, fad diets are often rooted in a grain of truth, some small scientific component in which the diet is based. However, and this is a crucial point, that grain of scientific truth often loses traction when applied to a real dieting person's situation. This is because people are not robots living in a laboratory. People are emotional beings living in a turbulent fallen world full of temptations, stress, and responsibilities. Many fad diets are based on a scientific concept that is true in a controlled laboratory environment, but when applied outside that laboratory context is doomed to fail because that original scientific truth can't provide success in this new, real-life environment. Unfortunately, this is the case with many fad diets.

Fad Diets in Real Life

Indeed, it would be wonderful if we only had to eat fat all day long to be guaranteed of losing all the body fat we want. It would be great if dieting were as easy as consuming 1–2 teaspoons of apple cider vinegar prior to meals, or snacking throughout the day on low-calorie cookies made with a secret "hunger-controlling" formula that kept us from feeling hungry, or if eating fruit cleaned out our gastrointestinal system and put us into fat-burn mode and made us lose all past food addictions. But in the real world, it is not as simple as these fad diets claim. Eating only fat gets boring and really difficult when you walk past the Cinnabon Bakery at the mall or get invited to a 5-year-old's birthday party. Eating only fat for any length of time is also dangerous, as many essential nutrients won't be consumed. Apple cider vinegar is great in salad dressing, but I don't know anybody who looks forward to two straight tablespoons. Is this where the phrase "no pain no gain" applies? While snacking during the day is often a good idea, there is no "secret hunger-controlling" formula. And, yes, fruit in the diet is good, but it doesn't put the metabolism into fat-burn mode. That would be nice!

Moreover, fad diets can be dangerous. For example, my colleague worked with a woman who was only 32 years old and ended up with permanent heart damage that could be attributed to the improper application and poor self-monitoring of a low-carb diet. She was not under the supervision of her physician; she simply wanted to experiment with the diet. In another case, I worked with a woman who bought "diet pills" because she wanted to lose weight. She had some success, but it was not long-lasting. During our discussion of her dieting history, she pulled the bottle of pills out of her purse. I read the directions, which instructed dieters to take one pill with 8 ounces of water 30 minutes before each meal. The pills claimed to be filled with fiber that would expand in the stomach to decrease hunger by the time the dieter began to eat. Interestingly, the package insert also directed the dieter to follow a specific diet the manufacturer provided. Well, my goodness! When I looked over the diet it was a 1,200-calorie diet! Nearly everyone would lose weight on a 1,200-calorie diet, even without taking the pills!

There are many fad diets available these days, so many that they can make our heads spin: diets that promise happiness through weight loss but deliver sorrow with regained weight. Diets that assure success but in actuality provide feelings of failure. Diets that tout more energy but result in a loss of well-being.

Tell-Tale Signs of a Fad Diet

"Behold, I am sending you out as sheep in the midst of wolves, so be wise as serpents and innocent as doves." —Matthew 10:16

Here are signs of a Fad Diet. If a client or patient describes any of the following in the diet they want to try, start waving a red flag and yell, "Halt!"

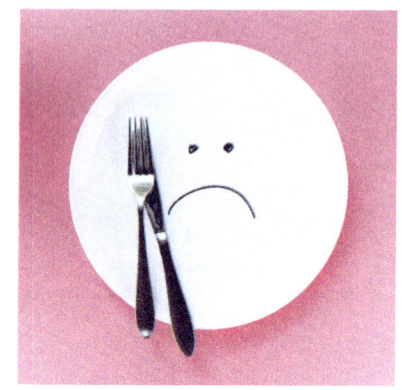

Limits food selections – Fad diets often focus on one research finding in an attempt to simplify science. In so doing, they become tunnel-visioned in their approach, ignoring all the other important scientific findings. Diets that eliminate entire food groups, such as carbs or dairy, can be labeled as nutritionally incomplete. If these diets are not completely avoided, they should at least be cautiously approached, and a physician should be consulted before subjecting one's health to such a diet. Variety in a diet is important.

Promotes rapid weight loss – Everyone who is trying to lose weight wants that excess fat gone now. We are an impatient population who does not like to wait for anything. Remember dial-up internet access? Now that people have experienced high-speed internet, it would be difficult to go back to dial-up. Overall, we are in an era where people don't wait well. From the Christian perspective, we need to learn to wait well. Jesus is coming back, and we need to be prepared…while we wait for his return. In my opinion, Satan has done a great job of manipulating this playground of his to make us a very impatient population that does not wait well.

In the initial stage of weight loss, water is lost. Water is heavy. So, a greater amount of "weight" loss in the first week can be expected. But after that first week, the recommended weight-loss rate should not exceed 1–2 pounds per week for most people. If someone is older and frail in stature, their recommended loss may be ¼ to ½ pound per week. But even small fractions show awesome progress! If any diet recommends or claims a weight loss greater than 2 pounds per week, chances are it is not body fat that is being lost. This is an important point to be conveyed to your patients and clients.

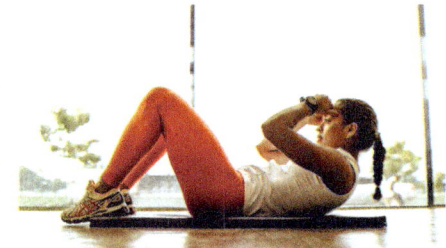

Advertises no exercise needed – My experience has been that people either love to get out and move their bodies or they hate it. But most people don't like being told they have to—well, fill in the blank with anything. Being told to exercise is a turn-off for many people, especially if they don't like to exercise. But exercise is the only guaranteed way to speed up our metabolism. Exercise burns calories and builds lean tissue, which then burns more calories. Exercise is essential to health, and it is essential to losing body fat. In this world of growing technology, we often must prioritize and schedule exercise, or else our bodies don't get worked and they simply waste away and gradually decline in vigor and function. Use it or lose it!

Requires a rigid menu and purchase of specific products (brand names) – Most people trying to lose weight are not test subjects in a laboratory. Most are out and about living life with friends, family, and co-workers. A diet plan that requires buying supplements or products instead of regular food from the local farmer's market or grocery store is simply trying to make money. Buying these extra products is a waste of money, and strictly eating prepackaged foods can be isolating. Eating the same prepared foods may be easy, as it removes all decision making, but it is monotonous and isn't helpful in learning how to eat better. Wasting money and eating monotonous food alone is usually not sustainable. People want flexibility and interactions with others during the day. Most enjoy the empowerment that accompanies knowing how to make wise choices. Many products sold involve shakes, liquid meals, and detox drinks. While more studies with larger sample sizes should be conducted on liquid versus solid meals and how they affect satiety and hunger, most research to date indicates that a meal's texture, viscosity, and the amount of chewing required all play a role in satiety. In other words, programs and fad diets that promote liquid drinks leave dieters hungry and less satisfied than if they were to eat real whole foods. This is true regardless of whether the liquid supplies protein, carbohydrates, or a mixture of macronutrients. A greater amount of oral processing has a statistically significant effect on reducing hunger.

Promises to speed up metabolism – Many diets promise to speed up our metabolism because that is what we want to hear. Foods don't really speed up metabolism. That is an exaggeration. This is discussed in more depth in the metabolism section. If this is a focal point of the diet, approach with caution. It is a great eye-catching selling point.

Requires expensive supplements – Supplements are not regulated by the Food and Drug Administration and therefore are susceptible to contamination through the global supply chain that involves many countries. The more we learn and discover, the more we realize how beneficial whole foods are when compared to supplements. While there are occasions that warrant supplement use—such as calcium for post-menopausal women, a prenatal vitamin for pregnant and lactating women, a multi-vitamin for some types of vegetarians, to name a few—eating a balanced diet will supply the body with the nutrients it needs. Scare tactics are often used with dieters to move them to buy non-essential supplements. Some fad diets even eliminate entire food groups then sell supplements to make up for missing nutrients not supplied. This makes no sense and doesn't help improve health or finances.

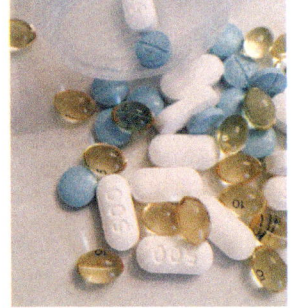

Relies on testimonials – Testimonials are remarkably interesting. We all love to gaze upon before-and-after pictures that portray a dream come true. The problem is that many of today's images have been photoshopped. I show one advertisement to my college students with an image of a young woman whose head is larger than her hips. This is anatomically impossible, but it is portrayed as an ideal body, one for which young women should strive. Due to technology, before-and-after pictures for testimonials can actually be produced on the same day. Programs or diet plans that rely heavily on testimonial promotion should be approached with caution.

Connects the diet with trendy places or celebrities – This technique is often used because it gets news coverage. That's it. This approach is meaningless, just popular and very visible. Carefully examine the food content and exercise recommendation with these types of diets.

Makes sensational claims – Fad diets exist because they tell us what we want to hear. They use words like "powerful," "breakthrough," "new," "secretes of the trade," "detoxify," "fat-burner," and "miracle cure." The basic belief in these claims is technology. Technological advances continue to occur in all areas of life from methods of transportation to approaches in communication to, yes, even procedures in health and weight management. Sensational claims bring hope. As we continue to look to the future, we need to do so wisely. And remember, if it seems too good to be true….it probably is.

> **RECAP:** Although fad diets may be based on a scientific truth, many cannot be sustained because they have impractical applications.

The Real Deal

Now that fad diets can be identified and their dangers recognized, what is the alternative? The alternative is a balanced eating plan that nourishes the body, keeps it healthy and functioning well, and promotes steady weight loss that is kept off. Some very good questions are asked in Isaiah 55:2: "Why spend your money on food that does not give you strength? Why pay for food that does you no good? Listen to me, and you will eat what is good. You will enjoy the finest food." Check out the amazing benefits that can occur with even a small weight loss.

Weight Lost	Resulting Heath Benefits
Losing 5-10 pounds	· Reduces risk of developing type 2 diabetes · Reduces triglycerides by 15 mg/dL · Reduces risk for non-alcoholic fatty liver disease · Improves liver function
Losing 10-20 pounds	· Decreases LDL (Low Density Lipoprotein) cholesterol by 5 mg/dL · Increases HDL (High Density Lipoprotein) cholesterol by 2-3 mg/dL · Improves ovulation frequency
Losing 20-30 pounds	· Reduces risk of dying from type 2 diabetes · Reduces sleep apnea events
Losing 2-5% of body weight	· Reduce fasting blood sugar · Lowers hemoglobin A1c by 0.2-0.3%
Losing 5% of body weight	· Reduces the need for new lipid-lowering medications · Reduces blood pressure · Reduces the need for new high blood pressure medications · Reduces arthritis disability
Losing 10 - 15% of body weight	· Lowers hemoglobin A1c by 0.6-1.0% · Reduces the need for diabetes medication · Increases HDL cholesterol by 2 mg/dL · Improves lung function and reduce need for rescue medication in those with asthma

As you can see, significant health benefits are realized from even small decreases in weight. The desire for fast weight loss is distinctly human: we are impatient. Moreover, it is heavily promoted and advertised as achievable by the diet industry. What they fail to share are the dangers and failures that accompany many fad diets.

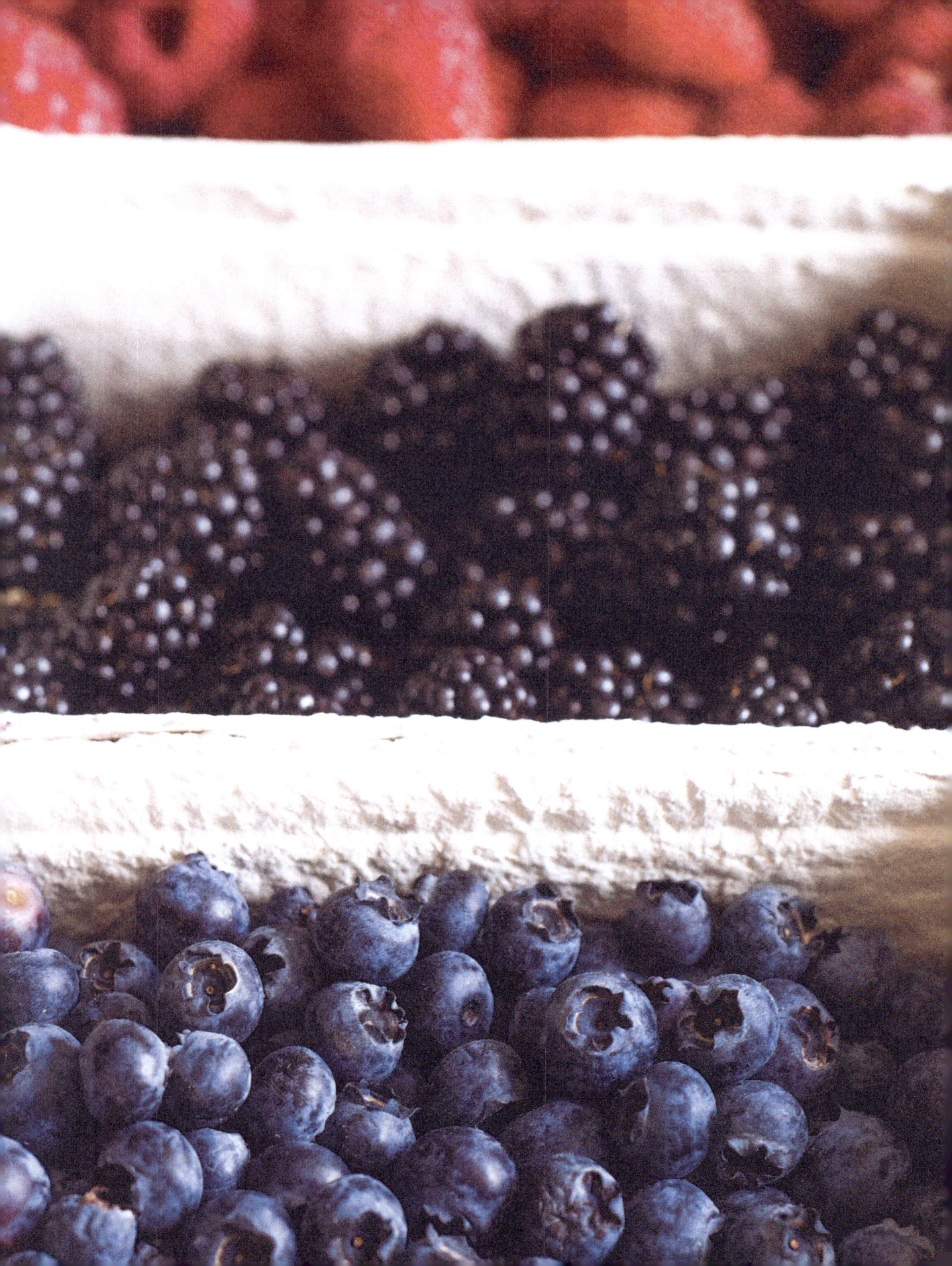

CHAPTER 3
Calories

"Let your eyes look directly forward, and your gaze be straight before you. Ponder the path of your feet; then all your ways will be sure." —Proverbs 4:25-26

I once had a graduate student who was scheduled to speak to a group of women in a church-based weight-management program tell me, "For my presentation, they want me to make a list and talk about foods they can eat and foods they shouldn't eat." I told him, "If you agree to that, you are on your own and I am not helping you makes those lists." Most people want a good food, bad food list. While this would make things quite easy, and some have attempted to create such lists, there has never been a complete list created that is applicable to everyone. There are too many variables. What is acceptable or even good for one person may not be good for another person. You already know this from working with your patients and clients. Yet it is possible to make food work for us to assist in weight loss. Let's first review where calories come from.

A calorie is a unit of energy. Therefore, when talking about weight loss, 100 calories is 100 calories, regardless of whether they come from a steak, a banana, or a candy bar. But not all calories are created equal. There are two reasons for this:

1. Food Source: The body uses energy to extract calories from food and process it. In other words, the body burns calories when it breaks down carbohydrates, fats, and protein. Immediately after eating, and for several hours after a meal, energy expenditure increases to generate adenosine triphosphate (ATP), the compound that provides energy for many body processes, such as muscle contraction. But in this case, it is providing energy to move food through the body, so it can be digested and absorbed, and nutrients can be transported. This burning of calories is called the Thermic Effect of Food (TEF). The type of nutrients consumed will influence the TEF. For example, a meal high in protein has the highest thermic effect, 20–30%. In other words, in a pure protein meal, 20–30% of the calories consumed would be used in metabolizing that protein. Carbohydrates have a TEF of 5 to 10%, which is greater than fat, which is 0–3%. The energy cost to convert dietary fat into stored fat or triglycerides is minimal. Fat is the most efficient: we eat it and much of it can get stored without much effort.

2. Health: When considering health, it is important to distinguish between quantity and quality. In fact, foods with the same quantity of calories can vary widely in their nutritional quality, which can ultimately affect health. For example, all fats contribute 9 calories per gram, but if those grams are coming from trans-fats in French fries versus the monounsaturated fats found in avocados, over time the first can harm the body and therefore should be avoided, while the second could be beneficial and is therefore recommended for consumption.

Calories Matter

Calories are a central part of weight loss. Metabolically speaking, when it comes to weight loss, a calorie deficit is always needed. I wish I could say calories don't matter, but there's no way around it: all calories count. Some weight-loss diets claim that what is eaten is more important than how much is eaten. I have had several family members, friends, and students claim that they lost more weight on low-carb diets than on high-carb diets, despite eating as many or even more total calories. And indeed, some studies seem to support this notion.

However, when examining these studies, we need to be cautious, and the following cannot be ignored:

1. Researchers of many studies do not directly measure foods eaten by the subjects in their studies but instead rely on participants keeping their own food and exercise records. Participants generally underestimate the amount of food they eat by as much as 45%. At the same time, people tend to overestimate how much they exercise, in some cases in excess of 50%!

2. By default, low-carbohydrate diets have to be higher in protein and fat. Both protein and fat digest slower than carbohydrates. This can help reduce hunger for longer periods of time, creating a greater feeling of fullness and therefore, for some, reducing eating. As noted above, protein also has a higher TEF, meaning it requires slightly more energy to digest than carbs and fat. This may contribute to an energy deficit and weight loss. However, it would be unwise to suggest eating more protein than the body needs based on this concept. Too much protein can be harmful to those with compromised kidneys or decreased bone health, and it can contribute to dehydration. High-protein diets tend to be low in fiber, which means all the benefits of fiber won't be realized. These diets also tend to be higher in fat if the protein source is not carefully selected. Moreover, the body will store excess protein as body fat, just like it will for excess dietary fat and carbohydrates.

3. Furthermore, if a study only reports total weight lost, without specifying if the weight lost was in the form of fat, muscle, or water, then the study results can't really be understood or applied because the data are ambiguous. When people are on a low-carb diet, they will deplete their glycogen stores within a short period of time. While the amount of glycogen varies from person to person, an overnight fast can deplete 50% of glycogen stores. For every one gram of carbohydrate stored in the body (as glycogen), 2.7 to 4 grams of water are stored. Therefore, much of the initial weight lost will be water weight. This fact immediately makes the fast weight-loss claims of many low-carbohydrate diets very unimpressive.

Therefore, when it comes to weight loss, only the studies that reflect these issues should really be considered. If we only examine these studies, we see that calorie amount matters. Fewer calories must be consumed than are expended.

Calorie counting works

Calorie counting is simply a tool that some may find useful. As a health care provider, it is important to familiarize yourself with the following:

Why calories matter:

1. *Identify Patterns* – Tracking calories helps to identify eating and exercise patterns that need modifying. Even if records are not exactly precise, tracking can begin the educational process of learning portion sizes.

2. *Assist with Accountability* – Food tracking can help with accountability.

3. *Identify Success* – Keeping food and exercise journals can help successes, achievements, and progress be comprehended and appreciated, which can ultimately help drive progress toward achieving goals.

How to monitor calories:

1. *Using Technology* – Tracking can be done either with paper and pencil or with an app. Both methods are helpful. Counting calories is one helpful tool, but it is not required for weight loss.

2. *Using Food* – Food groups can also be considered.

3. *Energy Deficit* – What is ultimately needed for weight loss is a sustained energy deficit. Some programs and diets do all the work by providing premade meals and snacks that, if followed, will create an energy deficit. Research does show that programs offering this approach do work. People do lose weight as long as they continue eating those predetermined portions of food. I tend to prefer educating people so they become empowered to make wise choices in all types of environments. I don't find it wise to be dependent on and limited to a product or a company.

4. *Feelings and Emotions* – In addition to counting calories, some people find it helpful to track the times they eat and their feelings before, during, and after eating. This additional endeavor can enlighten a dieter as to patterns and habits of which they might not be aware. The first step to changing behavior is being aware of the behavior.

RECAP: Tracking calories and food sources provides an overview of the food consumed. This type of activity, if consistently done, can bring to the surface an awareness of patterns, some which may need to be modified.

Portion sizes matter

Scripture is clear that portion sizes are important. The Word does not celebrate gluttony:

"One of Crete's own prophets has said it: 'Cretans are always liars, evil brutes, lazy gluttons.'" —Titus 1:12

"A discerning son heeds instruction, but a companion of gluttons disgraces his father." —Proverbs 28:7

"Listen, my son, and be wise, and set your heart on the right path: Do not join those who drink too much wine or gorge themselves on meat, for drunkards and gluttons become poor, and drowsiness clothes them in rags." —Psalm 23:19-21

God's word also talks about overeating and overindulgence:

"Their destiny is destruction, their god is their stomach, and their glory is in their shame. Their mind is set on earthly things." —Philippians 3:19

"They willfully put God to the test by demanding the food they craved." —Psalm 78:18

"If you find honey, eat just enough, too much of it, and you will vomit." —Proverbs 25:16

Christians need to tap into the Holy Spirit for self-control to guard against all forms of idolatry and temptations that can ultimately lead to treating our bodies poorly. These fleshly cravings are powerful. Think about the account of Esau in Genesis 25:29-34:

"Once when Jacob was cooking stew, Esau came in from the field, and he was exhausted. And Esau said to Jacob, 'Let me eat some of that red stew, for I am exhausted!' Jacob said, 'Sell me your birthright now.' Esau said, 'I am about to die; of what use is a birthright to me?' Jacob said, 'Swear to me now.' So he swore to him and sold his birthright to Jacob. Then Jacob gave Esau bread and lentil stew, and he ate and drank and rose and went his way. Thus Esau despised his birthright."

We have all been there—so hungry that we feel like we are going to die. Hunger and cravings can be very powerful.

When my sister was pregnant, she had cravings for butterscotch pudding. One day, when one of these cravings hit, she dumped the pudding packet into her favorite blue bowl, grabbed the milk out of the refrigerator, and started pouring it into the bowl. I raised my hand toward the bowl and asked, "Don't you need to measure the milk?" My question didn't cause her to flinch; she continued to pour the milk. She smiled and said, "I've made so much butterscotch pudding in this bowl I can accurately eye the right amount of milk needed." As you can tell from the above story about my sister, counting calories and using portion sizes only evaluates diet quantity. It says nothing about the diet's quality. Therefore, it is important not to choose foods based solely on how many calories they provide. To make this point, I simply need to retell the account of hearing some college women, in a Friday morning class, planning to fast all day so they could drink their calories that night. This approach only considers total calories. However, it is important to consider vitamin and mineral content too. This can be done by favoring whole, minimally processed foods. In order to not over- or underestimate how much is consumed, it is essential, at least when starting out, for your patients and clients to educate their eye to portion sizes. In other words, it is important to learn what serving sizes look like. There are many ways to do this. Scales can be used to weigh meats, and measuring cups and spoons can be used for other food items. If no scales or cups are available, other items can be used. (see table beside)

1 TEASPOON	The tip of your pointer finger, or a postage stamp	
1 TABLESPOON	Three fingertips, your thumb, a poker chip	
2 TABLESPOONS	A golf ball	
1 CUP	A baseball	
1.5 OUNCES	A lipstick tube, the size of an adult's thumb, pointer finger, 4 dice, or 3 dominos	
3 OUNCES	A deck of cards or the size and thickness of the palm of your hand	
4 OUNCES	A checkbook, or the size and thickness of your hand and fingers	
BAKED POTATO	A computer mouse	
1 PANCAKE	A CD	

RECAP: We need to develop an eye trained to serving sizes. We should choose nutrient-dense foods.

Calories and Exercise are Both Important in Weight Loss

There are many factors that go into weight loss and weight control. One of those factors includes calories consumed. In order to lose weight, fewer calories must be consumed than are burned. An obvious solution to aid in this process is to burn more calories.

In my years of working with people, I have seen that some people fall into one of two categories. Some have said, "I would rather run a marathon every day or climb a mountain daily than limit my food intake." Others have said, "I'll eat whatever you tell me to eat… just don't make me get up off the couch!" Undoubtedly some of your patients or clients fall into one of these categories. Most people lean to or favor one over the other, which is natural. However, to maximize health and weight maintenance, both diet and exercise should be incorporated. If only one area is addressed, the process will be slower and less efficient.

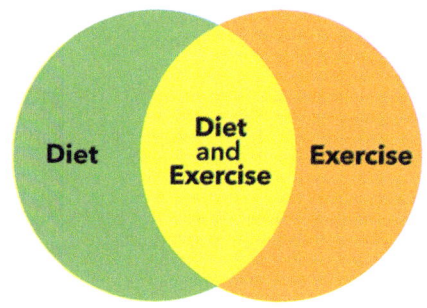

Different approaches are available for those who favor the diet category. Some people find counting calories reassuring and helpful, giving them confidence. Others prefer to monitor the number of portions of certain food groups eaten. It is important to remember that for continued success in weight loss, more than just total calories must be considered and monitored.

Nutrient-dense foods should fill meals and snacks. Nutrient-dense foods provide a lot of nutritional value but not a lot of calories. For example, fruits, vegetables, and nuts are nutrient-dense, meaning every calorie consumed is accompanied by many nutrients. Most whole foods are nutrient-dense. Nutrient density can be viewed on a continuum, with nutrient-dense foods on one end of the spectrum and calorie-dense foods on the other end. When a food is viewed this way, there is no exact or precise cutoff point when we cross over from nutrient-dense foods into calorie-dense foods. In fact, the application of this continuum could be personalized to different dieters with diverse needs. For example, when I introduce the terms "nutrient-dense foods" and "calorie-dense foods" to my students, after defining them I'll often ask the students, "Tell me your favorite calorie-dense food." My expectation is that they may respond with something like "ice cream, brownies, or a candy bar." To which I respond, "Yum, absolutely!" But sometimes a student may respond with "spaghetti" or "bread." It is less clear where these foods fall on the continuum. They are less clear because they come in various forms, and how they were prepared and made will determine where they fall on the continuum. One thing is for sure: spinach and kale are nutrient-dense foods, while cheesecake is at the other end of the spectrum.

While most of your patients and clients understand that kale and cheesecake won't equally contribute to their weight-loss efforts, many may not understand the concept of body composition or its role in weight loss.

What Is Body Composition?

"For You formed my inmost being; You knit me together in my mother's womb. I praise You, for I am fearfully and wonderfully made. Marvelous are Your works, and I know this very well. My frame was not hidden from You when I was made in secret, when I was woven together in the depths of the earth." —Psalm 139:13-15

As you know, the human body is made up of many types of cells, tissues, and organs. For the purpose of this discussion, we only need to talk about two types of tissue: fat tissue and lean tissue. Fat tissue is made up of adipose cells. This is the type of tissue people generally want less of on their body. Because adipose serves a number of different functions in the body like insulation, cushioning, and helping to absorb the fat-soluble vitamins A, D, E, and K, patients and clients often need reminding that we require some fat on our bodies. This is an especially important discussion with women, as they often need to be made aware that women need to have more fat on their bodies than men.

Below is a chart showing the recommended percentages of body fat derived by the American Council on Exercise.

Category	Males	Females
Essential Body Fat	2-5%	10-13%
Athletes	6-13%	14-20%
Fitness	14-17%	21-24%
Acceptable	18-24%	25-31%
Obesity	>25%	>32%

Source: Muth, ND. What are the guidelines for percentage of body fat loss? American Council on Exercise. https://www.acefitness.org/education-and-resources/lifestyle/blog/112/what-are-the-guidelines-for-percentage-of-body-fat-loss/. Published December 2009. Accessed April 8, 2020.

When looking at these numbers, it is important to keep in mind that these are approximate values of essential body fat to meet basic physiological needs. The athletic category may apply particularly to athletes who compete in events where excess body fat may be a disadvantage. Sometimes it is helpful to explain to clients and patients that lean tissue is often referred to as metabolically active tissue because it is the tissue that physically does work and burns calories. Just its existence on a body burns calories. Simply stated, lean tissue consists of our muscles, bones, connective tissue, blood cells, and organs (e.g., kidneys, heart, lungs)—any tissue that is doing work within the body. That is one of the reasons people with larger muscles need more calories than people with smaller muscles. This is an important concept for your patients and clients to embrace.

It is a concept that a woman I worked with many years ago did not understand. This client had a daughter who was engaged, and the wedding was 6 weeks away when she came to see me. We sat down, and this mother sheepishly revealed that she wished she had come months ago, as she had wanted to lose 75 pounds for her daughter's wedding that was now rapidly approaching. The question I pose to you is, "Do you think it would be possible for this or any other woman to lose 75 pounds in 6 weeks?" I hope you answered, "Yes – of course." This is possible because all we would need to do is amputate her legs. Right? Seventy-five pounds would be gone in an instant. But that is not what that woman really meant or wanted. What she specifically wanted was to lose was 75 pounds of body fat, and that is not possible in 6 weeks. It is not possible because we cannot lose fat quickly! This is another important concept that patients and clients need to understand. If "weight" is lost quickly, we can be guaranteed it is not body fat. But alas, we are impatient humans, so we want to hear that we can be 10–15 pounds lighter by the end of the week.

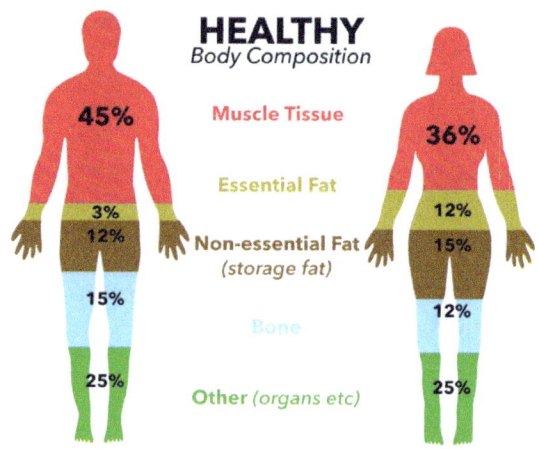

RECAP: Fat and lean tissues play different roles in the body and different roles in weight loss.

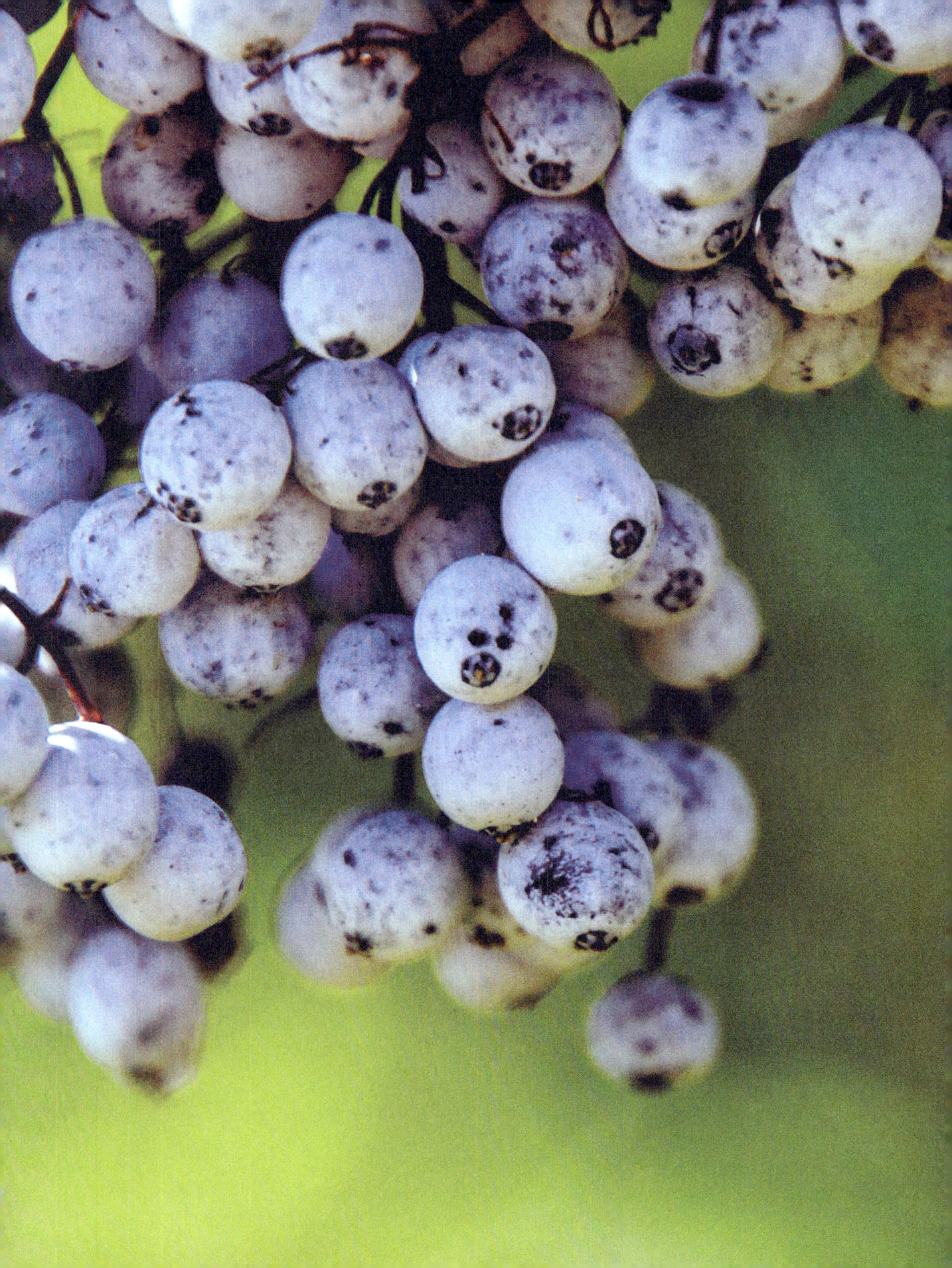

CHAPTER 4
Micronutrients

"But Daniel was determined not to defile himself by eating the food and wine given to them by the king. He asked the chief of staff for permission not to eat these unacceptable foods." —Daniel 1:8

Just as Daniel was resolved to eat only certain foods, we too must choose wisely what to eat.

Micronutrients are needed in small amounts but are essential to health. Diets that eliminate or severely restrict food groups have an increased risk of micronutrient deficiencies. This review of micronutrients serves as a reference for the deficiency risks associated with fad diets. Let's start with vitamins.

Vitamins

Vitamins are tasteless organic compounds that are essential in small amounts. The body requires small amounts for normal metabolic function. Because many diets cut out some foods or food groups, deficiencies of certain vitamins can develop. A deficiency in any vitamin can result in serious symptoms. Let's first look at how vitamins are classified.

A compound is classified as a vitamin when:

> 1. It cannot be synthesized in ample amounts in the body to meet the body's needs for it. For example, Vitamin K and two of the B vitamins (niacin and biotin) can be made in the body, but not in amounts sufficient to meet the body's metabolic needs.

> 2. Chronic deficiency can cause physical symptoms, and those symptoms will disappear once the vitamin has been sufficiently restored to the body.

There are 13 compounds classified as vitamins based on these criteria.

Traditionally, vitamins have been categorized into two groups based on their solubility in water or fat. This allows for generalizations to be made about how the vitamins are digested, absorbed, transported, excreted, and stored in the body.

> 1. Water-soluble vitamins include vitamins B and C. Collectively, the B vitamins are referred to as the "B complex." They consist of thiamine (B1), riboflavin (B2), niacin (B3), pantothenic acid, biotin, vitamin B6, folate, and vitamin B12.

> 2. The fat-soluble vitamins are A, D, E, and K.

All vitamins are defined as organic because they contain carbon. Vitamins also contain hydrogen and oxygen, and in some cases, nitrogen and sulfur. But the chemical structure of each vitamin is unique. Unlike the macronutrients, which are made up of units bonded together to form chains, vitamins are singular units. For this reason, there are no bonds for the body to hydrolyze during digestion. Vitamins are absorbed intact into the intestinal wall.

It is important when discussing diets to ensure that all vitamins (and minerals) are consumed in adequate amounts through a variety of whole foods. For example, a dieter may eliminate milk expecting to get adequate calcium through eating spinach which contains quite a bit of calcium. But only about 5% of the calcium in spinach is absorbed. Not all the vitamins consumed in foods are available to be used in the body. In other words, they are not 100% bioavailable. The body's ability to absorb and use these micronutrients is called bioavailability. Many fad diets promote various food groups while eliminating others. In doing this, many essential nutrients are often not consumed or may be consumed in forms that are poorly absorbed. Many dieters convince themselves that they are getting adequate vitamins through supplements. Most research indicates better health outcomes are achieved through eating a variety of whole foods instead of relying on supplements.

Factors that affect bioavailability:

1. Type of food – Minerals in animal products are absorbed better than from plants (plants have binders and dietary fiber that hinder digestion and absorption). In addition, animal products, as a rule, tend to have higher levels of minerals than plants.

2. Mineral-to-mineral interaction – Since many minerals have the same molecular weight, they compete for intestinal absorption. An excess of any one mineral can interfere with the absorption of other minerals.

3. Vitamin–mineral interactions – Vitamins interact with minerals in ways that affect mineral bioavailability. For example, vitamin D facilitates calcium absorption, and vitamin C enhances iron absorption.

4. Fiber–mineral interaction – Fiber can bind to minerals, causing them to pass unabsorbed. (This is true for calcium, iron, magnesium, and phosphorus.)

Bioavailability varies depending on conditions.

1. Fat-soluble vitamins are absorbed along with dietary fat. If the diet is very low in fat, absorption of these vitamins can be impaired. The bioavailability of fat-soluble vitamins is usually less than that of water-soluble vitamins, because fat-soluble vitamins require bile salts and rely on other working mechanisms. Thus, since fat-soluble vitamins are incorporated into other molecules for transport, their bioavailability depends in part on the availability of these transport systems.

2. The amount of vitamin in the food, considering its freshness or its age, influences bioavailability.

3. Whether a food is cooked or raw will affect its bioavailability. Generally, raw foods have more vitamins.

4. The efficiency with which food is absorbed is an individual factor.

5. One's nutritional status – In general, if the body needs more vitamins, a greater percentage will be absorbed. For example, a young growing child or a pregnant woman will absorb more ingested vitamins than will a non-pregnant adult.

Vitamins in plants are typically less bioavailable than those in animal foods, because plant fiber can trap vitamins, causing them to be excreted.

About 40 to 90% of the vitamins in food are absorbed, primarily in the small intestine.

Pro-vitamins and Vitamin Precursors

Some vitamins are absorbed in an inactive form called either pro-vitamin or vitamin precursor. These must be converted into active vitamin forms once they are inside the body. A well-known example of this is beta-carotene, which is split into two molecules of vitamin A in the liver cells. Vitamins found in foods that are already in the active form are called pre-formed vitamins.

Functions and Deficiencies

Let's look at each of the vitamins, their roles in the body, and what happens when we do not get enough supplied in our diet. Keep in mind that many diets limit food groups and increase the risk of various deficiencies. The stores of the water-soluble vitamins (B and C) do not last long. Let's start with them.

Water-Soluble Vitamins

The lack of water-soluble vitamins, except for B6 and B12, can be recognized within a few days.

THIAMIN (B1) was the first vitamin to be discovered. It is sensitive to pH; therefore, cooking with baking soda destroys its ability to function.

- *Sources:* Lean pork, enriched whole-grain foods such as breads, ready-to-eat cereals, pasta, and rice

- *Function:* Essential for the metabolism of carbohydrates and proteins

- *Deficiency:* Development of the disease beriberi, which involves swelling, damaged nerves, congestive heart failure, muscle wasting, and nerve degeneration

- *If too much is consumed:* No known adverse effects

RIBOFLAVIN (B2) is rather stable in cooking but degrades in the presence of ultraviolet light.

- *Sources:* Milk, yogurt, enriched cereals and grains, including quinoa, rice, and oats

- *Function:* Involved in the metabolism of several other vitamins, as well as energy and fat metabolism

- *Deficiency:* Causes the development of ariboflavinosis. In this disease the cells that line the throat, mouth, tongue, and lips become inflamed or swollen. Deficiency also affects enzyme systems.

- *If too much is consumed:* No known adverse effects

NIACIN (B3) is the generic term for the two active forms of this vitamin, nicotinic acid and nicotinamide, found in food. It is not destroyed by heat or ultraviolet light, but it can leach out if the food is soaked in water. Niacin found in plants is less bioavailable than niacin from animal sources. Prescription levels are used to treat high cholesterol.

- *Source:* Fish, poultry, meat, enriched whole-grain breads and fortified cereals

- *Function:* Needed for the metabolism of all three macronutrients (carbohydrates, protein, and fat). Keeps skin cells healthy and the digestive system functioning.

- *Deficiency:* Development of pellagra. This disease involves dermatitis, dementia, diarrhea, and death.

- *If too much is consumed:* Flushing, blurred vision, liver dysfunction, and glucose intolerance

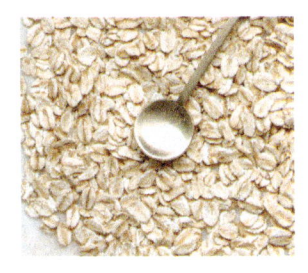

PANTOTHENIC ACID comes from the Greek word pantothen meaning "everywhere," and indeed, it is found in almost every food. Because it is destroyed by heat, foods that are processed may have less than their fresh counterparts.

- *Source:* Whole-grain products, nut meal, legumes, milk, eggs

- *Function:* Part of co-enzyme A, a gateway molecule in energy metabolism

- *Deficiency:* Vomiting, numbness, muscle cramps, nausea, fatigue

- *If too much is consumed:* No known adverse effects

BIOTIN – Raw eggs contain the protein avidin, which can bind biotin and render it useless.

- *Source:* Yeast, whole grains, peanuts, fish, liver and other organ meats

- *Function:* Essential for energy metabolism and DNA replication

- *Deficiency:* Dermatitis, especially around the nose, mouth, and eyes, conjunctivitis, hair loss, hallucinations

- *If too much is consumed:* No known adverse effects

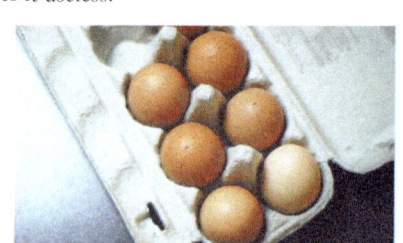

VITAMIN B_6 – The bioavailability of B_6 is about 75%. Alcohol depletes the body's B6.

- *Source:* Chickpeas and other legumes, chicken, ready-to-eat cereals, meat, nuts, peanut butter, vegetables and fruits

- *Function:* Protein and glucose metabolism, enzyme use, and red blood cell synthesis

- *Deficiency:* Sore tongue, inflammation of the skin, depression, confusion, and microcytic hypochromic anemia, which is anemia characterized by small, pale red blood cells.

- *If too much is consumed:* Nerve damage

FOLATE occurs naturally in foods. Its name is derived from the Latin word folium for "foliage." Its synthetic counterpart, folic acid, is a simpler molecule that is more bioavailable, more stable, and not as easily destroyed as the natural folate. Folic acid is the form in supplements and what is added to foods. Folic acid is required by law to be added to enriched cereals and grains.

- *Source:* Spinach, broccoli, asparagus, dried peas and beans, seeds, enriched breads, grains, and rice

- *Function:* Prevents birth defects, reduces the risk of cancer and heart disease, helps red blood cells divide and increase in number, and helps the body use amino acids

- *Deficiency:* Development of macrocytic anemia, which involves large red blood cells that have a diminished ability to carry oxygen, eventually leading to feeling tired and weak

- *If too much is consumed:* Can mask the symptoms of vitamin B12 deficiency

VITAMIN B12 is also called cobalamin because it contains the mineral cobalt. Naturally occurring B12 is found only in foods from animal sources. Using a microwave to cook foods with vitamin B12 can reduce its bioavailability by 30–40%.

- *Source:* Meat, fish, poultry, dairy, ready-to-eat cereals

- *Function:* Synthesis of new cells, needed to activate folate, needed for healthy nerve tissue, needed in fatty acid and amino acid metabolism

- *Deficiency:* Pernicious anemia, which is characterized by fatigue and nerve damage

- *If too much is consumed:* No known adverse effects

VITAMIN C – A few weeks without vitamin C can cause deficiency symptoms, and 20–30 weeks without vitamin C can result in death. Consuming too little vitamin C appears to inhibit the hormone leptin. Leptin sends the message that we are full and can stop eating.

- *Source:* Citrus fruits, tomatoes, peppers, broccoli, cantaloupe, and most berries

- *Function:* Acts as an antioxidant, needed to form collagen, helps iron be absorbed by the body, and needed for an effective immune system

- *Deficiency:* Development of scurvy, which is characterized by bleeding gums, wounds that can't heal, fragile blood vessel walls, and joint pain

- *If too much is consumed:* Nausea, diarrhea, insomnia, and fatigue

Fat-Soluble Vitamins

VITAMIN A occurs in animal tissues. It is also found in pro-vitamin form in vegetables pigmented by yellow and red carotenoids. It is sometimes referred to as the "anti-infection" vitamin. Consuming too little vitamin A also seems to inhibit the hormone leptin.

- *Sources:* Milk, cheese, cereals, egg yolks, liver, carrots, spinach, sweet potatoes, pumpkin

- *Functions:* Growth, rapid reproduction of different types of epithelial cells, and vision.

- *Deficiencies:* Vision problems, increased infections. Vitamin A is stored in the liver, and depending on the amount stored, may be sufficient to maintain a person for 5–10 months without any intake.

- *If too much is consumed:* Birth defects and poor bone health

VITAMIN D can also be stored in the liver, and this can suffice for 2–4 months before additional intake is needed. It is called the sunshine vitamin because it can be manufactured in the body with ultraviolet rays and cholesterol.

- *Sources:* Fortified milk, breakfast cereals, yogurt, fatty fish such as sardines and salmon

- *Functions:* Helps build and maintain bone mass, helps regulate the growth and differentiation of cells, reduces risk of developing certain autoimmune disorders, reduces hypertension

- *Deficiencies:* In children, rickets can develop as a result of bones not being adequately mineralized with calcium and phosphorus, causing them to become weakened "soft bones" and to bow. In adults, osteomalacia occurs when bones can't mineralize properly.

- *If too much is consumed:* Lack of appetite, nausea, vomiting, constipation, over-absorption of calcium to dangerous levels

VITAMIN E – There are 8 forms of vitamin E, but alpha-tocopherol is the most active in the body.

- *Sources:* Avocados, vegetables oils, nuts and seeds, wheat germ, safflower, corn and soybean oils

- *Function:* Neutralizes free radicals before they harm cell membranes, reduces the risk of atherosclerosis by protecting the LDL carrier from being oxidized, inhibits platelets from clumping together unnecessarily, and lessens the stickiness of cells that line the lymph and blood vessels, reducing plaque build-up

- *Deficiencies:* Nerve problems, muscle weakness, and increased susceptibility to cell membrane damage

- *If too much is consumed:* Increased risk of hemorrhage

VITAMIN K – Bacteria in the large intestine make vitamin K, but only about 10% is absorbed.

- *Source:* Kale, broccoli, Swiss chard, collard greens, asparagus, Brussels sprouts, spinach

- *Function:* Blood clotting, strengthening bones

- *Deficiencies:* Reduced blood clotting

- *If too much is consumed:* No known adverse effects

Phytochemicals

The term "phytochemical" literally means plant-chemical. Sometimes, these are called phytonutrients. While still being studied, research thus far indicates that phytochemicals work synergistically with vitamins, minerals, and fiber to promote health and lower disease risk. All of these are found in unprocessed, whole fruits, vegetables, and whole-grain products. Choosing a variety of foods continues to emerge as an important foundation to all diets. Below is a chart displaying this concept. Please notice the abundance of fruits, vegetables, and whole-grain sources. To provide the body with disease-fighting phytochemicals, vitamins, minerals, and fiber, consuming a variety of colorful fruits, vegetables, and whole grains daily is recommended.

A Guide to Phytochemicals by Color

Color	Phytochemical	Found in
White	Alliums/Allicin	Garlic, leeks, onion, scallions
Red	Anthocyanins	Apples, beets, cherries, red cabbage, red onions, red beans
Yellow/Orange	Beta-carotene	Apricots, butternut squash, cantaloupe, carrots, mangoes, peaches, pumpkin, sweet potatoes
	Flavonoids	Apricots, grapefruit, lemons, pears, pineapple, yellow raisins
Green	Lutein, zeaxanthin	Broccoli, collard greens, honeydew melon, kale, kiwi, lettuce, mustard greens, peas, spinach
	Indoles	Arugula, broccoli, bok choy, Brussels sprouts, cabbage, cauliflower, kale, Swiss chard, turnips
Blue/Purple	Anthocyanins	Blackberries, black currants, elderberries, purple grapes
	Phenolics	Eggplants, plums, prunes, raisins
Brown	Beta-glucan, lignans, phenols, plant sterols, phytoestrogens, saponins, tocotrienols	Barley, brown rice, oats, oatmeal, whole grains, whole-grain cereals, whole wheat

Source: Adapted from Fruits and Veggies – More Matters, Available at www.fruitsandveggiesmorematters.org.

Minerals

Minerals are inorganic elements needed by the body. Their bioavailability varies. They serve many functions and can be toxic if consumed in excess. The minerals needed by the body are sodium, chloride, potassium, calcium, phosphorus, magnesium, sulfate, iron, copper, zinc, selenium, fluoride, chromium, iodine, molybdenum, and manganese. Only the minerals identified in the various diets evaluated are elaborated on below.

CALCIUM is the most abundant mineral in the body. Over 99% of the calcium in the body can be found in bones and teeth. The bioavailability of calcium is worth discussing. Vitamin D and lactose improve calcium's absorption. Low-protein diets reduce calcium's absorption, while high-protein diets improve it. Foods with oxalates (spinach) and phytates (whole-wheat bread) reduce calcium's absorption. A person deficient in calcium will absorb it better than someone who is not deficient. Calcium is best absorbed in smaller, more frequent doses, rather than a large amount at one time. Seventy-five percent of women do not consume the recommended about of calcium; in fact, 50% consume less than half of the recommendation. With proper nutrition and regular weight-bearing physical activity, women normally show gains in bone mass throughout the early to mid-thirties. Adolescence serves as the prime bone-building years to maximize bone mass. In fact, 90% of bone mass accumulates by age 17! Do I have to repeat that? By the age of 17, you will have 90% of all the bone you will ever have! Yet, the average teenager consumes insufficient calcium to support growing bones. Men around age 50 experience a bone loss of about .4% each year. Women, on the other hand, begin to lose twice this amount at age 35. It is a big deal to consume adequate calcium through the growing years.

- *Sources:* Milk, yogurt, cheese, tofu, soy milk, salmon, orange juice fortified with calcium, leafy greens, broccoli
- *Functions:* Bone and teeth formation, muscle contraction, blood clotting, heart and nerve functioning
- *Deficiencies:* Less dense bones
- *If too much is consumed:* Constipation, impaired kidneys, and calcium deposits in tissues

IRON deficiency is the most common deficiency around the world. Iron deficiency anemia is common in children and women of childbearing age. Food provides two forms of iron. Animal tissue provides heme iron, which the body absorbs well. Non-heme iron is found in plants, but it is 2–3 times less bioavailable than heme iron. Bioavailability is impacted by oxalates found in vegetables and phenols found in tea and coffee. For example, phenols can reduce non-heme iron in a meal by 70%, but vitamin C enhances non-heme iron absorption. Adding heme iron foods to a meal with non-heme iron foods also enhances the absorption of the non-heme iron.

- *Sources:* Meat, fish, poultry, enriched and fortified breads and cereals
- *Functions:* Is a major component of hemoglobin, enhances the immune system, needed for brain function and energy metabolism
- *Deficiencies:* Poor immune function, inhibited growth in infants, reduced ability to fight infections, fatigue and weakness
- *If too much is consumed:* Vomiting, nausea, diarrhea, constipation, and kidney, heart, nerve, and liver damage

PHOSPHORUS is the second most abundant mineral in the body, most of which is bound with calcium in bones and teeth.

- *Sources:* Meat, fish, poultry, dairy products, nuts, beans, peas, yogurt, salmon, milk, seeds
- *Functions*: Needed for bone and teeth formation, is an important part of DNA and RNA, necessary for metabolism, transports lipids
- *Deficiencies:* Muscle weakness and bone pain
- *If too much is consumed:* Decrease in bone mass and formation of calcium deposits in soft tissue

POTASSIUM – About 85% of consumed potassium is absorbed. Over 95% of the body's potassium is found within cells. The kidney maintains potassium balance by excreting excess in urine.

- *Sources:* Fruits, vegetables, meat, dairy, nuts, watermelon, sweet potatoes, green leafy vegetables

- *Functions:* Regulates blood pressure, allows for the conduction of nerve impulses and muscle contractions, helps maintain fluid balance

- *Deficiencies:* Irregular heartbeat, muscle weaknesses and cramps, tiredness

- *If too much is consumed:* Irregular heartbeat, nausea, fatigue, muscle weakness, and tingling in feet and hands

ZINC is found in small amounts in almost every cell, but mostly in bone and muscle. Zinc supplements taken by obese individuals have been reported to lower leptin levels. Leptin is a hormone that tells us we are full.

- *Sources:* Red meats, oysters, whole grains and cereals

- *Functions:* Needed for DNA and RNA synthesis, supports the immune system, improves taste perception, and may prevent age-related macular degeneration

- *Deficiencies:* Hair loss, impaired taste, loss of appetite, diarrhea, skin rashes, delayed sexual maturation, impotence

- *If too much is consumed:* Stomach pains, nausea, vomiting, diarrhea, suppression of immune system, and lowering of HDL (good) cholesterol

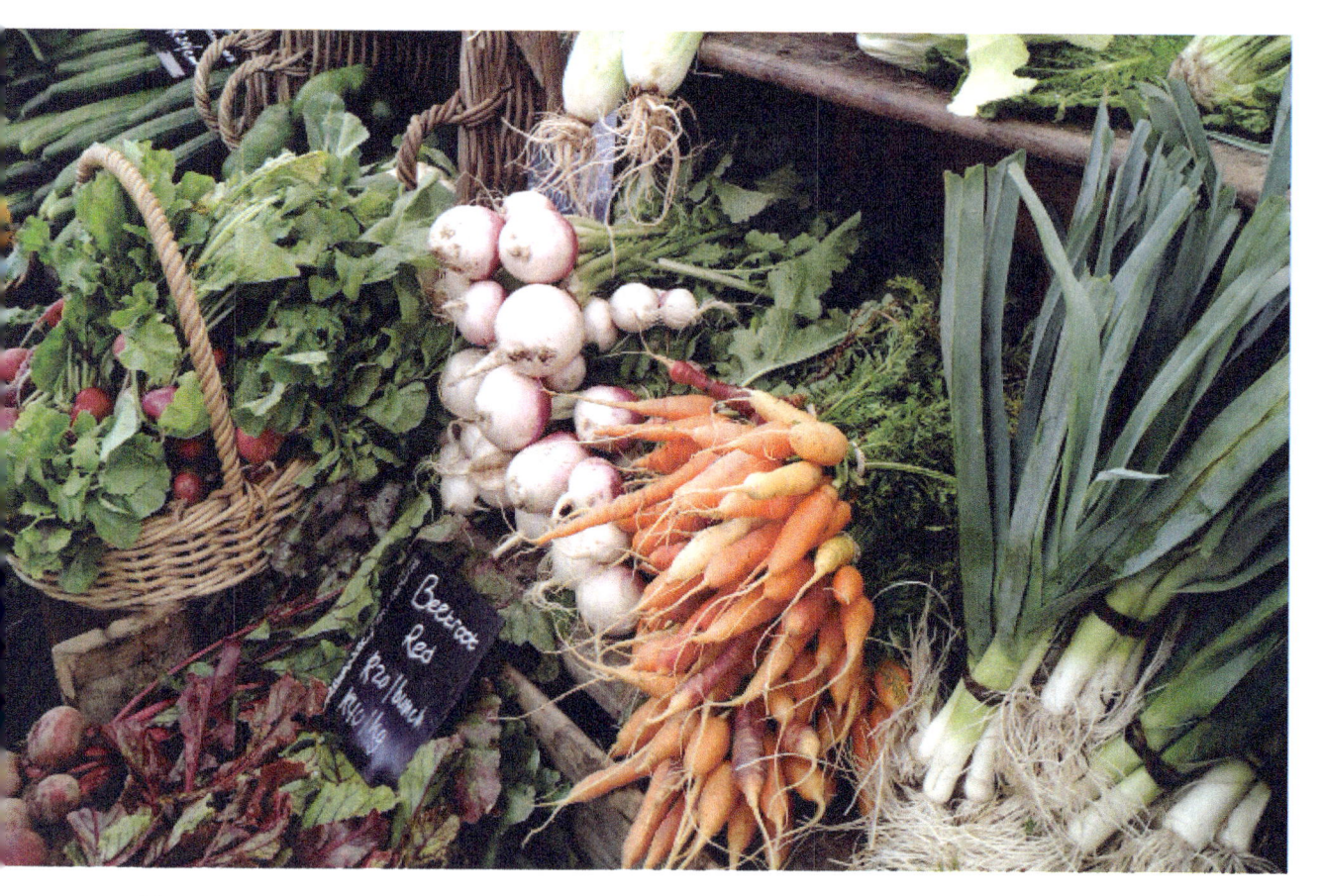

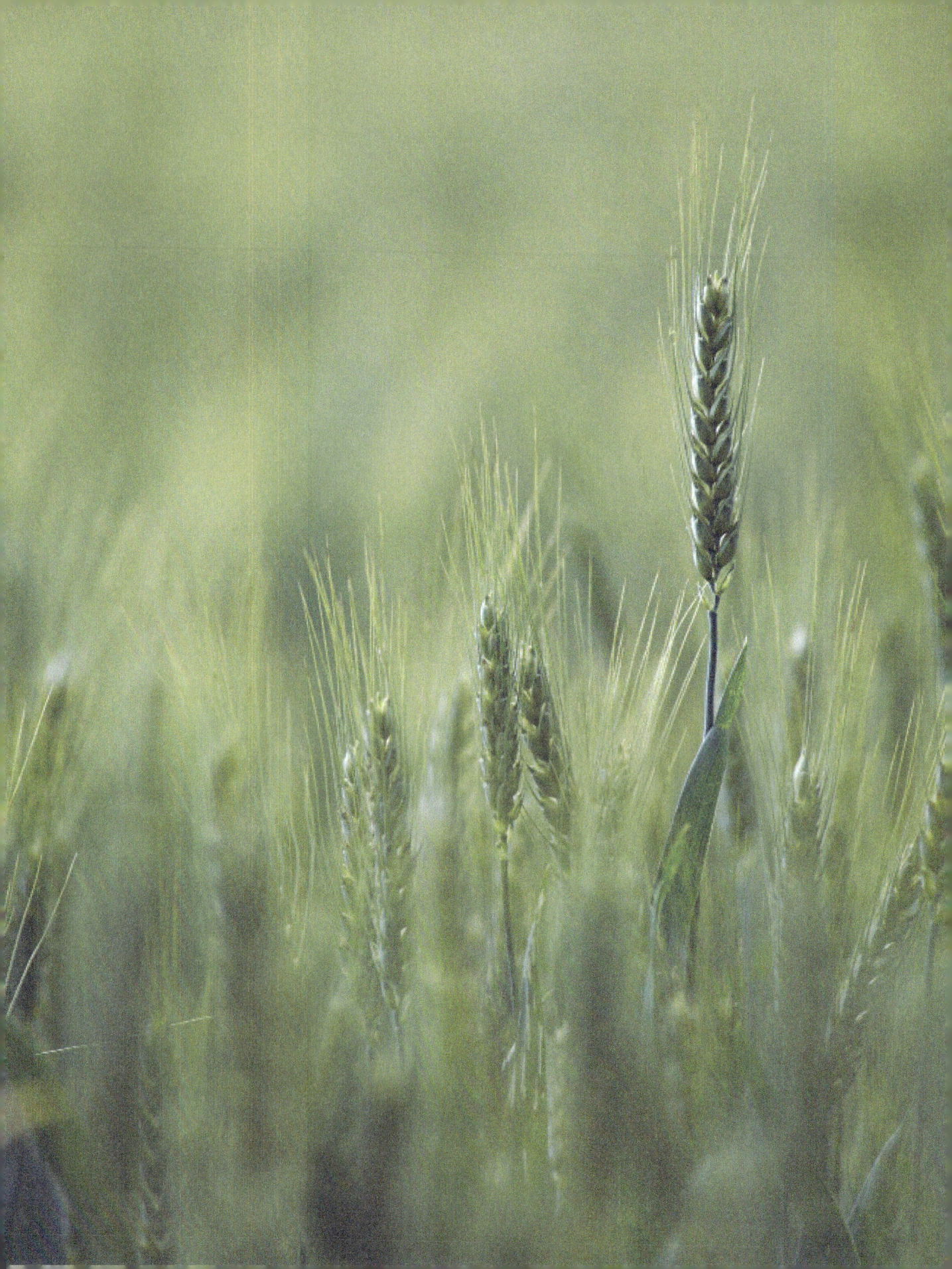

CHAPTER 5
Macronutrients

"For no one ever hated his own flesh, but nourishes and cherishes it, just as Christ does the church." —Ephesians 5:29

The above passage notes that Jesus cherishes and cares for us in a way similar to how we focus on our need for nourishing our bodies. In consideration of nourishing our bodies, let's look at the nutrients that provide calories. There are three of them: carbohydrates, proteins, and fat. Collectively, we call them macronutrients. (Alcohol also provides calories, but because it has no nutritional value and is not needed by the body, it is not called a macronutrient.)

- **Carbohydrates** provide 4 calories, or 4 units of energy, for every gram we consume.

- **Protein** also provides 4 calories, or 4 units of energy, for every gram we consume.

- **Fat,** on the other hand, provides 9 calories per gram, more than double the number of calories provided by carbohydrates and protein.

The Acceptable Macronutrient Distribution Range (AMDR) for each macronutrient is:

Carbohydrates: 45-65% of all calories

Protein: 10-35% of all calories

Fat: 20-35% of all calories

As we can see, the above guidelines provide a broad range of percentages for the calories that should come from each macronutrient. This means we can customize a meal plan with flexibility and still fall within the recommended ranges. Let's review each of these, beginning with carbohydrates.

Carbohydrates

"Jesus said to them, 'I am the bread of life; whoever comes to me shall not hunger, and whoever believes in me shall never thirst'." —John 6:35

"Truly, truly, I say to you, whoever believes has eternal life. I am the bread of life. Your fathers ate the manna in the wilderness, and they died. This is the bread that comes down from heaven, so that one may eat of it and not die. I am the living bread that came down from heaven. If anyone eats of this bread, he will live forever. And the bread that I will give for the life of the world is my flesh." —John 6:47-51

What powerful passages! Jesus tells us that He is what we need every day. We cannot spiritually survive without Him. Bread was and still is one of the most common forms of food. It is filling, satisfying, and enjoyable. Bread was essential for life in the Middle East and many, even today, would say they do not feel full or completely satisfied unless they have bread with meals. Bread is made of abundant carbohydrates. Carbohydrates are the preferred source of fuel for the body. This is especially true for the brain and red blood cells. When carbohydrates are in the body, the body will preferentially burn carbohydrates for fuel.

Carbohydrates are produced mainly in plants; they are found in rice, potatoes, corn, fruits, breads, beans, and cereals. Many diets have demonized carbohydrates, yet they are important to our health and energy. In fact, a study that followed men and women for over 20 years determined that a low-carbohydrate, high-animal-protein, high-fat diet is associated with higher all-cause mortality. This was true for both men and women. On the other hand, vegetable-based, low-carbohydrate diets were associated with lower all-cause and cardiovascular disease mortality rates. In other words, those who ate more animal proteins and fats (like on the keto and Atkins type diets) in place of carbohydrates were at a higher risk of dying prematurely, especially of cardiovascular disease. There appears to be less of a risk when the protein comes from plant sources. A study among men showed that consuming a low amount of carbohydrates was directly associated with higher rates of cancer. It appears from research that carbohydrates are valuable for health and well-being. Perhaps that is why Jesus likened our need for Him to bread, because it affects our well-being. A closer look at carbohydrates reveals they can be divided into two groups: simple sugars and complex carbohydrates.

Simple sugars can be natural (found in fruits) or they can be added by manufacturers. When they are added by manufacturers, they are just calories with no additional nutritional value included. However, when we eat things like fruit and other whole foods that come with sugar naturally in them, we get lots of needed nutrients. Glucose, fructose, and galactose are single sugar molecules; they are also called monosaccharides. Sucrose, lactose, and maltose are also classified as a simple sugar, but they have two sugar units and therefore are called disaccharides.

- **Glucose** (a.k.a. dextrose, blood sugar, sugar): simple sugar made by the body
- **Fructose**: the simple sugar found in fruit
- **Galactose**: along with glucose, this is a simple sugar found in milk
- **Sucrose (table sugar)**: a disaccharide of glucose and fructose
- **Lactose (milk sugar)**: a disaccharide of glucose and galactose
- **Maltose (malt sugar)**: a disaccharide of two glucose molecules

Complex carbohydrates, sometimes called polysaccharides, come in many forms and provide many health benefits.

As seen in the picture below, a kernel of grain is made up of three major parts.

The Bran is the outermost shell of a kernel of grain. It is a multi-layered outer skin that protects the inside of the kernel from pests and disease. Because it contains fiber, this portion of the kernel is important to a healthy diet. In addition to fiber, it contains antioxidants, iron, zinc, copper, magnesium, and many B vitamins.

The Germ is actually the embryo of the plant. If it is fertilized by pollen, it will sprout into a new plant. It contains many B vitamins, minerals, healthy fats, and some protein.

The Endosperm is the largest portion of the kernel. It is primarily starch. The endosperm is the germ's food supply; in other words, it provides essential energy to a young plant so it can put down roots for the water and nutrients found in the soil and send sprouts up for the sunlight's photosynthesizing power.

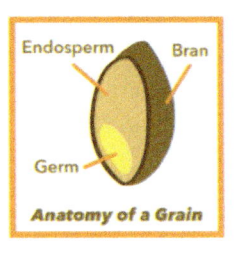

What is the big deal about whole grains?

The word "refined" refers to foods that have undergone processing to remove the coarse parts of the original grain. There has been an increase in the incidence of chronic diseases associated with the increased consumption of refined/processed foods; therefore, it is recommended that you consume unrefined foods.

As researchers have begun to look more closely at carbohydrates and health, they are discovering that the quality of the carbohydrates eaten is as important as the quantity. Most studies show a connection between eating whole grains and better health.

The invention of industrialized roller mills in the late 19th century changed how we ate grains. Milling strips away the bran and germ, making the grain easier to chew, easier to digest, and easier to keep without refrigeration, because the healthy oils in the germ have been removed so all chance of the oils turning rancid have been removed. Processing also pulverizes the endosperm, turning it from a small, solid nugget into millions of minuscule particles. Refining wheat creates fluffy flour that makes light, airy breads and pastries, which most of us love. But there's a nutritional price to be paid for eating refined grains: the process strips away more than half of the B vitamins, 90% of the vitamin E, and virtually all the fiber. It also makes the starch easily accessible to the body's starch-digesting enzymes, which can have an impact on health. When buying grain products, remember that the less processed they are, the better they are for health. One simple way to determine if a bread or cereal has had the healthy parts of the grain removed is to look at the ingredients list. If the first word on the list is "whole" grain, then all three parts of the kernel have been included in the product in large amounts. If the words "whole grain" are found lower on the ingredients list, it means all three parts of the kernel have been included in small amounts. If "whole grain" is not found in the ingredients list, look for another product.

Carbohydrates and Health

Many diets remove carbohydrates, villainizing them by suggesting they are not necessary and that all they do is make people gain weight. The truth is that carbohydrates are important and play a significant role in health and energy. In order to understand the importance of carbohydrates, we need to review a few terms.

- **Starch** is the storage form of carbohydrates in plants. It is called a polysaccharide (poly=many). These can be thousands of glucose units long. Two forms of starches are digestible, and one is not.

    - *Amylose* is the digestible starch in which the glucose units are a straight chain.

    - *Amylopectin* is the digestible starch that contains branched chains.

    Plants generally contain both amylose and amylopectin.

    - *Cellulose* is a plant starch that is resistant to the human digestive juices. We call this fiber, or resistant starch.

- **Glycogen** is the storage form of carbohydrates in the human body. When we eat extra carbohydrates that do not need to be used for energy right away, the body can store them as glycogen in the liver and in muscles. The amount stored varies from person to person. After the maximum amount of glycogen that can be stored is stored, the rest will be converted to body fat. Because carbohydrates are water-soluble, water is stored with the glycogen. Therefore, when carbohydrates are used for energy, weight is lost due to both the glycogen and the water being depleted.

- **Fiber** is sometimes called non-digestible carbohydrates or resistant starch. Fiber is found in the cell walls of plants. Animal foods do not provide any fiber. Humans can't digest fiber or resistant starch, so they basically pass through our bodies undigested and unabsorbed. This type of fiber, therefore, does not provide calories; instead it provides bulk, which can reduce hunger as well as bestow many other health benefits, including reduced serum cholesterol levels, suppressed appetite, improved blood glucose levels, relieved constipation, and even the stimulation of healthy gastrointestinal flora. Resistant starches are sometimes added to foods because they provide these health benefits.

- Fiber can be further subdivided based on its interaction with water:

  - **Insoluble Fiber** does not dissolve in water. Examples include cellulose, hemicellulose, and lignin. This type of fiber tends to move quickly through the GI tract. There are many health benefits to insoluble fiber:

    1. Helps reduce constipation – In other words, it moves quickly through the GI tract, contributing to bulk in the feces and stretching the circular muscles in the large intestine; as such, it reduces the likelihood of constipation and keeps the GI tract healthy. Fiber needs water to pass smoothly. If too much fiber is consumed too quickly without sufficient water also being consumed, nausea and constipation may result.

    2. Reduces cancer risk – When insoluble fiber is eaten, it increases the bulk of the stool, which can help the stool move more quickly through the GI tract. Thus, potential cancer-promoting substances may spend less time in contact with the colon's lining. Moreover, fiber can promote healthy gut flora (bacteria), which may have cancer-fighting properties.

    3. Reduces obesity risk – Insoluble fiber physically fills up space in the stomach and intestines, which can bring about the sensation of being full. This can reduce overeating, which helps with weight management.

    Some foods containing insoluble fiber: whole-grain breads, whole-grain cereals, bran, couscous, oats, brown rice, fruits, vegetables, and legumes.

  - **Soluble Fiber** does dissolve in water. Examples include pectin, beta-glucan, gums, and psyllium. These form thick gels that are fermented by intestinal bacteria and slow down food digestion and absorption. There are health benefits to consuming soluble fiber:

    1. Helps reduce cholesterol levels. In our bodies, we have bile acids that naturally have cholesterol. These bile acids are secreted by the gallbladder into the intestines, where they prepare fat for digestion. If soluble fiber has been eaten, it grabs or confiscates these bile acids and traps them, and out of the body they go, along with the fiber. To make up for this loss of bile, the liver makes more bile salts. The body uses cholesterol to make bile salts by pulling cholesterol out of low-density lipid (LDL), the "bad" type of cholesterol molecules in the bloodstream. The liver gets this new cholesterol from our blood, thus lowering the amount of cholesterol in our blood. Moreover, a diet high in fiber by its nature tends to be lower in fat.

    2. Helps manage diabetes. If someone has diabetes, they need to be careful of sugar highs and lows. The presence of this slow-moving, viscous, gel-like fiber can slow the digestion and absorption of glucose, which can help avoid large spikes in blood sugar levels after a meal. Instead, there will be a slower, steadier release of glucose from the GI tract, contributing to a slower, steadier rise in the bloodstream.

    3. Improves cardiovascular health. The presence of this slow-moving, viscous, gel-like fiber can reduce the rate dietary fats can be absorbed after a meal. When fat absorption is delayed, the rise of fats in the blood will be slower. Both lower blood lipid levels and being sensitive to insulin can result in improved cardiovascular health and circulatory conditions.

    4. Normalizes blood glucose. The presence of this slow-moving, viscous, gel-like fiber can slow the digestion and absorption of simple sugars, which can normalize blood glucose levels, even for those of us who do not have diabetes. Furthermore, those who struggle with hypoglycemia experience a rapid decline in blood glucose after a carbohydrate-rich meal, so consuming fiber-rich foods will lessen that effect.

5. *Reduces cancer risk.* Fiber binds to estrogen in bile, which then gets eliminated in feces, leading to lower blood estrogen levels. While this effect is still being researched, a number of studies have suggested that a diet high in fiber (even just 1 or 2 more servings a day) can help reduce the risk of cancer.

6. *Reduces risk of obesity.* Since soluble fiber slows down how quickly foods are digested, a feeling of fullness will last over time. This can reduce overeating, which helps with weight management.

Some foods containing soluble fiber: prunes, legumes, quinoa, flax seeds, barley, oats, Brussels sprouts, oranges, navy beans, white beans, and lima beans.

Functional Fiber: This is soluble or insoluble fiber that has been extracted or isolated from a plant and added to a food in an attempt to increase the health benefits of that food.

Note of Caution: Consuming too much fiber can reduce the absorption of several minerals, such as zinc and iron. In addition to causing mineral deficiencies, too much fiber too quickly may cause a fluid imbalance, gas, and bloating. It is recommended to gradually increase fiber content in your diet, along with increasing fluid consumption.

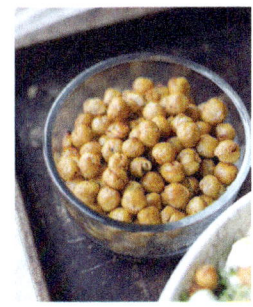

Recommended amount of fiber: According to the Academy of Nutrition and Dietetics, women should aim for 25 grams of fiber daily. Men should aim for 38 grams. According to the Institute of Medicine, the Adequate Intake for total fiber is 14g per 1,000 calories.

Fructose

Much discussion takes place in public arenas about the dangers of high-fructose corn syrup (HFCS).

HFCS is a sweetener produced from modified corn syrup. Remember from the above discussion that sucrose is a disaccharide, with a glucose and a fructose linked together. In contrast, the glucose and fructose molecules are not linked together in corn syrup. To increase the sweetness of corn syrup, the percentage of fructose in corn syrup is increased to levels between 45 and 55% to produce high-fructose corn syrup. This syrup is stable and easy to handle in food processing, and it is less expensive than sucrose (produced from sugar cane), making it a good choice for use in the food industry. It gives cookies and snacks their chewy, soft texture. It inhibits microbial growth by reducing the availability of water, which helps improve freshness and extends shelf life. It represents about 40% of added sugar in the food supply. It comes in two forms:

- HFCS 42 (42% fructose/58% glucose): used in baked products, jams, jellies, canned fruit, and dairy products.
- HFCS 55 (55% fructose/45% glucose): used in sweetened drinks, including soft drinks.

Because the amount of glucose and fructose consumed in sucrose is the same (50/50 glucose/fructose), while high-fructose corn syrup has more fructose (45/55 glucose/fructose), some researchers have suggested that HFCS may change our appetite-control mechanism, resulting in less satiation and ultimately, a greater calorie intake. But over time, studies that examined the effects of HFCS compared to other nutritive sweeteners have repeatedly found little to no evidence demonstrating that HFCS differs uniquely from sucrose or other nutritive sweeteners in metabolic effects, including levels of circulating glucose, insulin, leptin, or ghrelin. Research has also found little evidence on several subjective effects, such as hunger, satiety, and energy intake at subsequent meals. No convincing evidence has emerged that HFCS increases the risk of weight gain. Many randomized trials dealing specifically with HFCS had small subject numbers and were conducted for a short duration of time. Clearly, more research (including long-term data) is needed.

In the meantime, HFCS is found in many sweetened, processed foods. All health care professionals agree that the consumption of pre-sweetened foods and foods with lots of added sugar should be limited in your diet. Overall, yes, people should limit their consumption of foods sweetened with HFCS, but no more so than foods with any other type of added sugar. It is the excess empty calories of these foods that is concerning, not the specific ingredient of HFCS.

Although fructose tastes sweet like glucose, fructose is not metabolized or stored exactly the same as glucose. Glucose is the universal carbohydrate for cells in the body; in other words, every cell can use glucose for energy. Muscles store glucose as glycogen, and this glycogen is used as fuel when quick energy is needed. Muscles use fat for fuel during longer periods of energy demands. Athletes can train their muscles to store more and more glycogen, which is especially helpful in fueling their body during longer periods of physical activity. (More discussion on how fats and carbohydrates fuel the body together can be found in the metabolism section.) The glycogen stored in muscles can only be used by that particular muscle.

In addition to muscles storing glycogen, the liver stores glucose as glycogen, but unlike muscles, the liver doesn't hoard the glycogen for itself. Instead, the glycogen stored in the liver is shared with the entire body to supply it with glucose during times of fasting. It is important to note that both the muscles and liver have a maximum limit of glycogen storage.

Glucose consumed in excess of that maximum capacity is converted to fat. In other words, when glycogen stores are at their maximum capacity, the excess glucose becomes fat.

Fructose, on the other hand, is not used by all cells but is preferentially metabolized by the liver (see metabolism chapter).

Liver cells have special enzymes that other cells do not have. The action of these enzymes results in fructose being converted to fat rather than glycogen. This fat can be used for energy to fuel the body or stored, depending on the individual caloric demands. In other words, fructose and glucose are good at providing energy, but in excess, both will be stored as fat. So, in adequate amounts, carbohydrates are an important nutrient that supply the body with necessary energy for immediate demands and creates energy reserves. Diets that eliminate or minimize carbohydrates remove these health benefits.

Glycemic Index and Glycemic Load

Glycemic index and glycemic load are terms that classify the effect that foods with carbohydrates have on blood glucose. Not all carbohydrates impact blood glucose the same way. Some foods cause a sharp rise and a rapid fall in blood glucose, while other foods cause a gentler rise and fall of blood glucose levels. The amount of fat and fiber in foods can lower and slow the effect a carbohydrate will have on blood glucose.

- **Glycemic Index** is a scale that ranks food according to how that food item affects blood glucose; but it does not take into account the amount of carbohydrate eaten.

- **Glycemic Load** is a measure that considers the amount of carbohydrate usually eaten of a particular food, along with how quickly it raises blood glucose levels.

The usefulness of these tools in weight management and disease prevention is controversial. Some research findings suggest that high-glycemic-index foods do not raise blood glucose as quickly as it was once thought. Interestingly, following the dietary guidelines that include consuming whole-plant foods and limiting refined foods will result in consuming low-glycemic-index foods.

Research suggests that low-glycemic foods aid in satiety and therefore are helpful for weight loss. In fact, several studies found that subjects consuming low-glycemic foods lost more intra-abdominal fat when compared with those consuming a high-glycemic diet. However, when calorie levels were held constant, weight loss was similar. Two important takeaways from this are:

- Total calories still matter when it comes to weight loss.

- Low-glycemic foods are recommended because they tend to be satisfying and thus helpful in weight loss.

But the glycemic index rating of a certain food is not a sufficient basis for food selection. It is not that simple. Just because a food has a low glycemic index does not automatically mean it is always healthy. For example, potato chips have a lower glycemic index than oatmeal and about the same as green peas, but oatmeal and green peas are significantly more nutrient-dense.

RECAP: Carbohydrates are the preferred source of fuel for the body. They come in the form of simple sugars and complex carbohydrates. Complex carbohydrates provide many health benefits from the fiber in them. Eat plenty (3/4 of the plate) of whole grains, fruits, and vegetables, including the skin and peel. Seeds, like those found in strawberries, raspberries, blueberries, etc., add fiber to a diet. The bottom line is that the current recommendation is to eat both types of fiber (soluble and insoluble) for overall health. There is usually no need to split hairs and aim for a certain percentage of either. Just eat plenty of whole-grain foods, fruits, and vegetables.

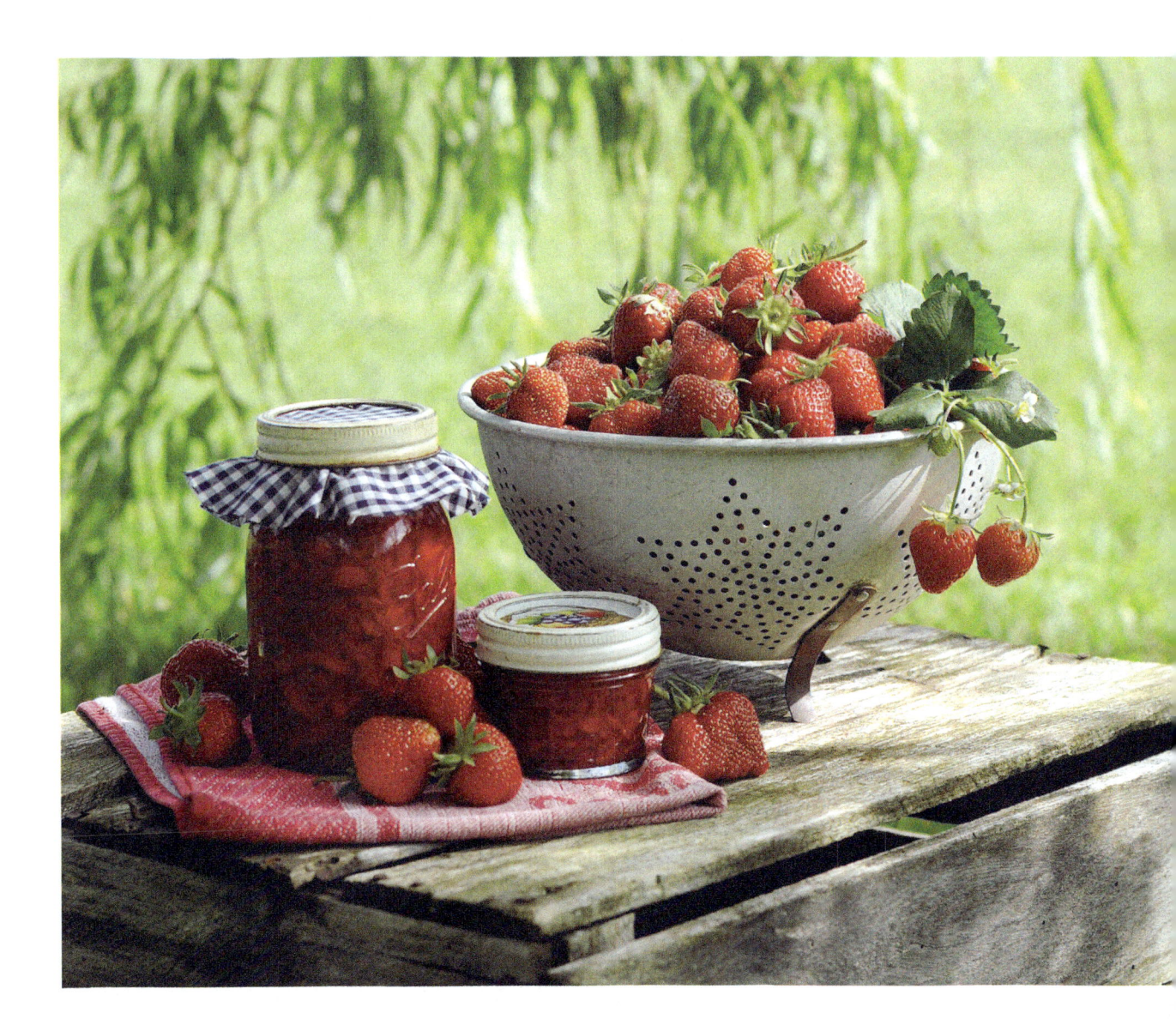

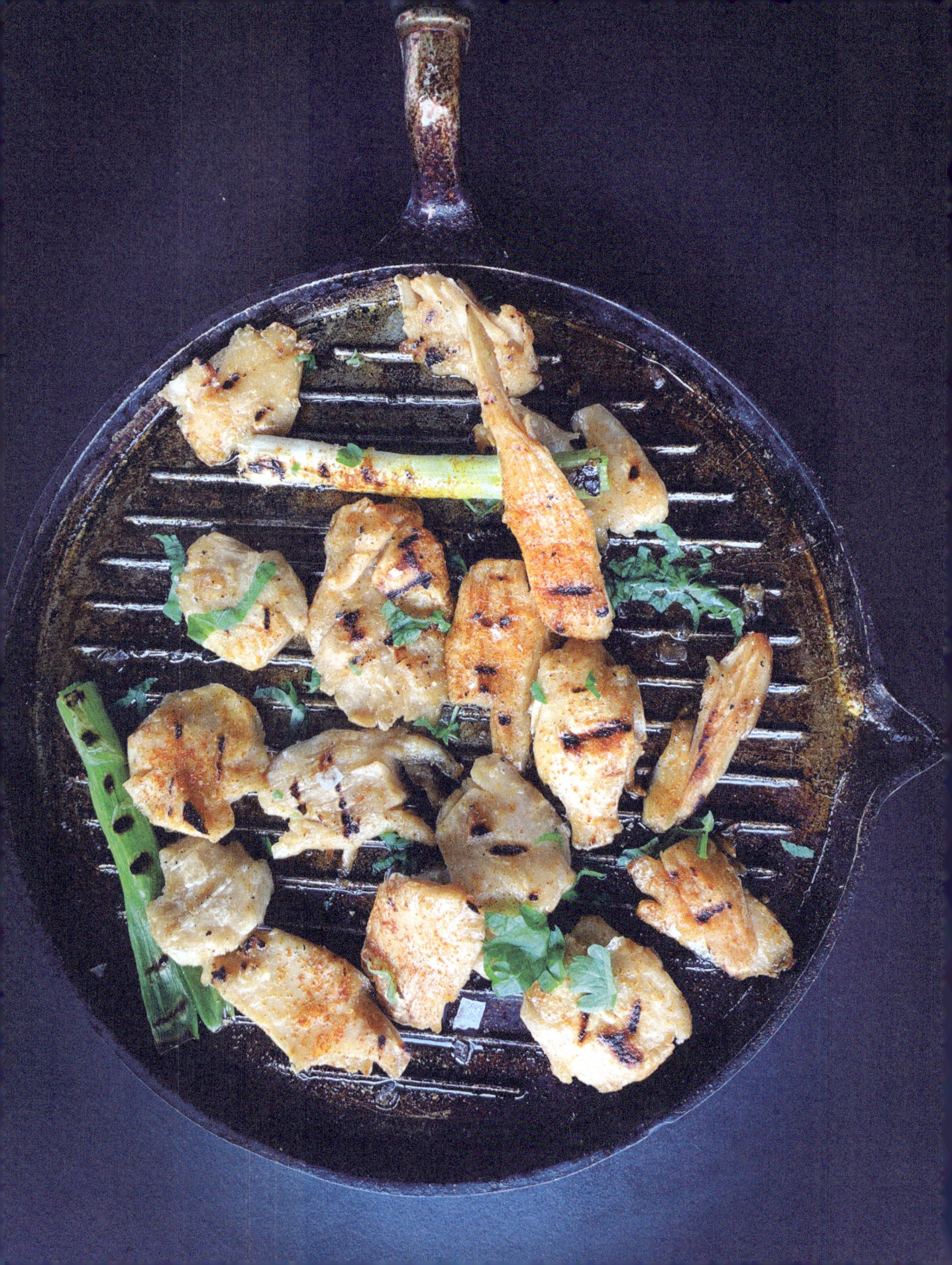

CHAPTER 6
Protein

"Everything that lives and moves about will be food for you. Just as I gave you the green plants, I now give you everything. But you must not eat meat that has its lifeblood still in it." —Genesis 9:3-4

The beginning of Genesis 9 notes God's blessings and commands to Noah and his sons. These instructions also apply to the generations that follow. God makes it clear that humanity is now free to eat any kind of creature that moves including mammals, birds, fish, and things that creep or crawl but notes that the blood of these creatures is not to be consumed along with their flesh. The verse depicts blood as the animal's life and is a first step in establishing the symbolism of Christ's sacrifice for human sin on the cross. While the blood of Jesus is vital to eternal life, protein is vital to life here on this Earth.

Protein is so vital it is found in every living cell in the body. In fact, protein makes up major structural components of our cells.

Protein is also the only macronutrient that has nitrogen (N). These are very important points that we will return to when we talk about ketogenic diets and low-calorie diets. Amino acids are often called the "building blocks" of protein because they come together to make proteins, and amino acids are made when proteins are broken down. Amino acids are categorized as essential amino acids and non-essential amino acids.

- **Essential Amino Acids** cannot be made by the body. Therefore, we need to eat them in our diet. They are essential in our diet. There are 9 essential amino acids.

- **Non-essential Amino Acids** can be made by the body if all the essential amino acids have been eaten in adequate amounts. As long as we have eaten sufficient amounts of all the essential amino acids, our body will make any non-essential amino acids needed. There are 11 non-essential amino acids.

Unlike carbohydrates and fats, our bodies generally don't have a specific storage molecule for stowing away protein for later use. We do have small amino acid pools throughout the body, but they are limited. These amino acid pools are how the non-essential amino acids can be made by the body.

Proteins are in constant fluctuation in the body; in other words, they are in constant turnover. Remember, every living cell has protein in its structure, and nearly all the enzymes in cells are proteins. So, when structural proteins in cells need to be repaired, or enzymes need to be recycled, the body will break down old proteins to create new proteins in order to maintain cellular function.

Roles of Protein

Protein has many different roles in the body. It is part of every cell and therefore it is part of body structures and functions.

> 1. It is found in all connective tissues, including bones, tendons, and ligaments. It forms the framework of bones and teeth. Structural proteins are also found in skin and hair, as well as all body tissues and organs.
>
> 2. They make up enzymes, hormones, and cell walls.
>
> 3. Proteins help maintain the acid-base balance.
>
> 4. Proteins are needed to regulate fluid balance by keeping water evenly dispersed in and outside cells.
>
> 5. Protein contributes to a healthy immune system. In addition to being part of the first line of defense, our skin, they make up antibodies.

Along with these multiple roles in our bodies, proteins serve many functions in our diet. So, ideally, you can see why eating the right amount and right kinds of protein is important. But what happens when we eat too much or too little protein?

The dangers of eating too little protein

When we don't eat enough protein, our bodies begin to prioritize the work that must be done, and in that process, it can strip, steal, or take away amino acids from various cells. Depending on where the amino acids are taken from, this can be very dangerous. Many years ago, while discussing weight management in a health class, a student who was attentively listening reflected on the discussion. After raising her hand, she asked, "So are you saying that if I don't eat enough protein, I will strip my muscle?" That was pretty close to what I had said, so I responded "Yes." To my surprise, with a laugh, she slapped her buttocks and replied, "Great, I always wanted a smaller gluteus maximus muscle." I quickly saw the error of my message and had to correct her view of this concept. Just like we cannot dictate where our body will store fat, we cannot dictate what skeletal muscles will be stripped for their protein. In general, skeletal muscle is prioritized over using proteins found in organ tissues. Organ tissues and other smooth muscles will be spared for as long as possible. On the other hand, our bodies will pull amino acids from the gluteus maximus muscle before breaking down the amino acids in our heart; however, unlike this student hoped, we cannot make our bodies strip lean tissue from our gluteus maximus instead of our deltoid muscle. Stripping lean tissue is a big deal, because when we decrease the amount of lean tissue in our body, our metabolic rate decreases, which makes it not only harder to lose weight but also more difficult to maintain weight.

The dangers of eating too much protein

When we eat more protein than we need, the body will take and use the amino acids it needs to function. It will then break apart the excess protein consumed into its amino acids. The body stores the excess throughout the body in amino acid pools. Once those pools become saturated, the body will remove the nitrogen component of the excess amino acids, and that nitrogen component will eventually get converted to urea by the liver and urinated out of the body by the kidneys. But the remaining (nitrogen-free) portion of the amino acid, which we will call the carbon skeleton, will be converted to body fat and stored in the adipose. So, the bottom line is excess protein consumed will result in added body fat.

> **RECAP:** Protein is found in every living cell. We need to eat sufficient essential amino acids in order to make the non-essential amino acids. If we eat too little protein, we can strip our lean tissue, or cells in other places. If we eat too much protein, the excess will be stored as body fat.

Protein plays a role in weight loss

Protein is important in weight loss in a number of ways. Remember when we previously talked about the carbon skeleton from excess protein? We said that when we eat too much protein, the excess amino acids are converted to fat and stored as fat in adipose tissue. When we strip lean tissue during a time of fasting, amino acids can either be used for energy by the skeletal muscle or a select few amino acids can be converted to glucose and the remaining amino acids can be converted to ketone bodies in the liver.

From a biochemistry perspective, carbohydrates can be used to make non-essential amino acids (protein parts) and fat.

Protein can be used to make fat, but only a select few amino acids can be used to make carbohydrates. Fat cannot be used to make either proteins or carbohydrates. In other words, if the necessary components are available in the body and the body is healthy, the body can make glucose (a form of carbohydrate) from proteins and non-essential amino acids (which are the building blocks of protein). Furthermore, both carbohydrates and protein can be used to make fat. Think about it: we eat too much of anything, we get fatter. The section on fat explains how triglycerides are a combination of a molecule of glycerol and three fatty acids. The majority of every triglyceride is fatty acids; in fact, about 95% of triglycerides are fatty acids. Only 5% of a triglyceride is made up of the glycerol molecule. While the small (5%) glycerol molecule can be used to make glucose, the fatty acids CANNOT be used to make carbohydrates or proteins. While fatty acids have other roles in the body, from a dietary perspective, fatty acids are ONLY used for energy production. Fatty acids can only be burned as fuel in Krebs cycles. (Remember, Krebs cycles are the factories in the body that turn fuel consumed into energy the body can use, i.e., ATP.) But fatty acids cannot be used to produce Krebs cycles. Krebs cycles can be produced by carbohydrates and protein, but not fatty acids. It is important to always remember that fatty acids CANNOT be used to make Krebs cycles, carbohydrates, or proteins.

Please do not walk away from this discussion thinking one can eat only carbohydrates and think the necessary proteins for healthy function will be made from these carbohydrates. Similarly, one shouldn't think they can eat only protein and think the necessary carbohydrates for healthy function will be made from these proteins. They are not exchangeable. Remember, there are essential amino acids the body can't make. They must be consumed within the proteins of one's diet. Therefore, every diet must provide the essential amino acids. In other words, every diet must provide the critical percentage of protein to supply those essential amino acids. If they are not provided, the body will be forced to use the amino acids already within the body to make the Krebs cycles needed to burn calories, regardless of the source, for fuel.

When fewer carbohydrates are available for energy production, our bodies have to convert more protein into carbon skeletons and eventually glucose. Limiting carbohydrate consumption may result in protein being broken down. This is not a good approach for weight loss. This idea of substituting proteins for carbohydrates is good in theory, except proteins are not stored for times of fasting like carbohydrates are. Therefore, during times of fasting, we must strip our lean tissues because carbohydrate stores are not maintained during fasting. This occurs in dieters on carbohydrate-limiting diets. In addition, this approach results in a lower metabolic rate, which makes it more difficult to lose and maintain weight. This is another case where diets can be based on facts but are limited in the application to actual dieters. In this case, the theory doesn't take into account multiple metabolic situations and long-term metabolic effect.

Some diets, like Atkins, promote eating mostly protein because the body uses more energy to digest and absorb proteins than carbs or fat. In fact, even 2.5 hours after eating a high-protein meal, thermogenesis is twofold higher than if lots of carbs were eaten. Thermogenesis simply means heat-producing, which is what happens when the body burns calories to generate heat as well as energy. These diets point to the fact that an increase in heat production may result in a slightly more rapid weight loss. Protein also brings about a greater feeling of fullness and satiation than either carbs or fats. Protein decreases the hunger hormone ghrelin, which may result in eating less.

If protein can do all this, it is no wonder there are many high-protein diets advertised. But we need to be cautious with how we apply this information. Just because protein digestion and absorption use more energy and keep us fuller longer doesn't mean we should load up on it or eliminate carbohydrates or fats. It means we need to make sure we get adequate amounts of protein: not too much and not too little. The principles of balance and moderation apply. Carbohydrates and fats are important, too. In fact, there is research to show that more total calories may be burned when fat and protein are both included in the diet. And, of course, carbohydrates provide fiber, phytonutrients, and many nutrients not found in most protein food sources. Thus, it is unwise, unnecessary, and even dangerous to eliminate any of the macronutrients from a diet.

High-Protein Diets

There is a lot of talk about high-protein diets. Atkins, Dukan, Ketogenic, and Paleo diets are a few that emphasize proteins. When we compare high-protein diets to high-carbohydrate diets, it is important to look at the definition of high protein and high carbohydrate. These diets do not use the same definitions. For example, the Atkins diet is actually a high-protein, high-fat diet that provides only 20 grams of carbohydrates. The Dukan diet allows for unlimited protein while nearly eliminating carbohydrates and fats, while some ketogenic diets allow up to 50 grams of carbohydrates. In fact, a diet can be considered a low-carbohydrate diet if carbohydrates provide 30% or less of all calories, or if it provides fewer than 100 grams of carbohydrates a day. The RDA for carbohydrates for adults is 130 grams per day. Even though most people need more than that, 130 grams is considered the minimum for the function of the brain and red blood cells. A diet can be considered a high-protein diet if protein contributes 20% of all the calories. That is pretty amazing, given the fact that the Acceptable Macronutrient Distribution Range (AMDR) for protein is 10–35%.

As protein intake increases, so does the production of the nitrogen breakdown product, urea. Urea must be eliminated from the body via the kidneys. In the past, it was thought that high-protein diets could cause kidney damage. It is now believed that high-protein diets aren't harmful to people with healthy, functioning kidneys, but people who tend to form kidney stones may see their condition worsen when a very high-protein diet is consumed. Furthermore, a high-protein diet may be detrimental for people with kidney disease, as it can speed the progression of renal failure. Additionally, in order to excrete more waste, more water must be lost in the urine, so high-protein diets increase water loss. Depending on one's health status, this can lead to dehydration. It is very important when on a high-protein diet to increase water consumption.

Another concern about high-protein diets is that they are often accompanied by a low carbohydrate intake. Having insufficient carbohydrates means that to maintain blood glucose levels, the body—specifically the liver—has to make glucose from glycogen stores or from the dietary protein. At the same time the liver is making glucose, it is converting dietary fats to ketone bodies. In other words, when the liver is forced to make glucose from protein (either skeletal tissue or dietary protein), dietary fat will be converted to ketone bodies by the liver. As one can see, dietary fat, in the absence of dietary carbohydrate, will lead to ketone body production. Glucose production and ketone body production by the liver go hand in hand.

Normally, one thinks of ketone bodies being produced in times of fasting; however, in the absence of dietary carbohydrates, ketone bodies will be produced when calories are consumed. This is what occurs in a keto diet, which reduces carbohydrates below the levels necessary to maintain glycogen storage and maintenance of blood glucose level.

Another concern with a keto diet arises when carbohydrates are insufficient, and inadequate protein is consumed. Protein needs are individual to each dieter. In other words, everyone needs different amounts of protein. If someone on the keto diet does not consume adequate protein for their needs, their cells will not have the essential amino acids needed to produce critical proteins like enzymes and other proteins necessary for cell function. Without these cellular functions, cells will be dysfunctional. The overall effect on health will depend on this dysfunction.

Another concern for some individuals is that high levels of ketones can build up in the blood and increase the blood's acidity. Severe ketosis can cause coma or death. If someone sustains a state of ketosis, especially if they are heavily exercising, their cells need to create a lot of Krebs cycles in order to use the ketone bodies for energy. As stated earlier, while Krebs cycles can burn fat, they cannot be created by fat. Krebs cycles can only be formed from carbohydrates or protein. Thus, the amount of protein consumed matters. This cannot be over-emphasized. If enough carbohydrates are not available, sufficient protein needs to be consumed to maintain all the body's needs and to create enough Krebs cycles to burn fat or ketone bodies.

If enough carbohydrates are not consumed, lean tissue will be lost. Lower amounts of lean tissue reduce the metabolism and the body's ability to lose weight. It will also make it more difficult for the body to maintain weight. Depending on the sources of the protein eaten, a high-protein diet can easily be accompanied by high fat. So, the risks of a high-protein diet may include heart disease, too.

When it comes to bones, regarding calcium and protein, there are mixed results in the literature. Overall, it appears that too much or too little protein is not healthy for bones. Historically it was thought that when too much protein was eaten then broken down, the amino acids could elevate the blood's acidity and that calcium would then be secreted into the blood to neutralize the acidity in the blood, leading to osteoporosis. In essence, calcium would be drawn out of the bone to balance the acidic levels in the blood. People have wondered if the effects of dietary protein may be greater as we age because aging kidneys may not function as well as younger ones. This traditional view is currently being called into question, as many epidemiological studies have found a significant positive relationship between protein intake and bone mineral density. Protein intake has been found to be inversely associated with hip fractures in postmenopausal women. In other words, as protein intake increased, hip fractures decreased. Other studies have found greater calcium retention and absorption among people consuming higher-protein diets when compared to people consuming lower-protein diets.

It is unwise to say that "high protein" diets are good, or "high carbohydrate" diets are bad. The truth is, we must be specific, and what is best or helpful for one person may not be best or even safe for another.

> **RECAP:** High-protein diets have many definitions, so it is important to make sure apples are being compared to apples. Too much or too little protein is not helpful or advised.

How much protein do we need?

Protein needs depend on several factors and therefore this quantity is highly individual. That is why it is important for a diet not to make blanket recommendations for everyone. There are actually a few ways to determine someone's protein needs.

> 1. It is recommended that 10–35% of total calories should come from protein in our diet.
>
> 2. For sedentary adults over the age of 18 years, the number used to determine how much protein is needed is: 0.8 grams of protein for every kilogram of body weight.

As you can see, the amount of protein that people need is not consistent. Both these methods consider weight. Neither directly considers the amount of lean tissue. Let's look at an example using the first method.

If 2,200 calories are needed and we want to know how many of those calories should come from protein, we need to take the total calories needed and make the following computations to determine calories from protein:

$$2,200 \text{ (total calories needed)} \times .10 = 220 \text{ calories (at the low end)}$$

$$2,200 \text{ (total calories needed)} \times .35 = 770 \text{ calories (at the high end)}$$

This tells us how many calories in our diet should come from protein. But it might be easier to determine how many grams of protein we need daily. Since every gram of protein provides 4 calories:

$$220 \div 4 = 55 \text{ grams of protein (at the low end)}$$

$$770 \div 4 = 193 \text{ grams of protein (at the high end)}$$

Let's look at an example using the second method. First, you need to determine how much you weigh in kilograms. To determine your weight in kg, you need to take your weight in pounds and divide that number by 2.2. This will give you your weight in kilograms. People who are trying to lose weight love to see their weight in kilograms because it is almost half their weight in pounds!

Example: Someone weighs 175 pounds.

$$175 \text{ divided by } 2.2 = 79.5 \text{ kg}$$

Once you know your weight in kilograms, the math is simple. Just multiply your weight in kilograms by .8. The answer will be the number the grams of protein you require every day.

$$79.5 \text{ kg} \times .8 = 64 \text{ grams of protein needed daily}$$

Notice the above answer (64 grams of protein) fits within the AMDR range of 55–193 grams. Now, remember the number .8 is used for sedentary people. But what about athletes or people who are regularly physically active? They do need more grams of protein per every kg of body weight. If your patient or client exercises regularly, use the following chart to determine which number should be plugged in instead of .8.

Category	Grams of protein/kg of body weight	Percent of total calories if adequate calories are being consumed
Sedentary Individuals	.8	10 - 35%
Athletes	1.4 - 2	15 - 35%
Injured Athletes	≥2	25 - 35%

Source: Campbell, B., Kreider, R.B., Ziegenfuss, T. et al. International Society of Sports Nutrition position stand: protein and exercise. J Int Soc Sports Nutr 4, 8 (2007). https://doi.org/10.1186/1550-2783-4-8

RECAP: Protein needs are individual.

Protein has many roles in the body, including providing structure to our bodies in our bones and other tissues, speeding up needed bodily processes by creating enzymes, signaling and controlling cells as hormones, and maintaining our fluid and acid-base balances. Since protein is found in every cell in our bodies, it is easy to see why we need to consume adequate amounts. However, just because protein is important, it doesn't mean more is better. In fact, there are some risks that accompany consuming too much protein, including storing excess body fat, the formation of kidney stones, and increased risk of dehydration. If carbohydrate consumption drops as a natural result of getting more of our calories from protein, all the benefits of fiber, phytochemicals, and the many nutrients found in carbohydrates will be lost. These are concerns when both carbohydrates and proteins are reduced to below recommended levels, such as in the keto diet.

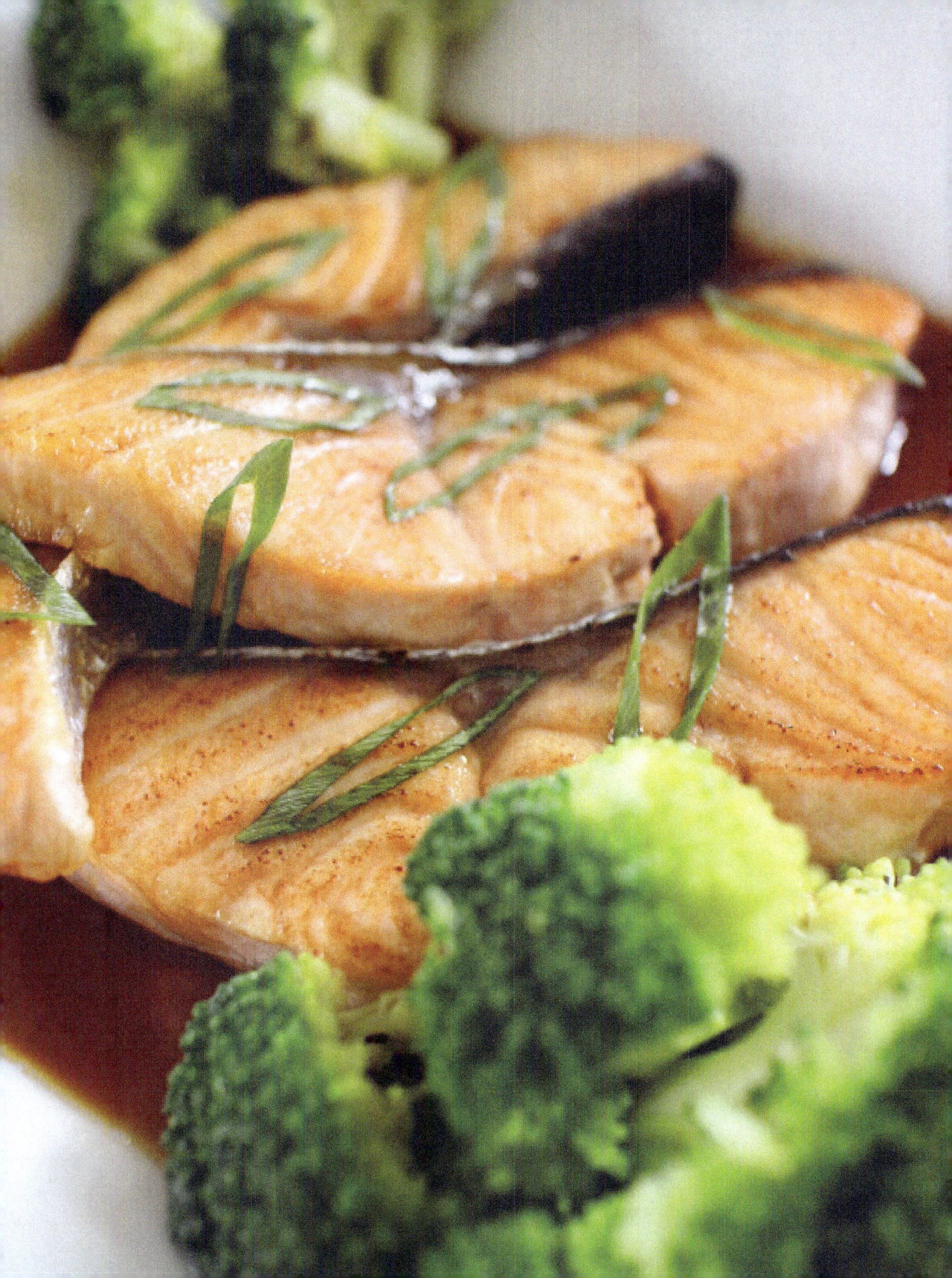

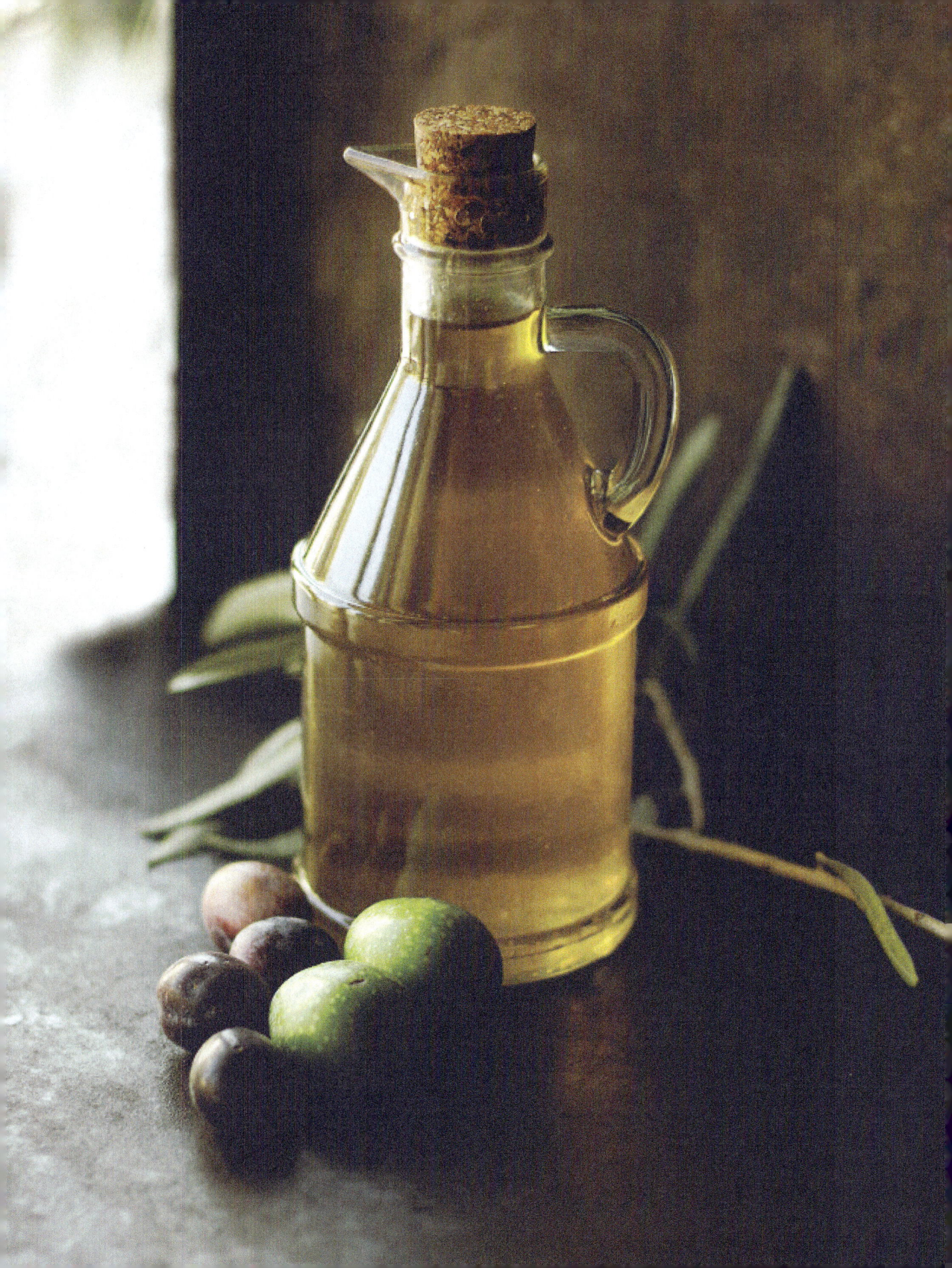

CHAPTER 7
Fat

"I will seek the lost, bring back the scattered, bind up the broken and strengthen the sick; but the fat and the strong I will destroy. I will feed them with judgment." —Ezekiel 34:16

The word "fat" conjures up different images for people. Previous encounters with the word and how it was used can sway and influence one's perception of how they feel about fat. The above scripture depicts a beautiful expression of God's love, support, and protection. It indicates that He will bring back those that stray and will bandage their injuries and help them heal. He strengthens those weakened or overwhelmed by anxiety and will bring back to Himself those who have strayed and who may struggle with negative feelings. Yet those who have taken great care of themselves and who were self-sufficient as evidenced by substantial weight will be judged. Historically, being fat was a sign of wealth and status. It was an indication someone didn't have to engage in manual labor. Most people couldn't afford to be fat and didn't have an abundance of food. A similar interpretation is made by the following passage.

"Therefore, thus says the Lord God to them, 'Behold, I, even I, will judge between the fat sheep and the lean sheep.'" —Ezekiel 34:20

The above scripture indicates that those who were "full of themselves," who were self-righteous, self-sufficient, and believed they did not need repentance, those who trusted in themselves while despising others and believed only in their own righteousness, represent the "fat sheep." The "lean sheep" represent the lowly, humble, meek, weary, and heavily laden who hunger for righteousness. Thus, it is again seen that fat is equated with wealth, abundance, overindulgence, and excess.

Fat isn't always depicted as something evil or contrary to God. In fact, fat represented the choicest pieces for sacrificing to God. This can be seen in Genesis 4:4 below:

"And Abel also brought an offering—fat portions from some of the firstborn of his flock. The LORD looked with favor on Abel and his offering."

Reflecting on the above passages, we see there are many views of fat. When we talk about fat, it can be confusing because we can talk about the fat in our diet or we can talk about the fat we store in our bodies. Let's first talk about the fat we eat.

Dietary Fat

There are many ways we can categorize fats, one of which is healthy fats versus unhealthy fats. But from a strict weight-management point of view, we need to point out that all fats provide 9 calories per gram, which is more than twice the calories per gram provided by carbohydrates or protein (4 calories per gram). Since 95% of all fats in the body and in foods are triglycerides, we do need to make special mention of them. Triglycerides are made up of 3 fatty acids and 1 molecule of glycerol. We want to make a distinction between these two different parts that make up a triglyceride because they are processed differently in the body for fuel.

- Fatty Acids: There are 20+ different fatty acids that vary in length. They are "fatty," which means they have a carbon chain that is not soluble in water. Some carbon chains are short (2–4 carbons), some are medium (6–10 carbons), and others are long-chain fatty acids (12+ carbons). Due to their chemical composition, they are acidic. These fatty acids make up about 95% of the triglyceride molecule.

- Glycerol: A glycerol molecule makes up only 5% of the triglyceride molecule and is water-soluble. The types of fatty acids in triglycerides determine the texture, taste, and physical characteristics in foods (as well as its function in the body). A few properties/functions of triglycerides in foods include adding texture to foods, giving flavor to food, and helping to make meat tender; and in various forms they can also preserve freshness.

As we said previously, a fatty acid is composed of two different parts. On one end, there is an acid group (called a carboxyl group, COOH). This is the alpha end and is considered the beginning of the chain. In the middle there is the chain of carbons and hydrogens. At the end of the chain is a methyl group, CH3, which is referred to as the omega end.

You have heard of the different terms saturated fat, monounsaturated, polyunsaturated, trans-fat, omega-3 fats, and omega-6 fats. These names/terms all stem from the structure of fatty acids. When we look at pictures of fatty acids, we see each carbon atom in the carbon chain is attached to up to 4 other atoms. At the methyl or omega end of the carbon chain, we see 3 hydrogen atoms are attached (CH3). At the other end is an acid group (COOH). Each of the carbons in between is attached to 2 carbons and either 1 or 2 hydrogen atoms, depending on whether the fatty acid is unsaturated or saturated.

Saturated Fats

One way to view saturated fats is to think of them as saturated with hydrogen (like a sponge that can hold no more water). Each of the carbons in the chain has 2 carbons and 2 hydrogens. In other words, it is saturated with hydrogens. The number of saturated and unsaturated fatty acids in the fat (triglyceride) of a food helps shape the food. Fats with a high number of saturated fatty acids tend to be solid at room temperature like:

- butter
- lard
- hard margarines
- fat from meat

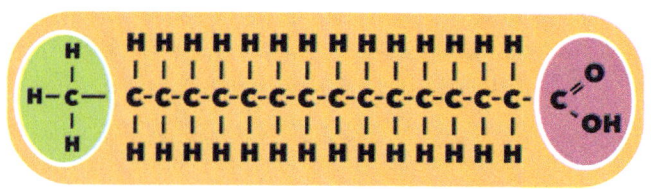

Saturated Fatty Acid

The straight chains of saturated fatty acids pack tightly together and are solid at room temperature. Two exceptions are coconut and palm oil (often called the tropical oils)—these can be liquid at room temperature due to the shorter length (less carbons) of their chain. While many saturated fats are from animal sources (meat, cheese, cream), they can also be from plants, as these oils demonstrate. Saturated plant oils are useful in food processing because they are less susceptible to spoilage. It is recommended that no more than 10% of fats consumed come from this type of fat, as it is associated with an increased risk of numerous chronic conditions.

Monounsaturated Fats

In an unsaturated fat, one or more of the carbons in the chain are not saturated with hydrogen. Instead, a double bond can be found, which is highlighted in purple in the following picture. The double bonds in unsaturated fatty acids cause kinks in the shape and prevent them from packing tightly together, so they tend to be liquid at room temperature. Fats that have a high number of unsaturated fatty acids tend to be liquid at room temperature and are called oils instead of fats. These include oils like:

- canola oil
- olive oil
- peanut oil
- sesame oil
- avocados
- many nuts and seeds

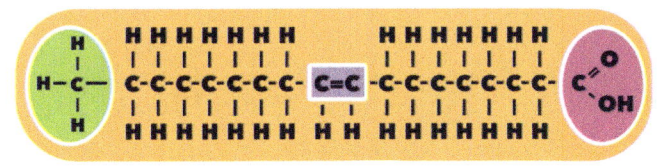

Monounsaturated Fatty Acid

These oils are NOT saturated with hydrogen atoms. The majority of the fats we consume should come from mono- and polyunsaturated fats. Monounsaturated fats can help reduce bad cholesterol levels in your blood, reducing your risk of heart disease and stroke.

Polyunsaturated Fats

Polyunsaturated fats are just like monounsaturated fats, except they contain more than one carbon-to-carbon double bond in their carbon chain. Oils that have a high number of unsaturated fatty acids are also liquid at room temperature. These include:

- fish oils
- walnut oil
- flaxseed oil
- corn oil
- safflower oil
- soybean oil
- canola oil

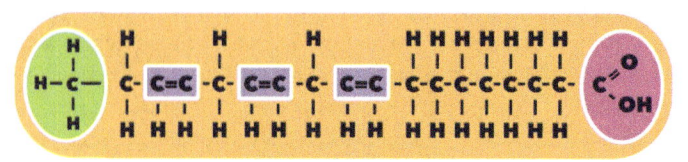

Polyunsaturated Fatty Acid

The presence and placement of the carbon-carbon double bonds contributes to the fatty acids' name and properties.

Beginning with the methyl carbon on the omega end, counting the number of carbons in the chain up to and including the first carbon of the double bond will classify the fatty acid as a certain "omega" fat.

This classification is where we find names like omega-3 and omega-6 fatty acids. The American Heart Association recommends people eat between 5 and 10% of their daily calories from omega-6 fatty acids. Most people already eat this amount of omega-6 fatty acids or more. These types of fats are recommended in the diet because they help reduce bad cholesterol levels, reducing the risk of heart disease and stroke. Some special polyunsaturated fatty acids are called essential fatty acids.

Omega-6 Fatty Acids and Omega-3 Fatty Acids: The Essential Fatty Acids

The body is capable of synthesizing most of the fatty acids it needs. However, humans are not able to synthesize fatty acids that have double bonds in the omega-6 and omega-3 positions. That's why these are called essential fatty acids, because we must consume them in our diet. The essential fatty acids are:

- Linoleic acid (omega-6)

- Alpha-linolenic acid (omega-3)

- Arachidonic acid is an omega-6 (found in both animals and vegetable oils). It becomes essential only it there is insufficient amounts of linoleic acid.

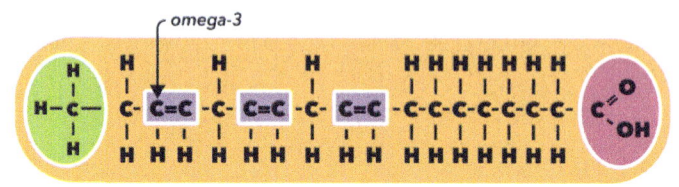

Polyunsaturated Fatty Acid

The above picture is an omega-3 fatty acid. We know this because of the placement of the double bonds, in purple. Starting on the omega end, the green end, if you count the number of carbons in the chain from left to right, up to and including the first carbon of the double bond, we see the double bond is on the third carbon from the omega end; thus, it is an omega-3 fatty acid.

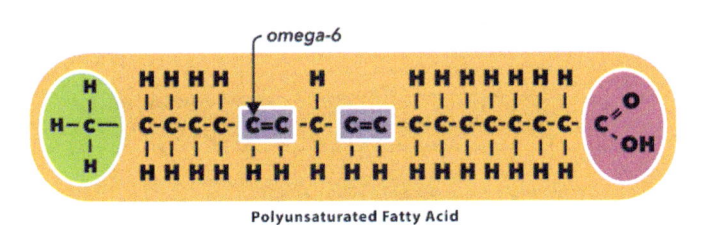

Polyunsaturated Fatty Acid

The above picture is an omega–6 fatty acid. We know this because of the placement of the double bonds, in purple. Starting on the omega end, the green end, if you count the number of carbons in the chain from left to right, up to and including the first carbon of the double bond, we see the double bond is on the sixth carbon from the omega end; thus, it is an omega-6 fatty acid.

Other fatty acids are formed from these. When fish high in omega-3 unsaturated fatty acids is substituted for saturated fatty acids, such as those in beef and pork, cholesterol and inflammation throughout the body may be lowered. Inflammation in the body can damage blood vessels and lead to heart disease. Omega-3 fatty acids may decrease serum triglycerides, lower blood pressure, reduce blood clotting, boost immunity, and improve arthritis symptoms. It may even improve learning ability in children. We often think of blood clotting as the process that stops us from bleeding out when we have a cut or injury; while this is true, a different kind of fatty, atherosclerotic clot can also form in our blood stream and cause blockages in blood vessels and, depending on the clot's location, lead to strokes, heart attacks, and deep vein thrombosis. The evidence is stronger for the benefits of eating fish rich in omega-3 fatty acids than for using supplements or for eating non-fish sources that do contain omega-3 fatty acids, such as flaxseed, flaxseed oil, walnuts, canola oil, soybeans, and soybean oil.

Your next question might be: Does it matter what kind of fish I eat? The answer is yes. Fatty fish, such as salmon, herring, and to a lesser extent tuna contain the most omega-3 fatty acids and therefore the most benefit. Most freshwater fish have less omega-3 fatty acids than do fatty saltwater fish. Some varieties of freshwater trout have relatively high levels of omega-3 fatty acids. Some fish, such as tilapia and catfish, don't appear to be as heart-healthy. Keep in mind that any fish can be unhealthy depending on how it's prepared. For example, broiling or baking fish is a healthier option than is deep-frying.

Rancidity and Hydrogenation

Rancidity occurs when unsaturated bonds are damaged by oxygen. When foods go rancid, they give an "off flavor." You can't always see a difference in the food. You probably will be able to smell it, but you will definitely taste it. In order to increase the shelf life of foods for sale, manufacturers often use a process called hydrogenation. This process makes the fatty acids in foods more saturated. This process improves the storage properties of oils by reducing the number of double bonds. This, consequently, makes the fat more saturated and solid at room temperature, because saturated carbon chains fit together more tightly than unsaturated carbon chains. While ruminant animals can make some trans-fatty acids, the majority of double bonds in food from animal and plant sources is in a cis configuration. During the process of hydrogenation, some of the double bonds can be changed into a trans-configuration. In food production, the goal is not to simply change the configuration of double bonds while maintaining the same ratios of hydrogen to carbon. Instead, the goal is to decrease the number of double bonds and increase the amount of hydrogen in the fatty acid. This changes the consistency of the fatty acid and makes it less prone to rancidity. Production of trans fatty acids is therefore a side-effect of partial hydrogenation. There has been movement to eliminate trans-fats from processed foods because they are no longer recognized as safe.

Our metabolic pathways don't recognize fatty acids with double bonds in the trans configuration, and trans-fats have been associated with an increased risk of developing heart disease. When it comes to fat, trans-fat is considered by most physicians to be the worst type of fat.

You may have noticed that some fats listed appeared in more than one category. That is because it contains more than one type of fatty acid. Remember, triglycerides have three fatty acids attached to a glycerol backbone. It is possible that the attached fatty acids do not all fall into the same category. The chart below provides the kind of fatty acids in various foods.

For example, 46% of the fatty acids in beef are saturated, while extra virgin olive oil only contains 13% saturated fatty acids.

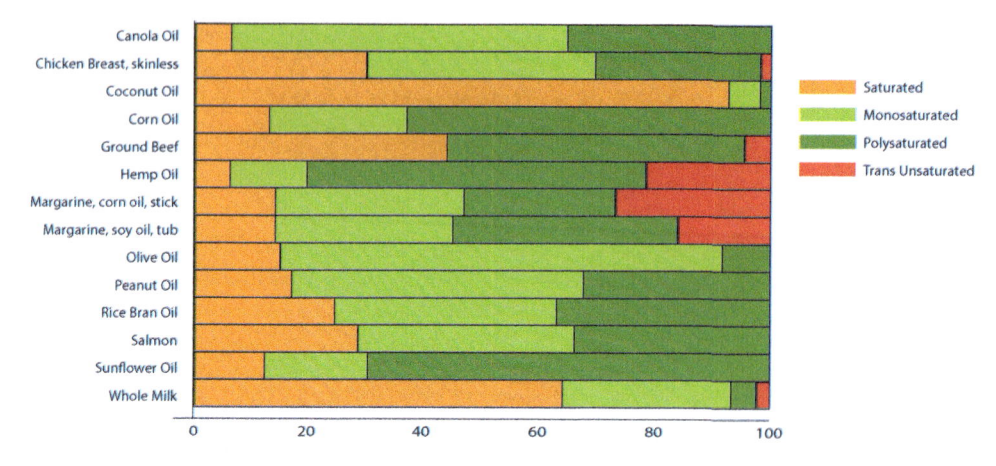

Adapted from: https://www.skillsyouneed.com/ps/fats-oils.html

Our bodies need only small amounts of fat. Thus, a diet that is rather low in fat can still provide sufficient fat for the body's needs. It is recommended that 20–35% of all our calories come from fats. Now that we have discussed dietary fat, let's take a look at the fat in our bodies.

Stored Body Fat

A fat cell is called an adipocyte. It is a roundish cell filled mainly with triglycerides. Adipocytes can occur in the body alone or in groups held together by connective tissue. We call it adipose tissue when many fat cells are found with fibrous connective tissue. Ninety percent of the body's energy reserves are found in adipose tissue. Fat serves many vital functions in the body; in addition to providing stored energy, fat provides thermal insulation, surrounds and protects internal organs, helps the absorption of fat-soluble vitamins, and cushions body areas like shoulders, hands, and feet.

There are different types of adipose tissue. There is white fat and brown fat, and some researchers also talk about beige fat.

- **White fat** is actually a light-yellow color, due to the carotenoids contained within it. These cells store triglycerides from the fats we eat and from the fat we make with excess carbohydrates and proteins we eat.

- **Brown fat** also derives its name from its color. Its brown color comes from the many mitochondria and blood vessels in the brown adipocyte. Brown fat is found predominately in fetuses, infants, and young children. It accounts for up to 6% of an infant's body weight. The primary purpose of brown fat is to generate heat in order to maintain body temperature. The amount of brown fat diminishes as we age. Adults have minimal amounts of brown fat; therefore, it has an insignificant effect on energy expenditure.

- **Beige fat** are adipocytes found within white adipocyte tissue but contain visibly more mitochondria than white adipocytes. The main difference between brown and beige fat is brown fat cells have higher levels of a protein called an uncoupling protein. This protein causes calories to be burned to generate heat without producing energy. Beige cells can, however, make high levels of the protein in response to cold. In addition, it has been noted that the hormone irisin, which is expressed during exercise, enables beige fat to burn calories nearly as effectively as brown fat. Great! Short of cool sculpting, this concept is only helpful if you relocated to one of the Arctic regions or you exercise. We do not recommend the procedure of cool sculpting without professional assistance.

How fat grows

Adipose tissue increases in two ways.

> **Hypertrophy** is when fat cells expand in size. Each cell stores more triglycerides. Research indicates that people with a Body Mass Index (BMI) of 25kg/m2–34.9kg/m2 (meaning they are overweight to moderately obese) experience this type of fat growth. If they lose weight, their cells empty and become smaller in size. Folks who fall into this category can experience more success at maintaining weight loss than people who have experienced hyperplasia.

> **Hyperplasia** is when fat cells increase in number. This can occur when immature adipocytes divide, producing more cells. When fat cells reach their maximum size, as is seen in people with a BMI >35 kg/m2, they experience hyperplasia. If these people lose weight, their fat cells will shrink in size, but the number of cells will not decrease. Achieving and maintaining a healthy body weight is more likely when fewer fat cells exist.

As you ponder these things, let's consider a few more facts. During the first year of life, body fat increases from around 15% at birth to about 30% at year one. Adipocytes undergo both hypertrophy and hyperplasia during this time. Differences are seen even at these early ages. Infants born with a high birth weight and to diabetic mothers tend to have a higher percentage of body fat and are at increased risk of being overweight in later childhood and adolescence.

Body fat percentage generally declines between ages 1 and 6 years but then increases between ages 6 and 8. This is called "adiposity rebound." Children who experience adiposity rebound earlier than this are at an increased risk of excess body fat early in life. Between 25% and 80% of overweight children remain overweight into adulthood. Thus, it is important to consider family genes, as well as weight-loss fluctuations. Factors mentioned here may make weight loss more difficult but not impossible. Considering these factors can help guide health care providers in making realistic weight-loss goals, as well as understanding the importance of a family-wide approach to health.

Belly Fat

Another way of looking at fat is by where it is stored on the body.

- **Subcutaneous Body Fat** is stored underneath the skin.

- **Visceral Body Fat** is stored around the abdominal area.

We make this distinction because when it comes to health and the focus of many diets, most attention is on visceral body fat because it is considered more dangerous than subcutaneous body fat. Abdominal fat also comes in two different forms. It can be subcutaneous fat, just beneath the skin, which is no more of a threat than subcutaneous fat anywhere else on the body, or visceral fat, which is inside the abdominal area. In essence, the difference is it is located around the internal organs, not just underneath the skin. While researchers are still not completely clear why this fat is more dangerous, one of the earliest explanations for the negative health impact was that visceral fat was linked to over-activity of the body's stress response mechanisms, resulting in raised blood pressure, blood sugar levels, and cardiac risk.

A more recent explanation is based on the concept of lipotoxicity. Lipotoxicity indicates that visceral fat cells have metabolic products, including free fatty acids, that are released into the bloodstream and carried directly to the liver. In other words, substrates from visceral fat cells are released directly into the portal circulation. Subcutaneous fat does not. As a result, visceral fat cells filled with excess triglycerides channel free fatty acids into the liver. But that is not the only problem; free fatty acids also begin to accumulate in the pancreas and heart, as well as other organs. These cells don't have the ability to make triglycerides for proper storage like adipose cells, nor do they have the normal stimulation to release these fatty acids like adipose cells. Fat that accumulates in tissues other than adipose cells is called "ectotopic fat." This "ectotopic fat" accumulates in cells that were never designed to store fat. This excess burden hinders organ function, including impaired heart function and diminished regulation of insulin, blood sugar, and cholesterol. The harmful effects of excess fatty acids, accompanied by their buildup in functioning cells of multiple tissues, including skeletal and cardiac, liver, and pancreatic cells, result in chronic cellular dysfunction and injury and is termed lipotoxicity. It can account for many indicators of metabolic syndrome.

Much evidence associates lipid accumulation in the liver with liver insulin resistance. But the mechanism of this association is not fully understood. In fact, it is quite controversial. The bottom line is that lipotoxicity leads to acute and chronic cell dysfunction and injury in many tissues. Furthermore, both clinical observations and basic research results agree that excessive fat inside the abdomen is a major contributor to cardiovascular disease.

A special word about alcohol and belly fat

The liver is vitally important, as it has about 500 functions in the body. A critical role of the liver is to act as a "filter" for foreign substances entering the body. Alcohol and drugs are foreign substances. The liver also plays important roles in the metabolism of fats, carbohydrates, and proteins. When fat builds up in the liver it is called fatty liver or hepatic steatosis. As discussed previously, too much visceral fat causes health problems. Too much fat in the liver can cause liver inflammation, leading to scarring. In severe cases, this scarring can lead to liver failure. A fatty liver in someone who drinks a lot of alcohol is known as alcoholic fatty liver disease (AFLD). In other words, drinking excess alcohol can lead to an overproduction of fat (remember that alcohol is converted to fat by the liver). An alcoholic fatty liver ultimately can negatively affect the way the body metabolizes and stores carbohydrates and fats, making it difficult to lose weight. There are currently no medications approved to treat fatty liver disease.

Alcohol can, in fact, contribute to excess belly fat. The phrase or concept of a "beer gut" is not a myth. Beer is high in simple sugars. Extra calories are converted to fat and stored in the body. In general, alcohol intake is associated with bigger waists, because when alcohol is available, the liver burns it instead of fat. Alcohol is metabolized into the same basic unit as fat, acetyl CoA, so it is burned in the same way as fat. When there is alcohol in the body, it is burned first. Because alcohol is burned in the same process as fat, alcohol in the system turns off the body's ability to burn fat. In fact, six hours after consuming 5.4 oz of 100-proof alcohol, our ability to burn fat is reduced by 595% because it is burning alcohol. Twenty hours after consuming 5.4 oz of 100-proof alcohol our ability to burn fat is decreased by 60%. The more frequently alcohol is consumed, the better the body is trained at burning it. When more calories are consumed than burned, the excess calories are stored as fat. Where a body stores that fat is determined in part by genes, age, sex, and hormones. Before puberty, boys and girls start out with similar fat storage patterns. In general, because women tend to have more subcutaneous fat than men, extra fat calories tend to be deposited in their arms, thighs, and buttocks, as well as their bellies. But because men tend to have less subcutaneous fat, their extra fat calories are stored more in their bellies.

You may have noticed that beer bellies in your patients tend to be more conspicuous in older people. As we age, calorie needs decrease and many people become less active. Plainly put, it is easier to gain weight as we age. Our metabolic rate decreases about 2% a decade. Furthermore, hormone levels decline in both men and women as they age, which results in a greater likelihood of storing fat around the middle. Even women who always had an hourglass figure when young and never struggled with belly fat their entire lives will start putting more fat in their abdominal area after menopause. Menopausal women taking hormone replacement therapy tend to experience less of this than women not taking therapy. Furthermore, when intoxicated, people find it difficult to make sound decisions. The lowering of inhibitions that accompanies drinking alcohol can lead to poor food decision-making (among other things). The Lord addresses this in Ephesians 5:18: "Don't be drunk with wine, because that will ruin your life. Instead, be filled with the Holy Spirit."

Determining abdominal obesity

Based on their past body weight, most people know if they are carrying excess body fat in their abdominal area. However, there are quantitative methods to determine abdominal obesity. Computed tomography (CT) or magnetic resonance imaging (MRI) are the most accurate methods of measuring the amount of visceral fat. These are both sophisticated pieces of equipment that can be costly to use.

A simpler and less expensive method is the waist-to-hip ratio. This requires measuring the waist at the navel while the abdomen is relaxed and measuring the hips at their widest point. Then, divide the waist size by the hip size:

Waist (in inches) / Hips (in inches) = ratio

The chance of a heart attack or stroke increases progressively as a man's ratio rises above 1.0; while a woman's risk begins to rise above 0.85.

Another simple method is waist circumference. To measure waist circumference, use a cloth measuring tape that can't be stretched, relax, exhale, and expose your bare belly. Keep the tape parallel to the ground while measuring the waist at the navel. Record the measurement to the nearest one-tenth of an inch. (Be sure not to use a stiff metal carpenters' tape from the toolbox.)

Risk	Men	Women
Low Risk	37 in. and below	31.5 in. and below
Intermediate Risk	37.1 - 39.9 in.	31.6 - 34.9 in.
High Risk	40 in. and above	35 in. and above

Just to clarify, waist measurement gives the best estimate of visceral fat and risk of obesity-related disease, while BMI provides the best estimate of total body fatness.

Losing belly fat

While much research and dieting interest are focused on belly fat, the only way to reduce visceral fat is to lose weight. This, of course, requires burning more calories with exercise than calories consumed from food. There is no magic bullet to losing belly fat. It comes down to cutting calories and getting more physical activity. This means monounsaturated fats and "belly fat" diets don't target belly fat or help to lose belly fat faster than any other healthy, low-calorie diet.

In many cases, lifestyle changes are in order for those with fatty liver disease. Suggestions for losing belly fat and any body fat include losing weight, following a balanced diet, limiting alcohol, and avoiding binge drinking. Current guidelines for health define moderate alcohol consumption for men as 2 drinks per day and for women 1 drink per day. Of course, when trying to lose body fat, it would be wise to only indulge on special occasions (not daily).

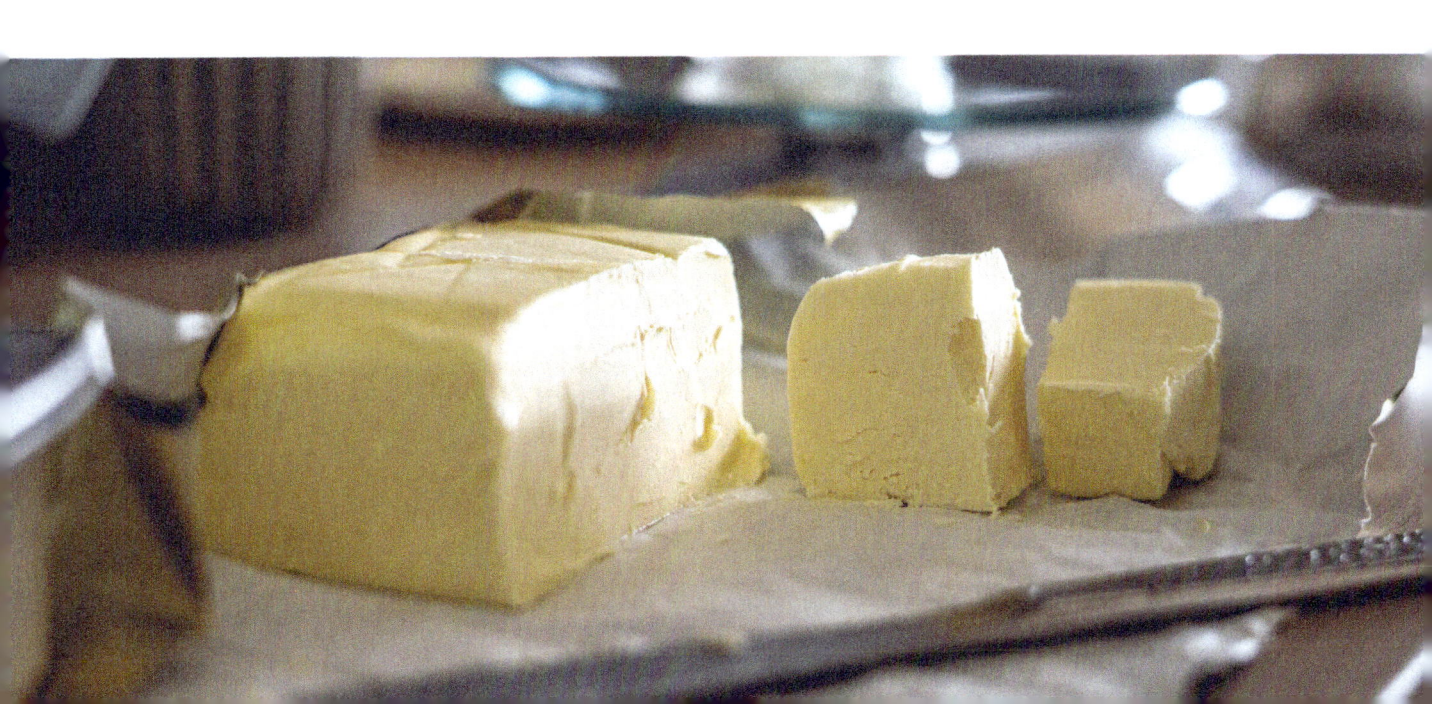

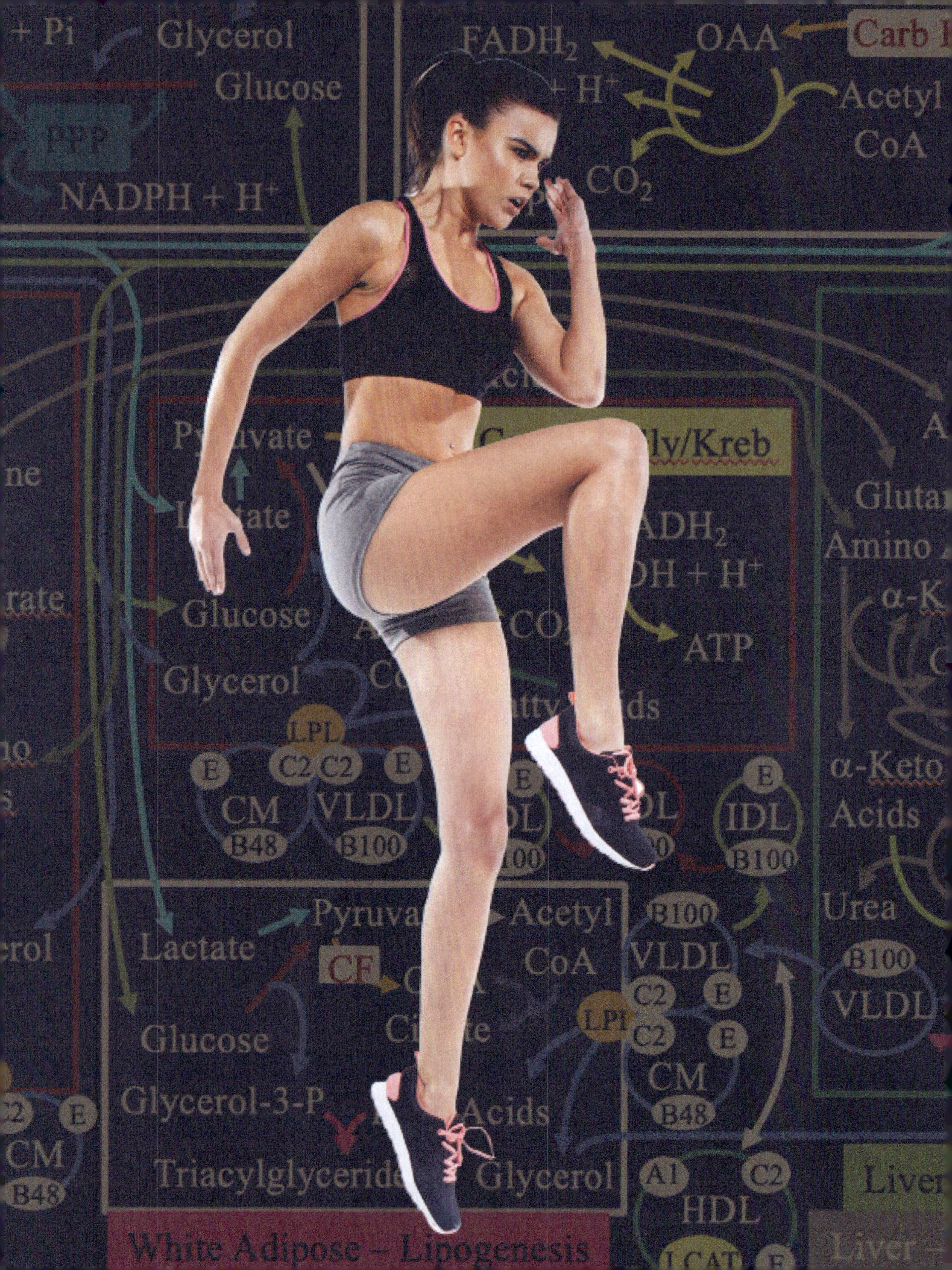

Glycerol
Glucose
PPP
NADPH + H+
FADH2
OAA
Carb
Acetyl
CoA
CO2
Kreb
Glucose
Glycerol
ATP
LPL
E
C2
CM
B48
VLDL
B100
IDL
α-Keto
Acids
Urea
Lactate
CF
Acetyl
CoA
Glucose
Glycerol-3-P
Acids
Triacylglycerides
Glycerol
LPL
HDL
A1
LCAT
Liver
White Adipose – Lipogenesis

CHAPTER 8
Metabolism

"I praise you because I am fearfully and wonderfully made; your works are wonderful, I know that full well."
—Psalm 139:14

The human body is certainly amazing! Modern discoveries involving the human body have proven this scripture true. Nothing is more brilliantly designed or breathtaking than the human body. The Lord included many unique and splendid design features from head to toe—features that go far beyond what is needed for survival. Contrary to evolutionist claims that apes are human ancestors, many human features are vastly different from apes. For example, humans see ten million colors and detect changes in hues just a few nanometers apart. As a result, humans are the only ones who stop to relish a sunset or admire the colors of autumn leaves. Humans have roughly fifty facial muscles that allow for 10,000 facial expressions. These include expressions of joy, pleasure, surprise, disapproval, confusion, grief, anger, boredom, and pain, to name a few. The ability to express emotions, combine expressions, and to make expressions of differing intensity is a remarkable, clever design, enabling humans to reveal feelings and passions quickly. In contrast, apes have fewer than thirty facial muscles and can make only a few expressions. Most of their muscles are for eating and closing their eyes, not communicating.

In a chapter devoted to metabolism, we don't have time to discuss the intricacies of human physiology. There is a whole host of examples, such as the complexity of human hands with fully opposable thumbs, or fingers with a full range of motion that allow for complex tasks such as sign-language and writing. We don't have room to fully discuss how human fingertips each contain thousands of touch sensors, or how the human body is lovingly wrapped in fine skin instead of fur. Think of all the things a fine sense of touch permits: sewing, playing music, surgery, and reading Braille. Of course, we could go on and on about the incomparable human speech and language ability, the human's upright stature and unrivaled arched foot design, the unique human genome and the unsurpassed human brain. On top of it all, we are imbued with the breath of life and an eternal soul from our Creator, making us distinct from animals. Suffice it to say, our Creator provided all we need to perceive the world so we can accomplish our unique callings of stewardship while bringing glory to Him.

Undoubtedly, many of your patients and clients don't have a mastery of all the ins and outs of their body functions. In fact, many may go on diets without understanding the metabolism behind the diet. For all intents and purposes, many may hold the perspective that they don't need to know anything about metabolism, even when they are "on a diet." This makes it all the more important for you, the health care professional, to understand the safety of diets as you guide your clients and patients. Let's examine this.

We Can Learn a Lot from the Disney Movie *Cars*®

Sometimes it helps to give your patients and clients an illustration using something they are familiar with to help convey complex concepts. Perhaps you can use the analogy of a car. Fueling the human body is like fueling a car. This is a concept I share with student athletes. In fact, I often refer to the popular Disney movie *Cars*® and say, "Mater and Lightning McQueen do not use the same fuel. Lightning McQueen uses high-test, high-speed fuel because he is a race car. Could you image how Lightning would perform if he fueled his body the same as his tow-truck friend, Mater?" The type of fuel we put into our bodies matters, and just as Lightning McQueen would not expect to perform his best on Mater's fuel, an athlete should not expect to perform at top levels with a poorly fueled "diet."

This isn't just true for athletes. While most people will not return to a mechanic who doesn't care well for their car, many will repeatedly return to bogus diet books and programs that can't and don't care for their body, which, unlike a car, can't be replaced or traded in for a newer version.

Understanding the Mechanics

When people have some understanding of how their body works, they can comprehend how to care for it and make wise choices. Having a foundational understanding of metabolism will help dieters recognize bogus or misguided information when they see it. As stated earlier, most fad diets have a grain of truth. The problem is that these truths that lay the foundation for many different diets lose their strength and impact when applied to human behavior, the body as a whole, or to reality. Therefore, many diets fall short of all their promises and expectations.

The Magnificent Metabolism

"For we are his workmanship, created in Christ Jesus for good works, which God prepared beforehand, that we should walk in them." —Ephesians 2:10

The human metabolism is truly a magnificent work of God. Metabolism is the total of all reactions that take place in the body. These reactions occur through various metabolic pathways. Because our bodies continually need energy, the metabolism doesn't, under any circumstances, rest or stop, even when we sleep. Our heart keeps pumping and our lungs keep inhaling oxygen as we breathe through the night. All body movement and actions need fuel. We can call this fuel "calories," or we can call it "energy." Obviously, our needs vary when we sleep versus when we are running, so these metabolic pathways and processes must continually adjust and change based on our circumstances. In fact, the body burns different fuels depending on what we are doing. For example, different percentages of different fuels are used if we are sprinting, jogging slowly, sleeping, if we recently ate or if we ate hours ago. Terms that are bolded in the text can be found in the glossary at the end of this chapter. Let's first review basal metabolic rate (BMR).

Basal Metabolic Rate

Basal Metabolic Rate (BMR) is the energy spent to meet the body's basic physiological needs when the body is at physical, emotional, and digestive rest but not asleep. It includes the functions of pumping blood, expanding the lungs, and firing nerve impulses during brain function. BMR is affected by a number of things:

- *Lean body mass* – Muscle mass is more metabolically active than fat tissue. So, the more lean tissue, the higher the metabolic rate.

- *Age* – BMR decreases 1–2% every decade after the early adult years, but it increases 15% during pregnancy.

- *Gender* – Women tend to have a BMR that is 10% lower than men.

- *Height* – Taller people will have a higher BMR, due to increased surface area (which means more heat is lost from the body, causing the metabolism to increase).

- *Genes* – One's genes obviously will influence BMR in various ways.

- *Ethnicity* – African Americans tend to have a BMR about 10% lower than Caucasians.

- *Nutritional state* – Nutritional state changes depending on when the last meal was consumed, activity level and in¬tensity, nutrient composition of meals, and individual metabolic rate. Sometimes the combination of these nutritional states is referred to as the Fed-Fast Cycle or the Feast or Famine Concept, which is discussed in more detail in the next section (under "States of Metabolism").

- *Hormones* – During periods of stress, the hypothalamus instructs the adrenal glands to release epinephrine (adrenaline), norepinephrine, and cortisol (hydrocortisone) into the bloodstream to speed up heart rate, respiration, blood pressure, and metabolism. Epinephrine breaks down glycogen into glucose in the liver. These hormones increase circulating free fatty acids. The extra glucose and fatty acids are used by the body as fuel in times of stress. Epinephrine, which is released during emotional stress, can increase BMR. An increase in thyroid hormone will increase BMR and vice versa. (This fluctuates during the menstrual cycle.) However, prolonged stress disrupts the digestive system. Such conditions serve to lower the BMR.

- *Injuries, fever, burns, infections* – These all will increase BMR, which means more calories should be consumed to aid in recovery.

- *Caffeine* increases BMR slightly when consumed regularly in moderate amounts.

- *Drugs* such as nicotine and amphetamines will increase BMR.

- *Environmental temperatures* – Being very cold or very hot can increase BMR. The change is minimal if clothing or air temperature is adjusted.

RECAP: Many factors can influence our BMR. Some can be controlled, others cannot.

States of Metabolism

"Watch and pray so that you will not fall into temptation. The spirit is willing, but the flesh is weak."   —Matthew 26:41

More goes into eating than our emotions and our past histories, and those factors account for a lot. In the previous discussion it was noted that the human body is powerfully magnificent, yet by God's standards, the flesh is weak. We have influences on our food intake from taste, temptation, gluttony, body image, and more. These can override our body's natural signals. God created many biological factors that influence food intake, and it's essential to be aware of them. These are often referred to as internal cues. These internal systems are complex and powerful. One aspect that increases complexity is the fed versus the fasted state. These conditions need to be discussed, as they will continually be referred to and addressed throughout this discussion of metabolism.

- **The fed state** is sometimes called the absorptive state because it occurs after a meal has been eaten (as the names imply). It is the state when the body is in the process of breaking food into component parts so the nutrients can be absorbed. Digestion begins the moment food enters the mouth, with the action of the saliva and teeth; the different elements are eventually absorbed through the intestine. These nutrients are then processed by different organ systems and used for energy or stored for later use.

- **The fasted state** occurs at least 3 hours and for up to 2 days after food has been digested, absorbed, and stored. Some researchers refer to the initial stage, 3–18 hours, as the post-absorptive state. During this time, the body draws upon its stored nutrients for energy. During a fast, the body relies initially on stored glycogen, lean tissue, and fat stores. Diets that promote "fasts," "cleanses," "very low calories," "detoxes," or "intermittent eating" are intentionally designed to put the body into this fasting state. Because water is stored with glycogen, when glycogen stores are used to fuel the body, the body also rids itself of water. This results in a decrease in total body weight and will be reflected on the scale. Although the number on the scale is lower, no fat has been lost. Moreover, as glycogen stores are depleted, lean tissue begins to be used to burn fat. Lean tissue is heavy compared to fat. Thus, when lean tissue is lost, the scale reflects a significant weight loss. Losing lean tissue can lower metabolism and damage the tissues or organs that are being degraded. In the long term, this makes losing weight and keeping it off more difficult.

- **The starvation state** occurs if fasting continues beyond 2 days. In this stage, there is a metabolic fuel shift to spare vitally important lean tissue protein. During the fasted state, the brain and other non-muscle tissues use ketone bodies made by the liver from fatty acids released from the adipose tissue. In addition, these non-muscle tissues use glucose made by the liver from the stripping of lean muscle. These two sources of fuel are liberally used by these non–muscle tissues. However, we see a change after 2 days.

The literature shows that in the time between 3 and 40 days of not eating, the brain transitions from using 100 grams of glucose daily to about 40 grams. During that same time period, the brain transitions from consuming about 50 grams of ketone bodies daily to about 100 grams. So, we see, as fasting continues, the brain begins to use more ketone bodies and less glucose. As we will soon discuss in detail, glucose can be used solely for fuel and is used to create Krebs cycles so ketone bodies can be used for fuel. Therefore, we see the brain limiting its use of glucose to only the amounts needed to create Krebs cycles so that ketone bodies will be used for fuel. In other words, the brain increases its use of ketone bodies and decreases its use of glucose in order to conserve the glucose being made by the liver. Ultimately, this conservation of glucose serves to slow the stripping of lean tissue, which is the source the liver is using to make glucose during starvation.

In essence, starvation reprograms one's metabolism. It may be difficult for the depressed metabolic rate of the starvation state to come back to normal levels. In addition, once feeding resumes, the body prepares for the possibility of another starvation state by storing calories in excess. We often see this in the typical fad dieter. While they may not fast for 40 days, they often severely restrict for numerous days in a row. The problem is most dieters can't continue this painful starvation process, especially when food is all around them. As a result, they "cheat." Cheating confuses the body—the metabolic rate remains depressed and the body rapidly stores everything eaten. As a result, the dieter ends up losing lean tissue and storing more fat. On top of that, he or she has a depressed metabolic rate.

ATP = Fuel Used by the Body

"Therefore, if anyone is in Christ, he is a new creation. The old has passed away; behold, the new has come."
—2 Corinthians 5:17

Just as we cannot directly enter heaven on our own merits, but only through the transformation of becoming a new creation through the acceptance of Jesus' sacrificial death for our sins, food can't enter cells without first undergoing change. Reactions in our body take energy, but we can't use carbohydrates, proteins, or fats directly as that energy. Each cell in the body must convert these macronutrients into a central molecule that can be used for all the reactions. In these magnificent human bodies, that central molecule is adenosine triphosphate (ATP). ATP is the only energy source all body cells can directly use. All the energy (calories) in carbohydrates, proteins, and fats is converted into energy in the form of ATP. The body can produce 4 calories of energy for every gram of carbohydrate or protein, and 9 calories of energy for every gram of fat.

> **RECAP:** Carbohydrates, proteins, and fats are "fuel" macromolecules delivered to each cell in the body by blood. Once delivered, these "fuel" macromolecules are converted into a central energy called ATP. ATP is the fuel that cells use for cellular function.

Metabolic Pathways Are Like Instruments

Our bodies are like an orchestra with the different tissues as sections of the orchestra. Each instrument produces a unique sound, and when all the sections combine their individual sounds, together they produce beautiful music that emphasizes the whole. An important difference between the sections of the orchestra and the tissues of the body is that the tissues of the body are dependent on each other. In other words, the strings in an orchestra can produce a sound without the woodwinds, but the brain can't function without the liver making glucose and ketone bodies for fuel so it can survive during times of fasting. For the processing of macronutrients in cells, there are a few basic pathways that need to be discussed. We will begin with common metabolic pathways found in all cell types (except red blood cells). These are glycolysis and the Krebs cycle. This discussion will be followed by a description of specialized pathways that aren't found in all cells.

1. Metabolic pathways common to all cell types (except red blood cells)

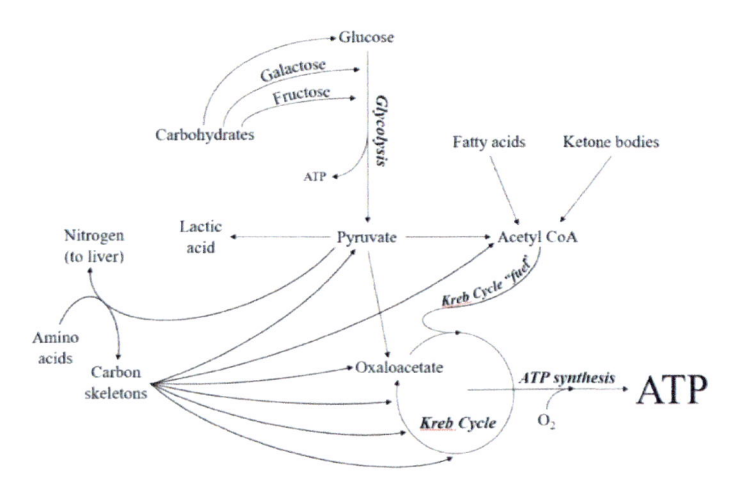

a. **Glycolysis.** This is a pathway where carbohydrates such as glucose, galactose, and fructose are converted to a single molecule called **pyruvate** and a small amount of ATP is made (small compared to what can be made from the Krebs cycle). Once pyruvate is made by glycolysis, the next step in metabolism will depend on the presence or absence of oxygen. Glycolysis will occur in the absence and/or presence of oxygen.

If there is sufficient oxygen to support the **Krebs cycle,** pyruvate will be transported into the **mitochondria** of the cell. Once inside the mitochondria, pyruvate can make Krebs cycles if sufficient fats or ketone bodies are available for fuel to be burned in those Krebs cycles. If fats and ketone bodies are not available for fuel, pyruvate can make Krebs cycles and become the fuel to be burned in the Krebs cycles. In other words, carbohydrates can create Krebs cycles and be used for fuel in Krebs cycles. The amino acids from proteins can create Krebs cycles, but only a few amino acids can be fuel for the Krebs cycles. Fats, on the other hand, cannot create Krebs cycles; they can only be used as fuel in the Krebs cycle.

If there is insufficient oxygen to support the Krebs cycle or the cell doesn't have mitochondria (as is the case with red blood cells), pyruvate will be converted to **lactic acid** and the lactic acid will be released into circulation. This is frequently called the **lactic acid metabolic system.**

b. **Krebs cycle.** This is a pathway found only in cells with mitochondria. Mitochondria are often called the "powerhouses" of the cell. This cycle is made by either pyruvate (from carbohydrates) or the **carbon skeletons** of amino acids (after their nitrogen has been removed). Note that fats and ketone bodies can only be used as fuel (for consumption) in this pathway and cannot create this pathway. The energy produced by Krebs is funneled into ATP synthesis by molecules made from vitamins. Both oxygen and vitamins are needed or no energy can be made.

2. Specialized metabolic pathways (these don't happen in all cells)

a. **Beta-oxidation of fatty acids** (muscle and liver cells)

Beta-oxidation is the chopping up of fatty acids into smaller units called acetyl CoA to be used for fuel in the Krebs cycle. Skeletal muscles use this pathway in both the fed and fasted states. In the fed state, skeletal muscles use dietary fats for fuel, and in the fasted state, they use fats released from adipose tissue for fuel. In the fasted state, liver cells use this pathway to produce ketone bodies from fats released from adipose tissue. Because liver cells are making glucose during the fasted state, the acetyl CoA produced during beta-oxidation is used to produce ketone bodies. The liver is doing these two things simultaneously, making ketone bodies and glucose. The ketone bodies and glucose made by the liver are sent to all tissues to be used for fuel during the fasted state.

b. **Synthesis of fatty acids** (adipose and liver cells)

Synthesis of fatty acids only occurs in the fed state. Excess carbohydrate and protein calories are made into fatty acids by liver cells. These fatty acids are sent to and stored in the adipose cells. Adipose tissue has the capability of making fatty acids from excess carbohydrates, but not from protein. All excess protein must go to the liver to be made into fatty acids. In other words, fat is made from excess calories in both liver and adipose cells, but all will be stored in the adipose tissue. Unfortunately, adipose cells have a maximum capacity, and as a result, as people get more and more obese, fatty acids get stored in tissues not designed to store fats. This can contribute to disease.

c. **Removing the nitrogen from amino acids** (skeletal muscle cells and liver cells)

Deamination is the scientific term that means removing the nitrogen from amino acids. In order to use protein for energy, the body must remove nitrogen from amino acids in both the fed and fasted state. Skeletal muscle cells remove the nitrogen from amino acids but must send the nitrogen to the liver cells for disposal. Liver cells receive nitrogen from the muscles and produce urea, which is then excreted from the body. Regardless of where amino acids come from, the liver is the only organ that can dispose of nitrogen as urea. In addition to receiving nitrogen from muscles, liver cells can remove the nitrogen from amino acids and can directly dispose of the nitrogen by producing urea. In contrast to the liver, skeletal muscle cells have large quantities of proteins (lean tissue) that can be stripped and used for fuel, in both the fed and fasted state.

d. **Gluconeogenesis** (liver cells)

Gluconeogenesis is the making of "new" glucose when blood glucose levels are low. During times of fasting, the liver will make "new" glucose from other substances in the blood. These substances include amino acids, lactic acid, and glycerol.

e. **Ketosis or ketone body production** (liver cells)

During times of fasting, the liver must make fuel molecules for the cells of the body. Unlike skeletal muscle cells, other cells do not have stored glycogen. Therefore, the liver must make glucose for these cells through the pathway of gluconeogenesis. At the same time it is making glucose, the liver is also chopping fatty acids received from the adipose and making acetyl CoA through beta-oxidation. This acetyl CoA is not used for fuel by the liver but to make ketone bodies that all cells (except red blood cells) can use for fuel. Therefore, one can see that during times of fasting, the liver makes both glucose and ketone bodies to be used as fuel by all body cells. For this to happen, the two pathways—gluconeogenesis and beta-oxidation—have to occur at the same time in the liver.

A ketone body is simply two acetyl CoA molecules linked together. Therefore, ketone bodies can be used by cells for energy by simply cutting the ketone body in half. All cells have the enzyme necessary to cut ketone bodies in half. Realize that a ketone body is considered and treated by the body as a very short fat. Therefore, all cells that can burn fat for fuel can use ketone bodies for fuel, too. Any cell that cannot burn fat for fuel will not be able to use ketone bodies for fuel. These include cells that do not have mitochondria, such as red blood cells.

f. Glycogen synthesis and degradation (liver and skeletal muscle)

Glycogen is simply many glucose molecules linked together and stored in the body. In other words, glycogen is stored "carbohydrates." They are stored in the liver and skeletal muscles. Skeletal muscles use their glycogen stores to produce energy for themselves. This occurs when blood glucose is insufficient to fuel their needs. In contrast, liver cells use their glycogen stores to supply glucose for the rest of the body when blood glucose levels are low.

Metabolic Coordination Is Like an Orchestra

"Now if the foot should say, 'Because I am not a hand, I do not belong to the body,' it would not for that reason stop being part of the body. And if the ear should say, 'Because I am not an eye, I do not belong to the body,' it would not for that reason stop being part of the body. If the whole body were an eye, where would the sense of hearing be? If the whole body were an ear, where would the sense of smell be? But in fact God has placed the parts in the body, every one of them, just as he wanted them to be. If they were all one part, where would the body be? As it is, there are many parts, but one body."
—1 Corinthians 12:15-20

Just as each body part is responsible for a function, and each instrument in an orchestra is responsible for a particular sound, each tissue is responsible for particular tasks. For simplicity, the terms "tissue" and "cell" are used interchangeably in this discussion. Let's look at these tissues and the fuel they use in the fed and fasted states. Their roles and functions will change based on if the body is in the fed or fasted state. In other words, tissues respond to the condition of the body and adjust accordingly. In fact, which fuel is available can determine what the tissue does.

Metabolism during the Fed State

Below is a diagram and discussion of what each tissue does and what fuel it uses during the fed state.

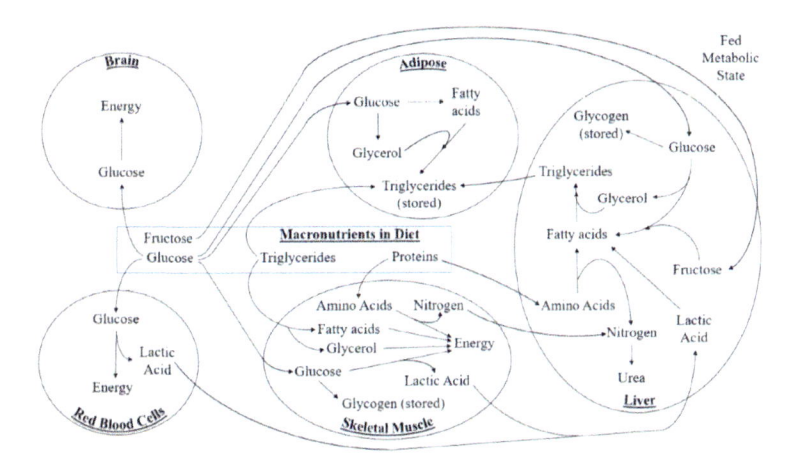

Liver: In the fed state, the liver is responsible for converting excess carbohydrate and protein calories into glycogen and fatty acids. Once liver glycogen stores are maxed out, if there are still excess carbohydrates, the liver will use them to make fatty acids. Three of these newly made fatty acids will be combined with one glycerol to make a triglyceride. The triglycerides will then be transported to and stored in the adipose tissue. The nitrogen of excess dietary amino acids is removed, and the carbon skeletons that remain are converted to fatty acids. Just like fatty acids made from carbohydrates, these fatty acids will be combined with glycerol to make triglycerides that will then be transported to and stored in the adipose tissue.

In contrast to other tissues, the liver is the only tissue that can process fructose. Other cells don't have the necessary enzymes to process it. Therefore, all fructose consumed goes to the liver to be processed. The liver will first convert it to fat before it can be used as fuel by other tissues. In other words, fructose will always be turned into fat initially; it is not directly used for fuel. That fat can then be used to fuel the body or stored as body fat, depending on energy expenditure. In contrast to glucose, fructose will not contribute to glycogen stores. Keep in mind sucrose is 50% glucose and 50% fructose, and high-fructose corn syrup can be 45% glucose, 55% fructose.

Adipose: In the fed state, the adipose tissues are responsible for storing triglycerides. Some of these triglycerides are delivered to the adipose from the liver. The remaining triglycerides are synthesized by the adipose from excess carbohydrates. In contrast to the liver, adipose cannot make triglycerides from excess amino acids because it doesn't have the enzyme necessary to remove the nitrogen from the amino acid.

Skeletal Muscle: In the fed state, the skeletal muscle will use available macronutrients for energy. It can use all three macronutrients: carbohydrates, fats, and proteins. Skeletal muscle stores excess glucose as glycogen or uses it for fuel if need be. Skeletal muscle breaks down fatty acids by beta-oxidation to acetyl CoA and then uses it for fuel. In contrast to other tissues, skeletal muscle can use amino acids for fuel because it can remove the nitrogen and send it to the liver, where the nitrogen is disposed of as urea.

Red Blood Cell: In the fed state, red blood cells can only use carbohydrates for energy. Because red blood cells do not have mitochondria, they cannot use fats or protein for energy.

Brain: In the fed state, the brain will use carbohydrates for energy. In contrast to the skeletal muscle, brain cells cannot use amino acids for energy because they don't have the enzyme necessary to remove the nitrogen from the amino acid. Also in contrast to skeletal muscle, brain cells cannot use fatty acids for energy because they do not have the enzymes necessary for beta-oxidation.

Metabolism during the Fasted State

Below is a diagram and discussion of what each tissue does and what fuel it uses during the fasted state.

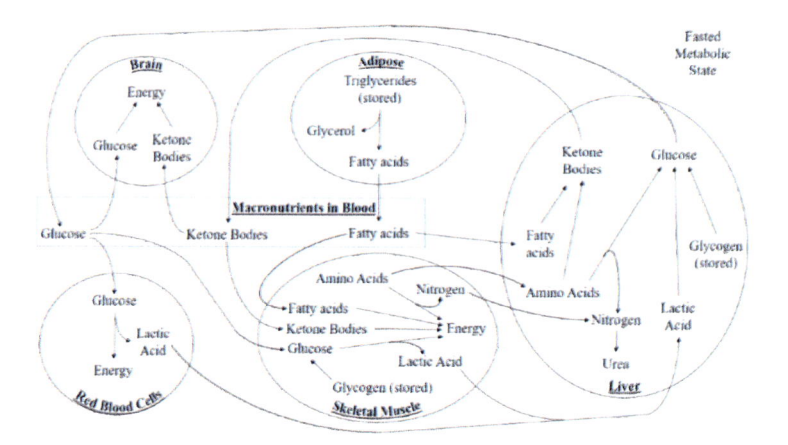

Liver: In the fasted state, the liver is responsible for making glucose in order to stabilize blood glucose levels. One way the liver makes glucose is by breaking down its stored glycogen. The liver makes "new" glucose from other substances in the blood by the gluconeogenesis pathway. These substances include amino acids, lactic acid, and glycerol. In the fasted state, the liver receives fatty acids from the adipose tissue and breaks them down to produce acetyl CoA. However, because in the fasting state liver cells are making glucose, the acetyl CoA produced during beta-oxidation is used to produce ketone bodies. The ketone bodies and glucose made by the liver are sent to all tissues to be used for fuel during the fasted state. In addition, the liver receives amino acids from the muscle, which it uses to make glucose (gluconeogenesis) and ketone bodies.

Adipose: In the fasted state, adipose tissue is responsible for supplying the liver and muscle with fatty acids. Stored triglycerides are broken down into fatty acids and glycerol and released into the blood. The fatty acids are used by the muscle for fuel; in contrast, the fatty acids are used by the liver to make ketone bodies. The glycerol can be used by other tissues for fuel. Remember, fatty acids make up 95% of a triglyceride, while glycerol accounts for only about 5%. Please note, the glycerol from triglycerides contributes a very small amount of carbohydrates necessary for cellular function. Therefore, a dieter in a fasted state must rely on gluconeogenesis to make glucose from lean tissue, due to diminishing glycogen stores.

Skeletal Muscle: In the fasted state, the skeletal muscle will use available macronutrients for energy. It can use all three macronutrients: carbohydrates, fats, and proteins. In contrast to other tissues, skeletal muscle has the luxury of having its own glycogen stores to use for fuel. Skeletal muscle receives fatty acids from the adipose tissue and breaks them down by beta-oxidation to acetyl CoA. In addition, skeletal muscle receives ketone bodies from the liver, and they break down into acetyl CoA. Skeletal muscle uses acetyl CoA for fuel. In contrast to other tissues, skeletal muscle can use amino acids for fuel too because it can remove the nitrogen and send it to the liver, where the nitrogen is disposed of as urea. Skeletal muscle cells have large quantities of proteins (lean tissue) that can be stripped and used for fuel.

Red Blood Cell: Just like in the fed state, in the fasted state red blood cells can only use carbohydrates for energy. Because red blood cells do not have mitochondria, they cannot use fats or protein for energy.

Brain: In the fasted state, the brain can use carbohydrates for energy. In contrast to the skeletal muscle, brain cells cannot use amino acids for energy because they don't have the enzyme necessary to remove the nitrogen. Also in contrast to skeletal muscle, brain cells cannot use fatty acids for energy because they do not have the enzymes necessary for beta-oxidation. However, in the fasted state, the brain can use acetyl CoA made from ketone bodies for energy. Remember, like most other cells, it has the enzyme necessary to cut the ketone body in half, producing two acetyl CoA molecules.

Metabolic Hormones Act like the Conductors in an Orchestra

"In the same way, the Spirit helps us in our weakness. We do not know what we ought to pray for, but the Spirit himself intercedes for us through wordless groans. And he who searches our hearts knows the mind of the Spirit because the Spirit intercedes for God's people in accordance with the will of God." —Romans 8:26-27

In times of weakness, Christians rely on the Holy Spirit for direction and help. The Holy Spirit has the power to intercede for us during those times and can also be compared to a musical conductor helping to direct the overall effect or result of the many separate parts. As part of God's orchestra, Christians should constantly seek to be under the direction of the Holy Spirit.

In the metabolism orchestra, the conductors are hormones. The conductor for the fed state is **insulin,** and the conductor for the fasted state is **glucagon.** These two conductors trade places as the orchestra changes back and forth between the fed and fasted states. Both insulin and glucagon are produced by the pancreas but different types of cells produce them. Insulin is produced by **beta cells.** Glucagon is produced by **alpha cells.** Many diets aim to keep insulin low; we will see that insulin and glucagon are balanced in their secretion.

Insulin's Role in the Fed State

Insulin is a hormone secreted from the beta cells of the pancreas. It is stimulated or summoned when macronutrients are available and need to be stored. We refer to this as the "fed metabolic state." Insulin secretion is stimulated by several very diverse signals.

    1. When blood glucose levels increase (after a meal), glucose enters the beta cell and ATP synthesis occurs. This, in turn, causes the beta cells to know that blood glucose levels are elevated, and insulin should be secreted.

    2. **Gastric Inhibitory Peptide (GIP)** and **Glucagon-like Peptide-1 (GLP-1)** are hormones released from the gut when macronutrients are present in the intestine. This stimulates pancreatic cells to secrete insulin.

3. Amino acids and fatty acids in the blood can also be recognized by beta cells and result in insulin secretion.

4. Signals from the brain can control insulin secretion.

    a. **Parasympathetic nerve** signals from the brain are thought to be "rest and digest" signals, so logically those signals would serve to increase insulin secretion to process and store the food consumed prior to the signals.

    b. **Sympathetic nerve** signals from the brain are thought to be "fight or flight" signals, so logically those signals would decrease insulin secretion so that more fuel molecules would be available for the fight or flight situation.

Insulin communicates with **insulin-dependent cells** (which we can think of as "target cells") by binding to a receptor (like a docking station) on the surface of a target cell and sending instructions (signals) into the cell that tell the cellular machinery what needs to be done. Insulin controls the storage of calories from dietary carbohydrates, fats, and proteins. Let's look at each of these.

A common misconception is that all cells need an insulin signal to take up glucose. Glucose is taken into cells by different glucose transporters. All cells have basic, "everyday" glucose transporters that allow glucose to enter the cells so they can use the glucose for energy. Insulin is secreted by the pancreas only when glucose levels are high, which indicates that there is excess glucose in the blood (usually after a meal) that needs to be stored for times when blood glucose levels are low (fasting).

Remember, some tissues store excess fuel. Muscles and the liver store glycogen, while adipose tissue stores fat. These are the tissues that take excess glucose and store those calories for times of fasting. Muscles, adipose, and liver cells have unique, insulin-stimulated, glucose transporters that work only when insulin tells them to work. Insulin doesn't stimulate other cells like brain cells to take up the excess glucose, because those cells can't store or make glycogen or fatty acids. Those non-insulin-responsive cells are counting on the liver to take up the excess glucose to make glycogen and to store it. The

liver will then break the glycogen down into glucose during fasting times to supply those non-insulin-responsive cells with glucose for fuel. Now that we have looked at carbohydrates, let's look at fat next.

Dietary fat is carried in the blood as triglycerides. They are transported inside carriers called **lipoproteins.** On the outside of muscle and adipose cells, a lipase enzyme is stimulated by insulin to cut the triglycerides into fatty acids and glycerol so that the dietary fatty acids can be stored in the adipose or used for energy by the muscles. Again, remember that non-insulin-responsive cells can store or degrade fatty acids (beta-oxidation), so there is no reason for them to have an insulin-stimulated lipase enzyme on the outside of their cells.

Finally, recall that dietary proteins are broken down in the intestines into amino acids. Those amino acids are absorbed into the blood. Insulin stimulates muscles to remove nitrogen from these dietary amino acids. The nitrogen is sent to the liver, while the resulting carbon skeletons are used for energy by the muscle. Liver cells also take these dietary amino acids in and remove their nitrogen. Liver cells combine the nitrogen from the skeletal muscle. But in contrast to skeletal muscle, the liver does not use the resulting carbon skeletons for energy; instead, the liver makes fatty acids from the carbon skeletons.

So, how does insulin help muscle and liver cells make glycogen and help liver and adipose cells make fatty acids? Remember that glycogen and fatty acids are made by specific metabolic pathways, which are a series of reactions that use enzymes to speed the reactions. Insulin tells the enzymes inside the muscle, adipose, and liver cells to work, and they use the excess glucose and amino acids that were transported into those cells to make glycogen and fatty acids. Other, non-insulin-responsive cells don't have these pathways or the enzymes to make glycogen or fatty acids, so there is no reason for insulin to communicate with them.

Here is a summary of what insulin tells muscle, liver, and adipose cells to do:

	Muscle	Liver	Adipose
Glucose uptake	Increase	Increase	Increase
Glycogen synthesis	Increase	Increase	
Fatty acid synthesis		Increase	Increase
Lipoprotein Lipase	Increase		Increase

In addition to directing muscle, liver, and adipose tissue to store excess macronutrients, insulin communicates with the **hypothalamus** to regulate hunger. Along with other molecules from adipose tissue (leptin), the stomach (ghrelin), and intestines (PYY, GIP, and GLP-1), insulin communicates with the **hypothalamus** to tell the brain that the body is "full." It's a feedback loop: you eat, food is processed, food macromolecules and the parasympathetic nervous system tell the pancreas to secrete insulin, and then secreted insulin tells the body to store what it has eaten and tells the brain to stop eating. This can take about 20 minutes. That is why eating slowly is recommended for weight loss. It can take 20 minutes for the brain to get and send the message "You are full, stop eating." No need to mention how much food can be eaten in 20 minutes if someone is eating quickly.

What if a muscle, liver, or adipose cell won't listen to insulin? This is called insulin resistance. There are two types of insulin resistance, peripheral and central. Peripheral insulin resistance is when muscles, liver, and adipose become resistant to insulin's signals. The second type is central insulin resistance, in which the brain becomes resistant to insulin's signals. There are multiple theories of what causes peripheral insulin resistance, and much research is being conducted on the subject. Even though the beta cells are secreting insulin in response to signals of available macronutrients, the insulin can't communicate with the skeletal muscle, liver, or adipose cells. Therefore, these insulin-responsive cells don't respond and remove the macronutrients from the blood for storage. As a result, the macronutrients continue to stimulate beta cells to secrete insulin and the beta cells continue to secrete insulin. This results in a condition called hyperinsulinemia. As it progresses, a diagnosis of type 2 diabetes is usually made.

Central insulin resistance is associated with peripheral insulin resistance in that insulin is being secreted, but the insulin can't communicate with its target cells, the hypothalamus. As a result, the regulation of appetite by insulin is disrupted, which can lead to overeating and weight gain. Thankfully, there are other signals to the hypothalamus, such as leptin, PYY, GLP-1, etc., which contribute to the suppression of hunger.

As can be seen, insulin is vital to health and metabolic processes. The goal of a diet should not be to eliminate insulin. Insulin is not the villain many fad diets make it out to be. While there are some conditions where insulin levels should be monitored, no diet should have as its goal the elimination of insulin. Eating a balanced, varied diet in moderation will fuel the body in such a way that insulin functions normally. This should be the goal of diets designed for weight loss.

Glucagon's Role in the Fasted State

Glucagon is a hormone secreted from the alpha cells of the pancreas. It is stimulated when macronutrients are unavailable, and the body starts crying out for storage molecules to be broken down to supply fuel. We refer to this as the "fasting metabolic state." While insulin secretion is stimulated by several very diverse signals, the secretion of glucagon appears to be dependent on blood glucose and insulin levels. As discussed earlier, when macronutrients are present in the blood, beta cells in the pancreas secrete insulin so that those macronutrients can be removed from the blood and stored for times of fasting. We also discussed how insulin stimulates the hypothalamus to tell the brain that macronutrients are high, and we don't need to eat more. What we haven't discussed yet is one additional, very important action that insulin does.

Insulin inhibits the release of glucagon from alpha cells. So, when macronutrients aren't available, insulin is NOT secreted. Insulin stops glucagon secretion.

Just like insulin, glucagon communicates with its target cell by binding to a receptor (like a docking station) on the surface of the target cell. It sends instructions (signals) into the cell that tell the cellular machinery what needs to be done.

Logically, one might think that glucagon would target cells that store macronutrients during the "fed" state. That is partially true. Glucagon communicates with adipose tissue and activates an enzyme inside the cell to cut the fatty acids from the stored triglycerides. These fatty acids are released into the blood so that muscle can use them to produce energy and the liver can use them to make ketone bodies that all cells can use for energy. Glucagon communicates with liver cells and activates the production of "new" glucose by a series of already discussed reactions called gluconeogenesis. In addition, glucagon activates the production of "old" glucose that was stored in the liver cells as glycogen. Remember glucose linked together into large strands and stored is called glycogen. The "old" and "new" glucose are released into the blood so that all cells can use it for energy or to create Krebs cycles that allow cells to use ketone bodies for energy.

Unlike insulin, glucagon does NOT communicate with skeletal muscle. It is not the responsibility of the skeletal muscle to supply the body with glucose; the liver does that. In contrast, the glycogen stored in skeletal muscle only supplies fuel to that skeletal muscle. In other words, skeletal muscle uses its glycogen to produce glucose for itself or to create Krebs cycles that allow the muscle cell to use fatty acids and ketone bodies for energy.

Here is a summary of what glucagon tells liver and adipose cells to do:

	Liver	Adipose
Gluconeogenesis	Increase	
Glycogen breakdown	Increase	
Triglyceride breakdown		Increase

Satiety

A specialized part of the brain, the hypothalamus, is a central component regarding relay signals that communicate energy needs. It integrates these signals and regulates hunger and satiety.

Hunger is a physiological response to the lack of food.

Satiety is more what you think—it is more emotional. In other words, satiation is the feeling of being satisfied after eating. While it can be both emotional and physical, it is mostly emotional.

The hypothalamus is an essential component in regulating **energy homeostasis.** It actually has a **hunger center.** In studies, when this part of the brain is overstimulated, it causes hyperphagia or an abnormally high intake of food. Destruction of this area causes a lack of desire for food and progressive weight loss, muscle weakness, and decreased metabolism.

The hypothalamus also has a **satiety center.** This center is believed to give a sense of nutritional satisfaction that inhibits the feeding center. Again, in research, electrical stimulation of this center causes complete satiety: subjects refuse to eat, even in the presence of appetizing food.

Together, these hypothalamic centers coordinate the processes that control eating behavior and the perception of satiety. But there is more to these centers; these feeding and satiety centers have a high density of receptors for neurotransmitters and hormones that help control feeding behavior. These neurotransmitters and hormones are the communication signals among the stomach, intestines, adipose tissue, pancreas, and the feeding and satiety centers in the hypothalamus. Some signals increase and some decrease feeding.

Substances That Increase Satiety (decrease hunger)

We have already discussed how insulin communicates with the hypothalamus to decrease hunger. It is important to discuss additional substances that decrease hunger.

Leptin is a hormone, made by fat cells, that decreases appetite. Also known as OB protein, leptin opposes adiponectin (which tells the body to store fat). Leptin levels rise as body fat increases and decrease when adipocytes (fat cells) shrink during weight loss. It has been shown that higher serum leptin levels correlate with greater feelings of fullness. The effect of leptin depends on how much of it is present. Since it is produced in the adipocytes, the amount produced is proportional to the number of adipocytes. Research findings suggest that leptin is a satiety hormone that reduces appetite. Obese individuals tend to have high levels of leptin, but these levels do not appear to be effective at reducing calorie intake or increasing energy expenditure. So why are people who have lots of fat and produce lots of leptin still fat? It is thought that weight gain in obese individuals is most likely due to other factors overriding this feedback regulation. When either the leptin hormone is not produced or the receptor for leptin is not recognizing the leptin, early onset of severe obesity in humans and animals can occur. Interestingly, leptin levels also appear to promote fertility when the body has the required amount of fat stores necessary for reproduction.

Cholecystokinin (CCK) is a hormone produced principally by the small intestine in response to the presence of fats and proteins. It causes contractions of the gallbladder to release bile and pancreatic digestive enzymes. It also activates receptors in nerves in the duodenum, which send messages to the brain to decrease feeding. Its effect is short-lived; therefore, it functions to mainly prevent overeating but doesn't necessarily play a role in the frequency of meals or total calories consumed.

Peptide Tyrosine Tyrosine (PYY) is a (36-amino-acid) peptide released by cells in the gastrointestinal tract in response to feeding. It travels through the circulation, with blood concentrations peaking 1–2 hours after eating a meal. The levels of PYY seem to be influenced by the number of calories consumed as well as the composition of the food a person is eating. Dietary fat seems to stimulate the highest levels. PYY appears to reduce appetite.

There are more neurotransmitters and hormones that influence the feeding and satiety centers in the hypothalamus. This complex area of feeding and satiety continues to be studied, and our understanding continues to evolve. The complexity of the body's mechanisms may explain why people respond differently to various stimuli and situations. It is not simple, clear, or fully understood.

There are also various oral factors related to feeding: chewing, salivating, swallowing, and tasting. All these sensations seem to measure the food as it passes through the mouth, which then contribute to inhibiting the feeding center. Animals with an esophageal fistula (hole in their esophagus), when fed, even though the food immediately exited the body through the fistula, stopped eating after a reasonable amount of food was tasted, chewed, and swallowed. However, they only seemed satisfied for 20–40 minutes, which is less than when gastrointestinal mechanisms are enacted. Regardless, it appears that chewing, tasting, and swallowing all help to satisfy hunger to some degree.

When the gastrointestinal tract becomes distended (especially the stomach and duodenum), "stretch inhibitory signals" are sent to suppress the feeding center. Fullness is the stretching sensation felt in the stomach.

It has been noted that decreased blood concentrations of glucose, amino acids, and lipids can also stimulate hunger. There are more studies on animals, but people are not animals. People can ignore the satiety center, especially when influenced by emotions, situations, socializing, and advertising. These environmental cues can influence consumption. Many of us can testify to eating when we are not hungry. And sure enough, research reports that even when there is no nutritional need and feelings of satiation exist, people still eat.

Substances That Decrease Satiety (increase hunger)

Just as there are substances that decrease hunger, there are substances released in the body that increase hunger.

Ghrelin is a hormone released mainly from the stomach cells when the stomach is empty (when your stomach growls, it releases "growlin"). It can stimulate the desire to eat. Blood levels of ghrelin change throughout the day, rising shortly before a meal and dropping afterward. More ghrelin is produced during sleep, during fasting, and between meals. Studies have shown that the composition of meals plays a role too. Proteins are the best suppressor of ghrelin. This is true in terms of depth and duration of suppression. In other words, proteins are satisfying. Eating carbohydrates results in a strong ghrelin suppression at first, but ghrelin levels rebound shortly thereafter. Fats are least effective in suppressing ghrelin release. It appears lean individuals have higher levels of ghrelin than those with more body fat. This seems particularly true in the morning. It should not come as a surprise that ghrelin levels increase when someone follows a low-calorie diet. Some theorize that the release of ghrelin requires feedback after eating, which might be regulated by insulin levels.

Adiponectin is a hormone produced by adipose tissue in the body. One function of adiponectin is to tell the body to store fat. Adiponectin levels increase as body fat decreases, a signal that the body might be starting a period of starvation. When adiponectin levels increase, the body becomes more sensitive to insulin. In other words, adiponectin, which wants the body to store fat (for survival purposes), enhances the body's ability to store fat. Higher adiponectin levels are associated with decreased risks of chronic health conditions that affect quality of life.

Cortisol is a glucocorticoid, a kind of steroid hormone produced from cholesterol in the two adrenal glands. During periods of stress, the hypothalamus instructs the adrenal glands to release epinephrine (adrenaline), norepinephrine, and cortisol into the bloodstream. This speeds up heart rate, respiration, blood pressure, and metabolism. Cortisol also stimulates the breakdown of muscle proteins to provide amino acids that can then be used for energy and to make glucose, so the body has fuel during fight or flight. This is done through liver gluconeogenesis. Epinephrine breaks down glycogen (stored carbohydrates in the liver and muscle) into glucose. Both hormones increase the breakdown of fat in the adipose to produce circulating free fatty acids. The extra glucose and fatty acids are made ready so they can be used by the body as fuel in times of stress. Prolonged stress, however, disrupts the digestive system, causing the stomach to produce excessive amounts of digestive acids. Irritable bowel syndrome can develop when the smooth muscular contractions that move food along the large intestine become spastic. Stress has also been related to increased flare-ups of ulcerative colitis. Such conditions serve to lower the basal metabolic rate (BMR).

Feast or Famine Concept

"That is why, for Christ's sake, I delight in weaknesses, in insults, in hardships, in persecutions, in difficulties. For when I am weak, then I am strong." —2 Corinthians 12:10

In the same way that it may not make sense to the unbeliever when a Christian says, "When I am weak, then I am strong," it may also seem confusing to an uninformed dieter if one were to say, "When you want to lose weight, you must eat." But that is exactly what the Feast or Famine Concept is about. This is an important foundational concept in understanding how metabolism changes in response to food. Simply stated, when we fuel our body with the calories and needed nutrients, it runs efficiently. When we starve our body of what it needs, it slows down in an attempt to conserve energy.

We were all born with a God-given metabolic range. Our genes help determine this range. We have a high end and we have a low end. We can fall anywhere within our God-given range. While we cannot change our metabolic range, we can influence where we fall within our range. A simple way of sharing this concept with your patients and clients is to say, "When we consistently fuel our bodies with what they need, they are happy, content and don't feel threatened. They have no fear or worry. They trust they will be fueled when hungry or in need because the track record has been one of assurance and constant fulfillment of needs. When we fuel our bodies this way, our metabolic rate rises to the top of our God-given range. This is the best place to be to lose weight. We want our bodies to burn calories freely."

On the other hand, when we starve our bodies or inconsistently provide adequate calories and nutrients, our bodies sense a famine beginning. To survive, the body's basal metabolism slows down to conserve calories because it is uncertain when or if there will be another meal. When signs of a famine continue, our bodies permanently conserve energy in order to survive. This is how our bodies respond when we go on crash diets and very low-calorie diets. People who eat very few calories daily experience a depression in metabolic rate and a stripping of lean tissue, both of which make losing weight very difficult. Additionally, they can experience dehydration, fatigue, and micronutrient deficiencies, which further make burning calories or exercise difficult.

Many fad diets put our bodies into the famine mode. Let's consider this concept more deeply and examine some metabolic specifics.

Concerns of Fasting, Starving, and Very Low-calorie Diets

"So after they had fasted and prayed, they placed their hands on them and sent them off." —Acts 13:3

Numerous biblical passages reference fasting. That must mean fasting is good, right? Well, no human, with certainty, can knowingly and honestly speak to the notion of fasting as it pertains to God's purposes. If God lays it on the hearts of his followers to fast and pray…so be it. But fasting for God's purposes is vastly different from fasting with the intent of gaining a sleeker, sexier body. Thus, we will only address fasting as it pertains to dieting.

There are many reasons why diets such as the ketogenic diet, Atkins, intermittent fasting, and very low-calorie diets all rank low when comprehensive criteria are used to assess them. They are all difficult to maintain over the long haul, and because they are so strict, they all lend themselves to "cheating." Nearly everyone who goes on one of these diets will struggle to sustain it. But cheating on some diets can actually be dangerous, as we will discuss. Let's begin by addressing fasting's effects on macronutrients and micronutrients.

Macronutrients

Blood glucose levels are maintained in the initial 10–14 hours of fasting by glucagon stimulation. Glucagon signals the liver to release glucose from glycogen stores and to produce "new" glucose from molecules in the blood (lactate and amino acids) through the process of gluconeogenesis. In addition, glucagon signals the adipose to cleave stored triglycerides into glycerol and fatty acids. The glycerol can be used by gluconeogenesis to make "new" glucose, and the fatty acids can be used by muscle for energy and by the liver to make ketone bodies for other cells to use for energy. Within the first 24 to 72 hours of fasting, blood glucose levels start declining, as liver glycogen stores begin to be depleted. After 72 hours of starvation, when glycogen stores in the liver have been depleted and the liver tries to maintain blood glucose level solely by gluconeogenesis, undesirable metabolic and hormonal changes occur so the body can conserve blood glucose.

This 72-hour timeframe assumes that glycogen stores are at maximum capacity at the outset. If glycogen stores have not been replenished between times of fasting, then they will be depleted earlier. Diets that promote short periods of intermittent fasting can jeopardize glycogen stores. Even if short periods of fasting involve excess carbohydrates, an insulin spike in response to the carbohydrates may actually result in fat storage, not complete restoration of glycogen stores.

Remember, the body loves to store calories as fat. This is because fat is stored without water (which means no water weight) and more calories are produced per gram of fat (compared to carbohydrates and proteins.)

Glucose from gluconeogenesis is predominantly made from the glycerol released from triglycerides (adipose fat) and from amino acids released from muscle as its protein breaks down (stripping of lean tissue). As the body begins to switch from using carbohydrate as its main fuel to using fat and protein as the main source of energy, the basal metabolic rate decreases by as much as 20–25% to conserve fuel resources.

During prolonged fasting, hormonal and metabolic changes occur to prevent protein muscle breakdown. Muscles decrease their use of ketone bodies and use fatty acids as the main energy source, which results in an increase of ketones in the blood. Non-muscle cells, like the brain, don't have the enzymes to use fatty acids for energy and must use ketone bodies or glucose. So, as muscles use fewer ketone bodies, there are more ketone bodies available for non-muscle cells to use instead of the depleting blood glucose. In fact, the brain switches from glucose to ketone bodies as its main energy source. Since less blood glucose is being used by the body for energy, the liver decreases its rate of gluconeogenesis to preserve muscle protein (decreasing the stripping of lean tissue). As one can see, restricting carbohydrates to a level that completely depletes liver glycogen results in a global change in metabolism, which creates an unhealthy condition and is not usually helpful for long-term weight management.

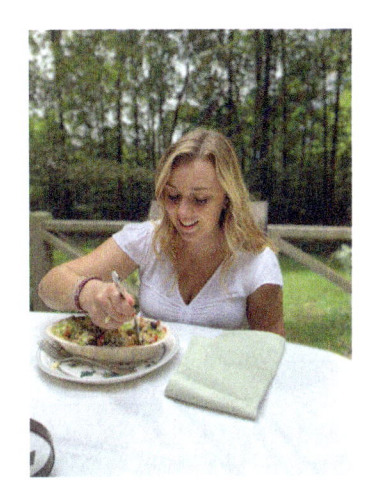

Gluconeogenesis uses energy to produce glucose from lactate, amino acids, and glycerol. In other words, it isn't "free" to switch from one molecule to another—it takes energy. For example, physician, biochemist and Nobel Prize winner Hans Krebs calculated that the synthesis of 1 g of glucose by gluconeogenesis using only amino acids as ingredients would require the breakdown of 1.75 g of protein. Clearly, such a contribution to gluconeogenesis cannot be sustained for long without a decline in muscle function. When someone is on a low-carbohydrate diet doesn't replenish glycogen supplies, or is on a diet that is too low in calories to replenish their body's stored resources, the body must use muscle protein to maintain blood glucose levels, which it does at an astonishing rate. In addition, studies consistently find that calorie restriction results in an energy expenditure drop greater than would be expected from the combined loss of lean tissue and fat mass. In addition to serious health consequences, this loss of metabolically active lean tissue reduces one's ability to maintain weight, to lose weight, and to perform athletically. Significant fat and muscle wasting are not the only results of these adaptations; there can be a total body depletion of electrolytes, magnesium, potassium, and phosphate. Let's take a look at these micronutrients.

Micronutrients (Vitamins and Minerals)

During starvation and fasting, even though serum concentrations of minerals (including phosphate) may remain normal, several intracellular minerals become depleted. This occurs because these minerals are mainly in the intracellular compartment, which contracts during starvation. These minerals are stored within the body over extended periods of time. They are slowly depleted due to their use for energy and a broad range of cellular functions in the body. In contrast to macronutrients—proteins, carbs, and fats—these micronutrients cannot be restored quickly. Their depletion and restoration are more complex than that of macronutrients. Let's consider the importance of these nutrients.

> **Phosphorus:** Phosphorus is essential for all intracellular processes, as well as the structural integrity of cell membranes. It is used to control enzymes and is required for storing energy. It regulates oxygen delivery to tissues and plays an important role in the acid-base buffer system. In refeeding syndrome, which is discussed later in this section, depletion of phosphorus occurs. Insulin surges cause an increased uptake and use of phosphate in the cells. This uptake can lead to a deficit in both intracellular (within the cells) and extracellular (outside the cells) phosphorus. In this scenario, even small decreases in serum (blood) phosphorus can lead to dysfunction of the cellular processes that affect every physiological system.

> **Potassium:** Potassium can be depleted in undernutrition. Upon refeeding, as a direct result of insulin secretion, potassium is taken up into cells, resulting in severe hypokalemia (low blood potassium). This causes dysfunction of the electrochemical membrane, which can result in arrhythmias (irregular heartbeat) and cardiac arrest.

> **Magnesium:** Magnesium is a predominantly intracellular cation that is important in most enzyme systems, including the production of energy. Magnesium is required for the structural integrity of DNA and RNA. It also influences membrane integrity. Deficiency can lead to cardiac dysfunction, weakness, depression, and high blood pressure, as well as problems in nerve stimulation.

The dangers don't end with these considerations about a few key minerals. A sudden swing from fat and protein breakdown to carbohydrate metabolism, as discussed earlier, stimulates a sudden and disastrous increase in insulin production. This increased insulin secretion results in intracellular shifts of glucose with necessary cellular uptakes of phosphate, magnesium, and potassium.

Sodium and Water

As yet another potential shift, changes in carbohydrate metabolism have a profound effect on sodium and water balance. The introduction of carbohydrate into the body after avoiding carbohydrates due to diet restrictions leads to a rapid decrease in kidney excretion of sodium and water. If fluid replacement is then instituted in an attempt to maintain a normal urine output, fluid overload may occur, potentially leading to congestive heart failure, pulmonary edema (fluid buildup in the lungs), and cardiac arrhythmia (irregular heartbeat).

Safe, healthy diets—diets that lead to success—are ones that can be maintained over the long term. Diets that are too low in calories and diets that eliminate certain food groups or certain macronutrients, like carbohydrates, cannot be sustained. Sometimes this is simply due to the nature of fad diets. Innocent dieters who go "on" strange new diets that claim to be miracle cures set themselves up for failure, and also danger. Most dieters do not understand the risks of "cheating" or going "off" the diet suddenly just because they want to take a break from it.

Vitamin deficiency is a concern any time a diet imposes restrictions. In the scenarios discussed above, of major concern is the B vitamin thiamine, an essential coenzyme in carbohydrate metabolism. Its deficiency can result in many problems, including coma.

Practical Aspects of Fasting

Many types of approaches to fasting exist. Many diets recommend various forms of fasting, detoxing, and intermittent fasting. These types of diets are very difficult to study for a number of reasons. There are many different time frames and variations, which makes it hard to categorize them in a study. Some diets are very difficult to maintain, which means most studies can only be conducted in the short term.

Difficulty in managing hunger sensations is one of the main reasons for unsuccessful dieting. Researchers advise caution in the interpretation of studies that rely on 24-hour dietary recalls and self-reported food diaries. This is because people tend to underestimate the amount of food eaten. There are many factors, such as intelligence, age, mood, attention, and outside stimulus, that can affect a person's ability to accurately remember and report past dietary intake. No well-constructed, repeatable, long-term studies have been conducted in this area of fasting effects Let's look at some of these fasting diets and "try" to attach definitions.

- Alternate day fasting (ADF) is not consuming food or consuming only a minimal number of calories at 1 meal for 2 or 3 days per week. These days should not be consecutive. During the remaining days of the week, food may be consumed as desired.

- Time restricted feeding (TRF) involves restricting the eating window to 4–13 hours.

- Intermittent energy restriction (IER) is defined broadly as at least 1 day per week with food consumption no more than 25% of a person's need.

- Continuous energy restriction (CER) is reducing daily calorie intake by 25% for a prolonged period without "cheat" days.

Proposed Benefits of Intermittent Fasting

Increasing interest in intermittent fasting may be attributable to news of rodent studies that reported benefits ranging from improved glycemic control, reduced cardiovascular disease risk, higher cancer survival rates, and increased lifespan. In these studies, rodents experienced these benefits without significant weight loss. It has been theorized that this result may be due to fasting's ability to increase stress resistance while reducing oxidative and cellular damage.

Based on animal models that include severe energy restriction plus high fat consumption, lean mass appeared to be preserved with greater reductions in fat mass. These models also observed a browning of white adipose tissue and greater insulin sensitivity, lower leptin and higher ghrelin levels, and lower levels of oxidative stress and inflammation. While this is interesting, people are not animals; and the leap that people can experience these benefits cannot be made. Furthermore, because it is unethical to impose this type of situation on human subjects, research in this area on humans is very limited.

The important topics to examine in this area are hunger, weight loss, lean tissue preservation, and metabolism. First, research shows that when someone is hungry, their ability to maintain their current diet decreases. In other words, they cannot sustain and will cheat or go "off" the diet. If they are able to maintain a fast, what happens to their lean tissue? Do they lose weight and if they do, is it fat weight? What happens to their metabolic rate? These and many other questions have yet to be answered with certainty.

Thus far, there do not appear to be any significant benefits consistently identified with intermittent fasting. Although many benefits have been suggested, intermittent fasting does not provide *more* benefits than balanced eating plans designed for weight loss. For example, between those engaged in intermittent energy restriction (IER) and those falling into the continuously energy restricted (CER) groups:

- No statistically significant differences in waist circumference reduction are observed
- No statistically significant differences in weight lost
- No statistically significant effect on serum triglyceride levels
- No statistically significant difference in LDL, total cholesterol, or blood pressure
- No statistically significant differences in blood glucose levels or HbA1c

While results are not consistent across all studies, most indicate that those engaging in time-oriented food restriction experience:

- Decreased sleep
- Decreased activity
- Decrease in both fat weight and lean tissue (nearly equal amounts); less lean tissue is lost when regimens provide adequate protein
- Decreased leptin (hormone that tells us we are full)
- Decreased testosterone in male athletes
- Decreased growth factors in male athletes
- Decreased adiponectin (low levels are associated with inflammation, lipid abnormalities, insulin resistance, and increased risk of diabetes, coronary heart disease, and cancer)
- Increased hunger that did not decline (even with healthy-weight individuals)
- Lower feelings of fullness on the first day of fasting that increased, possibly due to stomach's shrinking. When they did eat, they felt fuller as time on the diet continued.
- Higher drop-out rates from studies
- Decreased capacity to perform endurance exercise
- Decrease in fasting insulin
- When a high-fat diet (45% of calories from fat) was consumed on alternate day energy restriction, the high-fat group showed decreased brachial artery flow-mediated dilation, which may increase risk of hypertension and atherosclerosis. For those consuming balanced eating plans designed for weight loss:
- Lean body mass appears to be better preserved with more frequent meals when trying to lose weight.

Overall, the research does not show that intermittent fasting is better, promotes more fat loss, speeds up metabolism, or protects lean body mass more than balanced eating designed for weight loss. Intermittent fasting does increase hunger and may set the stage for developing a poor relationship with food. It is safe to say, the dieting method best tolerated long-term will be personal.

Refeeding Syndrome

Chronic fasting in association with low-calorie and very low-carbohydrate diets could lead to a phenomenon referred to as refeeding syndrome.

Refeeding syndrome was first described and reported during World War II when prisoners of war experienced cardiac failure after being rescued and fed food. Refeeding syndrome can be fatal. It is defined by dramatic shifts in fluids and electrolytes that may occur in people who have undergone prolonged fasting or low-energy diets, people who were morbidly obese and experienced a quick and profound weight loss, people medically classified as undergoing high stress and have been unfed for >7 days, long-term users of diuretics, and people with uncontrolled diabetes. Unfortunately, many fad diets promote fasting, low carbohydrate consumption, and dangerously low calorie consumption, which can potentially create a situation leading to refeeding syndrome.

Fasting, low-carbohydrate, and very low-calorie diets will deplete glucose and glycogen stores. In general, signs of refeeding syndrome are most apparent when carbohydrates are reintroduced. In other words, once the diet is "over" and carbohydrates are reintroduced, the release of insulin will suppress gluconeogenesis (the making of glucose from non-carbohydrate sources). Without careful monitoring and without being supervised by a physician, a number of problems can occur. The sudden introduction of carbohydrates can reduce water and sodium excretion. This can result in the expansion of the extracellular fluid compartment and fluid overload. It can also result in excess fluid in the lungs, making it difficult to breathe and creating an inefficiency within the heart, so it is no longer able to maintain efficient circulation.

Excessive intake of carbohydrates too soon may occur and lead to hyperglycemia. This, in turn, can lead to excessive urination, dehydration, metabolic acidosis, and ketoacidosis. Ketoacidosis is a dangerous situation in which the blood becomes acidic from excessive ketone production. It is also likely that overconsumption of glucose could lead to fat storage, especially since the metabolic rate has slowed during the fast. Other concerns may include fatty liver and increased carbon dioxide production, which can result in respiratory failure.

It's important to realize that micronutrients are used for more than just production of energy for the cell. These micronutrients are used for molecules that create cell structure, for enzyme function and regulation, and maintenance of cellular information. Therefore, when the cell becomes depleted of these micronutrients, it is depleted of important cellular functions. Just like depleting these important micronutrients occurs slowly, their restoration must be slow. Think about it: the body has to re-create many of the molecules and enzymes whose very structure and function depend on these micronutrients. It is not just a matter of calories; it is actually cell structure and function that have to be restored. Therefore, one can see that there can be detrimental effects at the cellular level when restoring these micronutrients too quickly.

Dangers of Naively Experimenting

People can be chronically undernourished for many reasons, including cancer, surgery, inflammatory bowel disease, and anorexia nervosa, just to name a few. People who have undergone prolonged fasting or low-energy diets, or people who were morbidly obese and experienced weight loss too quickly, or anyone with negligible food intake for more than five days are all at risk of developing refeeding problems. This is concerning because many diets on the market advertise a "do it alone" approach and don't require or mention the supervision of a physician. As you can see, many serious consequences can occur within the body when dieters haphazardly experiment with diets. In addition to the clear life-threatening dangers that can be experienced as a result of various diets, many people ascribe misery, short-term success, and long-term term failure at weight loss to these approaches.

> **RECAP:** Even in laboratory environments where external factors are controlled, the effects of short-term fasting are not clear. The benefits of intermittent fasting do not appear to outweigh the benefits of balanced eating designed to promote weight loss. Intermittent fasting may promote the development of unhealthy eating and a harmful relationship with food.

Thermic Effect of Food (TEF)

It doesn't matter if we are talking about carbohydrates, proteins, or fats, the body uses energy to extract calories from food. Calories are expended in the process of digestion, absorption, and metabolizing food (processing the macronutrients). The burning of these calories is called the thermic effect of food (TEF). Immediately after eating and for several hours after a meal, energy expenditure increases to provide ATP for peristalsis, digestion, and absorption and transportation of nutrients. The type of nutrient consumed will influence the TEF. For example: a meal high in protein has the highest thermic effect (20–30%); in other words, in a pure protein meal, 20–30% of the calories consumed would be "wasted" or used in metabolism. Carbohydrates have a greater TEF (5–10%) than fat, which is (0–3%). The energy cost to convert dietary fat into stored fat is minimal. Fat is the most efficient energy source. In a balanced diet, if excess fat is eaten, most of it can be stored.

Is this a reason to eat all protein and avoid fat, especially if it's going to be easily stored? No, all three macronutrients are important and essential. Eating too much protein means more nitrogen waste is produced and must be eliminated. A high-protein diet means more water must be consumed. In this scenario, insufficient consumption of water means an increased risk of dehydration and kidney stones.

Ketosis and the Ketogenic Approach to Weight Loss

Ketogenic diets are very popular, but they are quite complicated because there are many forms of ketogenic diets and they involve a lot of biochemistry. There are even many terms defining different kinds of ketosis. The definitions used are not all universally standardized or accepted. Below are a few examples of the different terms used:

- *Physiological ketosis* (sometimes called nutritional ketosis) occurs when carbohydrate resources are so low that the liver must produce glucose to support blood glucose levels. At the same time, the liver is converting fats (those stored in adipose tissue and dietary fats) into ketones that can be burned for energy by the body. This creates a metabolic state where the body is fueled mainly by ketones, instead of carbohydrates (glucose). This is what normally happens in an overnight fast, or on a very low-carbohydrate diet, or any time glucose levels drop, even on a normal diet.

- *Pathological diabetic ketosis* (aka diabetic ketoacidosis) occurs in a diabetic condition when either insulin is not secreted in sufficient amounts or target cells are resistant to the insulin signal. In either case, insulin is not signaling a "fed" metabolic state and not inhibiting glucagon secretion. Therefore, the body believes it is in a "fasted" state because of the glucagon signal. As a result, fatty acids are released from the adipose and broken down in the liver through beta-oxidation. Since glucagon is also signaling the liver to make glucose through gluconeogenesis, the product of beta-oxidation builds up and makes ketone bodies. Ketone bodies are released in the blood and are used for energy, since there is plenty of glucose for cells to use. However, without the signal of insulin in a diabetic condition, glucagon continues to signal a "fasted" state, even though the body appears to be in a fed state! So, the liver continues producing glucose through gluconeogenesis and ketone bodies from the beta-oxidation of fatty acids being released from the adipose. More ketone bodies are produced than the body can use for energy and so the ketone bodies build up in the blood. Because ketone bodies are acidic, their excess makes the blood treacherously acidic.

- *Deep ketosis* – This term is not clearly defined. It hints at the concept that since ketosis means burning fat, burning more fat must be better. Deep ketosis is a condition of constant circulating ketone bodies. To achieve this, carbohydrates are reduced to 5–10% and fats are increased to 70–80% of total calories. Since carbohydrate consumption is insufficient to maintain blood glucose levels, glucagon signals the liver to make glucose through gluconeogenesis and signals the adipose to release fatty acids. Ketone bodies are produced in the liver, since the liver is breaking down the fatty acids from adipose tissue while also making glucose. At this point, it appears to be just like physiological ketosis, which occurs in a fasting state. However, because of the consumption of high levels of fat, we would consider the dieter to be in a fed state, due to the presence of calories available from the fat being consumed. So, one can see that, ironically, deep ketosis is "fasting" in a "fed" state, due to limited carbohydrates. The key is keeping blood glucose low, which decreases insulin secretion and increases glucagon secretion. When not monitored by a health care professional, the risk of ketoacidosis may increase.

- *Ketone spectrum* refers to ketone levels or the levels of ketosis.

It seems as if new terms are continually invented to describe different stages, meanings, and purposes of ketosis. More terms are most likely on the horizon.

Definition of a Ketone Body

So, what is a ketone body? A ketone body is simply 2 acetyl CoA molecules put together, a 4-carbon fatty acid.

The Occurrence of Ketosis

After several days of fasting or a severe decrease in carbohydrates (usually below 20 g per day, but sometimes as high as 50 g per day), the body's glucose reserves (which are mostly stored as glycogen) get used up. This insufficiency does not allow for the production of **oxaloacetate,** which is required for two important things: normal fat oxidation in the Krebs cycle and supplying glucose to the central nervous system (CNS). The CNS cannot use fatty acids as an energy source because they do not cross the blood-brain barrier, and the brain does not have the enzymes to break down fat. Glucose is the preferred fuel for the brain. After 3–4 days of fasting or a very low-carbohydrate diet, the CNS needs an additional energy source to supplement for the glucose that is no longer there. This supplemental energy source is ketone bodies, which are derived from the breakdown of fat to acetyl CoA by the liver.

When there is underutilization of ketone bodies, they accumulate above normal levels, leading to higher levels in the blood (ketonemia) and in the urine (ketonuria). One characteristic often experienced is a "sweet breath odor." It is caused by acetone, which is a byproduct of ketone bodies and must be eliminated mainly through the lungs.

The Prevalence of the Keto Diet

Everybody and their brother is posting on the internet in all kinds of forums about ketosis, which is very typical when exciting new diet ideas emerge, even though they may not have been thoroughly researched. I recently read a blog on the topic of the keto diet. The only statements in the blog with any value were "I'm no doctor" and "the jury is out on whether or not being in a long-term state of ketosis is a good or healthy thing." It is unwise to "experiment" with diets without the supervision of a physician. However, posts like this blog are as equally accessible to the public as results from legitimate, reliable scientific studies. Blog-type posts are more inviting, though, because they are easier to read and understand, and they contain no big words.

A Look at the Macronutrients in the Keto Diet

A reduction of calories regardless of the source of those calories will result in weight loss. Interestingly, a number of studies demonstrate that subjects who follow a low-carbohydrate diet lose more weight during the first 3–6 months when compared with those following continuous balanced diets. But this is not surprising. The first stage of weight loss is water loss, and the first stage of weight loss in a ketogenic diet is loss of glycogen stores, along with the water that is stored with it. Of course, there is going to be more weight lost! But this does not mean more fat is lost.

On average, during the first phase of a low-carbohydrate diet, the body uses 60–65 g of glucose per day. About 16% of this glucose is obtained from the glycerol part of the triglyceride molecule. The remaining 85% must be derived from proteins of either dietary or tissue origin. So here is the concern: if a dieter is not consuming adequate protein, they must derive the remaining protein by stripping lean tissue, which lowers their metabolic rate. Another concern is when a dieter cheats on a ketogenic diet. Cheating keeps that dieter restarting this first phase over and over again. Each time this is done, they suppress their metabolic rate further and further. One of the primary goals of losing weight is gaining health benefits and having more energy. When carbohydrates are eliminated from the diet, all the health benefits of fiber go away, along with all the benefits of the good microbiome in the gut.

Keto Compliance

Most dieters do not behave like robots following a mechanical protocol, but are instead humans with all kinds of flaws, temptations, sins, and skill levels; thus, attempting to follow this diet sets them up for eventual failure. Even if a dieter could behave as though they were a robot while on this diet, most cannot stay on the diet without eventual health complications due to dietary deficiencies, since this diet eliminates many food groups and violates the rules of variety and balance. Since dieters on the keto diet do not learn how to eat a healthy, balanced diet, they will surely return to their old way of eating (but now with a lower metabolic rate) and regain the lost weight, which is what a number of studies have found.

Keto Controversy

To be fair, ketogenic diets have been found to have a positive impact on women with polycystic ovarian syndrome (PCOS). But a review of the literature shows limitations due to small sample sizes. If someone could follow a strict keto diet, there is some evidence that indicates no changes in resting energy expenditure after being on a ketogenic diet However, because this diet is so difficult to stay on, most studies are not long term. A review of the literature indicates that the low sustainability of a ketogenic diet can lead to weight regain. To date, there is no long-term sufficient data collected on the risks and benefits for cardiovascular health. Moreover, some practitioners have found the ketogenic diet to be helpful in limited circumstances involving type 2 diabetics. In these cases the diet lasts no more than 6 months and close monitoring by a physician and dietitian are required for the patient's safety.

We really don't have any solid long-term knowledge yet. Researchers theorize that ketones may have an appetite-suppressing effect, but no mechanism has been established. Some studies have found an increase in leptin levels, while others have found a decrease in leptin levels. Some studies have found an increase in ghrelin, while others have found a decrease in ghrelin.

Some theorize there is a reduction in appetite due to a higher satiety effect of proteins, along with the higher thermic effect of protein. But a ketogenic diet is high in fat, not protein.

Checking for Ketones

Other concerns about the ketogenic diet include the testing method. Ketone strips typically expire within 3–6 months after opening. Dieters are instructed to check urine ketones by daily adhering to specific times, especially during the first few weeks of starting the diet. In the beginning, the body of new dieters can't use ketones efficiently for energy, and thus many ketones are urinated out. As the body adjusts or, as some say, "you get deeper into ketosis," the body begins to adapt to using ketones for fuel. After adapting, months later, a ketone strip may indicate that urine contains only trace amounts of ketones, if any. Thus, people may need to test using blood ketone strips instead of urine for accurate results. These are more costly, and it is reasonable to ask if dieters really want to pay the higher price of the blood strips and prick their finger every time they want to measure ketone levels. It is also possible to measure ketones on the breath. The breath method is not as accurate as blood ketone tests, but it is better than urine test strips. This breath-testing option requires the purchase of a breathalyzer, with an up-front cost of about $150. Effectively following a ketone diet and adhering to all the requirements can be quite time-consuming and costly.

Ketone Spectrum

Some researchers think the keto diet is the silver bullet, suggesting it is good for disease prevention, weight loss, and exercise performance.

This is a small portion of the scientific community. I once attended a Sports Nutrition conference where researchers had a debate about which was the best way to fuel athletes: high fat – low carbohydrate (the keto diet) or high carbohydrates – moderate fat (Academy of Nutrition and Dietetics recommendations). Hands down, the winner was the high carbohydrate

– moderate fat team, who presented mounds of research spanning decades. The researchers touting the keto diet were citing their own research and citing studies with very small sample sizes. One study had a sample size of one subject!

This spectrum outlines nutritional ketosis as starting at molecular concentration levels of 0.5 mmol/L. Nutritional ketosis is considered "light" through 1.0 mmol/L, then becomes "optimal" in the 1.0 mmol/L through 3.0 mmol/L range. If you look at the spectrum there are lots of numbers. So, how does a dieter know for which level to aim? The few researchers supporting this idea state that dieters seeking to lose weight should try to achieve "optimal ketosis," which is when ketone levels are between 1.0 mmol/L and 3.0 mmol/L. Because supporters of this approach indicate the keto diet is the silver bullet, recommendations in the 3.0 mmol/L–5.0 mmol/L range are also made for people seeking therapeutic benefits for medical conditions such as epilepsy, cancer, or endocrine and metabolic disorders. Recommendations in the 3.0 mmol/L–8.0 mmol/L range are made for people who are fasting or eating a much higher fat-to-protein ratio. No recommendation is given for a "normal" healthy dieter who wants to eat healthy.

Certainly, people seeking therapeutic benefits for medical conditions such as epilepsy, cancer, or endocrine and metabolic disorders should regularly be working with their primary care providers and following their advice. It is not wise to experiment with a keto diet for self-treatment. People who are fasting cannot sustain this status for very long without stripping lean tissue or struggling with electrolyte imbalances, which can lead to death. This diet is not safe to "experiment" with for a while then go "off." The dieter cannot cheat! And yet, the majority of people going on this fad diet don't understand this or the dangers associated with it.

Deep Ketosis

If "ketosis" is fasting in a fed state, we might consider "deep ketosis" as starving in a fed state. Recall that in the starvation state, the brain changes its use of glucose and ketone bodies. It conserves blood glucose levels by only using enough glucose to support the burning of ketone bodies. There are not enough carbohydrates for any cell to use glucose for energy. Cells survive by using only enough glucose to support the burning of ketone bodies. In other words, the cells are starving for carbohydrates, and if carbohydrate resources drop even lower, cells will be forced to use even more lean tissue for the burning of ketone bodies. Eating lard all day long (which is unsustainable in itself) would not supply the body with sufficient carbohydrates or proteins to support cellular function. Remember, there are essential amino acids that must be obtained through the diet. Ketone bodies cannot be used for energy independent of carbohydrates and proteins. In other words, without adequate dietary carbohydrates and proteins, ketone bodies produced from dietary fat cannot produce sufficient energy to sustain cellular energy and function. This jeopardizes the dieter's life. The dieter can't produce all the molecules necessary for basic cellular functions, like necessary enzymes, hormones, neurotransmitters, and any other cellular molecule that requires amino acids for their synthesis. This deep ketosis perspective of "more is always better" is not applicable to health.

Ketones and Exercise

Every expert recommends exercise to maintain health and to assist in weight loss. Most dieters trying the ketogenic diet are doing so in an attempt to lose weight. Other keto followers think it will improve their physical performance. So, how does exercise affect ketone levels? The answer to this question will vary. It will depend on the individual and their diet composition, as well as their activities. This answer alone is concerning if a dieter is not under a physician's supervision.

Keto and High-Intensity Exercise

Exercise can be either aerobic or anaerobic. In general, anaerobic exercise consists of high-intensity activities for a short period of time. Can you sprint at maximum speed for a mile? No—nobody can. Sprinting is high-intensity. It is an all-out burst of energy. That is what anaerobic activity requires. People can only do it for short periods at a time and then they must slow down. Depending on the strength of their lungs and their legs, they will not be able to continue for very long. During an all-out burst, breathing changes and we don't get an adequate, steady flow of oxygen for the high demand of output taking place. Hence anaerobic!

Sprinting, or any type of short-term, high-intensity exercise, draws on glycogen stores and protein resources within the skeletal muscle. This is because this type of exercise is anaerobic, involving only glycolysis, which can occur without oxygen.

Remember, Krebs cycles must have oxygen to run. To be used for energy, fats and ketone bodies require Krebs cycles. Therefore, it is logical to see that fats and ketone bodies cannot be burned in anaerobic metabolism or during short-term high-intensity exercise. In other words, a keto diet does not support short-term high-intensity exercise. Keto dieters have no more of an advantage in short-term, high-intensity activities than if they were consuming a regular diet.

Keto and Low-Intensity Exercise

What about the keto diet and low-intensity activities? These are activities that are more aerobic in nature, such as jogging or long-distance running, where the majority of the activity allows for the steady flow of oxygen from the lungs to the muscles through steady breathing. In these situations, there are sufficient Krebs cycles to support burning ketone bodies for fuel. However, carbohydrate intake would have to be monitored so that glycogen stores can be maintained in order to support the burning of ketone bodies throughout the activity. If adequate carbohydrates are not consumed to maintain glycogen stores, then lean tissue must be stripped to support the burning of ketone bodies for fuel. This is less than ideal for athletes whose main focus is usually centered on performance.

Keto and Individual Needs

There are levels of the keto diet that might be able to support these low-intensity activities. The danger is when carbohydrate intake drops below the level needed to support the athlete's activity. Every athlete needs to know the level of glycogen stores needed to support their activity in order to optimally perform. If an athlete requires a high level of dietary carbohydrates to optimally perform, he or she can't do the keto diet. Most athletes don't know the answer to this without professional help. Moreover, this can only be determined through trial and error.

Maintaining Keto

The ketogenic diet is a high-fat (60 to 80% of calories), moderate-protein (10 to 15% of calories), and low-carbohydrate diet (less than 10% of your total daily calories). In the keto diet, carbohydrates and proteins are replaced by fat. In other words, carbohydrates and proteins are being reduced to critical levels. Therefore, without constant monitoring and professional guidance, dieters risk reducing carbohydrates and proteins below adequate levels, as we have discussed previously. Unfortunately, most people on the keto diet get no professional advice.

Even when professional advice is sought, health professionals are not all in agreement regarding the ketogenic diet. Many health care providers agree that the body is in desperation mode on keto; and without an adequate supply of carbohydrates, the body will start breaking down the amino acids in proteins to make necessary glucose. In other words, the body will strip lean tissue. Additionally, the high fat content in the diet, especially the saturated fats, can raise blood cholesterol levels and contribute to the development of chronic diseases like cardiovascular disease. Without the fiber from adequate whole grains and fruits, constipation and other digestive issues can occur. Even more importantly, without fiber, a healthy gut microbiome can't be supported.

Some researchers want to get out the message, "A keto diet isn't an approach that can safely be tried several days during the week but then discarded every weekend." Researchers and health care providers working in this field also indicate that staying in true ketosis is exceptionally challenging for adults. Some researchers have declared that getting an adult body into ketosis is difficult and point out this fact as the basis for why the keto diet is used as a treatment for epilepsy in children or infants but not adults. These same researchers are quick to point out that science has yet to identify the reasons for those differences, but they are adamant that it's so hard to get adults into deep ketosis that nearly all nutritionists won't suggest it as a therapy.

Others in favor of the keto diet indicate that the liver converts protein into glucose when we need more glucose. While this is true, this is only when protein is being consumed and not in between meals (fasting). Blood glucose in times of fasting is supplied from glycogen stores and stripping lean tissue.

Final Keto Thoughts

At this point, the only clear adult population that may benefit from a ketogenic diet, while under the care of a physician, is type-2 diabetics. In fact, very reputable clinics prescribe keto-like diets for patients whose risk of dying is higher if they keep the fat on their body than if they go on the keto diet. But of course, they closely monitor their patients. However, they also realize it is not a forever diet solution.

It is important to note there are no long-term studies on the ketogenic diet. We need to be very cautious with this diet. It is not clear what health effects this approach may have on the body if sustained. Renowned researchers and nutritionists still have many serious questions regarding the use of this diet, as well as its outcomes. The scientific community needs more answers before the ketogenic diet is promoted to the general public for weight loss. But this keto fad has taken off and now there is even a ketone spectrum. Think about it—now, the keto fad is even more confusing because it has become a "spectrum." In other words, it's all over the place, which makes it difficult for dieters to know what is healthy for them as an individual and what part of the spectrum might be dangerous for them. Maybe we need to recall 1 Timothy 4:4, which states, "For everything created by God is good, and nothing is to be rejected if it is received with thanksgiving."

Acid-Base Balance (Homeostasis) and Buffering

"My people have committed two sins: They have forsaken me, the spring of living water, and have dug their own cisterns, broken cisterns that cannot hold water." —Jeremiah 2:13

Homeostasis is when the body is in stable equilibrium so it can function properly. In homeostasis, the cells that make up the body's tissues and organs have the stability to function as God designed them to function—efficiently and in balance. Acid-base **homeostasis** and regulation of body pH are critically important for the body to function normally. In fact, everything about the human body revolves around buffering and homeostasis. Major problems including coma and death can occur as a result of the body not being in homeostasis.

Water is the most abundant liquid or component in our body. Therefore, when we talk about acids and bases and buffering, all this discussion about life is built around water. This fact makes it very clear why Jesus stated,

"Whoever believes in me, as Scripture has said, rivers of living water will flow from within them." —John 7:38

Many scientists refer to water as the "universal solvent" because many things can dissolve in water. It is also called "the solvent of life," perhaps because dissolved in the water of living beings are many other substances that support our lives. These substances interact with one another in the body's watery (aqueous) environment. These substances are changed as a result of their interactions, and that is a good thing because these interactions or reactions keep our bodies alive and functioning. We categorize substances in our body's aqueous solution as either acidic or basic.

- **Acids** are substances in the body that donate a proton to water, or to the aqueous environment.

- **Bases,** on the other hand, are substances that receive or accept a proton from water. Sometimes the word "alkaline" is used. It means basic.

- **Protons** are subatomic particles that go back and forth between body substances as they act acidic or basic.

In chemistry, the term "pH" is used to specify on a scale how acidic or basic a water-based solution is. pH is the unit used to measure acidity and alkalinity. It is the ratio of acids to bases. The pH of a substance ranges from 1(very acidic) to 14 (very basic).

- Acidic solutions have a lower pH.
- Basic solutions have a higher pH.

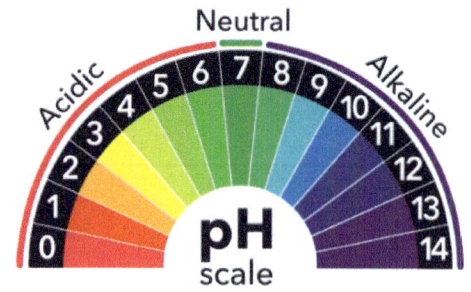

Even the pH scale is built on the assumption that you have an aqueous solution. As you can see from the graphic, the middle of the scale is neutral with a measurement of 7. Water has a pH of 7. That neutral pH changes as substances are dissolved in the water. If a substance is put in water and the pH of the water goes down, that substance must have donated a proton to the water, and it is referred to as acidic. If another substance is put into the water and the pH of the water goes up, that substance must have accepted a proton from water, and it is referred to as basic. That means in the body, homeostasis and harmony occur when the body is at a pH near 7. So, whenever we talk about pH in the body, we are always referring to what is happening to the water in our body liquids. Blood has a normal pH range of 7.35 to 7.45; it is naturally slightly alkaline or basic. But notice how close it is to 7!

Just as we discussed above, if we add something to our bodies, it is going to change the pH of the new, combined solution. If we add a substance to our body and the pH of our blood goes down, that substance must have donated a proton to the water in our body and the item added is acidic. For example, our liver produces ketone bodies during fasting times. When those ketone bodies are released into the blood, the pH of our blood decreases, because ketone bodies are acidic. Normally, the ketone bodies would be taken in by other cells and used for energy, but if the ketone bodies accumulate in the blood, the pH of our blood could continue to be acidic and create a condition called ketoacidosis.

The opposite is also true. If we add a substance to our body and the pH of our blood goes up, that substance must have accepted a proton from the water in our body and the item added is basic.

Since harmony, safety, and efficient functioning occur in the body when the pH is around 7, the body works endlessly to keep the pH of bodily fluid around 7 for us to stay alive and safe. How does the body keep the pH around 7? It does this through **buffer systems.** A buffer system is like an acrobat walking on the tightrope, where leaning to the left is acidic and leaning to the right is basic. Most acrobats hold a long pole in their hands to help them balance. The acrobat will adjust the position of the pole in their hands in order to maintain balance. If they are leaning left, they adjust the pole to the right; if they are leaning to the right, they will adjust the pole to the left. Maintaining balance is very important. Buffer systems in our bodies work to bring neutrality and balance back to the body when too much acid or base is introduced. The body's natural buffering systems keep it at healthy pH levels.

Let's look at this complex process of buffering a little more closely. In order to buffer or balance a change in pH, we must be able to "neutralize" any acid or base added to the solution. This "neutralization" cancels the change in the pH that would have occurred when the acid or base was added. In other words, we must be able to react with both sides. Furthermore, for a buffer system to react with both acids and bases that are added, it must have both acidic and basic characteristics. How can this be? To do this, the buffer system must be "weakly" acidic. Let's explain.

When an acid donates its proton, it becomes what is called its "conjugate base" because the "conjugate" base could accept the proton back and remake the original acid. In other words, an acid can go back and forth between its acid and "conjugate" base forms, as it donates and receives protons. If the acid is strong, it only wants to donate protons and become their "conjugate" base forms. So, if an acid is too strong, it can only react with a base but not another acid. Equally, if a base is too strong, it can only react with an acid but not another base.

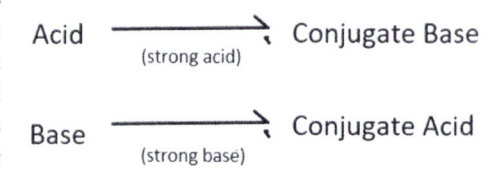

In contrast, if an acid is weak, only some of its molecules donate protons and become their "conjugate" base forms. So, the weak acid has some molecules in the acid form and some of its molecules in the "conjugate" base form. Thus, it can react with both an acid and a base that might be added to the solution! The same can be said for a weak base.

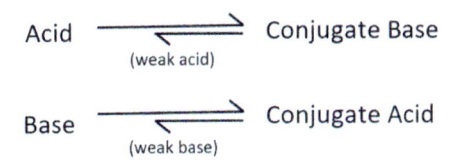

$$\text{Acid} \rightleftharpoons \text{Conjugate Base}$$
$$\text{(weak acid)}$$

$$\text{Base} \rightleftharpoons \text{Conjugate Acid}$$
$$\text{(weak base)}$$

To maximize buffering capacity, we want equal amounts of the acid form and the "conjugate" base form in the solution. Each acid has a different pH where it measures 50/50, depending on how strong an acid it is. For example, lactic acid is 50/50 at pH 3.85, but carbonic acid is 50/50 at 6.36. So, lactic acid is a stronger acid than carbonic acid. However, the closer the 50/50 pH is to water's pH, the more that acid can be a buffer for our body.

To examine this, we need to look at pKa values. Simply put, pKa is the term for the pH measure when an acid is 50/50. The pKa value (50/50 pH) indicates the strength of an acid. A lower pKa value indicates a stronger acid because it is 50/50 at a lower pH.

To help explain this, let's look at lactic acid for a moment, which has pKa value of 3.85. If we wanted to "buffer" our blood at pH 3.85, our bodies could have lots of lactic acid in the blood. But we need our blood to be close to pH 7. So we can't use lactic acid to buffer in the human body because it's trying to buffer at 3.85. When our muscles produce lactic acid during exercise, the lactic acid decreases the blood pH and we can get cramps if it accumulates in our muscles. In contrast, carboxylic acid has a pKa value of 6.36, and dihydrogen phosphate has a pKa value of 7.21. Thus, these two substances are great buffers for the body, because their pKa values are quite close to 7. Carbonic acid is created when the carbon dioxide that our cells produce dissolves in water (just like a carbonated beverage). Carbonic acid degrades quickly to carbon dioxide when blood enters the lungs. In addition, the pancreas makes and secretes sodium bicarbonate (the "conjugate" base of carbonic acid) to neutralize substances coming out of the very acidic stomach environment. Our kidneys will reabsorb bicarbonate in order to increase the pH. If necessary, we can urinate bicarbonate out of the body. One can see that carbonic acid, along with its "conjugate" base, sodium bicarbonate, is a buffer system that can be controlled by many parts of our body.

Dihydrogen phosphate is our dominant buffer inside our cells. Remember that we use ATP for energy. In ATP synthesis, ATP is made by putting a phosphate on an ADP. So, it is vital that we have a lot of phosphate in the body, since it is used to make the central currency of our cells, and it is the main buffering system inside our cells.

Thus, we can see that the body has natural buffering systems to maintain healthy pH levels. These include chemical buffers, the lungs, and the kidneys. In healthy individuals, these are powerful and successful systems. Chemical buffers are present in all bodily fluids, both in and out of the cell. They keep blood and other bodily fluids within the healthy, narrow pH range we require. In the body, these chemical buffering systems are very effective at preventing radical pH changes in liquids inside and outside our cells. While it only takes seconds for the chemical buffers in the blood to make adjustments to pH, lungs can adjust blood pH in minutes by exhaling CO_2. The most powerful of the buffering systems is the renal system. It can adjust blood pH by conserving bicarbonate and excreting hydrogen ions, but this process can take 12 to 24 hours before it begins to react.

Amino Acids as Buffers

Amino acids are often said to be great buffers in the body. Let's look at them. Every amino acid is made up of four parts: an amine group (which is basic), an acid group (which is acidic), a hydrogen group, and a side chain which is sometimes called an R group. Please note that amino acids have two competing parts. They have an acidic group and a basic group. Amino acids have both an acid and a base on their structure, so when they are added to water, they can "react" as both an acid and a base. This can get confusing, so let's look at the pKa values of these acid and basic groups. The pKa of the acid group of amino acids ranges from 1.7 to 2.4. That means that the acid groups would be good buffers for low pH, but they are too acidic to be buffers at physiological pH of 7. If this were true, then lactic acid (pKa = 3.85) released from the muscle would be considered a buffer. The pKa of the amino group of amino acids ranges from 8.8 to 10.8. Their pKa values are closer to 7 than the acid groups, but the amino groups of amino acids would still be better buffers for high pH. That means that the amino and acid groups of amino acids don't contribute significantly to the buffering of the blood.

One thing to consider is the balance of the acid group and the basic amine group when an amino acid is added to water (blood). The acid group reacts with water like an acid and the amine group reacts with water like a base. Although the acid group is slightly more acidic than the amine group is basic, their acid/base reactions cancel each other so that the amino acids don't make a considerable change in the pH like a molecule with a single acid or basic group (e.g., lactic acid or a ketone body).

What about the side chains of amino acids? Some of the groups attached to the amino acids have pKa values, meaning that they are acidic or basic and could be buffers. Only one of the amino acids has a side chain close to physiological pH, histidine. The pKa of histidine is 6.0. So, histidine can buffer blood pH much like carbonic acid, but it doesn't have the flexibility of carbonic acid (lungs breathing out CO2, pancreas producing sodium bicarbonate, and kidneys reabsorbing sodium bicarbonate).

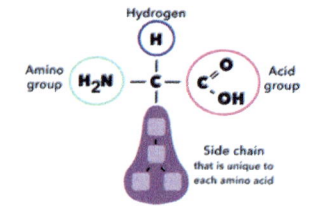

Amino acids are the building blocks of proteins, but we must be careful not to say that proteins are good buffers. When amino acids are joined together to make a protein, both the acid group and the amine group are used in making the peptide bond that joins the two amino acids. Those two competing acid/base parts actually create the peptide bond that holds proteins together. Thus, the acid and amine groups cancel each other and don't contribute to the buffering capacity of the blood. In a protein, the acidic and amine groups don't even exist to contribute to the buffering capacity of the blood. But, just like we saw with the amino acids, the histidine side groups in the protein have a pKa close to 7 so that they can contribute to the buffering capacity of the blood. Overall, proteins can provide a small buffering capacity, but not like bicarbonate and phosphate, which dominate intracellular buffering.

Obviously, these systems are very complex, and we have only hit upon the highlights, but it is important to note that good nutrition plays a role in keeping the body healthy enough to function properly. For example, proteins play many important roles in the body. Ideally it is clear why it is not possible to change blood pH by eating certain foods.

Food has to go through the acidic environment of the stomach, and the pancreas adjusts the amount of bicarbonate secreted to match that of the acidity of the chyme coming out of the stomach. So, acidity and basicity of the food is accounted for in the GI tract. The change in blood pH in response to the diet is small. Buffer systems kick in and make necessary adjustments. Thus, an alkaline diet, or any diet that results in the production of an acid or base, cannot raise blood pH to make it less acidic. All foods consumed simply allow the buffering systems to work. Blood acidity has to do with life and death and nothing with weight loss. Blood pH can change through disease and defects in metabolism. For example, there can be an overproduction of acidic ketone bodies in diabetes, an overproduction of pyruvic or lactic acid if there is a defect in pyruvate dehydrogenase enzyme, and the overconsumption of alcohol doesn't allow lactic acid to be cleared by the liver. Foods eaten have little impact on body pH levels. And thank goodness, with the self-control most of us exhibit, if it were up to us (and our choices), we would be in big trouble!

Glossary of Terms for Metabolism

Acetyl CoA – a molecule that participates in many reactions in protein, carbohydrate, and lipid metabolism. It delivers the acetyl group to the Krebs cycle for energy production. The liver can put 2 acetyl CoA's together, which makes a ketone body.

Adiponectin – a hormone produced by adipose tissue that tells the body to store fat. Adiponectin levels increase as body fat decreases, a signal that the body might be starting a period of starvation. When adiponectin levels increase, the body becomes more sensitive to insulin.

Adipose Tissue – fat tissue; it is made up of adipocytes.

Alpha Cells – a type of cell in the pancreas. Their main function is to produce and secrete glucagon, which functions in direct opposition to insulin. Alpha cells increase the amount of blood glucose in the blood by releasing stored fuel from the liver.

Aerobic – means "with oxygen" (air). Aerobic processes occur when oxygen is present.

Amino Acids – often called the building blocks of protein because they come together to make proteins, amino acids are made when proteins are broken down. They are categorized as essential amino acids and non-essential amino acids. Essential amino acids cannot be made by the body and must be eaten in the diet. Non-essential amino acids can be made by the body if all the essential amino acids have been eaten in adequate amounts.

Anaerobic – means "without oxygen" (air). Anaerobic processes occur when oxygen is not present or available.

ATP – stands for adenosine triphosphate, the only energy source all body cells can directly use. The energy (calories) in all food, whether from carbohydrates, proteins, or fats, must first be converted into ATP in order for the body to use that energy.

Basal Metabolic Rate (BMR) – the number of calories our bodies burn just to keep us alive (heart pumping, liver processing, lungs breathing, and brain functioning). Determining someone's exact BMR can be difficult without sophisticated equipment. As a result, formulas have been developed that take into account a person's age, sex, height, and weight to predict their BMR.

Beta Cells – a type of cell in the pancreas. Their main function is to produce and secrete insulin, the hormone responsible for regulating blood glucose levels.

Beta-Oxidation – the process of metabolizing fatty acids, i.e., the process by which fatty acid molecules are broken down. Free fatty acids in the body have an even number of carbon atoms ranging from 2 to 26. The metabolism of free fatty acids, regardless of chain length, is essentially the same. Free fatty acid is cleaved into separate two-carbon units of acetic acid. In essence, beta oxidation is the process of converting free fatty acids to multiple acetyl CoA molecules. As in glucose metabolism, one of the byproducts is ATP. However, the complete combustion of a free fatty acid requires more oxygen because it has many more carbon atoms than glucose. This means more energy (calories) is produced than by burning glucose.

Buffer Systems – these natural systems within the body bring neutrality and balance back to the body when too much acid or base is introduced. They keep the body at healthy pH levels.

Calories – the units most often used in nutrition to measure energy. It is the unit used to measure the energy released from food when it is digested by the human body. We use the word "calorie" in this text because it is the term with which most dieters are familiar. The "calorie" we refer to in food is actually kilocalorie, but most people are not familiar with that term. One kilocalorie is the same as one Calorie (note the uppercase C). Scientifically speaking, one kilocalorie is actually 1,000 calories or 1 kcal.

Carbon Skeletons – in the context of weight loss, this term refers to the "remaining parts" or the "the leftover parts" of an amino acid after the nitrogen has been removed from the molecule. These carbon "remains" can be used in the Krebs cycle to generate energy or to synthesize other biological molecules the cells need. Because the carbon skeletons can be used for energy, amino acids provide calories just like carbohydrates and fats.

Conjugate Base – when an acid donates its proton in water, it becomes what is called its "conjugate base," which can accept the proton back from water and remake the original acid. In other words, an acid can go back and forth between its acid and "conjugate" base forms, as it donates and receives protons.

Cortisol – a hormone produced from cholesterol. During periods of stress, the hypothalamus directs the release of numerous hormones including cortisol into the bloodstream. These speed up heart rate, respiration, blood pressure, and metabolism. Cortisol also stimulates the breakdown of muscle proteins to provide amino acids that can be used for energy and to make glucose, so the body has fuel during fight or flight. This is done through liver gluconeogenesis.

Deamination – the removal of the amine group from amino acids. Protein contains nitrogen. When protein is broken down to be used as fuel, the nitrogen group is cleaved off, ammonia is formed, converted to urea, and eventually urinated out of the body. This process is called deamination.

Energy Homeostasis – involves many processes that work in the body to balance food intake and energy expenditure. There can be negative or positive regulation of energy homeostasis. Another way to view this is there can be a positive energy balance when someone eats more than their body burns. In this case, the person would gain weight. There can also be a negative energy balance, where someone burns more calories than they consume. In this case, the person would lose weight.

Fatty Acids – made up of long chains of carbon and hydrogen atoms. If all the carbon atoms are linked by single bonds, the fatty acid is called saturated. If at least one pair of carbon atoms is linked by double bonds, the fatty acid is called unsaturated. These bonds help determine the name and classification of the fatty acid. Fatty acids provide 9 calories per gram and are burned aerobically in the body.

Gastric Inhibitory Peptide (GIP) – a hormone released from the mucosal epithelial cells in the first part of the small intestine when macronutrients are present in the intestine; the hormone stimulates pancreatic cells to secrete insulin.

Ghrelin – a hormone released mainly from the stomach cells when the stomach is empty. It can stimulate the desire to eat.

Glucagon – a hormone produced by the alpha cells in the pancreas. It signals the liver to break down stored glycogen and turn it back into glucose.

Glucagon-like Peptide-1 (GLP-1) – a hormone released from the gut when macronutrients are present in the intestine; it stimulates pancreatic cells to secrete insulin.

Gluconeogenesis – making glucose from something other than carbohydrate. Krebs calculated that the synthesis of 1 g of glucose by gluconeogenesis using only amino acids as precursors would require the breakdown of 1.75 g of protein. Contributions from amino acids to gluconeogenesis cannot be sustained for long without a loss of functional capacity.

Glucose – the most abundant simple sugar and primary energy source for the body.

Glycerol – triglycerides are made up of 3 free fatty acids and 1 molecule of glycerol. When fats are burned for fuel, the fatty acids are treated or metabolized differently than the glycerol molecule. Glycerol gets treated more like a carbohydrate and can make glucose. The fatty acids cannot make glucose.

Glycogen – stored glucose. It can be stored in the liver and in skeletal muscles. If it is stored in the liver, it can be released into the blood stream and used by any tissue. If it is stored in skeletal muscle, it can only be used by that muscle.

Glycogenesis – the process by which glycogen is synthesized from glucose, then stored in the liver or muscle.

Glycogenolysis – the process of breaking down glycogen into glucose. Glycogen is basically carbohydrates stored for later use. When "the time arrives" for it to be broken down, made into glucose, and used by the body, it goes through the process of glycogenolysis.

Glycolysis – the process of breaking down the carbohydrates (glucose) we eat and turning them into energy. It may be anaerobic or aerobic.

Hunger – discomfort, pain, or weakness caused by lack of food. It is usually accompanied by a strong desire to eat. It is a physiological response to the lack of food.

Hunger Center – a part of the brain also referred to as the lateral hypothalamus. It serves as a feeding center. When stimulated, the desire to eat emerges.

Hypothalamus – the region of the brain that controls food intake and body weight. It is an essential component in the regulatory system for energy balance.

Insulin – hormone secreted from the beta cells of the pancreas that stimulates the uptake of glucose from the blood and enables the glucose to enter cells so the glucose can be used as fuel.

Insulin-dependent Cells – store excess glucose as glycogen (skeletal muscle and liver) or convert glucose to fat (liver) to be stored in the adipose after a meal.

Ketone Bodies – created in the liver from fatty acids during times of fasting. As the liver produces glucose from amino acids and lactate, fatty acids are oxidized to acetyl CoA. Two acetyl CoA molecules are then linked together and are released for cells to use for energy. Ketone body production occurs during periods of low food intake, carbohydrate-restrictive diets, starvation, or prolonged intense exercise and fasting.

Ketosis – a condition of elevated ketone body concentrations in the blood. This accompanies low-calorie, low-carbohydrate diets and uncontrolled type-1 diabetes. Mild increase in ketone bodies is expected during fat loss and usually poses no harm.

Ketoacidosis – abnormally elevated ketone body concentrations in the blood that can occur in low-calorie, low-carbohydrate diets and uncontrolled type-1 diabetes. When the body has high levels of blood glucose but can't store (or "clear") that glucose for storage as glycogen (uncontrolled type-1 diabetes) or glycogen stores are depleted (low-calorie, low-carbohydrate diets), fatty acids are released from the adipose in response to this "fasting" metabolic state so that fats can be used for energy. However, fats can only be used for energy if there are sufficient Krebs cycles being produced from glycogen stores or protein degradation. Since glycogen stores are depleted in both of these "fasting" metabolic states, the ketone bodies that are being produced from fatty acids in the liver can't be used for energy and they build up in the body.

Krebs Cycle (aka the citric acid cycle and TCA cycle) – a series of chemical reactions that release energy from carbohydrates, fats, and proteins and other sources of calories such as alcohol and ketone bodies. The ultimate end product is energy (ATP) to fuel the body so it can do work.

Lactate (aka lactic acid) – lactate is basically lactic acid minus one proton. To be an acid, technically, a substance must be able to donate a hydrogen ion. If lactic acid donates its proton, it becomes lactate. When glucose is processed anaerobically (without oxygen), lactate is formed. In other words, the anaerobic breakdown of glucose results in lactic acid or lactate.

Lactic Acid System – a metabolic system the body uses if there is insufficient oxygen to support the Krebs cycle or if the cell doesn't have mitochondria, like red blood cells.

Lean Tissue – in the context of weight loss, lean tissue is considered the most metabolically active tissue. It consists of skeletal muscles, bones, organs, connective tissue, blood cells, and other tissues that are not adipose tissue.

Leptin – a hormone made by fat cells that decreases appetite.

Lipoproteins – because triglycerides and cholesterol are not water-soluble, they cannot move freely in the blood from one tissue to another. They are transported in phospholipid monolayer modules. They are hydrophobic in the middle (where the triglycerides and cholesterol are stored) and hydrophilic on the outside (where they interact with water).

Metabolism – the burning of calories in the body to do work such as disassembling food and converting it to energy to run cellular processes. All chemical reactions in the body are collectively called "metabolism."

Mitochondria (aka mitochondrion, which is just one—it's the single version. "Mitochondria" is used when talking about more than one mitochondrion). – often called "the powerhouse of the cell" because they take in nutrients from food, break it down, and turn it into energy for the body to use. They are found in the cytoplasm of most cells (but not in red blood cells.) While mitochondria are the location for ATP production, ATP can only be made if there is sufficient oxygen. A lack of or insufficient oxygen means the fuel can't be turned into ATP in the mitochondria. Proteins and fats need oxygen in order to be turned into ATP. Carbohydrates are more versatile and can make ATP with or without oxygen.

OAA (oxaloacetate) –the molecule made with pyruvate from glycolysis to create Krebs cycles.

Parasympathetic Nervous System – one of the two divisions of the autonomic nervous system; the other is the sympathetic nervous system. Signals from the brain are thought to include "rest and digest" and "feed and breed" activities, which occur when the body is at rest, such as after eating. Its action is complementary to that of the sympathetic nervous system. It increases insulin secretion.

Phospholipids – cell membranes are made up of a phospholipid bilayer. Triglycerides have 3 fatty acids attached to a glycerol, but phospholipids have 2 fatty acids and a phosphate group attached to a glycerol molecule. This allows them to have a hydrophobic end (fatty acids) to interact with nonpolar "stuff" like triglycerides, and a hydrophilic end (the phosphate) to interact with hydrophilic "stuff" like water. Thus, they can surround triglycerides and cholesterol and create a lipoprotein and carry that nonpolar "stuff" from one tissue to another tissue to use the triglycerides for energy or for storage. A cell needs to have a phospholipid bilayer so that it can surround polar "stuff" (things dissolved in water). The hydrophilic phosphate groups are on the outside of the bilayer, and the fatty acids are on the inside. This configuration allows a cell to have an inside of water and hydrophilic "stuff" in the water. Your diet contains cells (animal and/or plant), and those cells have phospholipid bilayer membranes. Therefore, a portion of the fat content of your diet is phospholipids.

Pyruvate (aka Pyruvic Acid) – the difference between pyruvic acid and pyruvate is one hydrogen atom. In the human body we find pyruvate, so that is the term we will use. Pyruvate is an important intermediate step in using glucose and fat to make energy. The presence or absence of oxygen determines the fate of the end product of pyruvic acid. In the presence of oxygen, pyruvic acid is converted into acetyl coenzyme A, which joins with acetic acid to make acetyl CoA, which then can enter the Krebs cycle. But oxygen must be present if this reaction is to continue in the mitochondria. If it doesn't go into the mitochondria, it must be converted to lactic acid.

Satiated – satisfied by one's fullness.

Satiety – the feeling of being sufficiently satisfied.

Satiety Center – a part of the brain also known as the ventromedial nuclei. This center is believed to give a sense of nutritional satisfaction. Electrical stimulation of this center causes complete satiety.

Skeletal Muscles – the three types of muscles are skeletal, cardiac, and smooth. Each has a unique structure and role in the body. Skeletal muscles move bones and other structures. Cardiac muscles contract the heart. Smooth muscle tissue forms organs. When we talk about stripping lean tissue, generally it is skeletal muscle that is stripped. If starvation continues, eventually smooth muscle will be stripped, and organ function will fail.

Sympathetic Nervous System – one of two divisions of the autonomic nervous system; the other is the parasympathetic nervous system. Signals from the brain are thought to be "fight or flight" signals. These signals decrease insulin secretion in order for more fuel molecules to be available for the fight or flight activities, like running.

Triglycerides – the major type of fat or lipid in our blood and in food. Triglycerides are stored in various places in the body, but especially in adipose cells, which are designed to store excess fat. Hormones release triglycerides for energy between meals. Triglycerides are made up of one glycerol molecule and three fatty acids.

Urea – a waste product that is the major organic component of human urine. It is naturally produced when nitrogen is removed by the liver in the process of breaking down amino acids. The liver converts ammonia to this non-toxic compound, which can then be safely transported in the blood to the kidneys and eliminated in urine.

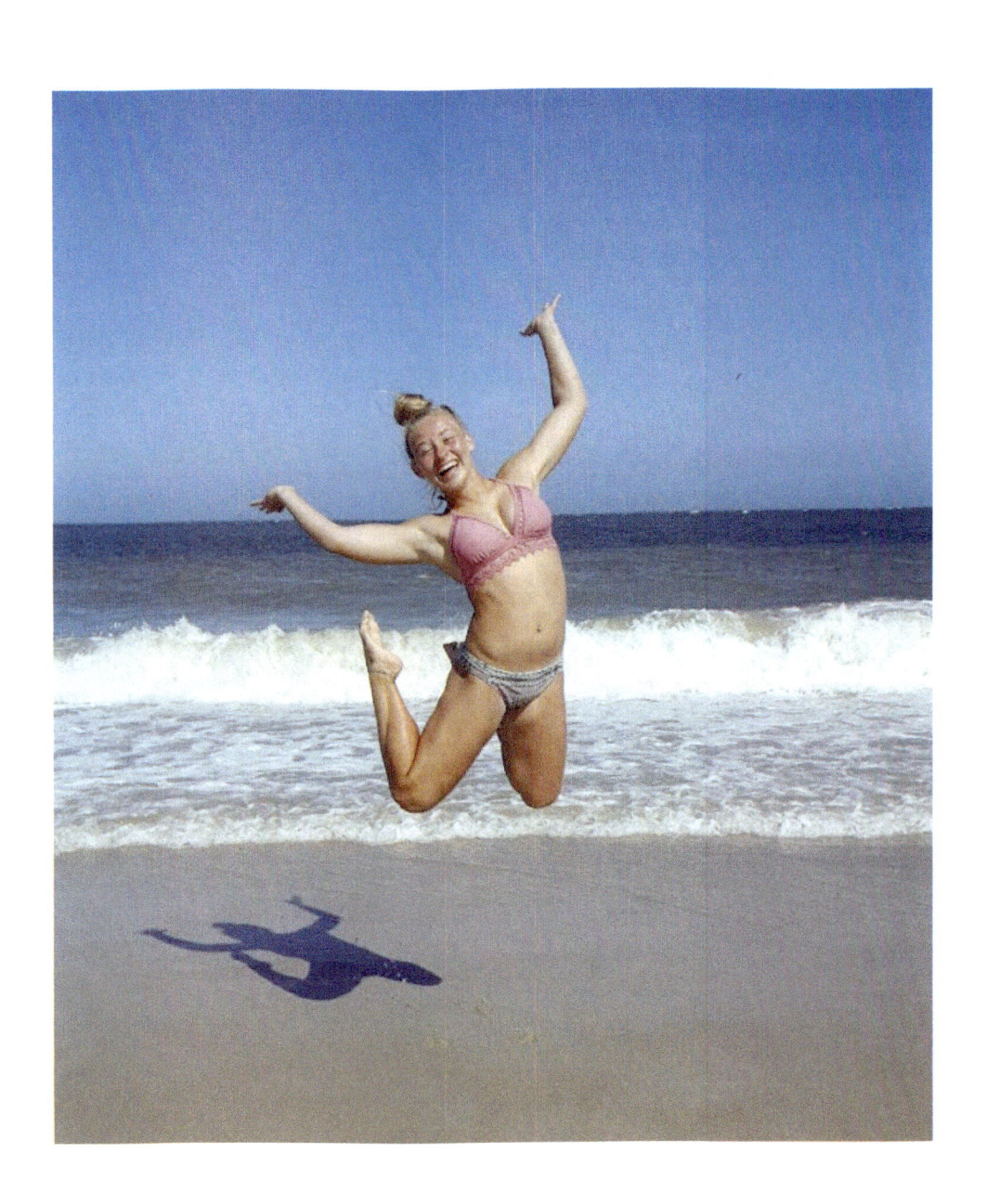

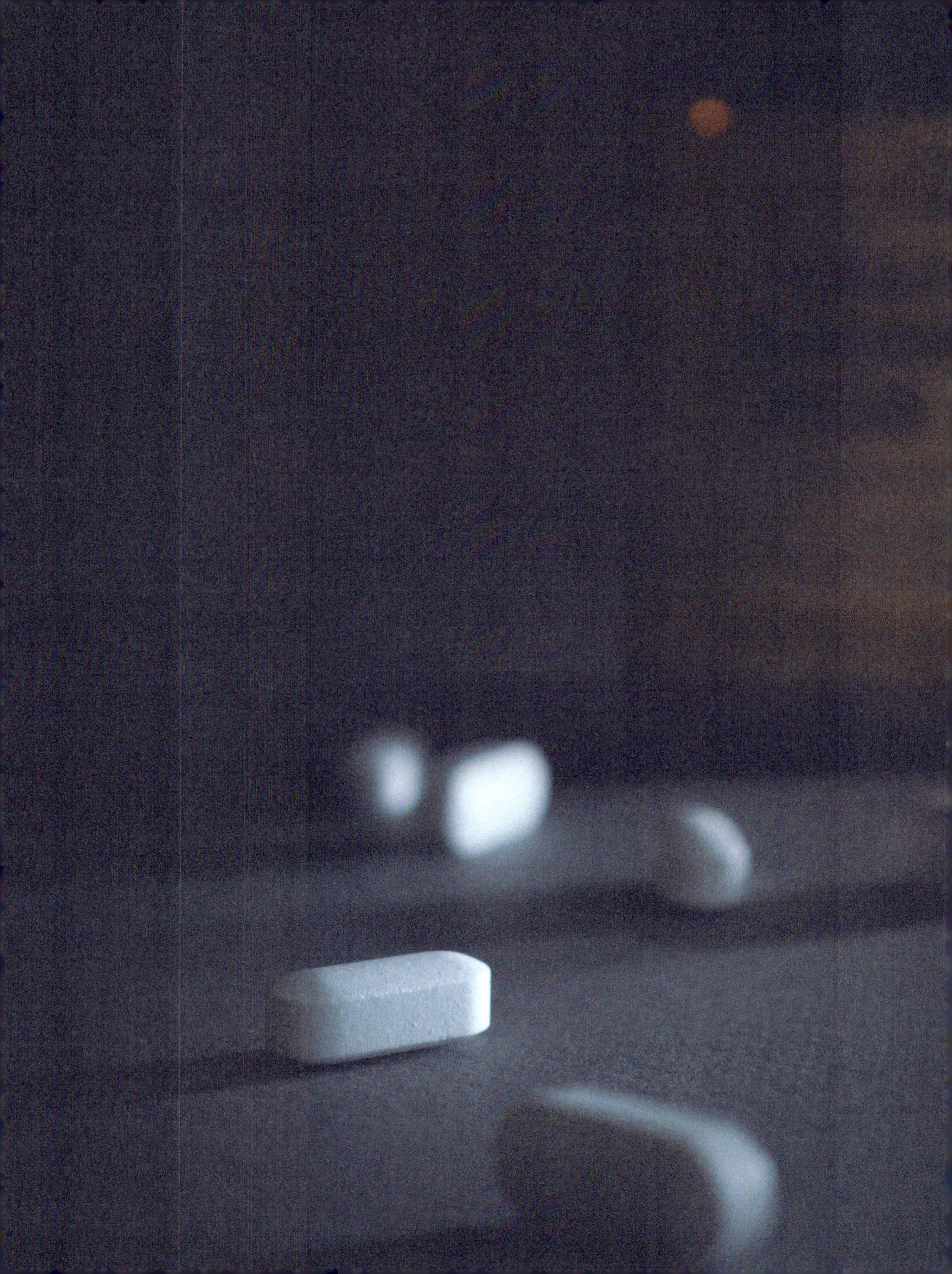

CHAPTER 9
Supplements

"Then God said, 'I give you every seed-bearing plant on the face of the whole earth and every tree that has fruit with seed in it. They will be yours for food'." —Genesis 1:29

"For He satisfies the thirsty and fills the hungry with good things." —Psalm 107:9

Supplements often falsely lead people to believe "health" can be bought if they only purchase the right products. Many also believe supplements are superior to food. Due to these beliefs, many ads encourage pill taking. One reason many people like to take pills and powders is that it's an easy way to feel that they are in control of their life and health; nobody likes feeling out of control. The reality is we are all truly "out of control," but thankfully the creator of the universe is not.

"Fear not, for I am with you; be not dismayed, for I am your God; I will strengthen you, I will help you, I will uphold you with my righteous right hand." —Isaiah 41:10

Quacks take advantage of our need for apparent control by giving their clients simple things to do, such as take vitamin pills or prepare special foods. These activities may, in fact, provide a temporary psychological lift. But they can be dangerous if they are substituted for better alternatives or if they delay pertinent changes that should be made.

Dietary supplements are products taken by mouth that contain a "dietary ingredient." Because supplements are considered food, the Food and Drug Administration (FDA) does not require proof of purity, safety, or effectiveness via clinical trials as it does for medications. The FDA's Good Manufacturing Practices (GMPs) for dietary supplements allow each manufacturer the freedom to determine the quality standards and analytical methods used in manufacturing their supplements. Some choose very low-quality raw materials, resulting in very low-quality supplements which are advertised as, and appear to be, high quality. For example, even the spice turmeric has been found to be contaminated with lead, as well as other toxic metals such as cadmium and arsenic. Plant extracts, as opposed to powders made from whole plant parts, are less likely to be contaminated, as the extraction process helps to remove contaminants. Supplement manufacturers do not have to guarantee ingredients on their labels.

Supplements were not always classified as foods. They used to be classified as drugs (which have safety and efficacy requirements). Their classification changed in 1994. At that time, supplement sales were about $5 billion per year. In 1997, sales doubled to about $10 billion. In 2011, sales jumped to about $29 billion. Consumers spent a total of $8.842 billion on herbal supplements in the United States alone in 2018. In 2019, worldwide supplement sales were $32 billion. According to research done in 2019, 77% of Americans consider themselves to be supplement users, with 35- to 54-year-olds reporting the highest percentage of use at 81%.

There are two main points that need to be made about supplements. The first is that the supplement industry is big business. There is a lot of money being made through the sale of supplements. Most of the sales are driven through people wanting assurance. They want to know they are well nourished. Consumers also buy supplements because they believe the claims made by the companies.

The second main point is manufacturers of supplements do not have to prove their product is effective, that it will do what it claims to do, or even that it is safe before it is marketed and sold to the public. It is up to the FDA to prove a supplement is not safe. The FDA cannot remove a supplement from the marketplace unless it has been shown to be unsafe or harmful to consume. Because of the large workload and numerous complaints about supplements, the FDA can have a 6-month lag time for investigating supplement complaints. This results in many useless supplements being consumed and some dangerous ones, too.

I had a college athlete in one of my nutrition classes a few years ago. He was not on an NCAA team and therefore was not eligible to receive guidance from the university's sports dietitian. He brought into class a canister of the supplement he was taking. Among other things, we talked about the fact that supplements are not pre-cleared for safety or efficacy by the FDA. About a week later, I received an email notification that the same product my student athlete was taking had been removed from the market because it was found to cause liver damage. I immediately forwarded the student the FDA's notice and suggested we talk again. Our second talk was not what I expected. I confirmed that the supplement was in fact what he was taking. He indicated it was, but then said, "But I only take half of the recommended dose. Do you think that is okay?" I was stunned. This comment proves how brainwashing the advertising can be for nutrition and performance supplements. I reiterated to the student that the product has been found to damage the liver and then proceeded to review several functions of the liver in an attempt to help him see the danger. In the end, it was his decision what he wanted to do with the information.

A few years ago, a fellow dietitian, who is also a Certified Specialist in Sports Dietetics, was so frustrated by the supplement industry that he began his own investigation. But no sooner did he open the door to the supplement industry world than he was blown away by its size. He realized quickly there was no way to grab this huge bull by the horns. There was too much money to be made. It involves a global supply chain with the raw ingredients coming from all over the world including countries without regulations for purity or cleanliness. After his investigation, he showed other dietitians the pictures he took of facilities where raw materials for supplements were housed. In the raw materials, he found things like bugs, hair, and metal shavings. Some raw materials even had unidentifiable substances. Diets that require or sell supplements as part of their program should be scrutinized. Companies and programs make a lot of money by instilling fear into the public and offering supplements as the solution.

USP

So, what is the consumer to do? Well, there is a non-profit organization, the US Pharmacopoeia (USP), that sets standards for dietary supplements:

- It does not endorse or validate health claims made by the manufacturer.

- It will test the supplement to ensure that it contains the ingredients in the amounts stated on the label, that those ingredients will disintegrate and dissolve in a reasonable amount of time in the body for proper digestion, and that the product is free of contaminants.

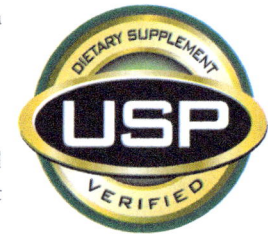

- It will verify that the supplement has been manufactured using safe and sanitary procedures.

NSF

Supplement manufacturers can voluntarily submit their products to the USP's staff of scientists for review. Products that meet the criteria can display the USP's seal on their label. I challenge you to look for this seal the next time you go to a pharmacy or grocery store. You will not see it often.

Another organization that can be helpful, especially for coaches, personal trainers, and sports dietitians, is the public health and safety company NSF International, located in Ann Arbor, Michigan. It will independently test dietary supplements. This company works to protects consumers by:

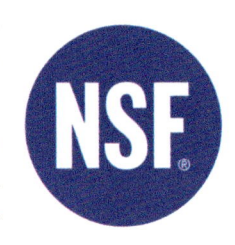

- Testing for harmful levels of contaminants.
- Certifying that supplements contain the ingredients listed on the label and nothing else.

There are three main components of the NSF dietary supplements certification program:

- They certify that what is on the label is, in fact, in the bottle.
- They run a toxicology review to certify the product formula.
- They run a contaminant review to ensure that the product contains no undeclared ingredients or unacceptable levels of contaminants.
- They will not test the product for efficacy. They will not test to see whether a product's claims are truthful or not.

Supplements specifically intended for use by athletes are evaluated under NSF Certified for Sport®. This program works to protect against the contamination of products and to verify product contents. Its scientists also screen supplements for the more than 270 substances banned by most major athletic organizations. The NSF Certified for Sport® is recognized by the NFL, NFL Players Association, MLB, MLB Players Association, PGA, LPGA, and Canadian Centre for Ethics in Sports. This is important because athletes may compete at levels where drug testing is involved. Athletes taking supplements with unidentified banned substances run the risk of potential positive drug tests. This is one of the few avenues that gives peace of mind for casual competitors, drug-tested athletes, and non-drug-tested athletes alike to have access to supplements free of banned substances.

To view NSF-certified dietary supplements go to: nsfsport.com. The NSF is accredited by the American National Standard Institute and gets input from the industry and from current regulating bodies, including the US Anti-Doping Agency.

Consumer Lab

Another consumer resource can be found at ConsumerLab.com. Their mission is to identify quality health and nutritional products through independent testing. Test results are published at www.consumerlab.com. When possible, products are tested in light of the following questions:

- Does the product meet the level of quality claimed on the label?
- Does the product contain the amount of ingredient claimed on the label?
- Is the product free of specified contaminants?
- Does the product break apart properly so that it may be used by the body?

If a manufacturer wishes to have the Consumer Lab's CL Seal of Approval on their product, the product must be tested for the above criteria every 12 months based on a random sample purchased on the open market.

Research continues to find that the cumulative, synergistic effect of different whole foods is what produces desired health benefits. Food is the solution, not supplements.

The bottom line is God made food and God made our bodies. He knew exactly what our bodies needed to function and bring about health, well-being, and satisfaction…and He put it in food. The unfortunate truth is we are sinful beings living in this fallen world. We are doing our best to get by and to discover this amazing world around us. And we have discovered many wondrous things about the human body, how it works, and what it needs. We have also discovered macronutrients and micronutrients in foods, and we continue to discover phytochemicals and deeper, more intricate mechanisms in the human body. But the truth is, we do not know what we don't know yet. We can give ourselves a pat on the back for being able to identify and extract vitamins from foods and put them in pill form. But extracting nutrients, isolating them, and putting them in a pill was not God's design for fueling these magnificent bodies He made. Pills are limited, incomplete, and not satisfying or filling. They may be helpful in certain situations, but they are inadequate and should not be thought of as a regular substitute for food or as the main source of nutrition. It should not be surprising that over and over again research finds that nutrients from whole foods—the foods God made—have greater health benefits than supplements. We don't know or understand all the mechanisms behind why these are the findings of research, but one can hypothesize that it has to do with the fact that we don't know what we don't know yet and that God (who is all-knowing) put other, as of yet unidentified, substances in foods to help with absorption and/or use of nutrients in foods. Praise be to the Lord God! Thus, it is important to encourage patients and clients to eat whole foods in order to fuel their bodies and not rely on supplements.

> **RECAP:** Supplements are not preapproved for safety or efficacy. It is best to get nutrients from food instead of powder or pills from a bottle.

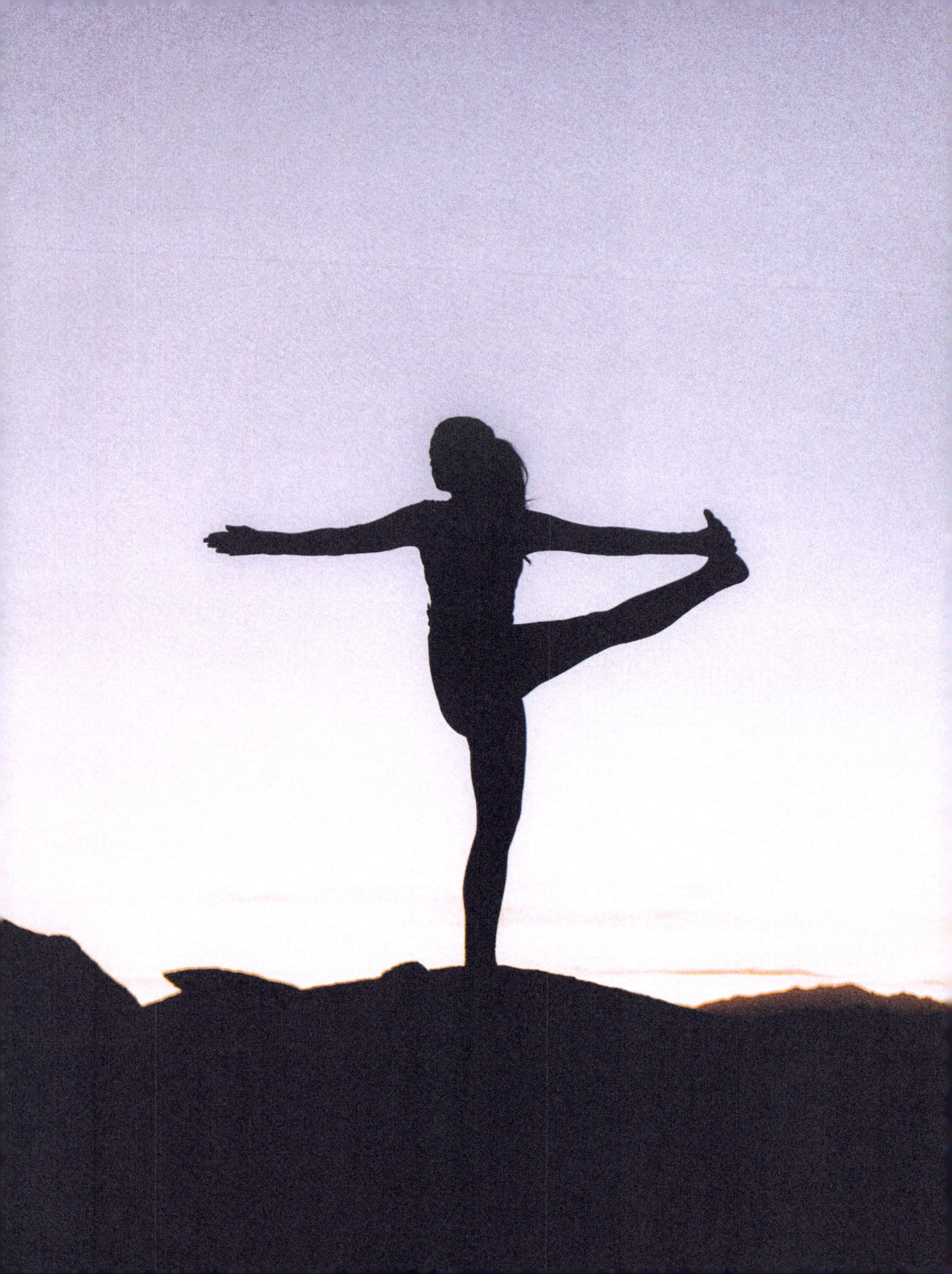

CHAPTER 10
Exercise

"For physical training is of some value, but godliness has value for all things, holding promise for both the present life and the life to come." —1 Timothy 4:8

Exercise is an essential component of weight management. It is also vital to overall health. In fact, the Scriptures frequently mention different physical positions in connection with worship: lying prostrate, standing, kneeling, lifting the hands, clapping the hands, lifting the head, bowing the head, and even dancing. God clearly states that our bodies should engage in action through the effort of work (Ephesians 4:28; 2 Thessalonians 3:10), even hard work (2 Timothy 2:6.) Like gluttony, idleness is a sin, and both are physical and spiritual dangers. Throughout history, humans had to physically labor on a regular basis; but we now live in an age of advanced technology, which has made for a much more sedentary lifestyle. This translates into the need to schedule regular physical activity if we are to experience the "value" mentioned in the above scripture.

Strong action words can be found in many passages if the scope of fitness is broadened to include obedient movements. This may include walking forward, turning back in repentance, lifting joyful hands, or bending grief-stricken knees. Regardless of the position or movement, these words involve bodies responding in obedience.

The point is, Worship is appropriately physical and along with everything else, we are called to offer God our bodies. Just because the health of the soul is the ultimate goal, it doesn't mean that the health of the body is inconsequential or unimportant. Bodily movement and physical exertion are necessary and good. If Christians are to be the hands and feet of Christ, we need to be able to put our bodies to work serving both our souls and the souls of others.

When I was a dietetic student, I did not have any room in my academic schedule for exercise science classes. Other than the general education requirements, every class I took was geared toward becoming a registered dietitian. Thus, upon graduating, I thought everything about health and weight revolved around food and nutrients. But once I started working with diverse members of the general public, I began to see a huge difference in the results of people's efforts. I started to see that the people who were faithfully exercising needed to eat more food to keep up their metabolic rate. Exercisers were losing weight faster, more consistently, and having less difficulty keeping it off. Like an explosion, I realized the importance of exercise and movement.

I retell that story in my college nutrition classes. I tell the students that we do not have time in class to discuss exercise in depth, but it is very important. I tell them that if nobody would get hurt and I wouldn't get fired, I would close the classroom door and set off a firecracker right in the middle of the classroom. They usually look at me as if I'm a few fries short of a Happy Meal!

I then explain to them that I would set off a firecracker right in class, so in 30 or 40 years, when they are sitting around talking about their life's adventures with their children and grandchildren, and the youngsters ask what college was like back in the day, this firecracker episode would come to mind, and they would have to tell their audience about the crazy time a firecracker went off right in class! Of course, their young kin will want to know why a firecracker was set off in a college classroom. And…voila, the importance of exercise would be recalled. I usually search their faces looking for acknowledgment that indeed, they would remember such an event. We then proceed to briefly talk about the importance of exercise.

A clear connection between good or improved health and physical activity is documented in research. And yet, problems arise when exercise is combined with a poor diet. Some of the risks associated with a poor diet and higher levels of exercise are an increased risk of inflammation, which can cause joint and tissue damage, increased risk of injury, and not enough fuel for exercise. Thus, it is critical to fuel the body well so that all the benefits of exercise can be realized.

Physical inactivity can increase one's risk for many chronic diseases, including the following:

- Increases risk of coronary artery disease by 45%
- Increases risk of stroke by 60%
- Increases risk of hypertension by 30%
- Increases risk of osteoporosis by 59%

When someone exercises, there is not an area of life left untouched. The quality of life is affected. The length of life is affected. Finances are affected. Mood is affected. Sleep is affected. Look at the health benefits accompanying regular physical activity:

- It lowers medical expenses
- It improves sleep
- It promotes healthy pregnancies
- It increases muscle mass, and therefore strength and metabolism
- It makes physical tasks easier
- It keeps older adults independent
- It improves the immune system
- It reduces stress and improves self-image
- It helps prevent or delay Alzheimer's disease
- It reduces the risk of heart attacks
- It reduces the risk of some cancers
- It reduces the risk of developing diabetes
- It reduces the risk of developing high blood pressure

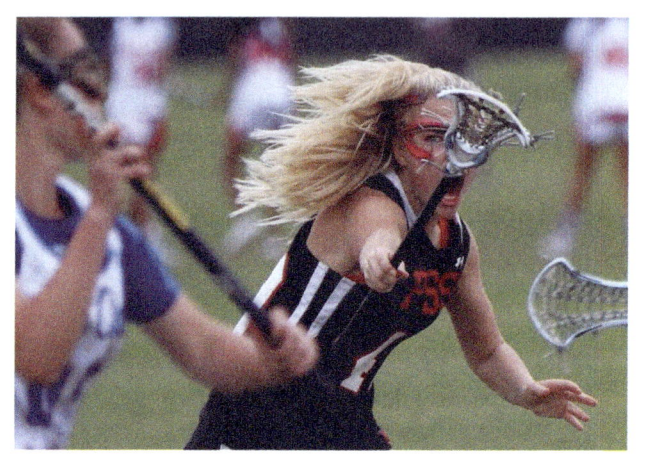

- It reduces the risk of having a stroke
- It reduces the likelihood of weight gain
- It reduces falls in the elderly
- It eases pain with arthritis
- It helps with symptoms of anxiety and depression
- It reduces hospitalizations
- It reduces physician visits
- It reduces the need for medications

But the previous list isn't even an exhaustive list. Exercise can also bring joy, strength, and stability to the soul.

The acknowledgment that "physical training is of some value" is two-edged. Your patients who are voluntarily sedentary may benefit from hearing that God designed our bodies to work and that our bodies feel best when they are moving. On the other hand, any clients who struggle with idolizing exercise and obsessing over it could benefit from hearing that it is only of some value, compared to pursuing godliness, which "is of value in every way."

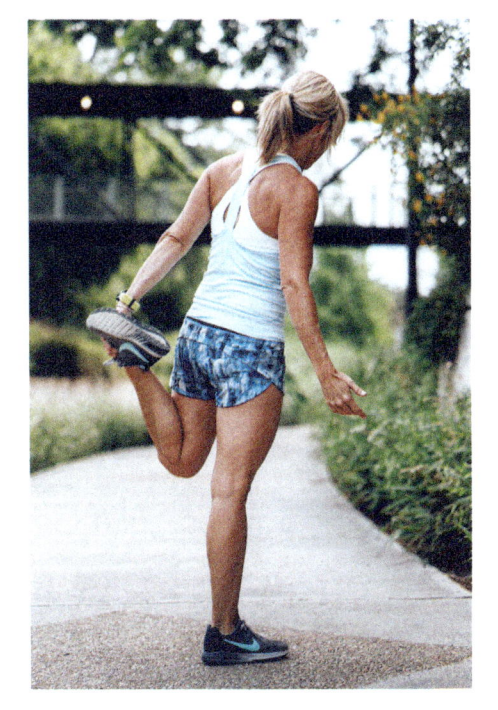

Pastor David Mathis of Cities Church in St. Paul MN puts it this way: "Regular exercise puts my body and soul—and their mysterious relationship—into better position to clearly see and deeply savor who God is." He goes on to note many spiritual benefits of exercise in addition to health benefits:

- The ability to exercise is a gift.

"Everything created by God is good, and nothing is to be rejected if it is received with thanksgiving." —1 Timothy 4:4

We need to thank the Lord that we can swing our arms, flex our legs, and bend and lift, and that our lungs, heart, brain, liver, and kidneys perpetually and endlessly meticulously function to keep us alive.

- Exercising honors God.

God made these amazing bodies so His work could be done. It pleases Him when we use them for doing things that honor Him. In fact, we are commanded to work.

- Exercise helps our mind.

Regular exercise can bring about better discernment and more mental energy, creativity, and mental stamina.

- Exercise can strengthen our will.

Over time exertion in exercise serves to strengthen confidence to push through elsewhere in life. In fact, exercise teaches that exertion produces reward and that there is often greater joy with greater work. One thing is certain, laziness is not satisfying.

- Exercise brings joy.

- Exercise releases endorphins, which can improve mood immediately, as well as help with long-term health. One vital truth is God wants us to desire Him. Many Christians believe enjoying God is essential to glorifying Him. Being indifferent or uninterested in Him dishonors him. In order to realize our purpose and the calling God has on our lives, it's essential to enjoy Him and be satisfied. Part of this is good stewardship of our bodies.

- Exercise makes us more fit to serve others.

Exercise creates strength to better serve others. When our worldview is "others-centered," as Christ asks of us, we are less likely to be passive and more likely to spring into action to help others. When we are fit, we are energetic and better able to serve others.

It is no wonder that those working in the medical profession consider exercise to be medicine. I have heard physicians say if they could only package the benefits of exercise in pill form, they would prescribe it for every one of their patients. The crazy thing is…the benefits are available to everyone—without a prescription! This is especially important for those who are in a "pre-disease" state. Health care providers have the challenge of finding out what motivates their patients and clients to exercise. It's always hardest in the beginning, before the benefits start to reinforce the desire to exercise.

Exercise Recommendations

For healthy adults, the U.S. Department of Health and Human Services recommends:

- At least 150 minutes of moderate aerobic activity or 75 minutes of vigorous aerobic activity a week (or a combination of moderate and vigorous activity). It is best to spread out this exercise throughout the course of a week. If someone can't do this at the start, it is encouraging to know that even small amounts of physical activity are helpful. Being active for short periods of time several times a day can add up and provide health benefits.

- Strength training is also important. All major muscle groups should be worked at least twice a week. A few appointments with a personal trainer can equip, educate, and bring confidence to anyone. For people who have never walked into a gym before, or those who cannot afford a personal trainer, viewing training videos on the internet can take away the mystery of the unknown.

Moderate aerobic exercise includes activities like brisk walking, swimming, and even mowing the lawn. Vigorous aerobic exercise includes activities such as running, working on the step machine, and aerobic dancing. Strength training can include using weight machines, one's own body weight, resistance bands, water activities, or activities such as rock climbing. Heart rate increases in proportion to exercise intensity. For moderate-intensity physical activity, a person's Target Heart Rate should be 50 to 70% of their maximum heart rate. An estimate of maximum heart rate is calculated as 220 beats per minute (bpm) minus age. It is important to remind patients and clients that they should consult with a physician before starting any exercise program. When starting a regular exercise program, heart rate should be kept at the lower end of the range, with the intensity of activity gradually increasing as fitness improves.

An easy way to determine exercise intensity is with the "Talk Test." Patients could benefit from applying this rule of thumb:

- If you can talk and sing without puffing at all, you're exercising at a low intensity level.

- If you can comfortably talk but find it hard to sing, you are in moderate-intensity activity.

- If you can't say more than a few words without gasping for breath, you're exercising at a vigorous intensity.

Burning calories throughout the day can be helpful. This can be done in many small ways. Since reducing the amount of sitting time is important, some people choose devices that raise their computers to chest height at work. This allows them to stand and do toe raises and squats easily throughout the day while they do computer work. Others choose to sit on an exercise/yoga ball instead of a chair while working on their computer. Slightly shifting weight while sitting makes core muscles work. Any activity is better than none. All activity will help with weight management. If schedules don't allow for a 30-minute walk, walk for 5 minutes. If your patient can't leave the house to go to a gym, have them run the steps at home several times.

If they can't afford expensive weights, use jars of tomato sauce. If they want to continue their evening routine of watching television, have them set a timer and every 10 minutes or during commercials stand up and do some squats right in place. When getting up from the dining room table, they can stand up and sit down 3 or 4 times in a row before actually leaving the table. Our bodies were designed to move, and many comforts of today's technology create an environment where we simply don't have to move much. So, we must be intentional about moving our bodies.

One pound of body fat equals 3,500 calories. For safe and effective weight loss, the American College of Sports Medicine (ACSM) and the Academy of Nutrition and Dietetics (AND) both recommend losing no more than 2 pounds per week. To lose this stored body fat, it must be burned by creating an energy deficit. To do this, 1,000 calories per day must be expended beyond what is eaten. To lose 1 pound a week, a 500-calorie deficit must be created each day (500 calories per day x 7 days per week = 3,500 calories). Losing 2 pounds a week can be achieved if exercise is added. The ACSM recommends striving to burn 300–400 calories per workout. For many reasons cited in this book, losing weight at a faster rate can be harmful and has been shown to be unsuccessful in the long run. Slow and steady does it best.

The Psalmist noted "My flesh and my heart may fail, but God is the strength of my heart and my portion forever." —Psalm 73:26

Until that time, God says, "…lift your drooping hands and strengthen your weak knees, and make straight paths for your feet, so that what is lame may not be put out of joint but rather be healed." —Hebrews 12:12-13

> **RECAP:** Exercise is important for weight loss and weight maintenance and should be scheduled and engaged in regularly.

References

Chapter 1: What shapes one's relationship with food?

Bes-Rastrollo M, Basterra-Gortari F, Sanchez-Villegas A, et al. A prospective study of eating away-from-home meals and weight gain in a Mediterranean population: the SUN (Seguimiento Universidad de Navarra) cohort. *Public Health Nutrition*. 2009;13(9). doi:10.1017/S1368980009992783.

Cason K. Family mealtimes: more than just eating together. *Journal of the American Dietetic Association*. 106(4):532-3. dOI:10.1016/j.jada.2006.01.012.

Eisenburg M, Olson R, Neumark-Sztainer D. Correlations between family meals and psychosocial well-being among adolescents. *Arch Pediatr Adolesc Med*. 2004;158(8):792–796. doi:10.1001/archpedi.158.8.792.

Franko D, Thompson D, Affenito S, et al. What mediates the relationship between family meals and adolescent health. *Health Psychol*. 2008;27(2S):S109-17. doi: 10.1037/0278-6133.27.2(Suppl.).S109.

Hennessy E, Hughes S, Goldberg J. Permissive parental feeding behavior is associated with an increase in intake of low- nutrient-dense foods among American children living in rural communities. *Journal of the Academy of Nutrition and Dietetics*. 2012;112(1):142-148. doi: 10.1016/j.jada.2011.08.030.

Internal Federation for Family Development. The crucial role of families. Accessed on October 6,2021. https://www.un.org/ecosoc/sites/www.un.org.ecosoc/files/files/en/integration/2017/IFFD.pdf.

Jansen A, Tenney N. Seeing mum drinking a 'light' product: Is social learning a stronger determinant of taste preference acquisition than caloric conditioning? *European Journal of Clinical Nutrition*. 55(6):418-22. doi:10.1038/sj.ejcn.1601175.

Loth K, Wall M, Choi C, et al. Family meals and disordered eating in adolescents: are the benefits the same for everyone? *Int J Eat Disorder*. 2015;48(1):100-110. doi:10.1002/eat.22339.

Macht M. Characteristics of eating in anger, fear, sadness, and joy. *Institute of Psychology (1), University of Würzburg, Germany*. 199;33:129-139. doi: 10.1016/j.jada.2011.08.030.

Moore E, Wilkie W, Desrochers D. All in the family? Parental roles in the epidemic of childhood obesity. *Journal of Consumer Research*. 2016;1-36. doi:10.1017/S1368980009992783.

Neumarksztainer D, Hannan PJ, Story M, et al. Family meal patterns: associations with sociodemographic characteristics and improved dietary intake among adolescents. *Journal of the American Dietetic Association*. 2003;103(3):317-322. doi: 10.1016/j.jada.2011.08.030.

Nicklas TA, Elkasabany A, Srinivasan SR, et al. Trends in nutrient intake of 10-year-old children over two decades (1973-1994); The Bogalusa heart study. *Am J Epidemiol*. 2001;153:969-977.

Saksensa M, Okrent A, Anekwe T, et al. America's eating habits: food away from home. *United States Department of Agriculture*. 2018;1-160. Accessed on October 11, 2021. www.ers.usda.gov.

Stewart H, Blisard N, Bhuyan S. et al. The demand for food away from home: full service or fast food? *United States Department of Agriculture*. Accessed on October 11, 2021. www.ers.usda.gov.

Wardle J, Carnell S, Cooke L. Parental control over feeding children's fruit and vegetable intake: how are they related? *Journal of the American Dietetic Association*. 2005;227-232. doi.10.1017/S1368980009992783.

Wardle J, Herrera ML, Cooke L, et al. Modifying children's food preferences: the effects of exposure and reward on acceptance of an unfamiliar vegetable. *Eur J Clin Nutr*. 2003;57(2):341-8. doi: 10.1038/sj.ejcn.1601541.

Chapter 2: Recognizing Fad Diets

Jensen MD, Ryan DH, Apovian CM, et al. 2013 AHA/ACC/TOS guideline for the management of overweight and obesity in adults: a report of the American College of Cardiology/American Heart Association Task Force on Practice Guidelines and The Obesity Society. Am J Cardiol. 2014;63(25):2985-3023. doi:10.1016/j.jacc.2013.11.004.

Krop EM, Hetherington MM, Nekitsing C, Miquel S, Postelnicu L, Sarkar A. Influence of oral processing on appetite and food intake – a systematic review and meta-analysis. Appetite. 2018;125:253-269. doi:10.1016/j.appet.2018.01.018.

Martens MJI, Lemmens SGT, Born JM, Westerterp-Plantenga MS. A solid high-protein meal evokes stronger hunger suppression than a liquefied high-protein meal. Obesity (Silver Spring). 2011;19(3):522-527. doi:10.1038/oby.2010.258.

Martens MJI, Lemmens SGT, Born JM, Westerterp-Plantenga MS. Satiating capacity and post-prandial relationships between appetite parameters and gut-peptide concentrations with solid and liquefied carbohydrate. PLoS One. 2012;7(7):e42110. doi:10.1371/journal.pone.0042110.

Mattes RD, Rothacker D. Beverage viscosity is inversely related to postprandial hunger in humans. Physiol Behav. 2001;74:551-557. doi:10.1016/s0031-9384(01)00597-2.

Rueda-Clausen CF, Ogunleye AA, Sharma AM. Health benefits of long-term weight-loss maintenance. Annu Rev Nutr. 2015;35:475-516. doi:10.1146/annurev-nutr-071714-034434.

Varkevisser R. D. M., van Stralen M, Kroeze W, Steenhuis I. H. M. Determinants of weight loss maintenance: a systematic review. *Obesity Reviews*. 2019;171-211. doi: 10.1111/obr.12772.

Chapter 3: Calories

Acharya SD, Eluci OU, Sereika SM, Music E, Styn MA, Turk MW, Burke LE. Adherence to a behavioral weight loss treatment program enhances weight loss and improvements in biomarkers. Patient Prefer Adherence. 2009;3:151-160. doi:10.2147/ppa.s5802.

Baker RC, Kirschenbaum DS. Self-monitoring may be necessary for successful weight control. Behav Ther. 1993;24(3):377-394. doi:10.1016/S0005-7894(05)80212-6.

Barnard ND, Cohen J, Jenkins DJ, et al. A low-fat vegan diet improves glycemic control and cardiovascular risk factors in a randomized clinical trial in individuals with type 2 diabetes. Diabetes Care. 2006;29(8):1777-1783. doi:10.2337/dc06-0606.

Boden G. Sargrad K, Homko C, Mozzoli M, Stein TP. Effects of a low-carbohydrate diet on appetite, blood glucose levels, and insulin resistance in obese patients with type 2 diabetes. Ann Intern Med. 2005;142(6):403-411. doi:10.7326/0003-4819-142-6-200503150-00006.

Bradley U, Spence M, Courtney CH, et al. Low-fat versus low-carbohydrate weight reduction diets. Diabetes. 2009;58(12):2741-2748.

Brehm BJ, Spang SE, Lattin BL, Seeley RJ, Daniels SR, D'Alessio DA. The role of energy expenditure in the differential weight loss in obese women on low-fat and low-carbohydrate diets. J Clin Endocrinol Metab. 2005;90(3):1475-1482. doi:10.1210/jc.2004-1540.

Buchholz AC, Schoeller DA. Is a calorie a calorie? Am J Clin Nutr. 2004;79(5):899S-906S. doi:10.1093/ajcn/79.5.899S.

Buhl KM, Gallagher D, Hoy K, Matthews DE, Heymsfield SB. Unexplained disturbance in body weight regulation: diagnostic outcome assessed by doubly labeled water and body composition analyses in obese patients reporting low energy intakes. J Am Diet Assoc. 1995;95(12):1393-1400. doi:10.1016/S0002-8223(95)00367-3.

Burke LE, Sereika SM, Music Edvin, Warziski M, Styn MA, Stone A. Using instrumented paper diaries to document self-monitoring patterns in weight-loss. Contemp Clin Trials. 2008;29(2):182-193. doi:10.1016/j.cct.2007.07.004.

Burke LE, Wang J, Sevick MA. Self-monitoring in weight loss: a systematic review of the literature. J Am Diet Assoc. 2011;111(1):92-102. doi:10.1016/j.jada.2010.10.008.

Burke LM, Styn MA, Sereika SM, et al. Using mHealth technology to enhance self-monitoring for weight loss a randomized trial. Am J Prev Med. 2012;43(1):20-26. doi:10.1016/j.amepre.2012.03.016.

Burrows TL, Martin RJ, Collins CE. A systematic review of the validity of dietary assessment methods in children when compared with the method of doubly labeled water. J Am Diet Assoc. 2010;110(10):1501-1510. doi:10.1016/j.jada.2010.07.008.

Butryn ML, Webb V, Wadden TA. Behavioral treatment of obesity. Pschiatr Clin North Am. 2011;34(4):841-859. doi:10.1016/j.psc.2011.08.006.

Davoodi SH, Ajami M, Ayatollahi SA, Dowlatshahi K, Javedan G, Pazoki-Toroudi HR. Calorie shifting diet versus calorie restriction diet: a comparative clinical trial study. Int J Prev Med. 2014;5(4):447-456.

Ellis E. Serving size vs portion size is there a difference. Eat Right. https://www.eatright.org/food/nutrition/nutrition-facts-and-food-labels/serving-size-vs-portion-size-is-there-a-difference. Reviewed February 2020. Accessed March 30, 2020.

Freedman MR, King J, Kennedy. Popular diets: a scientific review. Obes Res. 2001;9(S1):1S-5S. doi:10.1038/0by.2001.113.

Halton TL, Hu FB. The effects of high protein diets on thermogenesis, satiety and weight loss: a critical review. J Am Coll Nutr. 2004;23(5):373-385. doi:10.1080/07315724.2004.10719381.

Hartmann-Boyce J, Johns DJ, Jebb SA, Aveyard P, Behavioural Weight Management Review Group. Effect of behavioural techniques and delivery mode on effectiveness of weight management: systematic review, meta-analysis and meta-regression. Obes Rev. 2014;15(7):598-609. doi:10.1111/obr.12165.

Helsel DL, Jakicic JM, Otto AD. Comparison of techniques for self-monitoring eating and exercise behaviors on weight loss in a correspondence-based intervention. J Am Diet Assoc. 2007;107(10):1807-1810.

Hendrickson S, Mattes R. Financial incentive for diet recall accuracy does not affect reported energy intake or number of under reporters in a sample of overweight females. J Am Diet Assoc. 2007;107(1):118-121. doi:10.1016/j.jada.2006.10.003.

Hill, JO. Wyatt, H. Phelan, S. Wing, R. The National Weight Control Registry: Is it Useful in Helping Deal with Our Obesity Epidemic? https://digitalcommons.calpoly.edu/cgi/viewcontent.cgi?referer=https://www.google.com/&httpsredir=1&article=1018&context=kine_fac. Accessed July 29, 2020

Hu T, Mills KT, Yao L, et al. Effects of low-carbohydrate diets versus low-fat diets on metabolic risk factors: a meta-analysis of randomized controlled clinical trials. Am J Epidemiol. 2012;176(S7):S44-S54. doi:10.1093/aje/kws264.

Kinsell LW, Gunning B, Michaels GD, et al. Metab. 1964;13(3):195-204. doi:10.1016/0026-0495(64)90098-8.

Kong A, Beresford SAA, Alfano CM, et al. Self-monitoring and eating-related behaviors associated with 12-month weight loss in postmenopausal overweight-to-obese women. J Acad Nutr Diet. 2012;112(9):1428-1435. doi:10.1016/j.jand.2012.05.014.

Kreitzman SN, Coxon AY, Szaz KF. Glycogen storage: illusions of easy weight loss, excessive weight regain, and distortions in estimates of body composition. Am J Clin Nutr. 1992;56(S1):292S-293S. doi:10.1093/ajcn.56.1.292S.

Layman DK, Boileau RA, Erickson DJ, et al. A reduced ratio of dietary carbohydrate to protein improves body composition and blood lipid profiles during weight loss in adult women. J Nutr. 2003;133(2):411-417. doi:10.1093/jn/133.2.411.

Lichtman SW, Pisarska K, Berman ER, et al. Discrepancy between self-reported and actual caloric intake and exercise in obese subjects. N Engl J Med. 327(27):1893-1898. doi:10.1056/NEJM199212313272701.

Manninen AH. Is a calorie really a calorie? Metabolic advantage of low-carbohydrate diets. J Int Soc Sports Nutr. 2004; 1(2);21-26. doi:10.1186/1550-2783-1-2-21.

Mawer R. 13 easy ways to lose water weight (fast and safely). Healthline. https://www.healthline.com/nutrition/13-ways-to-lose-water-weight. Published August 2018. Accessed March 30, 2020.

Mockus DS, Macera CA, Wingard DL, Peddecord M, Thomas RG, Wilfley DE. Dietary self-monitoring and its impact on weight loss in overweight children. Int J Pediatr Obes. 2011;6(0):197-205. doi:10.3109/17477166.2011.590196.

Noakes M, Foster PR, Keogh JB, James AP, Mamo JC, Clifton PM. Comparison of isocaloric very low carbohydrate/high saturated fat and high carbohydrate/low saturated fat diets on body composition and cardiovascular risk. Nutr Metab (Lond). 2006;3(7). doi:10.1186/1743-7075-3-7.

Nordmann AJ, Nordman A, Briel M, et al. Effects of low-carbohydrate vs. low-fat diets on weight loss and cardiovascular risk factors: a meta-analysis of randomized controlled trials. Arch Intern Med. 2006; 166(3):285-293. doi:10.1001/archinte.166.3.285.

Schoeller DA, Buchholz AC. Energetics of obesity and weight control: does diet composition matter? J Am Diet Assoc. 2005;105(5-1):S24-28. doi:10.1016/j.jada.2005.02.025.

Schoeller DA, Buchholz AC. Energetics of obesity and weight control: does diet composition matter? J Am Diet Assoc. 2005;105(5-1):S24-28. doi:10.1016/j.jada.2005.02.025.

Shay LE, Siebert D, Watts D, Sbrocco T, Pagliara C. Adherene and weight loss outcomes associated with food-exercise dietary preference in a military weight management program. Eat Behavior. 2009;10(4):220-227. doi:10.1016/j.eatbeh.2009.07.004.

Soenen S, Westerterp-Plantenga MS. Proteins and satiety: implications for weight management. Curr Opin Clin Nutr Metab Care. 2008;11(6):747-751. doi:10.1097/MCO.0b013e328311a8c4.

Turk MW, Elci OU, Wang J, et al. Self-monitoring as a mediator of weight loss in the SMART randomized clinical trial. Int J Behav Med. 2013;20(4). doi:10.1007/s12529-012-9259-9.

Varady KA. Intermittent versus daily calorie restriction: which diet regimen is more effective for weight loss? Obes Rev. 2011;12(7):e593-601. doi:10.1111/j.1467-789X.2011.00873.x.Epub.

Veldhorst MA, Westerterp KR, van Vught AJ, Westerterp-Plantenga MS. Presence or absence of carbohydrates and the proportion of fat in a high-protein diet affect appetite suppresion but not energy expenditure in normal-weight human subjects fed in energy balance. Br J Nutr. 2010;104(9):1395-1405. doi:10.1017/S0007114510002060.

Volek JS, Sharman MJ, Love DM, et al. Body composition and hormonal responses to a carbohydrate-restricted diet. Metab. 2002;51(7):864-870. doi:10.1053/meta.2002.32037.

Westerterp KR. Diet induced thermogenesis. Nutr Metab (Lond). 2004;1(5). doi:10.1186/1743-7075-1-5.

Yon BA, Johnson RK, Harvey-Berino J, Gold BC, Howard AB. Personal digital assistants are comparable to traditional diaries for dietary self-monitoring during a weight loss program. J Behav Med. 2007;30(2):165-175. doi:10.1007/s10865-006-9092-1.

Chapter 5: Carbohydrates

Baskin DG, Porte D, Schwartz MW. Insulin signaling in the central nervous system: a critical role in metabolic homeostasis and disease from C. elegans to humans. Diabetes. 2005;54:1264-1276.

Blake JS, Munoz KD, Volpe S. Nutrition: From Science to You. 3rd ed. New York City: Pearson Education; 2016.

Blazquez E, Velazquez E, Hurtado-Carneiro V, Ruiz-Albusac JM. Insulin in the brain: its pathophysiological implications for states related with central insulin resistance, type 2 diabetes and Alzheimer's disease. Front Endocrinol (Lausanne). 2014;5:161. doi:10.3389/fendo.2014.00161.

Craft S. Insulin resistance and Alzheimer's disease pathogenesis: potential mechanisms and implications for treatment. Curr Alzheimer Res. 2007;4(2):147-152. doi: 10.2174/156720507780362137.

Craft S. Insulin resistance syndrome and Alzheimer disease: pathophysiologic mechanisms and therapeutic implications. Alzheimer Dis Assoc Discord. 2006;20(4):298-301.

Diabetes.co.uk. Glycemic load. Diabetes.co.uk. Updated January 2019. Accessed July 14, 2020. https://www.diabetes.co.uk/diet/glycemic-load.html.

Flint A, Gregersen NT, Gluud LL, et al. Associations between postprandial insulin and blood glucose responses, appetite sensations and energy intake in normal weight and overweight individuals: a meta-analysis of test meal studies. Br J Nutr. 2007;98:17-25. doi: 10.1017/S000711450768297X.

Fun TT, van Dam RM, Hankisnson SE, Stampfer M, Willett WC, Hu FB. Low-carbohydrate diets and all-cause and cause-specific mortality: two cohort studies. Ann Intern Med. 2010;153(5):289-298. doi:10.1059/0003-4819-153-5-201009070-00003.

Goss AM, Goree LL, Ellis AC, et al. Effects of diet macronutrient composition on body composition and fat distribution during weight maintenance and weight loss. Obesity (Silver Spring). 2013;21(6):1133-1138. doi:10.1002/oby.20191.

Halkjaer J, Sorensen TIA, Tjonneland A, Togo P, Holst C, Heitmann BL. Food and drinking patterns as predictors of 6-year BMI-adjusted changes in waist circumference. Br J Nutr. 2004;92(4):735-738. doi:10.1079/BJN20041246.

Neth BJ, Craft S. Insulin resistance and Alzheimer's disease: bioenergetic linkages. Front Aging Neurosci. 2017;9:345. doi: 10.3389/fnagi.2017.00345.

Neumann KF, Rojo L, Navarrete LP, Farias G, Reyes P, Maccioni RB. Insulin resistance and Alzheimer's disease: molecular links & clinical implications. Curr Alzheimer Res. 2008;5:000-000. doi: 10.2174/1567205087859019.

Noakes M, Foster PR, Keogh JB, James AP, Mamo JC, Clifton PM. Comparison of isocaloric very low carbohydrate/high saturated fat and high carbohydrate/low saturated fat diets on body composition and cardiovascular risk. Nutr Metab. 2006;3(7). doi:10.1186/1743-7075-3-7.

Park S. Hong SM, Sung SR, Junk HK. Long-term effects of central leptin and resistin on body weight, insulin resistance, and b-cell function and mass by the modulation of hypothalamic leptin and insulin signaling. Endocrinol. 2008;149(2):445-454. doi: 10.1210/en.2007-0754.

Porte D. Central regulation of energy homeostasis: the key role of insulin. Diabetes. 2006;55(2):S155-S160. doi: 10.2337/db06-S019.

Roberts SB. High-glycemic index foods, hunger, and obesity: is there a connection? Nutr Rev. 2000;58(6):163-169. doi:10.1111/j.1753-4887.2000.tb01855.x.

Sharma MD, Garber AJ, Farmer JA. Role of insulin signaling in maintaining energy homeostasis. Endocr Pract. 2008;14(3):373-380.

Sluijs I, Beulens JWJ, van der Schouw YT, et al. Dietary glycemic index, glycemic load, and digestible carbohydrate intake are not associated with risk of type 2 diabetes in eight European countries. J Nutr. 2013;143(1):93-99. doi:10.3945/jn.112.165605.

Trichopoulou A, Psaltopoulou T, Orfanos P, Hsieh CC, Trichopoulos D. Low-carbohydrate–high protein diet and long-term survival in a general population cohort. Eur J Clin Nutr. 2007; 61:575–581.

Willett G. Sweet talk: the insulin connection. Institute for Natural Resources. February 2013-K.

Chapter 6: Proteins

Abete I, Parra D, De Morentin BM, Alfredo Martinez J. Effects of two energy-restricted diets differing in the carbohydrate/protein ratio on weight loss and oxidative changes of obese men. Int J Food Sci Nutr. 2009;60(S3):1-13. doi:10.1080/09637480802232625.

Astrup A, Raben A, Geiker N. The role of higher protein diets in weight control and obesity-related comorbidities. Int J Obes (Lond). 2015;39(5):721-726. doi:10.1038/ijo.2014.216.

Barzel US, Massey LK. Excess dietary protein can adversely affect bone. J Nutr. 1998;128(6):1051-1053. doi:10.1093/jn/128.6.1051.

Blom WA, Lluch A, Stafleu A, et al. Effect of a high-protein breakfast on the postprandial ghrelin response. Am J Clin Nutr. 2006;83(2):211-220. doi:10.1093/ajcn/83.2.211.

Campbell, B., Kreider, R.B., Ziegenfuss, T. et al. International Society of Sports Nutrition position stand: protein and exercise. J Int Soc Sports Nutr 4, 8 (2007). https://doi.org/10.1186/1550-2783-4-8

Crovetti R, Porrini M, Santangelo A, Testolin G. The influence of thermic effect of food on satiety. Eur J Clin Nutr. 1998;52(7):482-488. doi:10.1038/sj.ejcn.1600578.

Cuenca-Sanchez M, Navas-Carrillo D, Orenes-Pinero E. Controversies surrounding high-protein diet intake: satiating effect and kidney and bone health. Adv Nutr. 2015;6(3):260-266. doi:10.3945/an.114.007716.

Delimaris, I. Adverse effects associated with protein intake above the recommended dietary allowance for adults. ISRN Nutr. 2013. doi.org/10.5402/2013/126929

Foltz M, Ansems P, Schwarz J, Tasker MC, Lourbakos A, Gerhardt CC. Protein hydrolysates induce CCK release from enteroendocrine cells and act as partial agonists of the CCK1 receptor. J Agric Food Chem. 2008;56(3):837-843. doi:10.1021/jf072611h.

Foster GD, Wyatt HR, Hill JO, et al. Weight and metabolic outcomes after 2 years on a low-carbohydrate versus low-fat diet: a randomized trial. Ann Intern Med. 2010;153(3):147-157. doi:10.7326/0003-4819-153-3-201008030-00005.

Friedman AN, Ogden LG, Foster GD, et al. Comparative effects of low-carbohydrate high-protein versus low-fat diets on the kidney. Clin J Am Soc Nephrol. 2012;7(7):1103-1111. doi:10.2215/CJN.11741111.

Gillespie AL, Calderwood D, Hobson L, Green BD. Whey proteins have beneficial effects on intestinal enteroendocrine cells stimulating cell growth and increasing the production and secretion of incretin hormones. Food Chem. 2015;189:120-128. doi:10.1016/j.foodchem.2015.02.002.

Halton TL, Hu FB. The effects of high protein diets on thermogenesis, satiety and weight loss: a critical review. J Am Coll Nutr. 2004;23(5):373-85. doi:10.1080/07315724.2004.10719381.

Hession M, Rolland C, Kulkarni U, Wise A, Broom J. Systematic review of randomized controlled trials of low-carbohydrate vs. low-fat/low-calorie diets int eh management of obesity and its comorbidities. Obes Rev. 2009;10(1):36-50. doi:10.1111/j.1467-789X.2008.00518.x.

Jesudason DR, Pedersen E, Clifton PM. Weight-loss diets in people with type 2 diabetes and renal disease: a randomized controlled trial of the effect of different dietary protein amounts. Am J Clin Nutr. 2013;98(2):494-501. doi:10.3945/ajcn.113.060889.

Johnston CS, Day CS, Swan PD. Postprandial thermogenesis is increased 100% on a high-protein, low-fat diet versus a high-carbohydrate, low-fat diet in healthy, young women. J Am Coll Nutr. 2002;21(1):55-61. doi:10.1080/07315724.2002.10719194.

Kerstetter JE, Kenny Am, Insogna KL. Dietary protein and skeletal health: a review of recent human research. Curr Opin Lipidol. 2011;22(1):16-20. doi:10.1097/MOL.0b013e3283419441.

Lomenick JP, Melguizo MS, Mitchell SL, Summar ML< Anderson JW. Effects of meals high in carbohydrate, protein, and fat on ghrelin and peptide YY secretion in prepubertal children. J CLin Endocrinol Metab. 2009;94(11):4463-4471. doi:10.1210/jc.2009-0949.

Martens EA, Gonnissen HK, Gatta-Cerifi B, Janssens PL, Westerterp-Plantenga MS. Maintenance of energy expenditure on high-protein vs. high-carbohydrate diets at a constant body weight may prevent a positive energy balance. Clin Nutr. 2015;34(5):968-975. doi:10.1016/j.clnu.2014.10.007.

Martin WF, Armstrong LE, Rodriguez NR. Dietary protein intake and renal function. Nutr Metab (Lond). 2005;2(25). doi:10.1186/1743-7075-2-25.

Mawer R. Ghrelin: the "hunger hormone" explained. Healthline. https://www.healthline.com/nutrition/ghrelin. Published June 2016. Accessed March 31, 2020.

Nouvenne A, Ticinesi A, Morelli I, Guida L, Borghi L, Meschi T. Fad diets and their effect on urinary stone formation. Transl Androl Urol. 2014;3(3)303-312. doi:10.3978/j.issn.2223-4683.2014.06.01.

Pesta DH, Samuel VT. A high-protein diet for reducing body fat: mechanisms and possible caveats. Nutr Metab (Lond). 2014;11(1):53. doi:10.1186/1743-7075-11-53.

Riggs AJ, White BD, Gropper SS. Changes in energy expenditure associated with ingestion of high protein, high fat versus high protein, low fat meals among underweight, normal weight, and overweight females. Nutr J. 2007;6(40). doi:10.1186/1475-2891-6-40.

Spritzler F. 10 natural ways to build healthy bones. Healthline. https://www.healthline.com/nutrition/build-healthy-bones. Published January 2017. Accessed March 31, 2020.

Sukumar D, Ambia-Sobhan H, Zurfluh R, et al. Areal and volumetric bone mineral density and geometry at two levels of protein intake during caloric restriction: a randomized, controlled trial. J Bone Miner Res. 2011;26(6):1339-1348. doi:10.1002/jbmr.318.

Tang M, Armstrong CL, Leidy HJ, Campbell WW. Normal vs. high-protein weight loss diets in men: effects on body composition and indices of metabolic syndrome. Obesity (Silver Spring). 2013;21(3):E204-210. doi:10.1002/oby.20078.

Veldhorst MA, Westerterp-Plantenga MS. Westerterp KR. Gluconeogenesis and energy expenditure after a high-protein, carbohydrate-free diet. Am J Clin Nutr. 2009;90(3):519-526. doi:10.3945/ajcn.2009.27834.

Chapter 7: Fat

Blake JS, Munoz KD, Volpe S. Nutrition from Science to You. 3rd ed. New York: Pearson Education; 2016.

Carobbio S, Guenatin A, Samuelson I, Bahri M, Vidal-Puig A. Brown and beige fat: from molecules to physiology and pathophysiology. Biochim Biophys Acta Mol Cell Biol Lipids. 2019;1864(1):37.50. doi:10.1016/j.bbalip.2018.05.013.

ECLINPATH. Production and metabolism of non-esterified fatty acids. Cornell University College of Veterinary Medicine. http://eclinpath.com/chemistry/energy-metabolism/non-esterified-fatty-acids/print-2/. Accessed July 14, 2020.

Engin AB. What is lipotoxicity? Adv Exp Med Biol. 2017;960:197-220. doi:10.1007/978-3-319-48382-5_8.

Hall JE. Guyton and Hall Textbook of Medical Physiology. 12th ed. Philadelphia: Saunders Elsevier; 2011.

Harvard Medical School. Abdominal obesity and your health. Harvard Health Publishing. Updated January 2017. Accessed July 14, 2020. https://www.health.harvard.edu/staying-healthy/abdominal-obesity-and-your-health.

Moon J. Metabolic control and the impact of body composition, nutrition, and lifestyle. Eat 2 Win webinar. April 28, 2020. Accessed April 28, 2020. https://exsci.cuchicago.edu/free-sports-nutrition-webinar-4-2020/

Nelms M, Sucher KP, Lacey K, Roth SL. Nutrition Therapy & Pathophysiology. 2nd ed. Belmont, CA: Brooks/Cole Cengage Learning; 2011.

Petersen MC, Shulman GI. Roles of diacylglycerols and ceramides in hepatic insulin resistance. Trends Parmacol Sci. 2017;38(7):649-665. doi:10.1016/j.tips.2017.04.004.

Sethi S. Everything you need to know about fatty liver. Healthline. https://www.healthline.com/health/fatty-liver. Updated February 2020. Accessed July 14, 2020.

Weinberg JM. Lipotoxicity. Kidney Int. 2006;70(9):1560-1566. doi:10.1038/sj.ki.5001834.

Zelman KM. The truth about beer and your belly. WebMD. https://www.webmd.com/diet/features/the-truth-about-beer-and-your-belly#1. Accessed July 14, 2020.

Chapter 8: Metabolism

Amboss. Glycolysis and gluconeogenesis. Amboss. https://www.amboss.com/us/knowledge/Glycolysis_and_gluconeogenesis. Accessed July 14, 2020.

Blazquez E, Velazquez E, Hurtado-Carneiro V, Ruiz-Albusac JM. Insulin in the brain: its pathophysiological implications for states related with central insulin resistance, type 2 diabetes and Alzheimer's disease. Front Endocrinol (Lausanne). 2014;5:161. doi:10.3389/fendo.2014.00161.

Burgess, S. In God's image. *Creation Points*. 2008. Pages 4-31.

Burgess S. Humans: Purposely designed. Answers in Genesis. Published July 1, 2007. Updated February 13, 2017. Accessed November 15, 2021. https://answersingenesis.org/what-is-the-meaning-of-life/humans-purposely-designed/.

Burgess S. An eye for every occasion. Answers in Genesis. Published October 9, 2019. Accessed November 15, 2021. https://answersingenesis.org/biology/eye-every-occasion/.

Bruce H. Nerve distribution- a sensitive topic. Answers in Genesis. Published on March 1, 2018. Accessed November 15, 2021. https://answersingenesis.org/human-body/nerve-distribution-sensitive-topic/.

Brehm BJ, Seeley RJ, Daniels SR, D'Alessio DA. A randomized trial comparing every low carbohydrate diet and a calorie-restricted low fat diet on body weight and cardiovascular risk factors in healthy women. J Clin Endocrinol Metab. 2003;88: 1617–1623.

Cahill GF Jr, Herrera MG, Morgan AP, et al. Hormone-fuel interrelationships during fasting. J Clin Invest. 1966;45:1751–69.

Cahill GF. Fuel metabolism in starvation. Annu Rev Nutr. 2006;26:1-22.

Castle J, Indy CL. Family Dinner Statistics. The Scramble. https://www.thescramble.com/family-dinner/family-dinner-statistics/. Published March 30, 2019. Accessed April 30, 2020.

Chodosh S. Sorry, keto fans, you're probably not in ketosis. Popular Science. https://www.popsci.com/not-in-ketosis/. Published June 2018. Accessed July 14, 2020.

Coiffi I, Evangelista A, Ponzo V, Ciccone G, Soldati L, Santarpia L. Intermittent versus continuous energy restriction on weight loss and cardiometabolic outcomes: a systematic review and meta-analysis of randomized controlled trials. J Transl Med. 2018;16(1):371. doi:10.1186/s12967-018-1748-4.

Comstock JP, Garber AJ. Ketonuria. In: Clinical Methods: The History, Physical, and Laboratory Examinations. 3rd ed. Boston: Butterworths;1990:Chapter 140.

Cooperman MT, Davidoff F, Spark R, Pallotta J. Clinical studies of alcoholic ketoacidosis. Diabetes. 1974;23(5):433-439. doi:10.2337/diab.23.5.433.

Craft S. Insulin resistance and Alzheimer's disease pathogenesis: potential mechanisms and implications for treatment. Curr Alzheimer Res. 2007;4(2):147-152. doi: 10.2174/156720507780362137.

Dhillon KK, Gupta S. Biochemistry, Ketogenesis. Treasure Island, FL: StatPearls Publishing; 2020.

Durrer C, Lewis N, Wan Z, Ainslie P, Jenkins N, Jonathan Little, J. Short-term low-carbohydrate high-fat diet in healthy young males renders the endothelium susceptible to hyperglycemia-induced damage, an exploratory analysis. Nutrients, 2019;11(3):489. doi:10.3390/nu11030489.

El-rashidy OF, Nassar MF, Abdel-hamid IA, et al. Modified Atkins diet vs classic ketogenic formula in intractable epilepsy. Acta Neurol Scand. 2013;128(6):402-8.

Fine EJ, Feinman RD. Thermodynamics of weight loss diets. Nutr Metab (Lond). 2004;1:15.

Flint A, Gregersen NT, Gluud LL, et al. Associations between postprandial insulin and blood glucose responses, appetite sensations and energy intake in normal weight and overweight individuals: a meta-analysis of test meal studies. Br J Nutr. 2007;98:17-25. doi: 10.1017/S000711450768297X.

Fromentin C, Tomé D, Nau F, et al. Dietary Proteins Contribute Little to Glucose Production, Even Under Optimal Gluconeogenic Conditions in Healthy Humans. Diabetes. 2013;62(5):1435-1442.

Gardner CD, Kiazand A, Alhassan S, et al.Comparison of the Atkins, zone, Ornish, and LEARN diets for change in weight and related risk factors among overweight premenopausal women: The A TO Z weight loss study: a randomized trial. JAMA. 2007;297:969-977.

Halton TL, Hu FB. The effects of high protein diets on thermogenesis, satiety and weight loss: a critical review. J Am Coll Nutr. 2004;23: 373–385.

Harvie M, Howell A. Potential benefits and harms of intermittent energy restriction and intermittent fasting amongst obese, overweight and normal weight subjects – a narrative review of human and animal evidence. Behav Sci. 2017;7(4). doi:10.3390/bs7010004.

Hetherington MM, Cunningham K, Dye L, et al. Potential benefits of satiety to the consumer: scientific considerations. Nutr Res Rev. 2013;26:22e38.

Hutchinson AT, Heilbronn LK. Metabolic impacts of alternate meal frequency and timing – Does when we eat matter? Biochimi. 2016;124:187-197. doi:10.1016/j.biochi.2015.07.025.

Johnstone AM, Horgan GW, Murison SD, Bremner DM, Lobley GE. Effects of a high-protein ketogenic diet on hunger, appetite, and weight loss in obese men feeding ad libitum. Am J Clin Nutr. 2008;87(1):44-55.

Keys A. The residues of malnutrition and starvation. Science. 1950;112:371-373.

Kilbourne J, Jhally S. Killing Us Softly: Advertising's Image of Women. Cambridge Documentary Films; 2010. Accessed July 13, 2020. https://thoughtmaybe.com/killing-us-softly/#top

Klein CJ, Stanek GS, Wiles CE. Overfeeding macronutrients to critically ill adults: metabolic complications. J Am Diet Assoc. 1998;98:795-806.

Knochel JP. The pathophysiology and clinical characteristics of severe hypophosphatemia. Arch Intern Med.1977;137:203-220. doi:10.1001/archinte.1977.03630140051013.

Krall EA, Dwyer JT, Coleman A. Factors influencing accuracy of dietary recall. Nutr Res. 1988;8(7):829-841. doi:10.1016/S0271-5317(88)80162-3.

Krebs HA. The regulation of the release of ketone bodies by the liver. Adv Enzyme Regul. 1966;4:339–335.

Krebs KA. The metabolic fate of amino acids. In: Munro HN, Allison JB, eds. Mammalian protein metabolism. Vol 1. New York: Academic Press; 1964:125–177.

Lessan N, Saadane I, Alkaf B, et al. The effects of Ramadan fasting on activity and energy expenditure. Am J Clin Nutr. 2018;107(1):54-61. doi:10.1093/ajcn/nqx016.

McCray S, Walker S, Parrish CR. Much ado about refeeding. Pract Gasteroenterol. 2005;28(12):26-44.

Mehanna HM, Moledina J, Travis J. Refeeding syndrome: what it is, and how to prevent and treat it. BMJ. 2008;336:1495-1498. doi:10.1136/bmj.a301.

Moro T, Tinsley G, Bianco A, et al. Effects of eight weeks of time-restricted feeding (16/8) on basal metabolism, maximal strength, body composition, inflammation, and cardiovascular risk factors in resistance-trained males. J Transl Med. 2016;14:290. doi:10.1186/s12967-016-1044-0.

Most, J, Redman, LM. Impact of calorie restriction on energy metabolism in humans. Experimental Gerontology. 2020; Volume 133, May 2020, 110875 https://doi.org/10.1016/j.exger.2020.110875 -- https://www.sciencedirect.com/science/article/abs/pii/S0531556519308642

National Clinical Guideline Centre (UK). Ketone monitoring and management of diabetic ketoacidosis (DKA). In: Type 1 Diabetes in Adults: Diagnosis and Management. London: National Institute for Health and Care Excellence (UK);2015:Chapter 12.

Neth BJ, Craft S. Insulin resistance and Alzheimer's disease: bioenergetic linkages. Front Aging Neurosci. 2017;9:345. doi: 10.3389/fnagi.2017.00345.

Nilsson LH, Hultman E. Liver glycogen in man—the effect of total starvation or a carbohydrate-poor diet followed by carbohydrate refeeding. Scand J Clin Lab Invest. 1973;32:325–330.

Nilsson LH. Liver glycogen content in man in the postabsorptive state. Scand J Clin Lab Sci. 1973;32:317–323.

Owen OE, Morgan AP, Kemp HG, Sullivan JM, Herrera MG, Cahill GF., Jr Brain metabolism during fasting. J Clin Invest. 1967;46:1589–1595.

Paoli A, Grimaldi K, Toniolo L, Canato M, Bianco A, Fratter A. Nutrition and acne: therapeutic potential of ketogenic diets. Skin Pharmacol Physiol. 2012;25:111–1174.

Paoli A, Rubini A, Volek JS, Grimaldi KA. Beyond weight loss: a review of the therapeutic uses of very-low-carbohydrate (ketogenic) diets. Eur J Clin Nutr. 2013;67:789-796. doi: 10.1038/ejcn.2013.116.

Paoli A, Canato M, Toniolo L, et al.The ketogenic diet: an underappreciated therapeutic option? Clin Ter. 2011;162: e145–e153.10

Park S. Hong SM, Sung SR, Junk HK. Long-term effects of central leptin and resistin on body weight, insulin resistance, and b-cell function and mass by the modulation of hypothalamic leptin and insulin signaling. Endocrinol. 2008;149(2):445-454. doi: 10.1210/en.2007-0754.

Reuler JB, Girard DE, Cooney TG. Wernicke's encephalopathy. N Engl J Med.1985;312:1035-1039.

Schnitker M, Mattman P, Bliss T. A clinical study of malnutrition in Japanese prisoners of war. Ann Intern Med. 1951;35:69-96 .

Shai I, Schwarzfuchs D, Henkin Y, et al. Weightloss with a low-carbohydrate, Mediterranean, or low-fat diet. N Engl J Med. 2008;359:229-241.

Sharma MD, Garber AJ, Farmer JA. Role of insulin signaling in maintaining energy homeostasis. Endocr Pract. 2008;14(3):373-380.

Song B, Thomas DM. Dynamics of starvation in humans. J Math Biol. 2007;54:27-43. doi:10.1007/s00285-006-0037-7.

Stock MJ. Effects of fasting and refeeding on the metabolic response to a standard meal in man. Eur J Appl Physiol Occup Physiol. 1980;43(1):35-40. doi:10.1007/bf00421353.

Stubbs J, Brogeli D, Pallisoter C, Avery A, McConnon A, Lavin J. Behavioural and motivational factors associated with weight loss and maintenance in a commercial weight management programme. Open Obes J. 2012;4:35e43.

Taboulet P, Deconinck N, Thurel A, et al. Correlation between urine ketones (acetoacetate) and capillary blood ketones (3-beta-hydroxybutyrate) in hyperglycaemic patients. Diabetes Metab. 2007;33(2):135-139. doi:10.1016/j.diabet.2006.11.006.

Takaoka A, Sasaki M, Kurihara M, et al. Comparison of energy metabolism and nutritional status of hospitalized patients with Crohn's disease and those with ulcerative colitis. J Clin Biochem Nutr. 2015;56(3):208-214. doi:10.3164/jcbn.14-95.

Urbain P, Berts H. Monitoring for compliance with a ketogenic diet: what is the best time of day to test for urinary ketosis? Nutr Metabl (Lond). 2016;13:77. doi:10.1186/s12986-016-0136-4.

Veverbrants E, Arky RA. Effects of fasting and refeeding: I. Studies on sodium, potassium and water excretion on a constant electrolyte and fluid intake. J Clin Endocrinol Metab. 1969;29(1):55-62. doi:10.1210/jcem-29-1-55.

Volek JS, Noakes T, Phinney SD. Rethinking fat as a fuel for endurance exercise. Eur J Sport Sci. 2015;15(1):13-20. doi:10.1080/17461391.2014.959564.

Volek JS, Phinney SD. The art and science of low carbohydrate living. Coral Gables, FL:Beyond Obesity;2011.

Wacker WEC, Parisi AF. Magnesium metabolism. N Engl J Med. 1968;278:658-663.

Westerterp-Plantenga MS, Nieuwenhuizen A, Tome D, Soenen S, Westerterp KR. Dietary protein, weight loss, and weight maintenance. Annu Rev Nutr. 2009;29:21–41.

Willett G. Sweet talk: the insulin connection. Institute for Natural Resources. February 2013-K.

Chapter 9: Supplements

Adar S, Boldbourt U. Nutritional recommendations for preventing coronary heart disease in women: Evidence concerning whole foods and supplements. *NMCD*. 2010;20(6):459-466. https://doi.org/10.1016/j.numecd.2010.01.011.

ConsumberLab.com. Question: Which dietary supplements and health foods contain high levels of lead? ConsumberLab.com. https://www.consumerlab.com/answers/supplements-and-foods-that-may-be-contaminated-with-lead/lead-contamination-supplements/. Published October 5, 2019. Accessed April 15, 2020.

Council for Responsible Nutrition. Dietary supplement use reaches all time high. Council for Responsible Nutrition. https://www.crnusa.org/newsroom/dietary-supplement-use-reaches-all-time-high. Published September 2019. Accessed April 15, 2020.

Fito M, Konstantinidou V. Nutritional genomics and the Mediterranean diet's effects on human cardiovascular health. Nutrients. 2016;8(4):218. doi:10.3390/nu8040218.

Polak E, Stepien A, Gol O, et al. Potential Immunomodulatory effects from consumption of nutrients in whole foods and supplements on the frequency and course of infection: Preliminary results. *Nutrients*. 2021;13(4). doi.org/10.3390/nu13041157.

Smith T, Gillespie M, Eckl V, Knepper J, Morton-Reynolds C. Herbal supplement sales in US increase by 8.4% in 2018. HerbalGram. 2019;123:62-73.

Statista. Revenue of vitamins & nutritional supplements production in the United States from 2018 and 2019 (in billion U.S. dollars). Statista. https://www.statista.com/statistics/235801/retail-sales-of-vitamins-and-nutritional-supplements-in-the-us/. Published February 2019. Accessed April 15, 2020.

Chapter 10: Exercise

Better Health Channel. Exercise intensity. Better Health Channel. https://www.betterhealth.vic.gov.au/health/HealthyLiving/exercise-intensity. Updated June 2015. Accessed April 14, 2020.

Mathas D. A little theology of exercise. DesiringGod.org. 2020. Accessed September 28, 2021. https://www.desiringgod.org/messages/a-little-theology-of-exercise.

President's Council on Sports, Fitness & Nutrition. Physical activity guidelines for Americans. U.S. Department of Health & Human Services. https://www.hhs.gov/fitness/be-active/physical-activity-guidelines-for-americans/index.html. Reviewed February 2019. Accessed April 14, 2020.

Riebe D, Ehrman JK, Liguori G, Magal M, eds. ACSM's Guidelines for Exercise Testing and Prescription. 10th ed. Philadelphia: Wolters Kluwer; 2018.

Shuler K. What does the Bible say about exercise? 34 fitness and exercise Bible verses. KaseybShuler.com. 2020. Accessed September 28, 2021. https://www.kaseybshuler.com/blog/fitnessverses

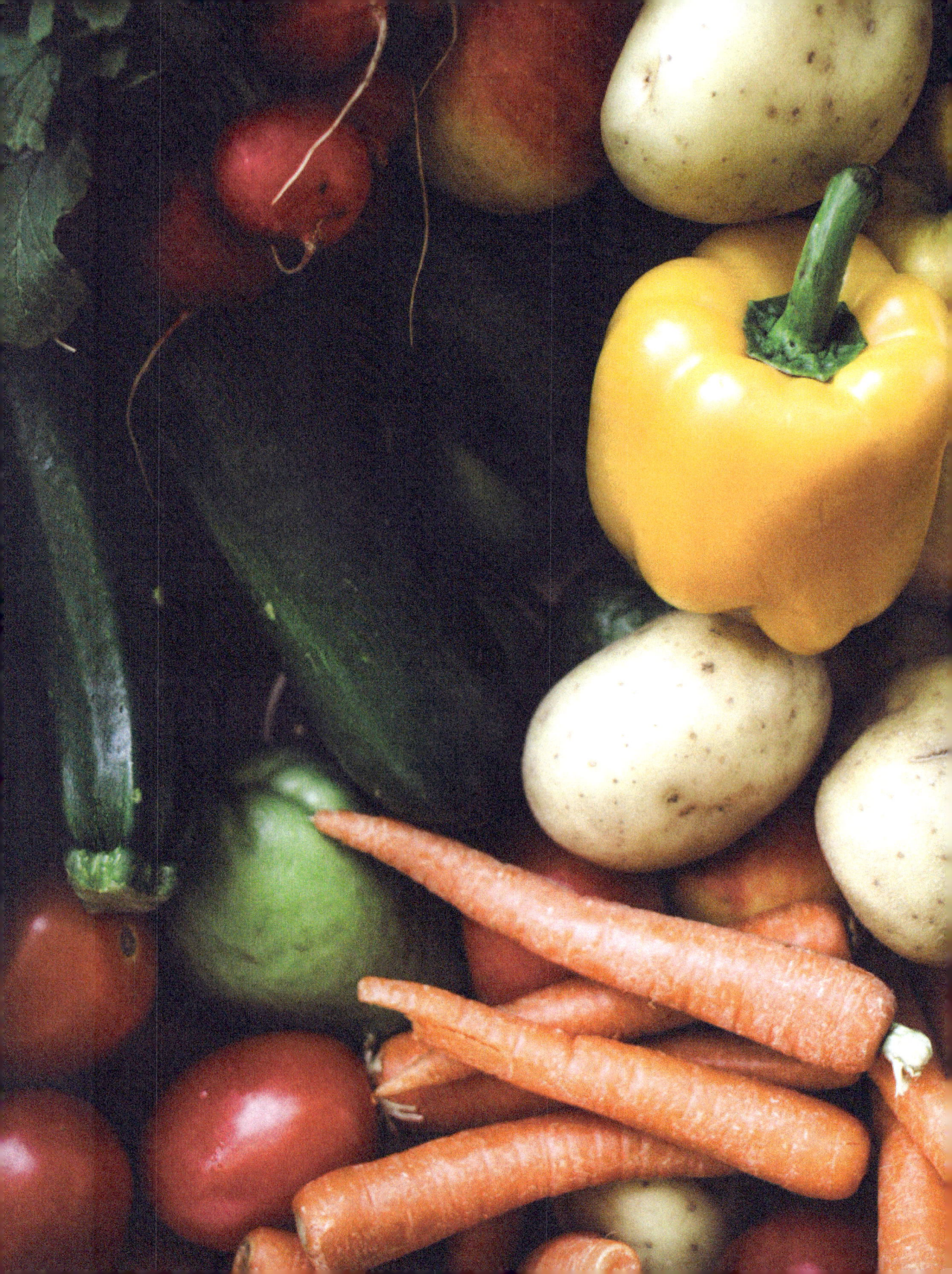

PART 2: CHAPTER 11

Rating the Diets

Rating popular diets

There are so many diets out there that it can make our heads spin. How do we know which diet is best to choose? The answer is: It depends. Not all diets are safe. Not all diets are based on science. Not all diets work. Not all diets were designed for weight loss. This section assesses diets based on their ability to deliver safe, effective weight loss that will last.

The Criteria and Rankings

Each diet in this section is assessed as poor, fair, good or excellent, based on 17 criteria. Those criteria and rankings are listed and defined below.

1. Variety - Food variety means eating foods from all of the food groups (starches, vegetables, fruits, fats, meats, and dairy) in recommended amounts. Eating many different kinds of foods from various food groups helps ensure a range of different nutrients to help the body stay healthy. It is also important to choose a variety of foods from within each food group. Eating a variety of foods can promote good health and help reduce the risk of disease. Different foods provide different types and amounts of essential nutrients, phytonutrients and adds interest, different flavors, aromas and color to the diet which can reduce monotony. It is important to not get bored with the food or meals eaten. After all, for many, it is an event that occurs three times each day. Eating the same food over and over again takes a psychological toll. This is especially true when other types of food are available, seen and within reach.

Poor	Fair	Good	Excellent
2 or more food groups eliminated or 3 or more food groups severely restricted	Eliminates 1 food group or severely restricts 2 or more food groups while emphasizing variety in other groups	Restrictions placed on 1 food group that have not been adequately, scientifically documented	Variety emphasized within each group (e.g., eating the rainbow)

2. Balance - A balanced diet includes combining the nutrients (protein, fat, carbohydrates, water, vitamins and minerals) at each meal and involves consuming them throughout the day. Providing these nutrients in each meal can help with satiety (the feeling of fullness) and help keep the body healthy. Recommendations for a balanced diet include 45-65% of calories coming from carbohydrates, 20-35% from fat, 10-35% from protein, sufficient fluids to stay well hydrated, and adequate vitamins, minerals and fiber.

Poor	Fair	Good	Excellent
Diet eliminates 2 or more food groups or severely restricts 1 or more macronutrients, leading to profound deficiency; diet has days that could be considered extreme (e.g., uncontrolled eating, severe restriction, or overemphasis of 1 macronutrient)	Diet eliminates 1 food group or restricts 1 macronutrient, leading to moderate deficiency	Diet leans too heavily on 1 food group or macronutrient, leading to mild deficiency	Diet provides all food groups and macronutrients at recommended levels

3. Fiber - Women should consume 25 grams of fiber daily. Men should aim for 38 grams of fiber daily. Sources of fiber should come from a variety of foods, including whole grains and cereals, fruits, vegetables and nuts.

Poor	Fair	Good	Excellent
Eliminates many high fiber foods; constipation on this diet is likely	Includes some high fiber foods, but will not meet the recommendation	Meets or exceeds recommendations for fiber (women: 25g & men: 38g) with use of fiber supplements or will be close to recommendation	Meets or exceeds recommendations for fiber (women: 25g & men: 38g) without use of supplements

4. Micronutrients – Micronutrients refers to all the vitamins and minerals needed by the body. A diet that is balanced and has variety should adequately provide these. It is difficult for diets that eliminate entire food groups to provide all the necessary vitamins and minerals. Research has demonstrated that different micronutrients are absorbed with different efficiency. For example, vitamins from animal sources tend to be absorbed better than the same vitamins provided by plant sources. Research also points out that vitamins are better absorbed when the whole food is consumed versus attempting to get them from a pill or dietary supplement.

Poor	Fair	Good	Excellent
Diet eliminates 2 or more food categories and will lead to severe and/or many micronutrient deficiencies	Diet eliminates 1 food category without addressing how to ensure micronutrient adequacy (e.g., eliminates dairy without addressing calcium and vitamin D needs)	Diet will provide all micronutrients through pre-packaged foods or recommends less absorbable forms/sources of micronutrients	Diet will provide all micronutrients without use of supplements or pre-packaged foods

5. Carbohydrates – Carbohydrates are one of the 3 essential macronutrients. It is the body's preferred source of fuel and it provides the health benefits of fiber. Our brain needs a minimum of 130 grams of carbohydrates a day. Our diet should provide adequate amounts of carbohydrates for fuel, health and proper function.

Poor	Fair	Good	Excellent
Recommends eliminating or reducing carbs to 65g or less per day (half of RDA)	Eliminates many healthy sources of carbs or recommends 65-129g of carbs per day	Carbs fall within AMDR or at least meet RDA	Emphasizes complex carbohydrates and making at least half of the grains consumed whole, while overall carb intake remains within AMDR

6. Protein – Protein is one of the 3 essential macronutrients. It is the only macronutrient that can help with the growth and repair of body tissue. We cannot make up for not eating enough protein by overeating on carbohydrates or fats, because they are incapable of doing what protein does. Our need for protein depends on our weight, our goals and our current health status. Our diet needs to provide the unique amount for each of us and needs to provide the 9 essential amino acids in the foods we consume.

Poor	Fair	Good	Excellent
Protein exceeds AMDR by 10% or is recommended to provide 10% or less of calories. Protein recommended is dangerous, leading to muscle wasting or taxing of kidneys	Recommends healthy proteins but at an inappropriate level (exceeds or is less than the AMDR by 5%); or recommends high-fat protein sources while maintaining a percent of calories within the AMDR	Protein falls within AMDR with some healthy sources recommended	Healthy proteins (e.g., lean, plant-based, fish) recommended at appropriate levels rotein falls within AMDR with some healthy sources recommended

7. Fat – Fat is one of the 3 essential macronutrients. While all fats have 9 calories per gram, not all fats are created equal when it comes to health. Our diet needs to provide adequate healthy fats while minimizing unhealthy fats.

Poor	Fair	Good	Excellent
Fat exceeds AMDR by 10% or is recommended to provide 10% or less of calories.	Recommends healthy fats but at an inappropriate level (exceeds or is less than the AMDR by 5%), or recommends high saturated fat while maintaining a percent of calories within the AMDR	Fat falls within AMDR, with some healthy sources recommended	Healthy fats (omega-3s, monounsaturated) recommended at appropriate levels; unhealthy fats (trans fats, saturated fats) recommended at or below appropriate levels

8. Moderation – Moderation is a subjective term. It is relative and individual. In some cases, moderation may include restraint and self-control. It can be defined as the avoidance of excess or extremes or within reasonable limits. In the field of nutrition and eating, it can apply to behaviors, habits and food frequency or amounts. This may translate to occasional, ie., not every day, if we are talking about junk food or eating out. It may translate to reasonable, enough or adequate amounts when it comes to portion sizes. Once familiar with serving sizes, this term may take on more precise meaning.

Poor	Fair	Good	Excellent
Serving sizes are not addressed or are not appropriate for weight loss; foods are permanently labeled "off-limits"	Specific serving sizes are not recommended but general guidelines are provided; "unhealthy foods" are considered off-limits except on rare occasions	Serving sizes are appropriate for most but take a 1 size fits all approach; occasional dessert, junk food, or eating out is allowed but with some restrictions	Diet includes appropriate serving sizes for each calorie level and allows for occasional dessert, junk food, or eating out (i.e., does not take an all or nothing approach)

9.. Calories – Calories matter in weight loss. We need to know how many calories are needed to maintain and lose weight. Diets designed for weight loss need to provide all the nutrients our bodies need while staying within the necessary calories. For example, if a diet provides too few calories based on recommendations (fewer than 1200 calories a day), it was ranked poorly, due to increased risk of lowering basal metabolic rate, decreasing the likelihood of adherence, and increased risk of muscle loss and nutrient deficient. On the other hand, if a diet recommended too many calories for most people to lose weight, it was also ranked poorly. If a diet did not address calories at all, it also received a low score.

Poor	Fair	Good	Excellent
Diet severely restricts calories (<1,200kcals per day), recommends a meal plan that severely restricts calories, or does not address calories	Diet does not directly address calories but provides a menu that will be adequate for most. Discussion of calories is vague. Calories may not promote weight loss in some. Recommends 1,200 to 1,400 Calories.	Diet does not involve a calorie calculation but makes a recommendation that is not below the BMR of most (e.g., 1,200 or 1,400 kcals per day)	Diet considers individual calorie differences and involves a specific calorie calculation

10. Individualized plans – People are unique. We have different schedules, different histories, different tastes, different budgets, different calorie requirements, and different foods available to us. In order for a diet to work, it must be flexible enough to accommodate our differences and different needs. A healthy diet should allow individuals the flexibility to eat with their families and friends. Nobody should feel ostracized or singled out during mealtimes because they have to eat "special/different foods" because they are trying to lose body fat. A successful weight loss program must consider individual needs.

Poor	Fair	Good	Excellent
Has a 1 size fits all approach	Accounts for male/female differences or amount of weight a person has to lose or a fair amount of flexibility	Plan has a multi-level or category approach or allows for some flexibility	Plan can be tailored to person's dietary needs, involves a calorie calculation, and considers other lifestyle factors.

11. Exercise is recommended – Exercise is an important component of weight management and weight loss. Ideally, adults should aim to participate in moderate-intensity physical activity 3 to 5 days each week, for a total of 150 minutes each week. This base should be supplemented with lifting weights, flexibility, and balance training.

Poor	Fair	Good	Excellent
Not recommended while on the diet	Recommended but no plan given	Recommended with plan given, but does not account for individual differences or is inaccurate/ inadequate	Recommended with an accurate plan that can be tailored to each person

12. Enjoyable food – While food nourishes our body, food is also a central part of our social lives. We go out for dinner, we celebrate birthdays, holidays and homecomings. We have around 10,000 taste buds with which to enjoy a variety of flavors. A diet should be flexible enough to accommodate these aspects of our lives. If it does not incorporate the flexibility for us to live and enjoy life's special moments or the unforeseen circumstances that arise, the likelihood of staying on the diet is not good.

Poor	Fair	Good	Excellent
Far too restrictive; makes person feel very deprived; foods recommended are prepared in distasteful ways and/or involve no chewing	Diet is somewhat restrictive; does not include a mindful approach to eating	Mindfulness approach to eating is mentioned but not incorporated into diet; foods are mildly pleasing	Includes mindfulness approach to eating, allows eating to be social/something the whole family can enjoy, and recommends foods that are tasty and appealing

13. Easy to understand – Eating is natural. A diet should not make it so complicated that we are confused or constantly having to think about what we can and can't eat.

Poor	Fair	Good	Excellent
Very complicated diet; based on poorly-explained scientific principles	Diet uses a system that does not fully explain 1 or more aspects	Diet uses an easy-to-use system but has room for improvement	Diet uses a user-friendly system and excellently explains scientific principles that back the diet

14. Sustainability – This is the ability to remain on the diet. If a diet is too strict, too low in calories, unhealthy, monotonous, or too confusing, the likelihood of being able to stay on the diet decreases. Diets that can't be sustained usually claim to speed up the metabolism or quick weight loss. Diets that can't be sustained can lead to yo-yo dieting, binge eating or returning to previous poor eating habits. A diet that is sustainable generally translates into slow, steady, weight loss and slow, consistent behavioral changes which lead to victorious long-term weight loss.

Poor	Fair	Good	Excellent
Diet recommends too few calories or macronutrients to be safely maintained long-term	Diet is too restrictive of food or monotonous to be maintained long-term	Diet is sustainable during weight loss but provides few or no suggestions for maintenance or is moderately restrictive for long-term maintenance	Diet includes a sustainable maintenance or transition phase and builds skills that are helpful in weight maintenance

15. Long-term weight loss – The perspective of "long term" is subjective. Long-term weight loss in research often translates to maintaining weight loss from 1 to 5 years. Weight loss may mean being able to keep even 10% of the lost weight off for a length of time. Most people desire to never regain the weight they lose back. In order to do this, they cannot go "on and off" diets. Keeping weight off long term means consuming a sustainable, well balanced diet filled with flexibility and variety. It also requires patience and a lifestyle change.

Poor	Fair	Good	Excellent
Diet promotes weight loss faster than recommendations of 1-2 pounds per week, which reduces likelihood that weight loss will be maintained	Diet promotes 1 or more healthy skills or slow weight loss that promotes maintenance of weight loss	Diet promotes 2 healthy skills and slow weight loss that promote maintenance of weight loss	Diet promotes 3 or more healthy skills and slow weight loss that promote maintenance of weight loss

16. Educates the consumer – It is easier to follow a diet if we understand why we eat what we eat, why certain preparation methods are used in the kitchen, what nutrients are provided by various foods and how the body functions. Because many diets state false claims based on either false scientific facts or scientific facts twisted to the point they are not applicable in real life, it can be difficult to distinguish between truth and myth.

Poor	Fair	Good	Excellent
Requires many expensive supplements or packaged foods; grocery bill will be significantly more expensive than average grocery bill	Contains some accurate information but either twists that information, resulting in false statements, or scientific unknowns; information is incomplete	Information provided is accurate but based on experiential knowledge	Information provided is accurate and based on scientific knowledge

17. Cost – Obviously, cost matters. What is the point if we can't afford to follow the diet? Diets that require supplements can be very expensive, which may make the diet unsustainable. We should be able to buy food from regular grocery stores nearby.

Poor	Fair	Good	Excellent
Requires many expensive supplements or packaged foods; grocery bill will be significantly more expensive than average grocery bill	Requires purchase of organic only or grass-fed only	Most foods recommended are inexpensive, but recommends some expensive "superfoods" or specialty items	Cost is close to average or even below average grocery bill

Additional Information and Comments

In addition to the specific 17 criteria, more general comments are also provided.

Positive and Negative Aspects of each Diet

Most diets will score high in some areas and low in others. This next portion describes the overall positive and negative aspects of the diet, allowing the dieter to make informed choices in various areas.

Truths and Myths of each Diet

Most diets claim to be based on scientific facts. But since most diets exist to sell books, supplements, programs, or memberships, the claims made may be sensationalized, exaggerated or hyped up. This section discusses statements made by the diet as well as concepts for which the diet is based. This section is provided to help guide dieters to a better understanding of the science behind how a diet works (or doesn't work.) Some diets will have magnifying glass icons in this section. This icon is provided for dieters who want to know more about a specific topic or concept. The icon provides page numbers that direct the dieter to the relevant foundational scientific information on which the diet of interest is based.

Final Decision (Thumbs Up or Thumps Down)

Lastly, an overall final decision of thumbs up or thumbs down is made. This decision is based on the likelihood that I would agree to or encourage a loved one (my mother, my sisters, my children) to go on this diet. This decision takes into account the 17 criteria, the pain and or suffering likely to be experienced, the reasonableness and safety of the methods used for weight loss, the likelihood of damaging body and the, likelihood of long-term success. I hate to watch loved ones suffer needlessly while dieting, only to regain the weight and be worse off than when they started. And I don't want this for you either!

Suggestions for Improvement

While some diets are so far off the mark nothing can be done to improve them, other diets could be made better with some tweaking. Suggestions for how each diet can be improved are also provided.

Blank Templates

Please keep in mind that diets are like fashion. They come and they go. They recycle and experience name changes. The truth is, nobody will ever be able to "know" all the diets that exist. Even if we know a diet by one name, the same diet could go underground and reemerge with a new name years later, but in essence it is the same diet.

When a student asks for my opinion about a weight loss diet I have never heard of, I simply ask them to describe the diet. Depending on their answers to the above criteria, a thumbs up or a thumbs down can be determined.

While many of the popular diets are rated here, new weight loss diets will come along. That is why blank templates are provided at the end of this section. Using the recommendations and scientific facts provided in the first section, along with the 17 criteria, as you encounter new diets, use the blank templates to assess them. The ultimate goal behind me, a registered dietitian, rating the diets is for you to learn the process of how to assess diets so you can continue to practice the procedures as a way to keep yourself healthy and safe.

Just a reminder to use the "more information" icons for quick and useful information regarding the diets which interest you most.

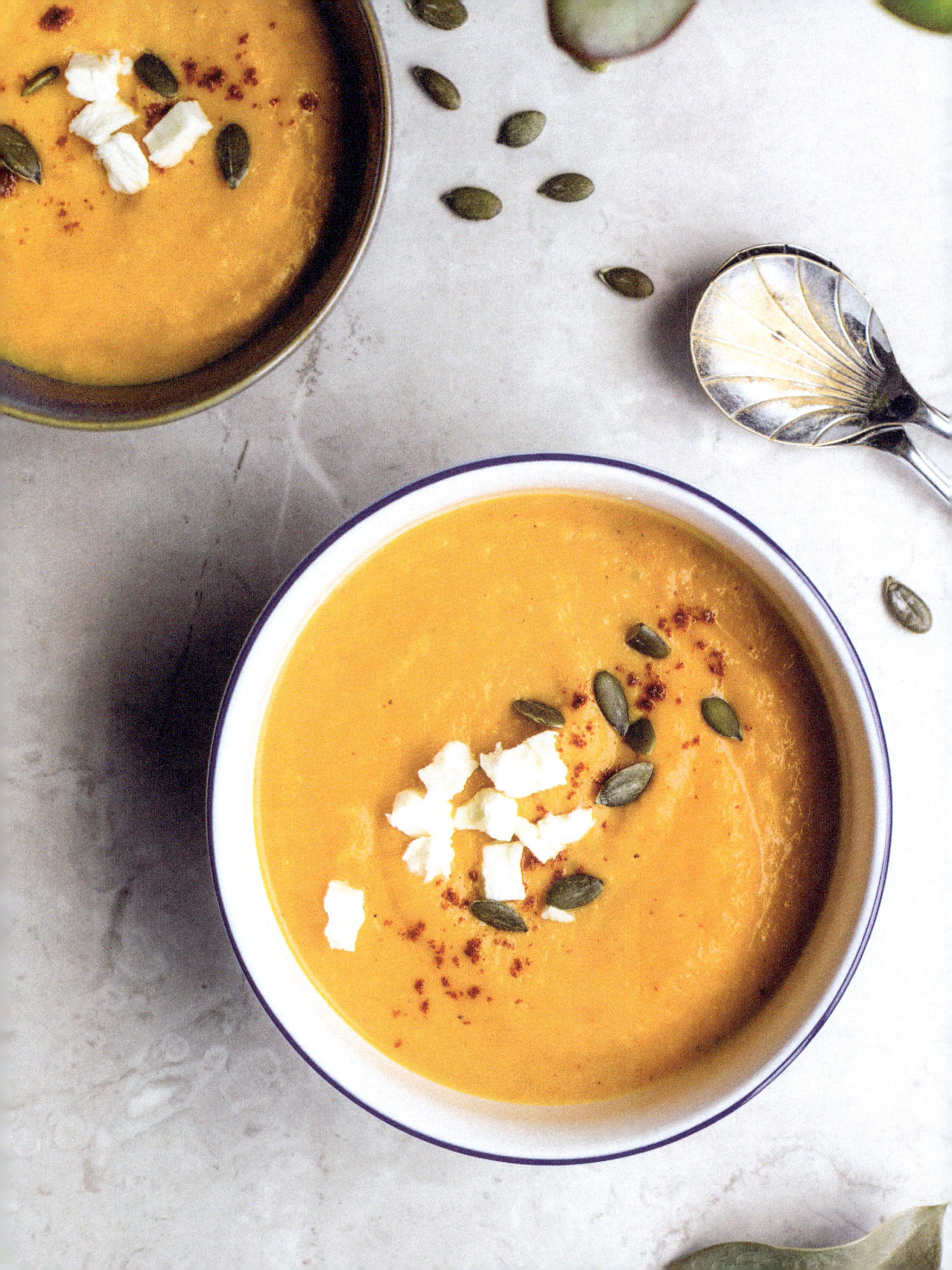

Diets Listed in Alphabetical Order

02 Diet

310 Diet Plan

Alkaline Diet

Apple Cider Vinegar Diet

Atkins Diet

Baby Food Diet

Beachbody – The 21 Day Fix

Belly Fat Cure Diet

Best Life Diet

The Big Breakfast Diet

Biggest Loser Diet

Biggest Loser Simple Swaps Diet

Body for Life Diet

Body Reset Diet

Brown Fat Revolution Diet

Bullet Proof Diet

Cabbage Soup Diet

Carb Lovers Diet

Caveman Diet (aka: Paleo, Stone Age diet, Hunter-gatherer diet)

Cheater's Diet

Clean and Lean Diet: 30 Days, 30 Foods, A New You.

Cookie Diet

Cruise Control Diet

DASH Diet Weight Loss Solution (aka Dietary Approaches to Stop Hypertension)

Diet Solution (aka The Beyond Diet)

Diet-to-go

Dr. Andrew Weil Diet

Dr. Phil's Ultimate Weight Solution (aka: Dr. Phil's 20/20 Ultimate Weight Solution)

Dukan Diet

Eat Clean Diet

Eat More Weigh Less Diet

Eat Right for Your Type Diet

Eat This, Not That Diet

Eat to Live Diet (aka Nutritarian Diet)

Eat What You Love, Love What You Eat Diet

Eco Atkins Diet

Engine 2 Diet

F-Factor Diet

Fast Diet

Fast Food Diet

Fast Metabolism Diet

Faster Way to Fat Loss Program

Fat Smash Diet

Five Factor Diet

Flat Belly Diet

Flavor Point Diet

Flexitarian Diet

Four Day Diet

French Women Don't Get Fat Diet: The Secretes of Eating for Pleasure

Fruit Flush Diet

FullBar Diet

Gene Smart Diet

Genotype Diet

Gluten Free Diet

Glycemic Index Diet

GOLO Diet

Good Calories Bad Calories

Grapefruit Diet

Hallelujah Diet

hCG Diet

High School Reunion Diet

Hormone Diet

Instinct Diet

Intermittent Fasting Diet

Jenny Craig Diet

Keto Fast Diet

Keto Cycle

Keto Diet Hypnosis

Ketogenic Diet

Kind Diet

LA Weight Loss Diet

Lemonade Diet

Living Low Carb Diet
Macrobiotic Diet
Maker's Diet
Martha's Vineyard Diet
Master you Metabolism Diet
Mayo Clinic Diet
Medifast Diet
Mediterranean Diet
Morning Banana Diet
Naturally Thin Diet
New Beverly Hill Diet
Noom
NutriSystem Diet
Obesity Code
Omega-Z Diet
Optavia Diet
Park Avenue Diet
Perricone Diet
Personality Type Diet
Potato Hack Diet
Pritikin Principle
Protein Power Diet
Raw Food Diet
Rice Diet
Senza Diet
Seventeen Day Diet
Shangri-La Diet
Skinny Bastard Diet
Skinny Vegan Diet

Slim Fast Diet
Sonoma Diet
South Beach Diet
Special K Diet
Spectrum Diet
Step Diet
Sugar Busters
The Trinity Diet
Thin for Life Diet
This is Why You're Fat Diet
Three Day Diet
Three Hour Diet
Ultrametabolism Diet
Volumetrics
Warrior Diet
Weigh Down Diet
Weight Loss Cure Diet
Weight Watchers Diet
Werewolf Diet
What Color is Your Diet
Wheat Belly Diet
Whole 30 Diet
Zone Diet
Zero Belly Diet

02 Diet

Premise of the Diet: Based on the ORAC Scale.

Claims of the Diet: Slows down aging, provides more energy, and promotes weight loss.

Diet Description: A 32-day plan that provides the ORAC (oxygen radical absorbance capacity) scale and counts ORAC points. This scale measures how well a food protects against free radicals by identifying antioxidant concentration in foods. The higher the ORAC score, the better. Top-rated foods include leafy greens, prunes, blueberries, and nuts, while fried foods, baked goods, sugar- and fat-free processed foods, processed meats, and soda are off limits.

Phase 1, which lasts 4 days, is a "cleanse" and consists of 50,000 ORAC points per day on very few calories. Drink water and green tea.

Phase 2 consists of 2 weeks of 30,000 ORAC points daily; portions are controlled and lots of fresh fruits and vegetables are eaten.

Phase 3 lasts for 2 weeks and continues with 30,000 ORAC points daily, adding one indulgence per week.

Phase 4 is ongoing, uses Phase 3 guidelines, and adds one more indulgence per week and one more high-ORAC fruit per day.

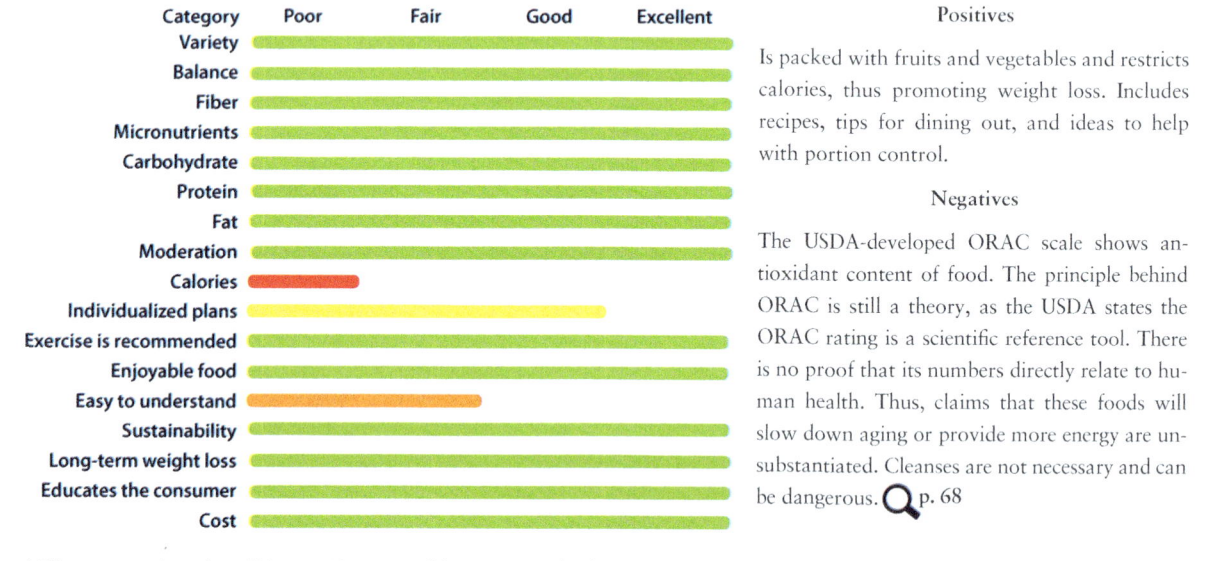

Category	Rating
Variety	Excellent
Balance	Excellent
Fiber	Excellent
Micronutrients	Excellent
Carbohydrate	Excellent
Protein	Excellent
Fat	Excellent
Moderation	Excellent
Calories	Poor
Individualized plans	Good
Exercise is recommended	Excellent
Enjoyable food	Excellent
Easy to understand	Fair
Sustainability	Excellent
Long-term weight loss	Excellent
Educates the consumer	Excellent
Cost	Excellent

Positives

Is packed with fruits and vegetables and restricts calories, thus promoting weight loss. Includes recipes, tips for dining out, and ideas to help with portion control.

Negatives

The USDA-developed ORAC scale shows antioxidant content of food. The principle behind ORAC is still a theory, as the USDA states the ORAC rating is a scientific reference tool. There is no proof that its numbers directly relate to human health. Thus, claims that these foods will slow down aging or provide more energy are unsubstantiated. Cleanses are not necessary and can be dangerous. 🔍 p. 68

*All scores are based on Skipping Phase 1 and beginning with Phase 2.

The hook/catch or brilliant selling point: Popularized by author Keri Glassman, a nationally renowned healthy living expert.

Truths/Myths: None worth noting.

Final decision: Thumbs up 👍

How to improve this diet: Skip Phase 1 and begin with Phase 2.

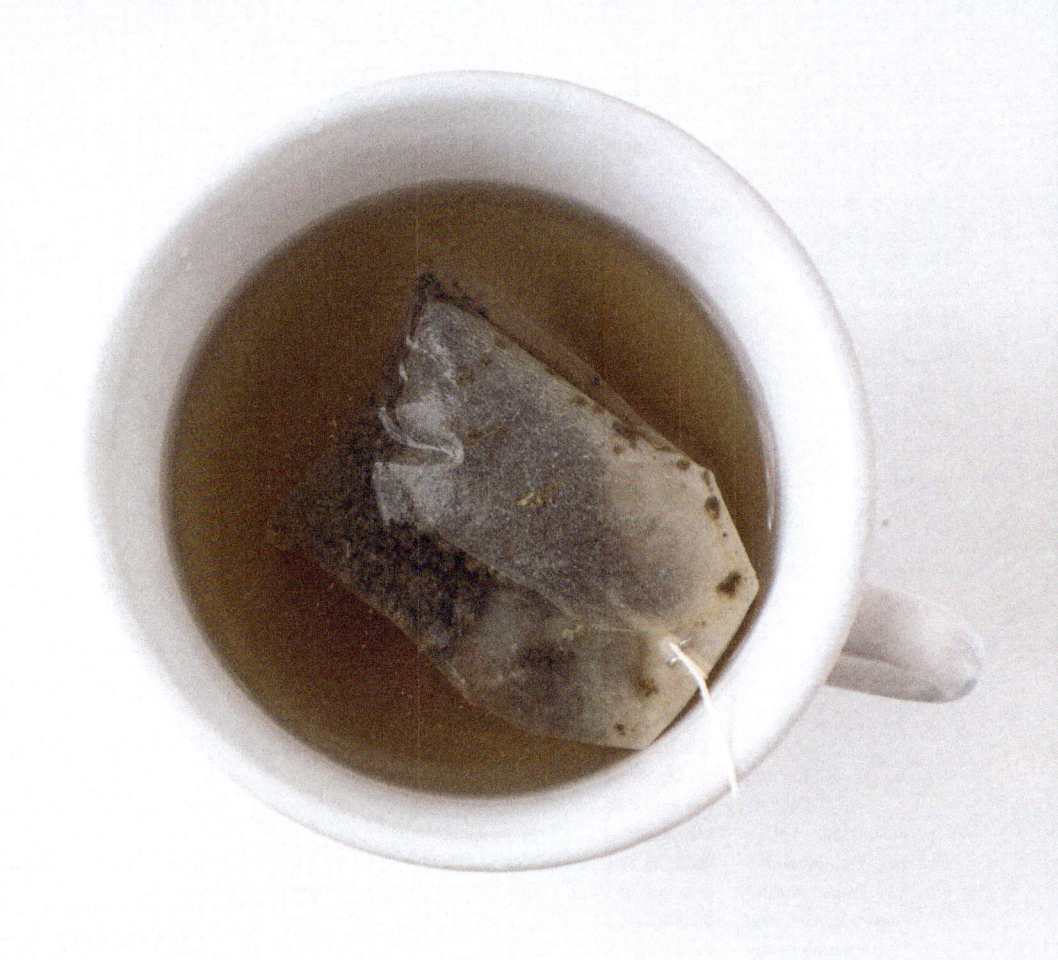

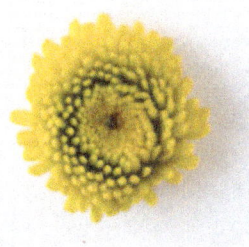

You will always live happy if you live with heart.

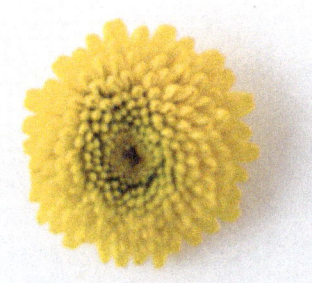

310 Diet Plan

Premise of the Diet: Replace meals with the company's products and lose weight.

Claims of the Diet: The ingredient lists are so good that your doctor will be thoroughly impressed.

Diet Description: The 310 Diet Plan consists of a 90-calorie powdered drink mix designed to replace two meals. A clean, healthy, balanced meal is to be consumed in the evening. A bottle or bag of 310 Shake costs $68 and contains 28 single-scoop servings lasting about 14 days. Shakes are dairy-free, gluten-free, soy-free, and sugar-free. Each serving contains approximately 15g of protein, 8g of carbs, and 5g of fiber. A newly available formulation claims to contain three types of protein, versus one in the original shake. The plan also sells 310 Tea (to be consumed hot or iced) for a full-body cleanse, which the company indicates can energize the body, assist with digestion, control appetite, and replace unhealthy snacking. Also offered are 310 Lemonades to replace sugary drinks; they help to alkalize the body, support a healthy metabolism, and satisfy a sweet tooth. And 310 Berry Greens, a mix of 70 fruits and vegetables containing enzymes and probiotics, can also be purchased.

Category	Poor	Fair	Good	Excellent
Variety	●			
Balance	●			
Fiber	●			
Micronutrients	●			
Carbohydrate	●			
Protein	●			
Fat	●			
Moderation	●			
Calories	●			
Individualized plans	●			
Exercise is recommended	●			
Enjoyable food	●			
Easy to understand	●			
Sustainability	●			
Long-term weight loss	●			
Educates the consumer	●			
Cost	●			

Positives

Simple, convenient, and easy to follow. Products are high in protein, which can help maintain lean tissue and curb hunger. Products are easily accessible. Offers vegetarian products and recipes too. Provides the "My 310" App enabling connection with others in the 310 Community, access to recipe ideas, and connection with a health coach.

Negatives

Does not emphasize or promote exercise. Once off this diet, going back to regular eating habits can result in weight regain. Can be costly. Because it emphasizes calories rather than nutrients, following a healthy diet is never really learned. This program is missing education about behavioral modifications and the development of other healthy habits that are needed for long-term success, such as portion control. Studies have shown dieting with changing behaviors to be effective only short-term. Recommended foods are primarily processed foods. Does not provide a structured transition or maintenance plan. Does not meet the USDA's definition of a healthy meal plan.

The hook/catch or brilliant selling point: Simple and Easy.

Truths/Myths

- **Myth:** This is a healthy method to lose weight.

- **Truth:** Because diets that promote eating processed prepackaged foods like bars and shakes instead of real foods aren't sustainable or nutritious, they are not healthy and won't result in long-lasting, satisfying results.

Final decision: Thumbs down

How to improve this diet: Instead of eating a few prepackaged meals and one "real" meal, go ahead and make all your meals "real"—meaning they are fresh, satisfying, full of variety, meet the US Dietary Guidelines, and adhere to a calorie level necessary for slow and steady weight loss.

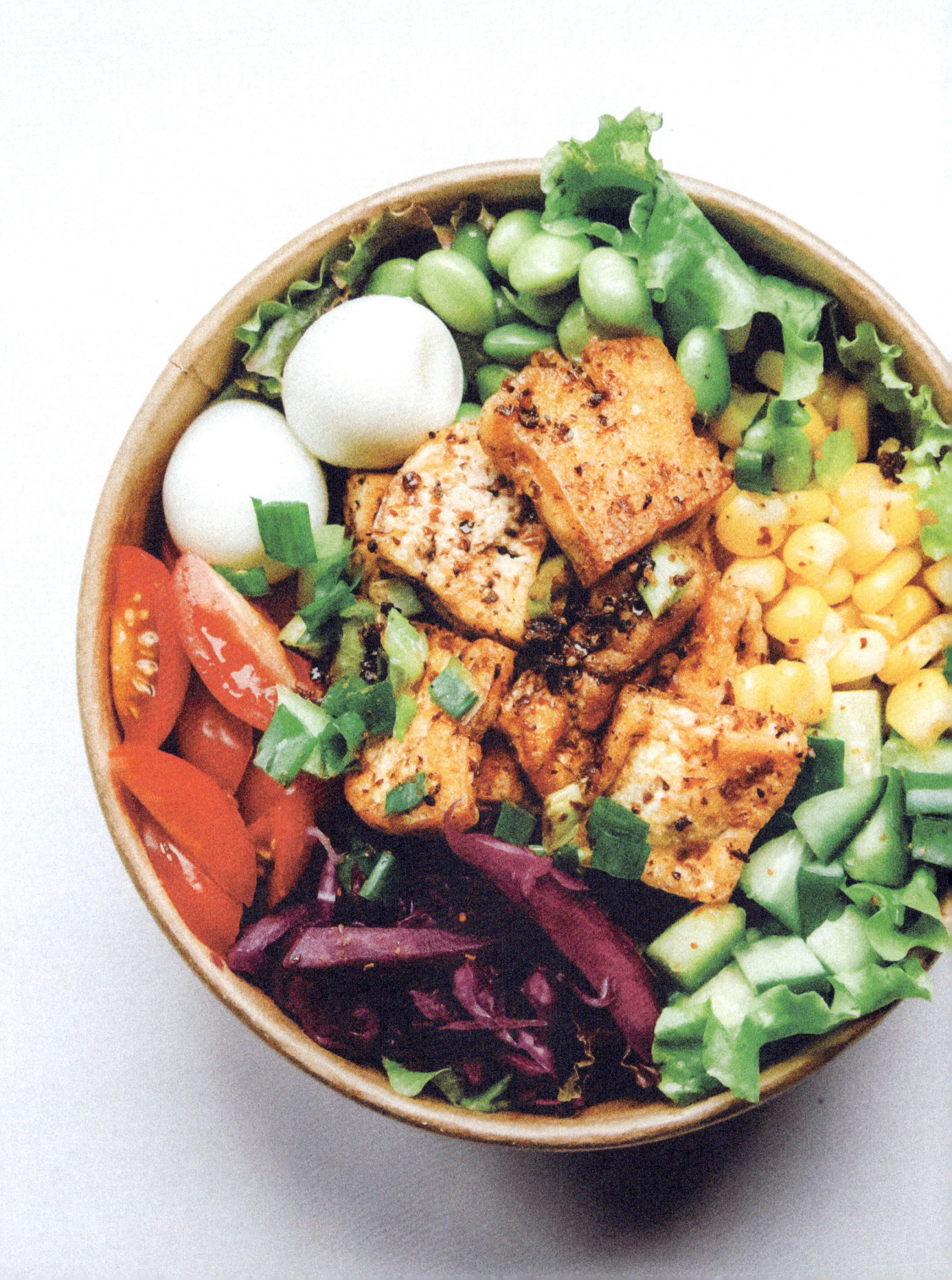

The Alkaline Diet (aka Acid-Alkaline Diet or Alkaline Ash diet)

Premise of the Diet: Foods eaten can change body pH levels. Eating acidic foods makes blood more acidic. Eating alkaline foods makes blood more alkaline.

Claims of the Diet: Having acidic blood makes us more vulnerable to illness and disease. Choosing foods that are more alkaline improves health.

Diet Description: Eat foods that are alkaline, like fruits, vegetables, nuts, and legumes, while avoiding acidic foods like meat, fish, poultry, eggs, dairy, grains, and alcohol. Neutral foods include natural fats, starches, and sugars.

The hook/catch or brilliant selling point: We have total control over our health, all we need to do is choose the "right" foods.

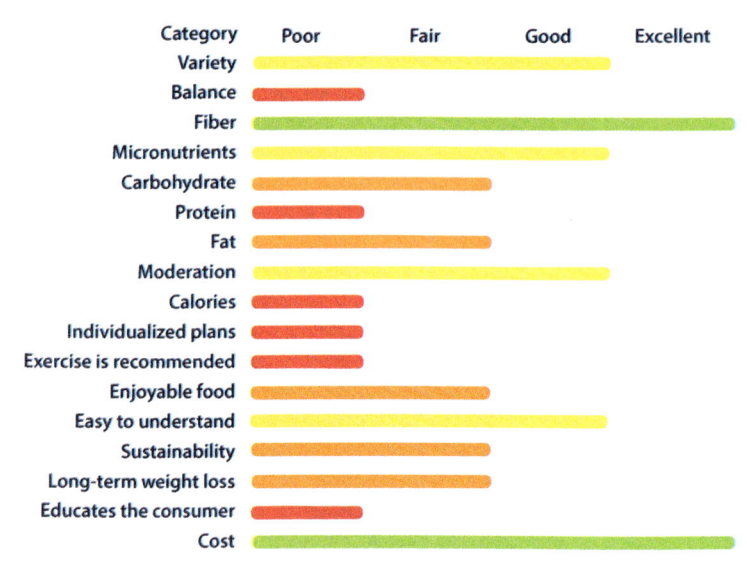

Category	Rating
Variety	Good
Balance	Poor
Fiber	Excellent
Micronutrients	Good
Carbohydrate	Fair
Protein	Poor
Fat	Fair
Moderation	Good
Calories	Poor
Individualized plans	Poor
Exercise is recommended	Poor
Enjoyable food	Fair
Easy to understand	Good
Sustainability	Fair
Long-term weight loss	Fair
Educates the consumer	Poor
Cost	Excellent

Positives

Encourages nutrient-dense fruits, vegetables, legumes, and nuts. Focuses on health, not "getting skinny."

Negatives

Eliminates three major food groups (meats, grain, and dairy). Requires careful planning to ensure adequate protein is consumed. Overconsumption of neutral foods like fat and sugar is associated with many chronic health conditions, including obesity. May become deficient in micronutrients found in meat and animal products. Because meat, grain, and dairy are eliminated, many complementary proteins will also be eliminated, which can result in specific amino acid deficiencies.

Truths/Myths:

• Myth - The alkaline diet raises blood pH to make it less acidic, which promotes weight loss and decreases the likelihood of disease.

• Truth - This diet encourages eating more fruits and vegetables and fewer processed meats and high-fat dairy, and years of research indicate these are nutrient-dense foods that are healthy for the body. Thus, health is not achieved by changing blood pH.

• Myth - It is possible to change blood pH by eating certain foods. 🔍 p. 89

• Truth - While a change in the pH of urine and saliva is possible by manipulating the diet and one's metabolism, the pH of blood remains the same.

• Myth - It is important to drink alkaline water.

• Truth - Most alkaline water brands are is just like other bottled water, with a slightly different mineral content. It cannot change blood pH.

• Myth - Foods eaten have a tremendous impact on body pH levels. Acid-forming diets have an impact on body or bone calcium levels and make the body more susceptible to illness.

• Truth - The pH value ranges from 0 to14. Acidic is considered 0.0–6.9. Neutral is 7.0. Alkaline (aka basic) is 7.1–14. Within the body, pH values vary. Some parts are acidic, others are alkaline. The stomach secretes and contains hydrochloric acid, making it a very acidic environment with a pH around 2–3.5. Normal blood pH is tightly regulated. It is kept between 7.35 and 7.45. If blood pH falls out of this normal range, it can be fatal. This can occur during ketoacidosis caused by diabetes, starvation, and excessive alcohol consumption. Osteoporosis is characterized by reduced density and quality of bone mineral content, and it results in porous and fragile bones. This diet speaks to the "Acid—Ash Hypothesis of Osteoporosis," claiming this progressive bone disease may result because the body seeps alkaline minerals, like calcium from bones, in order to buffer acidic foods eaten. However, this idea discounts the fact that the kidneys and other organs work to carefully monitor pH. Kidneys produce bicarbonate ions that neutralize acids in blood. Bicarbonate ions from kidneys bind to acids in the blood, forming carbon dioxide, which we can either exhale or urinate out of the body. While scientific evidence is mixed, and more research needs to be done on the relationship of bone density and dietary acid, eating a variety of foods including lean proteins is recommended.

• Myth - This diet can reverse cancer.

• Truth - While in vitro studies show that cancer grows in an acidic environment, no scientific evidence directly supports this claim to be true in the complex human body. A diet high in fruits, vegetables, and whole grains, which provide vitamins C, A, and fiber, might reduce cancer risk, especially when combined with avoiding processed high-fat foods and soft drinks.

• Myth - This alkaline diet can change a highly acidic environment.

• Truth - Correcting a highly acidic environment with supplements such as bicarbonate can promote alkalinity, but this does not mean the alkaline diet will have the same effect.

• Truth - Raising the pH of urine (making it less acidic) may improve health for those with kidney disease, as a lower-acid diet may slow the disease's course and improve some symptoms.

Final decision: Thumbs down

How to improve this diet: Incorporate meat, grain, and dairy in moderation.

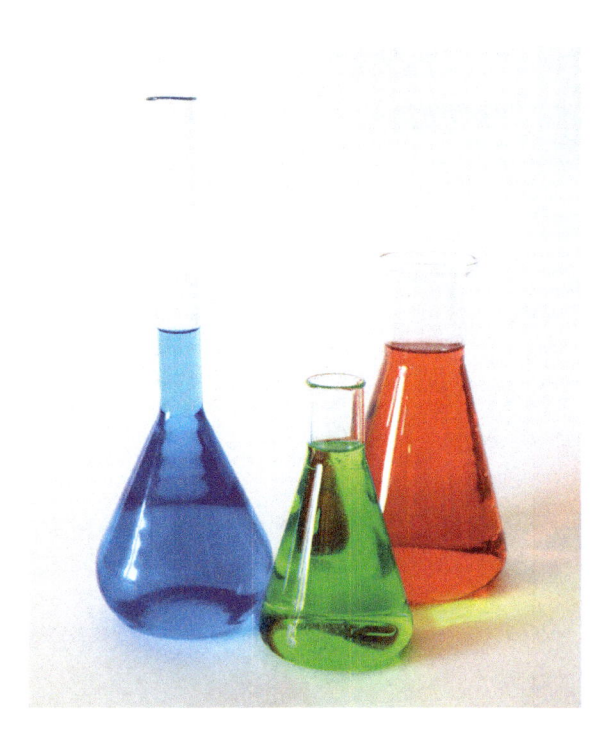

Apple Cider Vinegar Diet

Premise of the Diet: Compounds containing vinegar have been used for their "presumed" healing properties for a long time. In spite of the lack of scientific evidence, it has been used to improve strength, detoxify, treat sore throats, acne, wounds, dandruff, and varicose veins. So why not try it for weight loss, too?

Claims of the Diet: Among other compounds, apple cider vinegar contains high levels of acetic acid, which may be responsible for its supposed health benefits. Although recommendations for "dosing" vary, most recommend 1 to 2 teaspoons before or with meals.

Diet Description: While different recommendations exist, in general the diet recommends consuming 1-2 teaspoons of apple cider vinegar prior to meals or at least once a day.

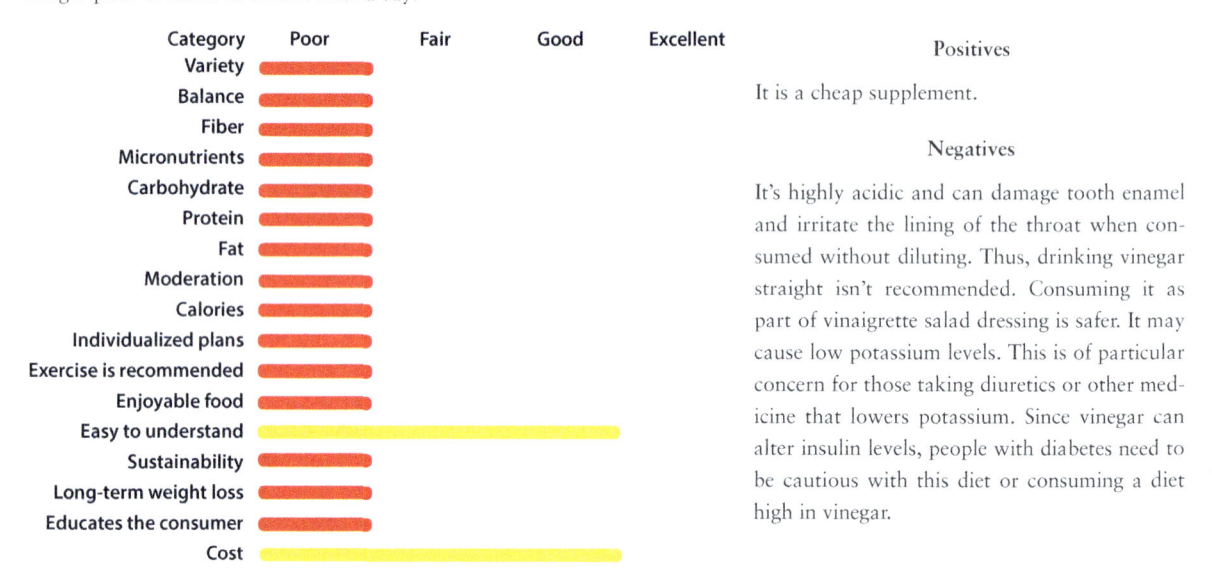

Category	Rating
Variety	Poor
Balance	Poor
Fiber	Poor
Micronutrients	Poor
Carbohydrate	Poor
Protein	Poor
Fat	Poor
Moderation	Poor
Calories	Poor
Individualized plans	Poor
Exercise is recommended	Poor
Enjoyable food	Poor
Easy to understand	Excellent
Sustainability	Poor
Long-term weight loss	Poor
Educates the consumer	Poor
Cost	Excellent

Positives

It is a cheap supplement.

Negatives

It's highly acidic and can damage tooth enamel and irritate the lining of the throat when consumed without diluting. Thus, drinking vinegar straight isn't recommended. Consuming it as part of vinaigrette salad dressing is safer. It may cause low potassium levels. This is of particular concern for those taking diuretics or other medicine that lowers potassium. Since vinegar can alter insulin levels, people with diabetes need to be cautious with this diet or consuming a diet high in vinegar.

*This diet rated poorly in most categories because it provides no guidance related to food consumption. It is treated as a supplement, as opposed to modifying one's diet for healthy weight loss.

The hook/catch or brilliant selling point: Natural remedies must be safe. If there is no risk, why not try it?

Truths/Myths

- Myth - When it comes to weight loss, the Apple Cider Vinegar diet is a good solution.

- Truth - While some study results examining obese rats and mice suggest acetic acid may prevent fat deposition and improve their metabolism, human studies are lacking. One study found a 2-4 pound weight loss after 3 months of taking apple cider vinegar. But studies of apple cider vinegar for weight loss have not shown to be significant or sustainable for humans. In fact, one study found consuming vinegar brought about feelings of fullness after eating, but it did so by causing nausea.

- Truth - Though some studies have been promising, there's still little evidence to prove drinking apple cider vinegar helps with weight loss.

- Truth - Organic apple cider vinegar may contain harmful bacteria due to the lack of pasteurization or distillation.

Final decision: Thumbs down

How to improve this diet: Cannot be improved. Apple cider vinegar most likely won't be harmful; it is calorie-free and adds flavor

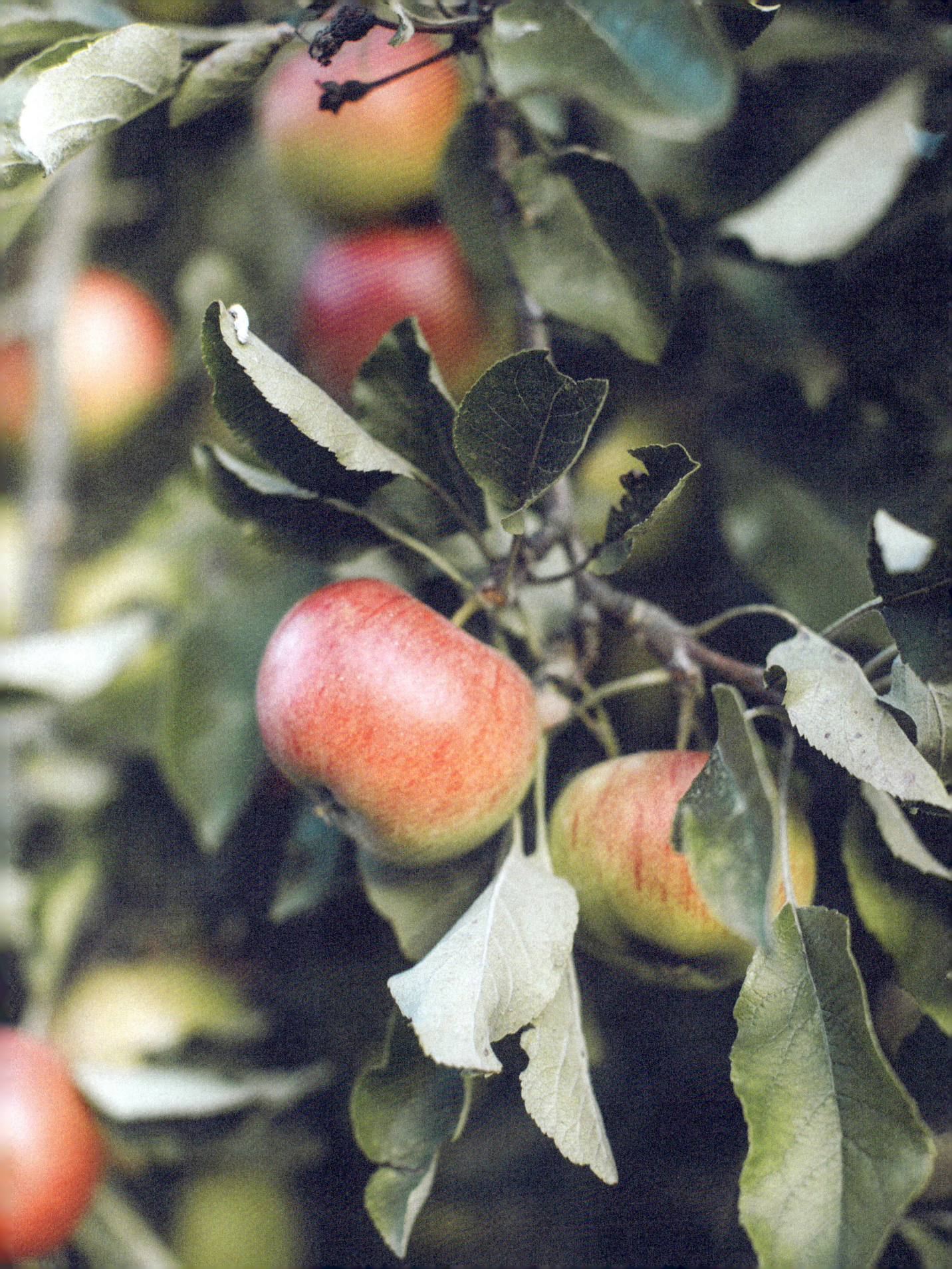

Original Atkins Diet
(aka Atkins 20; Atkins 40; Atkins 100)

Premise of the Diet: When there is too much sugar in the bloodstream, the body stores it as fat. A low-carb diet will help the body burn fat instead of sugar for fuel.

Claims of the Diet: Expect to lose 1-2 lbs. per week. Will help improve health. Improves health markers for heart disease, insulin resistance, and diabetes. Will "flip the body's metabolic switch" from burning carbs to burning fat. Limits blood sugar and insulin spikes. Dieter will not experience hunger or cravings.

Diet Description: This diet provides 3 different plans. For those who have over 40 pounds to lose and/or are diabetic, begin with 20 grams of carbs. Those who have less than 40 pounds to lose, who desire a wider variety of food choices at the start of their diet, or who are breastfeeding with the goal to lose weight should begin with 40 grams of carbohydrates. Those who want to maintain their current weight should consume 100 grams of carbs. The diet plan a person goes on, 20, 40, or 100, will affect the category rankings below.

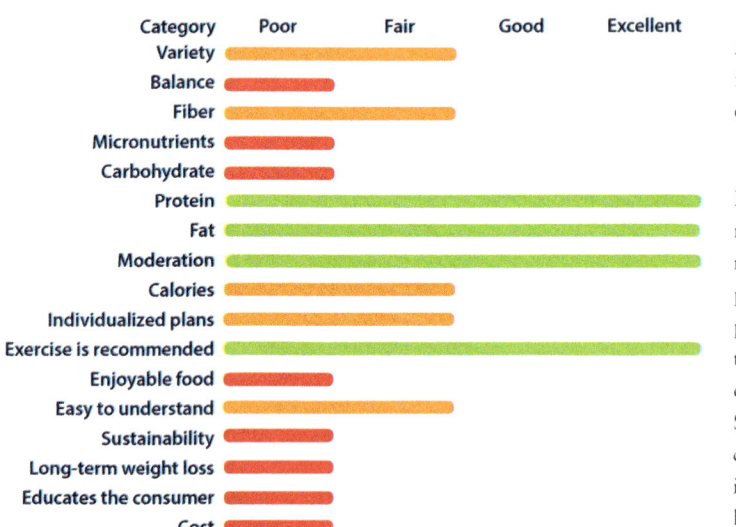

Category	Poor	Fair	Good	Excellent
Variety		Fair		
Balance	Poor			
Fiber		Fair		
Micronutrients	Poor			
Carbohydrate	Poor			
Protein				Excellent
Fat				Excellent
Moderation				Excellent
Calories		Fair		
Individualized plans		Fair		
Exercise is recommended				Excellent
Enjoyable food	Poor			
Easy to understand		Fair		
Sustainability	Poor			
Long-term weight loss	Poor			
Educates the consumer	Poor			
Cost	Poor			

Positives

Adequate protein is consumed. Limits sugary foods and processed grains. Recommends eating every 3-4 hours.

Negatives

Does not provide sufficient complex carbs. Does not provide the health benefits that accompany fiber in complex carbohydrates. With the prevalence of carbohydrates in society, it is not practical to think someone will be able to avoid them long term. Carbohydrates are the foundation of all diets in every country and nation. Suggests pricy branded snacks and foods. When cheaper foods like rice and potatoes are removed in lieu of more pricy foods, cost of this diet can be prohibitive.

The hook/catch or brilliant selling point: It is easy to point the finger at one villain. Eliminate that one and we are home free!

Truths/Myths

- **Myth** - Carbs and weight loss are closely related.

- **Truth** - Actually, reducing calories and weight loss are closely related. 🔍 p. 21

- **Myth** - Everyone's metabolism can use two different types of fuel for energy: either sugar (and carbs that are quickly turned into sugar by the body) or fat. But the type of fuel burned can have a big difference in losing or maintaining weight. A typical diet reduces calories, but is still high in carbohydrates (and thus sugar).

- **Truth** - Actually, everyone's metabolism can use varying components of carbohydrates, fats, proteins and alcohol for fuel, depending on what is available and what the demands of the body are at any given moment. Simple sugars can turn into glucose quickly and are therefore a rather immediate source of fuel, while consumed complex carbohydrates, fat and protein have to undergo more processes, but this is not bad. A combination of a variety of complex carbohydrates is recommended for a sustained feeling of satisfaction and many health benefits accompany consuming complex carbohydrates. 🔍 p. 65

- **Myth** - Many people constantly cycle between sugar "highs" (where excess sugar is actually stored as fat in the body) and sugar "lows" (where you feel fatigued and ravenously hungry – for more carbs and sugar). 🔍 p. 75

- **Truth** - Candy bars and foods with simple sugars can cause an immediate rise in blood sugar and then a potential crash, depending on if any other food sources are consumed. Therefore, eating a candy bar or other sugary food (especially alone and with no other "healthy" food) is not recommended. The body can quickly turn consumed carbohydrates into glucose (blood sugar). Fat and protein do have to go through more metabolic processes in order to be used as fuel.

- **Myth** - limiting carbohydrates (sugar) means the body will burn fat, including body fat, for fuel.

- **Truth** - Limiting calories (regardless of their source) means the body may have to tap into body fat for fuel. Eating calories that provide carbs, proteins and fats in recommended amounts and in sufficient amounts to meet BMR while exercising is the best way to burn body fat.

- **Myth** - Weight is lost, even when more calories are consumed. 🔍 p. 21

- **Truth** - If more calories are consumed than the body burns, the body will store excess calories as fat.

- **Truth** - Steady fueling also means more constant energy levels all day long and less hunger and cravings! Consuming healthy foods more frequently, like the 3-4 hour window Atkins recommends, would have the same effect as consuming Akins-approved foods with that frequency.

- **Myth** - There are no dangers associated with this style of eating. 🔍 p. 13

- **Truth** - This type of diet should only be conducted under the close supervision of a physician. Attempting to try this diet without a physician's supervision can be dangerous because of the likelihood of "cheating." Breaking ketosis by eating carbohydrates (cheating) can be dangerous. 🔍 p. 84

Final decision: Thumbs down 👎

How to improve this diet: Add adequate carbohydrates in the form of complex carbohydrates. Carbohydrates should be at least 45-65% of all calories consumed. Continue to eat a variety of fruits, vegetables and lean meats, and consume no more than 35% of calories from fat sources.

Baby Food Diet

Premise of the Diet: Eating baby food as a meal replacement will help with portion control and therefore assist in losing weight or maintaining the weight already lost.

Claims of the Diet: Swapping meals for baby food promises quick weight loss.

Diet Description: Replace two meals and snacks every day with 14 jars of baby food. Eat a regular evening meal. Jars of baby food might range from 20 to 100 calories.

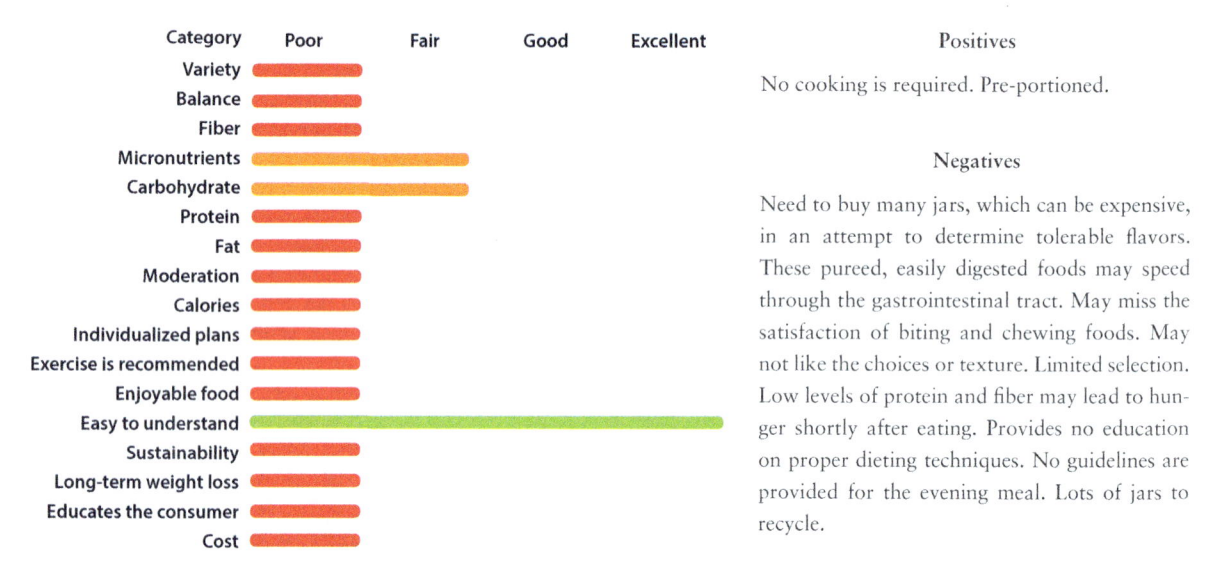

Category	Poor	Fair	Good	Excellent
Variety	▬			
Balance	▬			
Fiber	▬			
Micronutrients	▬▬▬▬			
Carbohydrate	▬▬▬▬			
Protein	▬			
Fat	▬			
Moderation	▬			
Calories	▬			
Individualized plans	▬			
Exercise is recommended	▬			
Enjoyable food	▬			
Easy to understand				▬▬▬▬▬▬▬▬
Sustainability	▬			
Long-term weight loss	▬			
Educates the consumer	▬			
Cost	▬			

Positives

No cooking is required. Pre-portioned.

Negatives

Need to buy many jars, which can be expensive, in an attempt to determine tolerable flavors. These pureed, easily digested foods may speed through the gastrointestinal tract. May miss the satisfaction of biting and chewing foods. May not like the choices or texture. Limited selection. Low levels of protein and fiber may lead to hunger shortly after eating. Provides no education on proper dieting techniques. No guidelines are provided for the evening meal. Lots of jars to recycle.

The hook/catch or brilliant selling point: So easy to use! These are prepackaged, tiny portioned meal replacements. Anyone can lose weight with this method.

Truths/Myths

- **Truth** - Adults can't live healthily on infant-sized portions. Will quickly become bored with this diet. It is not sustainable; therefore, any weight lost will be regained once off the diet. Biting and chewing foods provide satisfaction, and this has been removed from this diet.

- **Myth** - Eating baby food is a good way to lose weight.

Final decision: Thumbs down 👎

How to improve this diet: Can't be improved.

Beachbody Diet (aka The 21 Day Fix)

Premise of the Diet: Uses portion-controlled, color-coded food containers combined with daily exercises designed to promote weight loss.

Claims of the Diet: Lose up to 15 pounds in 3 weeks

Diet Description: This diet involves a portion-controlled diet plan with different calorie target ranges: Plan A: 1,200–1,499 calories, Plan B: 1,500–1,799 calories, Plan C: 1,800–2,099 calories, Plan D: 2,100–2,300 calories. The diet consists of 40% of calories from carbohydrates, 30% from protein, and 30% from fat. The plan also includes a workout guide of home exercises that use either a DVD or the company's streaming service. The exercises target six areas: Upper Fix for the upper body; Lower Fix for the lower body parts; Total Body Cardio Fix, a cardiovascular workout with weights; Cardio Fix, a second cardiovascular workout with no weights; Pilates Fix, which focuses on abdominal and thigh muscles; and Yoga Fix, which focuses on flexibility and balance. The plan culminates in a "3-Day Quick-Fix" guide to use during the last 3 of the 21 days.

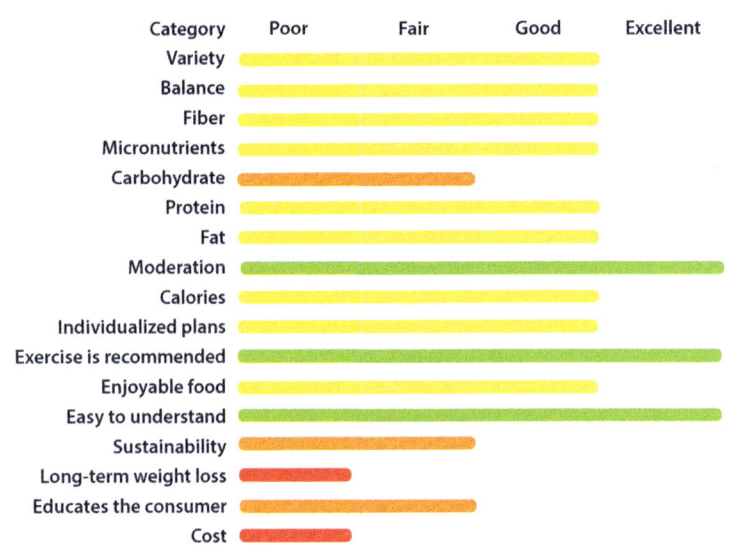

Category	Rating
Variety	Good
Balance	Good
Fiber	Good
Micronutrients	Good
Carbohydrate	Fair
Protein	Good
Fat	Good
Moderation	Excellent
Calories	Good
Individualized plans	Good
Exercise is recommended	Excellent
Enjoyable food	Good
Easy to understand	Excellent
Sustainability	Fair
Long-term weight loss	Poor
Educates the consumer	Fair
Cost	Poor

Positives

Provides 24/7 online support. Does not recommend eating fewer than 1,200 calories per day, even if estimated needs fall below that number. Provides tally sheets for tracking food. Encourages lean proteins, vegetables and healthy fats. Discourages sugary beverages and emphasizes nutrient-dense foods. Encourages preparing meals at home. Teaches and practices portion control. Recommends 3 meals and 3 snacks.

Negatives

Encourages only eating 21-Day Fix approved foods, which can eliminate other healthy options. Focuses on short-term weight loss, which increases the chance of a quick weight regain. Does not focus on slow, consistent changes over time and thus is not a realistic way to eat for permanent weight loss. Recommends and sells expensive supplements. Because dieters determine their calorie level, there is an increased potential for unsafe calorie restriction by certain dieters. Moreover, this multilevel marketing system does not employ professionals trained in exercise or nutrition; instead, advice comes from coaches who could also be identified as commission-motivated sales representatives.

The hook/catch or brilliant selling point: Everyone want a "Beach Body"

Truths/Myths

- Myth - Losing 15 pounds in 3 weeks is safe. p. 13

- Truth - Losing weight quickly results in a quick weight regain and cannot ensure that the weight lost was fat.

Final decision: Thumbs down for weight loss. (Great exercise format for those wanting to increase fitness.)

How to improve this diet: Be sure to consume an adequate number of calories so weight loss does not exceed 1-2 pounds per week. Do not purchase supplements. p. 99

Belly Fat Cure Diet

Premise of the Diet: Keeping insulin levels in balance by avoiding all simple sugars, including sugars in fruit, will prevent the liver from converting excess sugars into fat that specifically gets stored in the belly.

Claims of the Diet: Don't count calories. Count carbs and sugar. Promises a weight loss of four to nine pounds every week. The Carb Swap System provides "the one critical key."

Diet Description: Consume 15 grams of sugar daily, along with 6 servings, or between 5-20 grams, of healthy, unprocessed carbohydrates for a total of 120 grams. Carbohydrate servings are based on the total number of carbohydrates in a food item. Foods with 0 to 4 grams of sugar are not counted. Foods with 5 to 30 grams equals one serving; 21 to 40 grams equals two servings and 41 to 60 grams equals three servings. The planner in the book is used to mark off each day's 15 sugar/6 carbohydrates formula.

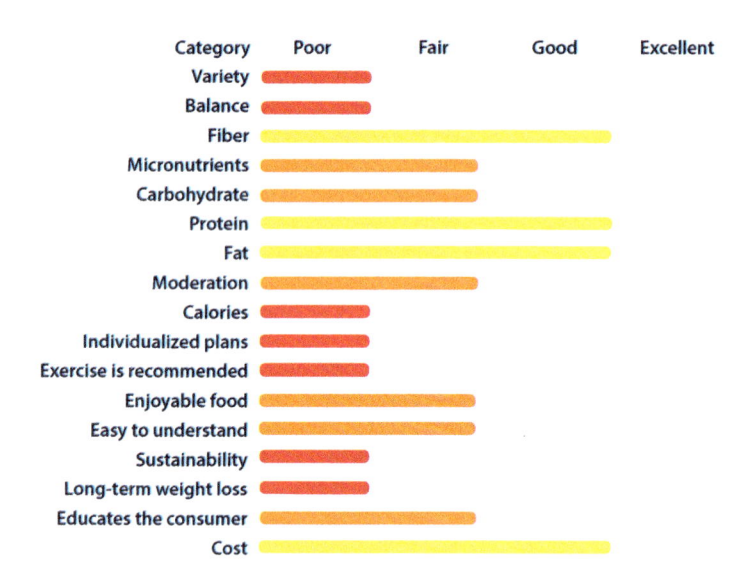

Category	Poor	Fair	Good	Excellent
Variety	■			
Balance	■			
Fiber			■	
Micronutrients		■		
Carbohydrate		■		
Protein			■	
Fat			■	
Moderation		■		
Calories	■			
Individualized plans	■			
Exercise is recommended	■			
Enjoyable food		■		
Easy to understand		■		
Sustainability	■			
Long-term weight loss	■			
Educates the consumer		■		
Cost			■	

Positives

Teaches participants to read labels for hidden sugars and look for whole grain alternatives. Reference guide is rather easy to use. Advises developing a support team of friends or family to help along the weight-loss journey. Recommends eating breakfast. Recommends not allowing yourself to get hungry. Emphasizes planning ahead and packing meals.

Negatives

Doesn't encourage exercise. Limits fruits for the long term. Limiting fruit and dairy may cause nutritional deficiencies, especially if they are not exchanged for nutrient-rich vegetables. Calorie content for suggested meals is lacking. Does not address portion control.

The hook/catch or brilliant selling point: So many diets demonize carbohydrates; it is easy to point the finger at this well-known villain and remind us how bad carbohydrates are while loosely referencing insulin's role. Everyone with fat in their abdominal area wants to believe we can target fat loss there.

Truths/Myths

- Myth - The secret to dropping belly fat is eliminating sugar and processed carbs. 🔍 p. 61

- Truth - Short of liposuction, we cannot target where we will lose body fat. Our bodies store body fat in different places. For some, it's the back and neck, for others it's the belly, and for some, it is the hips or thighs. The first place we lose weight will be the last place we stored it. The last place we lose body fat will be the first place we stored it.

- Truth - Limiting calories (regardless of their source) means the body may tap into body fat for fuel. Eating calories that provide carbs, proteins, and fats in recommended amounts and in sufficient amounts to meet BMR while exercising is the best way to burn body fat. It is wise to minimize highly-processed foods that are high in added sugar.

- Myth - Belly bad foods include foods naturally high in sugars, like carrots, beets, and most fruits.

- Truth - Carrots, beets and most fruits are nutrient-dense foods that should not be eliminated from the diet due to the carbohydrates they contain. In fact, half our meal's plate should consist of fruits and vegetables like these. 🔍 p. 40

• Myth - Insulin is the culprit that increases belly fat. 🔍 p. 73

• Truth - Insulin is a necessary hormone that moves sugar from the blood into cells/tissues that store the excess sugar as glycogen or fat.

• Myth - Insulin manages blood sugar levels and controls the accumulation of fat, especially around the waistline.

• Truth - While insulin does assist in managing blood sugar levels, it is too simple to state it controls the accumulation of fat. The number of excess calories consumed (regardless of their source) gives insulin more excess calories to store and has a greater impact on the accumulation of fat.

• Myth - Since protein and fat do not affect insulin levels, they are allowed in unlimited quantities while following the plan and weight can still be lost. 🔍 p. 21

• Truth - Protein and fat do not affect insulin levels as much as carbohydrates do, but they do have an impact, as they are sources of calories that insulin will tell the body to store. Unlimited amounts of protein or fat are dangerous and can cause significant weight gain, especially considering fats contribute 9 calories per every gram consumed compared to the 4 calories per gram for protein and carbohydrates.

• Myth - Natural sugars, such as those found in milk and fruit, contribute to belly fat. 🔍 p. 41

• Truth - Any excess calories (regardless of the calorie source) can add to body fat. Fat will be deposited based on genetics.

Final decision: Thumbs down 👎

How to improve this diet: Add exercise to a well-rounded diet that consists of lean meat and poultry, whole grains, fish, and healthy oils. Add low-fat dairy products and fruits to the diet.

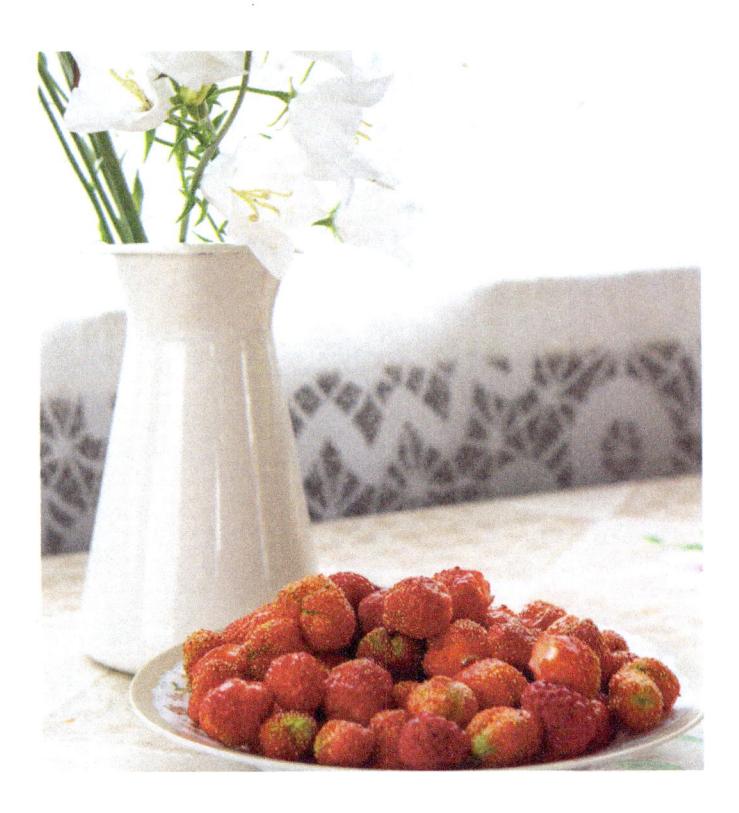

Best Life Diet

Premise of the Diet: A way of eating and living that promotes a gradual change in eating habits that can last a lifetime.

Claims of the Diet: Will break the cycle of going on and off one diet after another by permanently revamping the approach to healthy eating and exercise.

Diet Description: There are three phases to this diet. 1) Baby Steps, which lasts 4 weeks, prepares the body for weight loss by being more active and waking up the metabolism. In this stage, six "problem foods" are avoided. These are alcohol, soda, trans-fats, fried foods, white bread, full-fat milk and yogurt. 2) The Get Moving stage lasts at least 4 weeks. It suggests keeping calories in check by increasing activity at least one level. In this stage, the diet recommends understanding the emotional reasons for eating, introducing "anything-goes calories," and portion control. 3) The Your Best Life stage is ongoing. Add even more activity while cutting back on saturated fat, sodium, and added sugar and eliminating trans-fats.

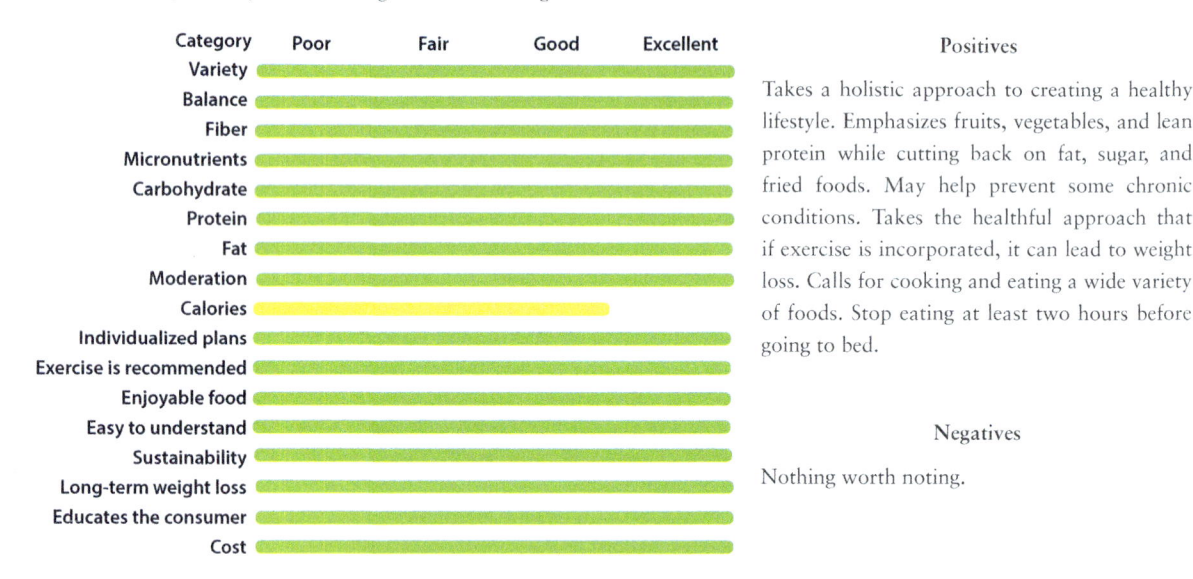

Category	Poor	Fair	Good	Excellent
Variety				✓
Balance				✓
Fiber				✓
Micronutrients				✓
Carbohydrate				✓
Protein				✓
Fat				✓
Moderation				✓
Calories			✓	
Individualized plans				✓
Exercise is recommended				✓
Enjoyable food				✓
Easy to understand				✓
Sustainability				✓
Long-term weight loss				✓
Educates the consumer				✓
Cost				✓

Positives

Takes a holistic approach to creating a healthy lifestyle. Emphasizes fruits, vegetables, and lean protein while cutting back on fat, sugar, and fried foods. May help prevent some chronic conditions. Takes the healthful approach that if exercise is incorporated, it can lead to weight loss. Calls for cooking and eating a wide variety of foods. Stop eating at least two hours before going to bed.

Negatives

Nothing worth noting.

The hook/catch or brilliant selling point: Looks to reach people using common sense. Celebrity endorsement.

Truths/Myths: None worth noting.

Final decision: Thumbs up 👍

How to improve this diet: No recommendations

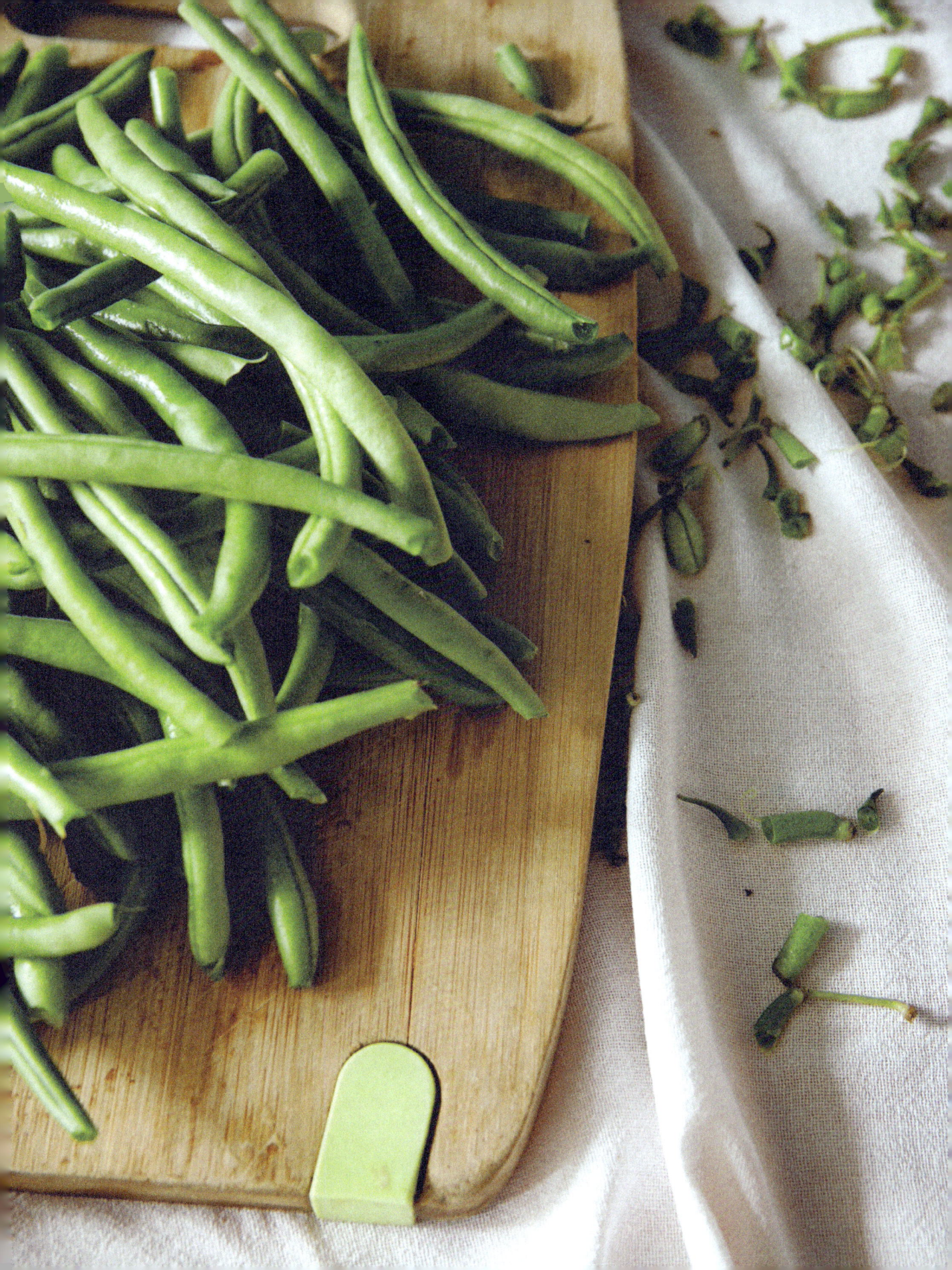

Big Breakfast Diet

Premise of the Diet: Because our appetite, energy, and metabolism vary based on the time of day, what matters most is when we eat.

Claims of the Diet: Eating the biggest meal of the day in the morning can curb our appetite for the rest of the day, leading to weight loss.

Diet Description: Eat within 15 minutes of waking up in the morning. Breakfast should be big, consisting of 7 servings of protein, 2 servings of carbohydrates, 2 servings of fat, and one sweet, such as a doughnut or a piece of cake. No carbohydrates or sweets are allowed for the next two meals. Sugar-free drinks, gum, and bouillon can be consumed at any time of day. After a month, alcohol can be consumed with a meal occasionally. Should be combined with 20 minutes of exercise.

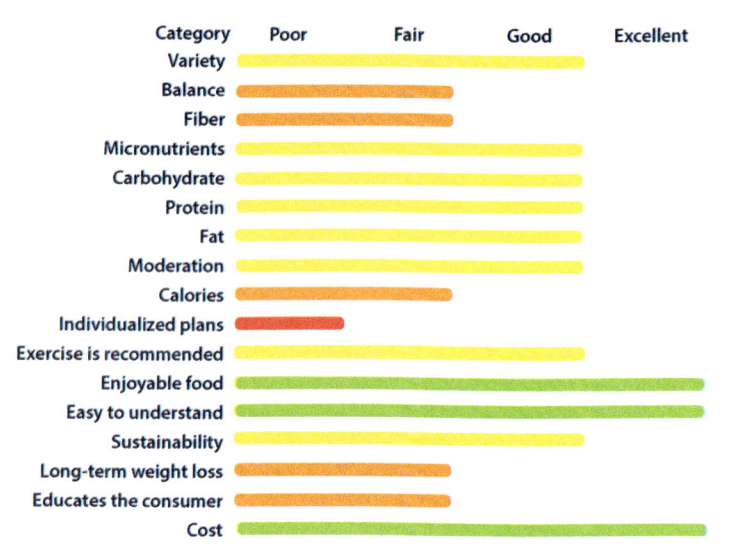

Category	Poor	Fair	Good	Excellent
Variety			▬	
Balance		▬		
Fiber		▬		
Micronutrients			▬	
Carbohydrate			▬	
Protein			▬	
Fat			▬	
Moderation			▬	
Calories		▬		
Individualized plans	▬			
Exercise is recommended			▬	
Enjoyable food				▬
Easy to understand				▬
Sustainability			▬	
Long-term weight loss		▬		
Educates the consumer		▬		
Cost				▬

Positives

Most foods can be consumed, which adds variety to the diet. Eating out is fine, too. The diet breaks down fast food items such as pizza, hamburgers, and wings into serving sizes of proteins, carbs, and fat that fit into the diet.

Negatives

Nearly 1,000 calories are consumed for breakfast, leaving few calories for the remainder of the day. This can lead to very skimpy meals for lunch and dinner. Practically speaking, eating the recommended food within 15 minutes of waking up in the morning is challenging. No concrete suggestions or guidelines are provided for the rest of the day.

The hook/catch or brilliant selling point: Hones in on the concept that we should eat most foods early in the day and less as the day continues.

Truths/Myths

- Myth - We should have nearly 1,000 calories for breakfast.

- Truth - Breakfast is the most important meal of the day. Starting each day with a healthy, satisfying meal makes us less apt to seek out less nutritious foods during the day. Overnight, our bodies are considered to be in a "fasting" mode. Overnight is a long time to go without fueling our bodies. Starting right into the day without fueling up in the morning means our bodies don't get the energy needed for the day, which affects concentration, mood, and weight maintenance. Eating breakfast can help maintain blood glucose levels, which can promote weight maintenance and weight loss. It can also keep our metabolism up as we start our day. We are more likely to overeat if we are very hungry, which often happens if we skip breakfast.

- Myth - We should consume 7 servings of protein for breakfast. 🔍 p. 48

- Truth - We should consume 1 or 2 servings of lean protein for breakfast. Protein is slow to digest, so it keeps us fuller longer than if we only consume carbohydrates which can digest quickly, especially if they are simple sugars. 🔍 p. 84

- Myth - Eating a sweet food in the morning will prevent us from eating them later in the day.

- Truth - Everyone is different. Some of us will still crave sweets at different times of the day, even if we have a sweet in the morning.

Final decision: Thumbs down 👎

How to improve this diet: Determine how many calories your body needs and divide those calories up more evenly throughout the day between breakfast, a morning snack if desired, an afternoon meal, an afternoon snack if desired, an evening meal and a small evening snack if it is desired (but not eaten too late).

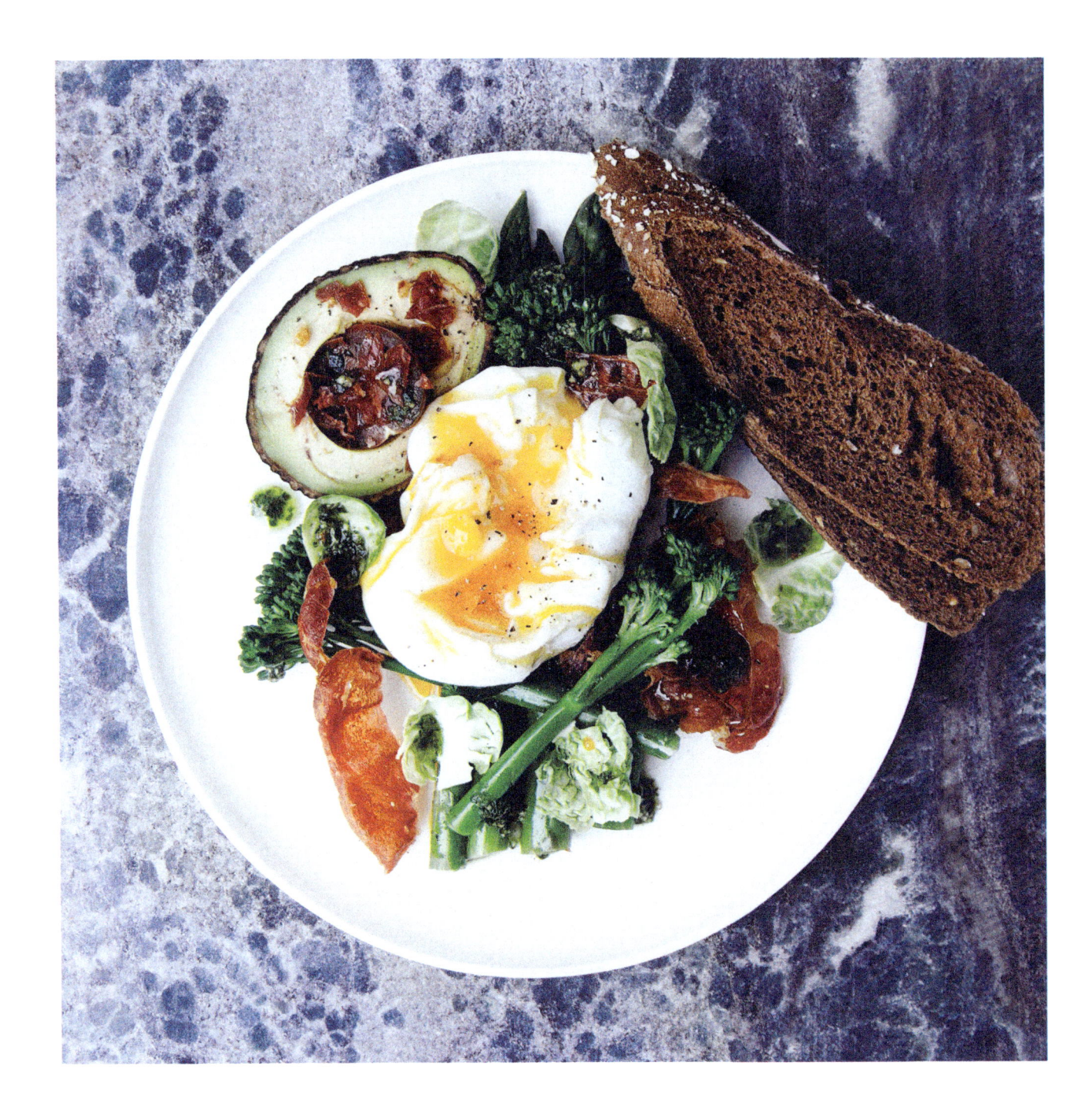

Biggest Loser Diet

Premise of the Diet: Eat a lot less, move a lot more.

Claims of the Diet: Lose 1% of body weight per week. Helps prevent or reverse diabetes. Reduces the risk for cancer, dementia, and Alzheimer's Disease. Improves heart health and boosts the immune system.

Diet Description: Calorie requirements range from 1,050 to 2,100, depending on starting weight. Food choices are consumed in 3 meals and 2 snacks and are guided by a "4-3-2-1" Biggest Loser Pyramid. Consume 4 servings of fruits and vegetables, 3 servings of protein, 2 servings of whole grains, and about 200 calories from sweets.

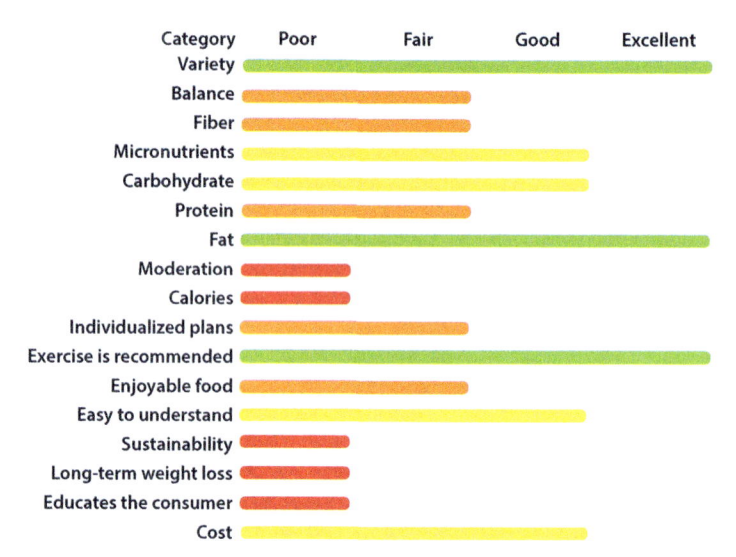

Category	Rating
Variety	Excellent
Balance	Fair
Fiber	Fair
Micronutrients	Good
Carbohydrate	Good
Protein	Fair
Fat	Excellent
Moderation	Poor
Calories	Poor
Individualized plans	Fair
Exercise is recommended	Excellent
Enjoyable food	Fair
Easy to understand	Good
Sustainability	Poor
Long-term weight loss	Poor
Educates the consumer	Poor
Cost	Good

Positives

Encourages exercise. No food group is eliminated. Carbohydrates, proteins, and fats do fall within the recommended ranges. Recommends keeping a journal. Encourages preparing foods and eating at home.

Negatives

Too low in calories to keep metabolic rate from dropping or to provide for heavy exercise. May not provide enough protein to keep the body from stripping lean tissue. Limits whole grain consumption to two servings a day. When consuming such low levels of calories, 200 calories from sweets is a rather significant contribution. While portions do vary depending on calorie needs, overall, the total consumed may still be too low to promote a healthy fat loss. Most adults cannot devote the huge time commitment to maximizing their fat loss like those on the TV show. Healthy fats should not be lumped in the same category as the "extras" budget or the 200 calories of sweets. 🔍 p. 48, 55

The hook/catch or brilliant selling point: Capitalizes on the hit TV show.

Truths/Myths

• **Myth** - It is healthy to lose 1% body weight in a week's time. 🔍 p. 16

• **Truth** - Rate of weight loss varies depending on the amount of excess body fat to be lost. In general, the more body fat, the faster someone will lose it, at least in the beginning. The first stage of fat loss is water loss, so the first week or so is generally the largest amount lost. However, it is not all fat that is lost. It is not healthy for everyone to lose 1% of their body weight period, much less to do so every week. Competitors from the TV show have shared they needed to spend many hours of the day working out. This schedule is nearly impossible to maintain for most adults who work a full-time job or have family obligations. Former contestants have also revealed that the length of time between 'weekly' weigh-ins could be as much as 25 days, which makes it look like people are losing weight a lot faster than they are in reality.

Final decision: Thumbs down 👎

How to improve this diet: Determine how many calories are needed to maintain your current weight, then subtract 500-1,000 calories from that total for a slow (1-2 pound a week) weight loss. If vast amounts of weight need to be lost, physician supervision is recommended.

Biggest Loser Simple Swaps Diet

Premise of the Diet: Getting healthy is less daunting when small manageable steps are taken. Not all changes need to be made at once.

Claims of the Diet: People who may be overwhelmed by really big changes, and therefore not try to lose weight, can start with small baby steps.

Diet Description: Swap daily habits and choices for healthier versions. (Example: swap your daily glass of fruit juice for a piece of whole fruit, or swap sugary cereals for whole-grain options.) Provides 100 "Simple Swaps" and many recipes.

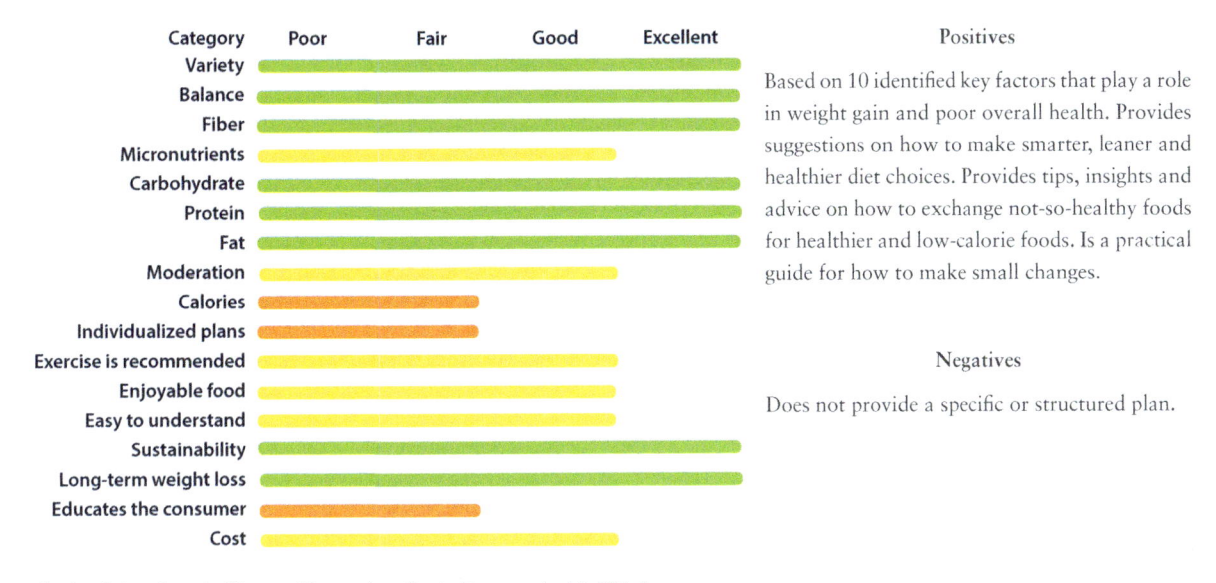

Category	Poor	Fair	Good	Excellent
Variety				✓
Balance				✓
Fiber				✓
Micronutrients			✓	
Carbohydrate				✓
Protein				✓
Fat				✓
Moderation			✓	
Calories		✓		
Individualized plans		✓		
Exercise is recommended			✓	
Enjoyable food			✓	
Easy to understand			✓	
Sustainability				✓
Long-term weight loss				✓
Educates the consumer	✓			
Cost			✓	

Positives

Based on 10 identified key factors that play a role in weight gain and poor overall health. Provides suggestions on how to make smarter, leaner and healthier diet choices. Provides tips, insights and advice on how to exchange not-so-healthy foods for healthier and low-calorie foods. Is a practical guide for how to make small changes.

Negatives

Does not provide a specific or structured plan.

The hook/catch or brilliant selling point: Capitalizes on the hit TV show.

Truths/Myths: None worth noting.

Final decision: Thumbs up 👍

How to improve this diet: For people who want more structure, become educated on the number of calories needed to lose weight so the tips provided can be fitted into your goals.

Body for Life Diet

Premise of the Diet: Combines the two proven elements: fewer calories in and more calories out leads to weight loss.

Claims of the Diet: In 12 weeks, we will have the lean, healthy body we always wanted and not have to turn our life upside down to get it. We will have the energy to be at our peak from dawn to dusk. We will have the confidence to do all the things we have been putting off and know that we really do have the power to change—not just our body, but anything in the world to which we set our mind.

Diet Description: A 12-week nutrition and exercise program. It promotes eating small meals of lean protein and healthy carbohydrates every few hours, up to six times a day. The exercise component includes 45 minutes of weight training three days a week, alternating with 20 minutes of aerobic exercise three days a week. On the seventh day, you can eat whatever you want and take a break from workouts.

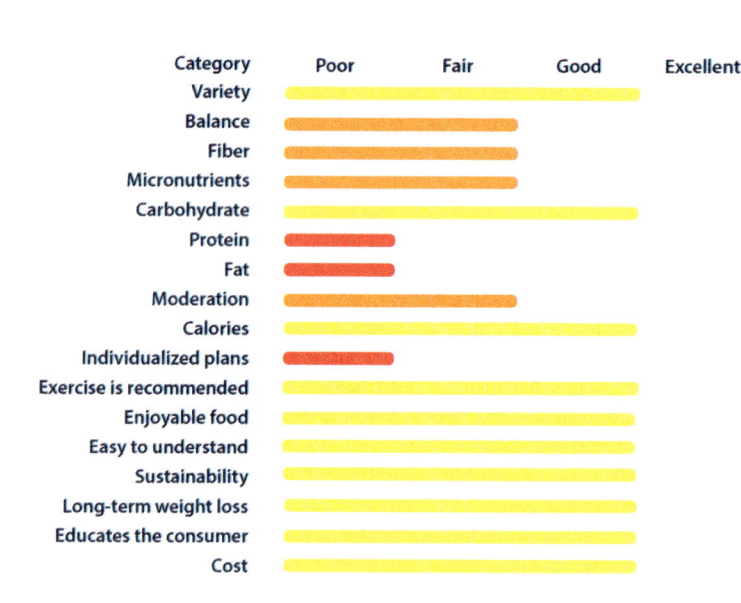

Category	Poor	Fair	Good	Excellent
Variety				●
Balance			●	
Fiber			●	
Micronutrients			●	
Carbohydrate				●
Protein	●			
Fat	●			
Moderation			●	
Calories				●
Individualized plans	●			
Exercise is recommended				●
Enjoyable food				●
Easy to understand				●
Sustainability				●
Long-term weight loss				●
Educates the consumer				●
Cost				●

Positives

Recommends smaller, frequently consumed meals to help speed up metabolism and help maintain steady energy levels throughout the day. Stresses balancing protein and carbohydrates. Is high in vegetables and whole grains. Offers variety, so we are less likely to get bored; therefore, we may be more likely to stay on it long term.

Negatives

Recommends too much protein, 40 to 50% of all daily calories. The acceptable recommended amount is 10-35% of all calories. If this protein is consumed mostly from animal proteins, excessive amounts have been linked to a number of chronic diseases including diabetes, cancer, and heart disease. Intense exercise training may be too much for some; they should first consult their physician before engaging. The plan suggests consuming powders, shakes, supplements, and nutrition bars sold on their website. Requires only 2 servings of vegetables, which may lead to a lack of certain vitamins, minerals, and fiber. Need to be careful not to overdo it on the free day.

The hook/catch or brilliant selling point: Capitalizes on the connection often made between protein – exercise and youthful energy.

Truths/Myths

- Myth - Eating frequent, small meals is a direct link to weight loss success.

- Truth - Fueling the body throughout the day can help keep metabolism up throughout the day. So, in essence, when we eat, we do get a little metabolic boost. When we graze, we don't have a lot of time between meals for our metabolism to drop.

- Truth - Exercise does increase our metabolic rate while we exercise and for a while after exercise. Exercise can change the shape of a body to some extent through toning muscles.

- **Truth** - Protein may help stabilize insulin levels, as it is slower to digest than simple sugars, and it therefore may help keep energy levels steadier throughout the day, which may result in curbing appetite.

Final decision: Thumbs down

How to improve this diet: Add healthy fats to reach the recommended range of 20-35% of all daily calories. Decrease protein to the recommended range of 10-35% of all calories. Exercise is important, just get physician clearance prior to starting.

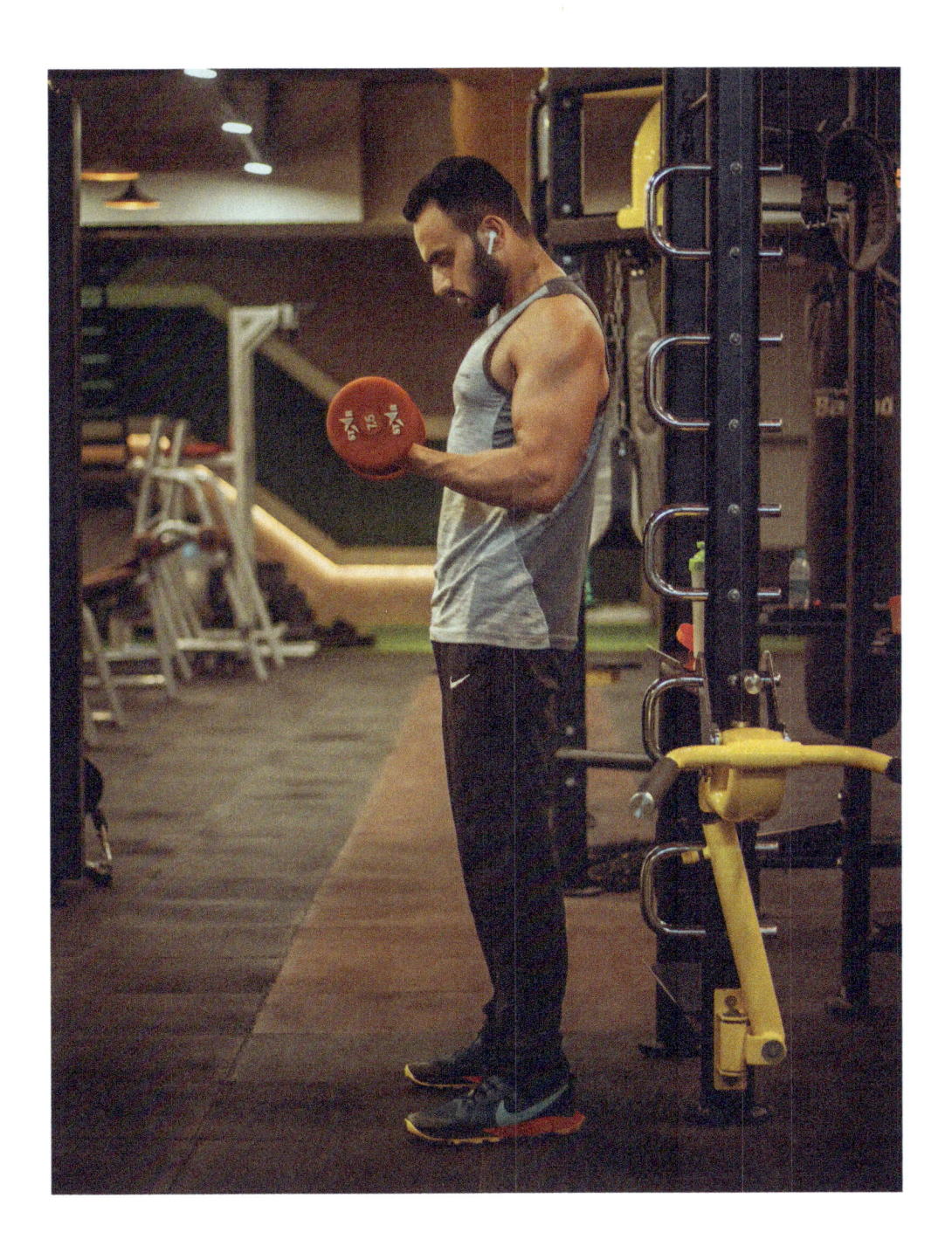

Body Reset Diet

Premise of the Diet: Gradual change makes for lasting change.

Claims of the Diet: No real claims, other than Jessica Simpson's announcement of losing 100 pounds in the six months after giving birth.

Diet Description: Has 3 phases lasting 5 days each, with the first phase starting with 3 smoothies and 2 snacks. The diet progresses to phase two so that on days 6 through 10, 2 smoothies and 1 solid meal and 2 snacks per day are consumed. In phase three, days 11 through 15, smoothies are reduced to one a day and 2 meals and 2 snacks. The diet continues to increase the number of meals to result in 3 meals and 2 snacks daily. Each meal provides protein, fiber, and fat. Each snack contributes either protein and fiber or protein and fat. All snacks should be about 150 calories and contain at least 5 grams of fiber, 5 grams of protein, and less than 10 grams of sugar.

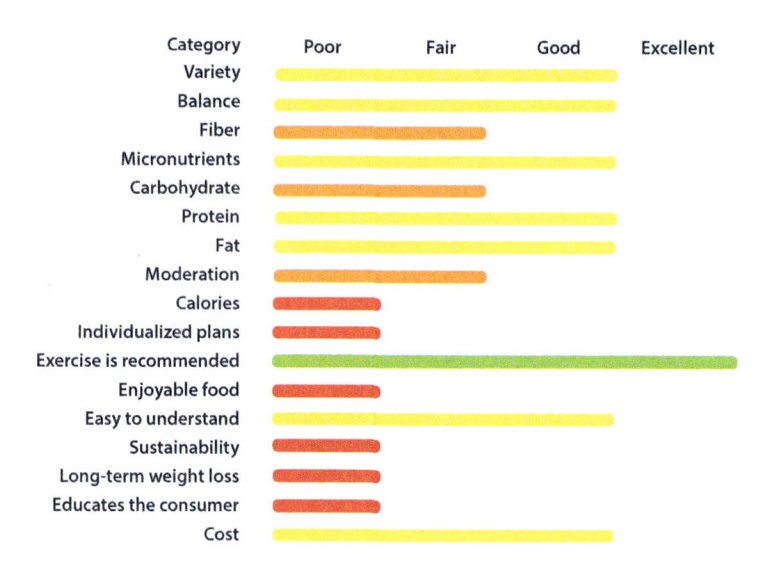

Category	Poor	Fair	Good	Excellent
Variety			Good	
Balance			Good	
Fiber		Fair		
Micronutrients			Good	
Carbohydrate		Fair		
Protein			Good	
Fat			Good	
Moderation		Fair		
Calories	Poor			
Individualized plans	Poor			
Exercise is recommended				Excellent
Enjoyable food	Poor			
Easy to understand			Good	
Sustainability	Poor			
Long-term weight loss	Poor			
Educates the consumer	Poor			
Cost			Good	

Positives

Recommends eating five times a day. Provides a structured plan of balanced meals at regular times. Encourages making healthy choices and developing lifestyle habits. Recommends exercise, 10,000 daily steps and resistance training. Recommended smoothies are healthy in composition. Diets high in fruits and vegetables are associated with better overall health.

Negatives

Can be difficult to transition from consuming a smoothie as a meal to a real meal. Calorie level is too low for most, which leads to fast weight loss, a slower metabolism, and stripping of lean tissue.

The hook/catch or brilliant selling point: Rides on the coattails of a celebrity.

Truths/Myths

- Myth - Will train your body to use energy more efficiently and burn calories faster, even while you're asleep. 🔍 p. 13, 66

- Truth - Only exercise makes us burn calories faster.

- Myth - Smoothies are a good meal substitution.

- Truth - Smoothies several times a day, day after day, can get boring, which leads to inability to follow it long term. 🔍 p. 16

Final decision: Thumbs down 👎

How to improve this diet: Instead of consuming smoothies, consume a variety of interesting nutrient-dense foods for all meals and snacks. Incorporate more complex carbohydrates. Increase calorie consumption to a level near BMR and increase/keep exercise level up to burn more calories.

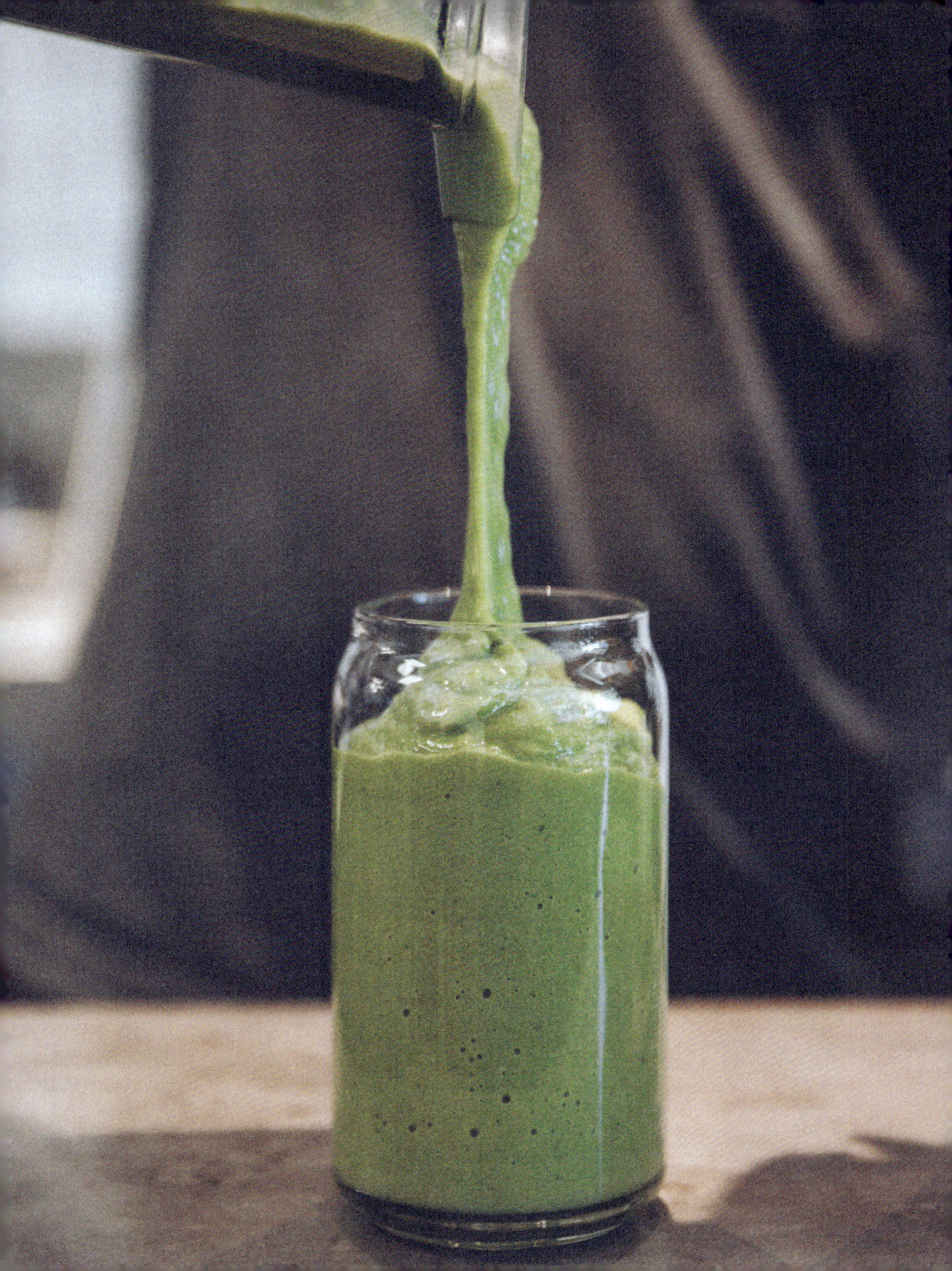

Brown Fat Revolution Diet

Premise of the Diet: This 4-week diet and exercise program focuses on developing lean muscle, boosting metabolism, and building more brown fat. It's based on the idea that when stimulated, brown fat in the body can burn calories than white fat.

Claims of the Diet: As we age, brown fat turns into white fat. Focusing on eating healthier and exercising more will cause weight loss and a more toned and youthful body.

Diet Description: Eat almost any food six times a day, while avoiding processed foods and foods that contain empty calories. There are "Carb Days" and "Protein Days" and one free day. Several core exercises are engaged in but not daily. Encourages weight training.

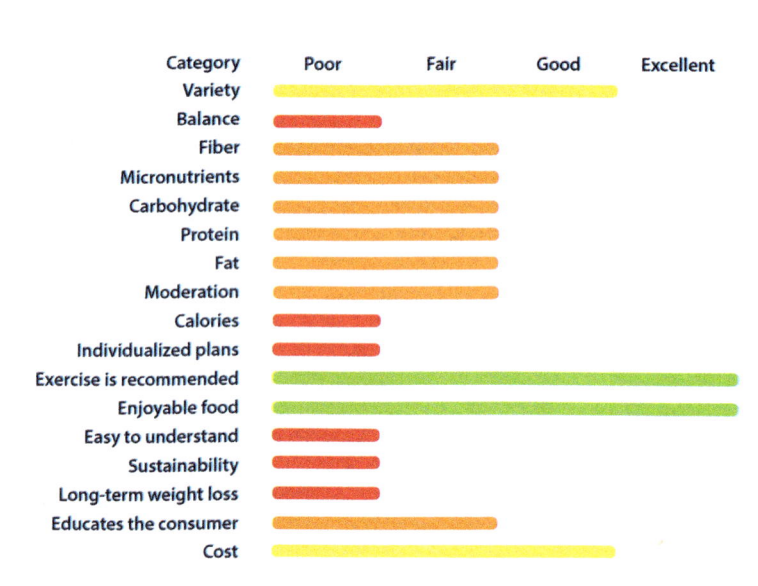

Category	Poor	Fair	Good	Excellent
Variety				■
Balance	■			
Fiber		■		
Micronutrients		■		
Carbohydrate		■		
Protein		■		
Fat		■		
Moderation		■		
Calories	■			
Individualized plans	■			
Exercise is recommended				■
Enjoyable food				■
Easy to understand	■			
Sustainability	■			
Long-term weight loss	■			
Educates the consumer		■		
Cost				■

Positives

Recommends eating six times a day to keep metabolism up. Avoid processed foods. Includes many types of foods, including whole grains, starchy vegetables, fresh and lean protein, and unsaturated fats. Recommends avoiding many foods that contain empty calories. No food group is eliminated.

Negatives

It is risky to have one day a week as a free day to eat whatever is wanted, within reason. There are "Carb Days" and "Protein Days", which may be problematic for many people, particularly those with diabetes. Avoiding all foods that contain artificial flavors, sweeteners, colors, and preservatives may be difficult.

The hook/catch or brilliant selling point: Sometimes the more weird something sounds, the more often people believe it must be true. (A mystery has finally been revealed.)

Truths/Myths

- **Myth** - Yellow fat makes us look soft, flabby, and old. 🔍 p. 60

- **Myth** - Brown fat is a good, healthy fat that keeps our body firm and youthful.

- **Truth** - Brown fats have more mitochondria, which causes it to be brown in color. Brown fat converts calories to heat instead of storing them.

- **Myth** - focusing on changing "bad" yellow fat into "good" brown is a good goal in weight loss. 🔍 p. 81

- **Truth** - Some studies have shown 12 weeks of exercise caused a browning of some body fat, making it more like a beige fat. Beige fat is white adipocytes that have responded to some type of stress, like cold or exercise, then undergo a process making them more like brown fat. Exercise creates more mitochondria that create energy/ATP for working muscles to use. However, if exercise is stopped, those mitochondria will no longer be needed. When exercise is stopped, mitochondria and their corresponding Krebs cycles will be reabsorbed by the body. There are also no studies showing that we can build brown fat long term.

- Myth - It is important to emphasize protein on some days and carbohydrates on other days.

- Truth - Alternating days of eating proteins and carbs has not been scientifically proven to be an effective weight-loss strategy and may prove dangerous for people with diabetes.

- Myth - A "free day" is important for weight loss.

- Truth - While it is a good idea to not be too restrictive, we should lose weight as long as we don't give into too much temptation on our "free" day each week.

- Myth - As we age, brown fat gets converted to yellow/white fat. 🔍 p. 85

- Truth - Infants do have the most brown fat, as it helps keep them warm. They have small surface areas and thus their core temperature can cool off easily. As infants grow, they will lose the need for warming insulation. In other words, as we get older and bigger, we no longer need to be heated. As an adult, the only substantial way to create more mitochondria in fat is to exercise.

- Myth - Eating frequent, small meals is a direct link to weight loss success. 🔍 p. 15

- Truth - Fueling the body throughout the day can help keep metabolism up throughout the day. So, in essence, when we eat, we do get a little metabolic boost. When we graze, we don't have a lot of time between meals for our metabolism to drop.

Final decision: Thumbs down 👎

How to improve this diet: Provide more structure regarding what to eat and emphasize a slow, steady fat loss that lasts for a lifetime, not just for 4 weeks while on the program. Take the focus off the type of fat, as it has little to no relevance for weight loss.

Bullet Proof Diet

Premise of the Diet: Get 50 to 60% of your daily calories from healthy fats (such as coconut oil, avocado, and grass-fed and/or pastured animals), 20% from protein, and the remaining 20 to 30% from vegetables.

Claims of the Diet: Eating the "right" foods makes for a lean, muscular, energetic body. It also helps prevent disease and improves mental sharpness.

Diet Description: Grains and legumes are to be avoided. Eliminate sugar and replace it with the "right" fats. Switch to grass-fed meat and wild-caught seafood. Eliminate synthetic additives, colorings, flavorings, pasteurized dairy, industrially raised meats, sodas and juices, farmed seafood, dried fruit, and anything fried or cooked in a microwave. Switch to organic fruits and vegetables but have no more than 2 servings of fruits daily.

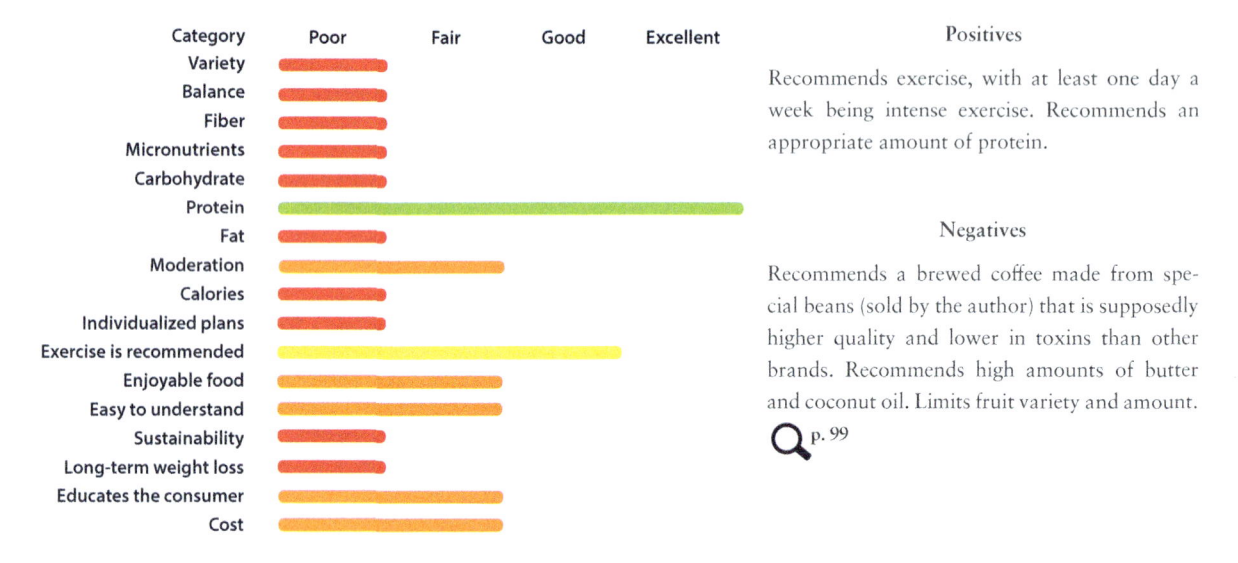

Category	Rating
Variety	Poor
Balance	Poor
Fiber	Poor
Micronutrients	Poor
Carbohydrate	Poor
Protein	Excellent
Fat	Poor
Moderation	Fair
Calories	Poor
Individualized plans	Poor
Exercise is recommended	Good
Enjoyable food	Fair
Easy to understand	Fair
Sustainability	Poor
Long-term weight loss	Poor
Educates the consumer	Fair
Cost	Fair

Positives

Recommends exercise, with at least one day a week being intense exercise. Recommends an appropriate amount of protein.

Negatives

Recommends a brewed coffee made from special beans (sold by the author) that is supposedly higher quality and lower in toxins than other brands. Recommends high amounts of butter and coconut oil. Limits fruit variety and amount. p. 99

The hook/catch or brilliant selling point: When a 300-pound man shares how he lost weight... people listen.

Truths/Myths

- **Myth** - All hormones are made out of saturated fat.

- **Truth** - Hormones are actually made out of proteins, not fat. Cholesterol is necessary for the formation of some hormones. Cholesterol can be consumed in animal products, but our livers also manufacture cholesterol. p. 47

Final decision: Thumbs down

How to improve this diet: Incorporate grains, legumes and low-fat pasteurized dairy.

Cabbage Soup Diet

Premise of the Diet: Eat a very low-calorie diet to lose weight fast.

Claims of the Diet: Lose up to 10 pounds in a week.

Diet Description: This diet provides less than 1,000 calories, which come mostly from cabbage soup, along with 1-2 servings of other fruits and vegetables. No other substitutions are allowed. Drink only water or other calorie-free beverages. Take a daily multivitamin. Follow the 7-day schedule, which consists of unlimited cabbage soup along with random rules about which fruit is acceptable to eat on certain days. It includes one day that allows for unlimited consumption of bananas, and a few other days that allow for a baked potato. Go on the diet for no more than 7 days at a time. Can be repeated again after 2 weeks of being off the diet.

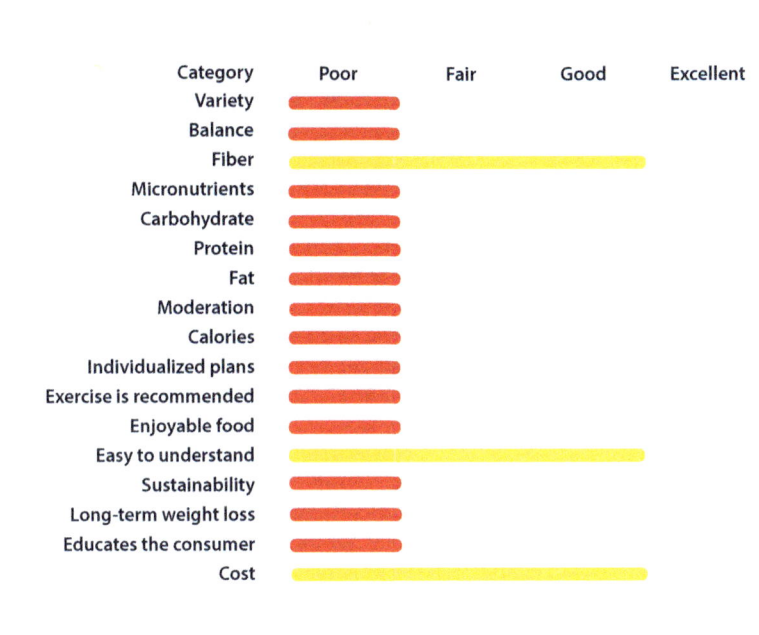

Category	Poor	Fair	Good	Excellent
Variety	▬			
Balance	▬			
Fiber	▬	▬	▬	
Micronutrients	▬			
Carbohydrate	▬			
Protein	▬			
Fat	▬			
Moderation	▬			
Calories	▬			
Individualized plans	▬			
Exercise is recommended	▬			
Enjoyable food	▬			
Easy to understand	▬	▬	▬	
Sustainability	▬			
Long-term weight loss	▬			
Educates the consumer	▬			
Cost	▬	▬	▬	

Positives

Provides plenty of fruits and vegetables, which are high in fiber. Inexpensive ingredients. Eat frequently throughout the day.

Negatives

Even with the inclusion of a daily multivitamin, it's deficient in numerous vitamins and minerals. Insufficient protein is provided. Bland. Very low calorie level may lead to dizziness, weakness, or lightheadedness. The high fiber may cause flatulence and cramping and other GI distress. It contains a very limited menu. A majority of initial weight lost will be water weight, not fat loss. Due to entering a starvation metabolic state, weight will be regained as soon as diet is over, and a low-normal metabolic state will be resumed as the body prepares for another possible starvation metabolism state.

The hook/catch or brilliant selling point: Everyone loves to hear we can lose weight fast.

Truths/Myths

- Myth - Fat can be lost quickly. 🔍 p. 13

- Truth - When weight is lost quickly (like 10 pounds in a week) it is mostly water weight and lean tissue that is lost, not fat.

- Myth - This is a good method to kick-start weight loss or to trim a few pounds for a special event. 🔍 p. 84

- Truth - This is a terrible approach to weight loss because the very low calorie level will result in stripping lean tissue and a lowering of the metabolic rate which, immediately after the diet, will result in weight gain in the form of fat. 🔍 p. 81

- Myth - This approach is fine because it only lasts for 7 days.

- Truth - It doesn't provide the nutrients needed to stay healthy. The diet does not encourage the necessary lifestyle changes needed to sustain long lasting weight loss.

Final decision: Thumbs down 👎

The Carb Lovers Diet

Premise of the Diet: Resistant starches will fill up the stomach, causing less food to be consumed and weight loss to result.

Claims of the Diet: Drop up to 8 pounds in 30 days.

Diet Description: Fill one-quarter of the plate with resistant starches, such as: lentils, garbanzo beans, brown rice. The first week on the diet, eat 1,200 calories per day. After that eat 1,600 calories in 3 meals and 2 snacks per day. Have a "carb star" at each meal. The rest of the plate should contain lean meats, low-fat dairy, good fats, fruits, and vegetables.

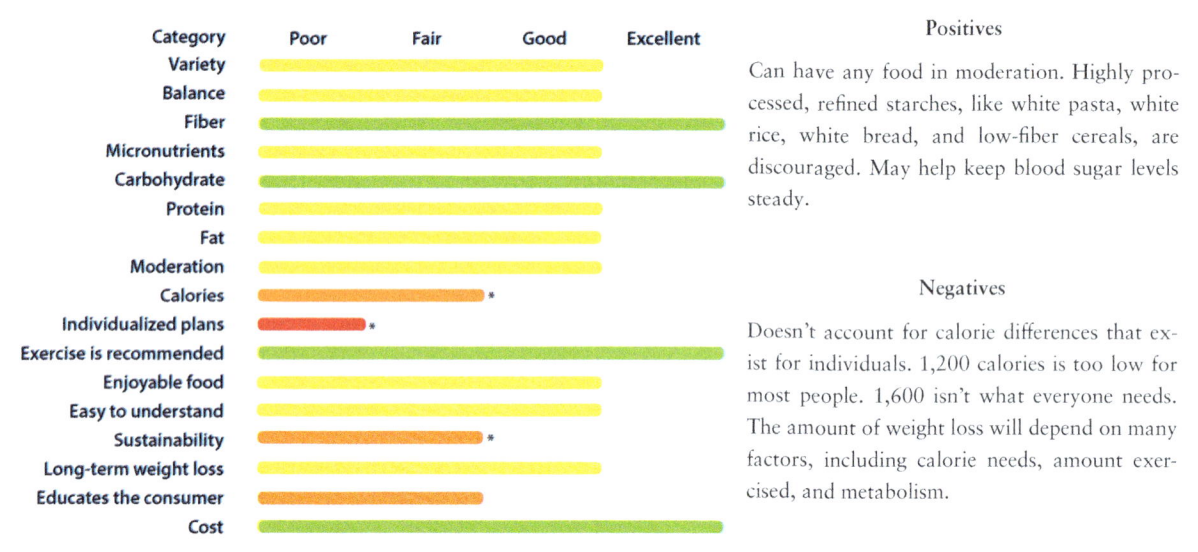

Category	Poor	Fair	Good	Excellent
Variety				
Balance				
Fiber				✓
Micronutrients				
Carbohydrate				✓
Protein				
Fat				
Moderation				
Calories		✓*		
Individualized plans	✓*			
Exercise is recommended				✓
Enjoyable food				
Easy to understand				
Sustainability		✓*		
Long-term weight loss				
Educates the consumer		✓		
Cost				✓

Positives

Can have any food in moderation. Highly processed, refined starches, like white pasta, white rice, white bread, and low-fiber cereals, are discouraged. May help keep blood sugar levels steady.

Negatives

Doesn't account for calorie differences that exist for individuals. 1,200 calories is too low for most people. 1,600 isn't what everyone needs. The amount of weight loss will depend on many factors, including calorie needs, amount exercised, and metabolism.

Please note*- These will vary depending on the number of calories needed. Currently, the diet has a set standard for everyone and doesn't take into account individual needs.

The hook/catch or brilliant selling point: Hope is provided for those who hate the idea of giving up carbohydrates, which is what many diets have demonized.

Truths/Myths

- Myth - It promotes fat-burning

- Truth - Exercise burns fat. Eating various foods has really no impact on burning fat. p. 16, 105

- Truth - There is evidence that eating a diet high in complex carbs and fiber can help lose weight, mostly through creating a feeling of fullness and satiation.

Final decision: Thumbs up 👍

How to improve this diet: Individuals should determine the number of calories they need to maintain weight, then, in most cases, subtract -500 calories from that number. The resulting answer is the suggested number of calories needed to lose weight. Incorporate sufficient fiber-rich foods into the diet so as to consume the recommended amount (women – 25 grams; men – 38 grams). All calories consumed should supply the AMDR (Carbohydrates 45-65% of calories; Protein 10-35%; Fat 20-35% of all calories).

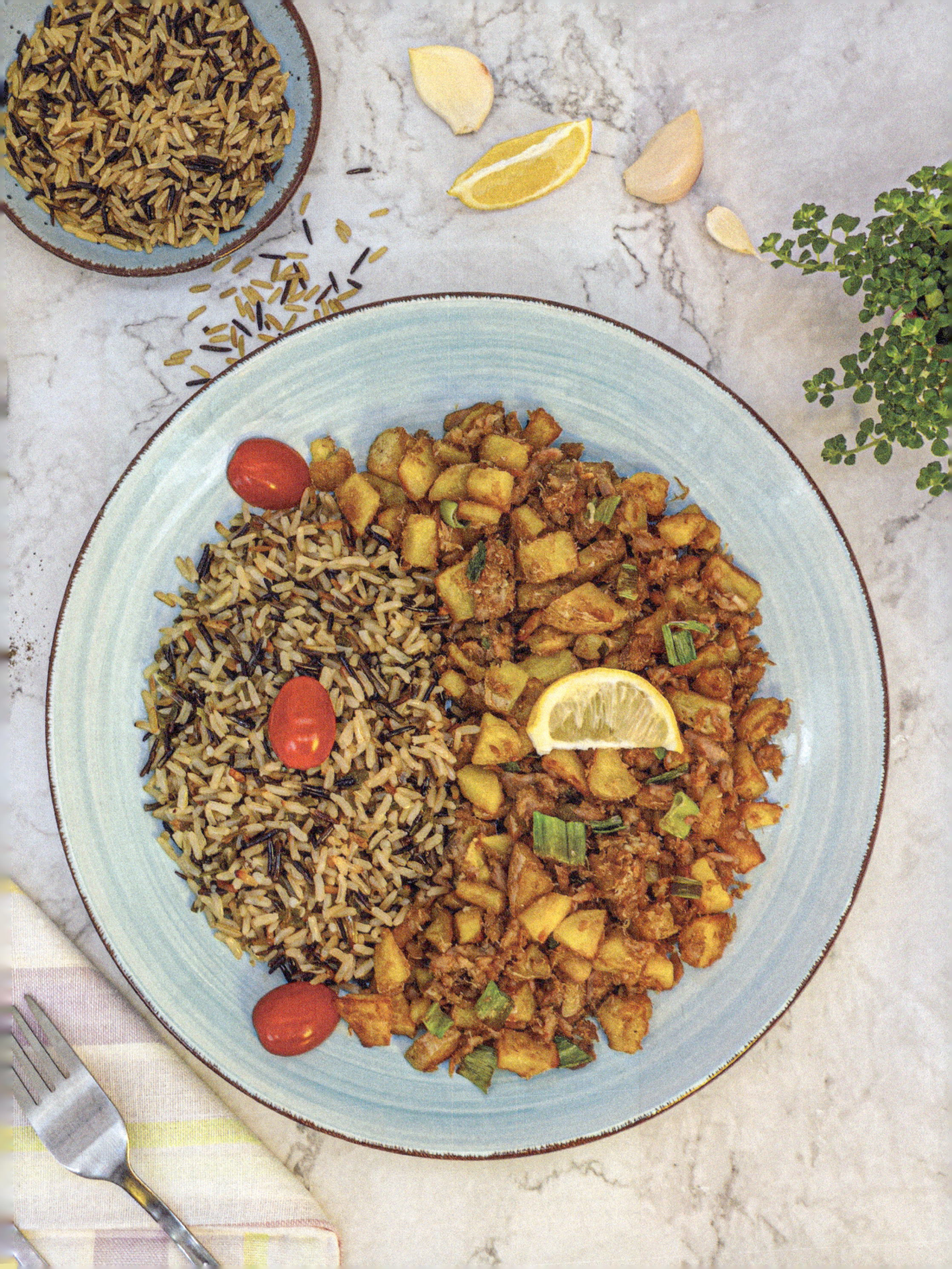

Caveman Diet
(aka Paleo, Stone Age diet, Hunter-Gatherer diet)

Please note: Over the years, this diet has evolved and now has several different versions.

Premise of the Diet: Eating like our prehistoric ancestors will lessen the likelihood of chronic diseases.

Claims of the Diet: Promises weight loss without cutting calories. Lowers the risk of heart disease, blood pressure, inflammation, and acne, all while promoting optimum health and athletic performance.

Diet Description: Eat fresh lean meats, fish, fruit, vegetables, healthy fats, coconut oil, eggs, most nuts and seeds. Can't eat any processed foods, wheat, beans, peanuts, dairy, refined sugar, potatoes, salt, or refined vegetable oils like canola oil. If possible, choose grass-fed and organic products.

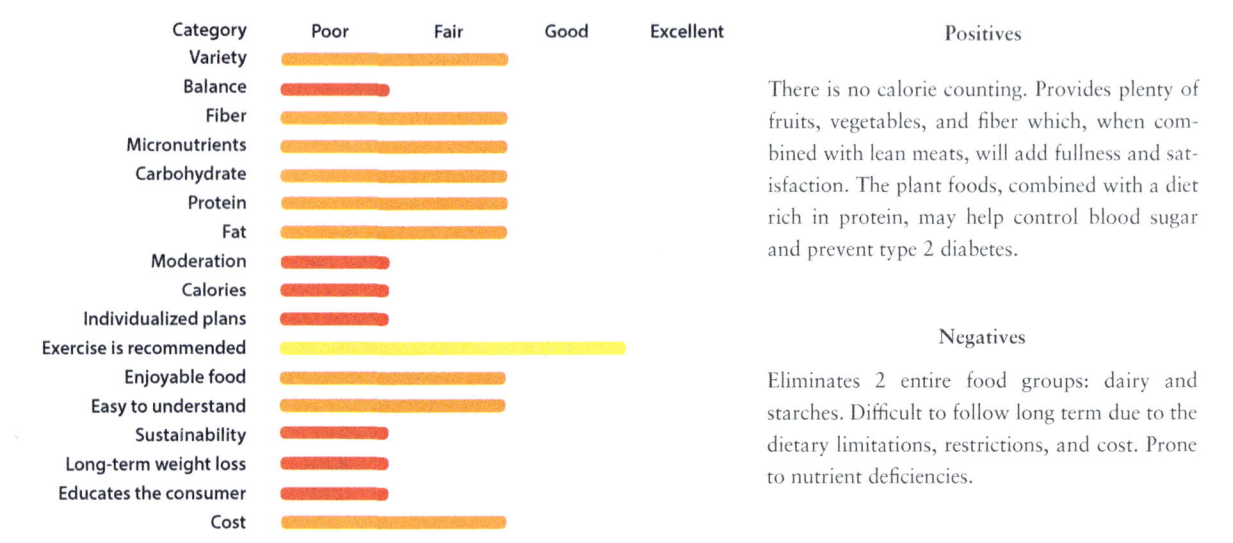

Category	Poor	Fair	Good	Excellent
Variety		▬▬		
Balance	▬			
Fiber		▬▬		
Micronutrients		▬▬		
Carbohydrate		▬▬		
Protein		▬▬		
Fat		▬▬		
Moderation	▬			
Calories	▬			
Individualized plans	▬			
Exercise is recommended			▬▬▬	
Enjoyable food		▬▬		
Easy to understand		▬▬		
Sustainability	▬			
Long-term weight loss	▬			
Educates the consumer	▬			
Cost		▬▬		

Positives

There is no calorie counting. Provides plenty of fruits, vegetables, and fiber which, when combined with lean meats, will add fullness and satisfaction. The plant foods, combined with a diet rich in protein, may help control blood sugar and prevent type 2 diabetes.

Negatives

Eliminates 2 entire food groups: dairy and starches. Difficult to follow long term due to the dietary limitations, restrictions, and cost. Prone to nutrient deficiencies.

The hook/catch or brilliant selling point: Sometimes the weirder something sounds, the more often people believe it must be true. (A mystery has finally been revealed.)

Truths/Myths

- **Myth** - It is possible to eat like our ancestors.

- **Truth** - Foods today are different from the foods our ancestors ate. For example, carrots and most fruits and vegetables have been genetically modified and cultivated at some point in time. Wild game is not readily available now. In fact, most of the meat we consume has been domesticated and is produced in mass. Moreover, it is impossible to know exactly what our human ancestors ate in different parts of the world. There really is NO Paleo diet.

- **Myth** - Lowers the risk of heart disease, blood pressure, inflammation, and acne, all while promoting optimum health, just like our historic ancestors.

- **Truth** - Years ago, people didn't live long enough to die from chronic diseases.

- **Myth** - This is a healthy diet to follow because it eliminates processed foods.

• Truth - Whole grains, legumes and dairy are nutrient-rich foods that contain important vitamins and minerals, yet they are excluded from this plan. 🔍 p. 16

• Myth - Eliminating grains will stop the development of disease.

• Truth - Whole grains contain dietary fiber, which may help reduce the risk of heart disease, cancer, diabetes, and other health complications. 🔍 p. 40

Final decision: Thumbs down 👎

How to improve this diet: Because this plan may exceed the Dietary Guidelines for fat and protein intake and definitely falls short on carbohydrate recommendations, it is important to incorporate the missing food groups in moderation and monitor amounts of fat and lean meats to meet the AMDR.

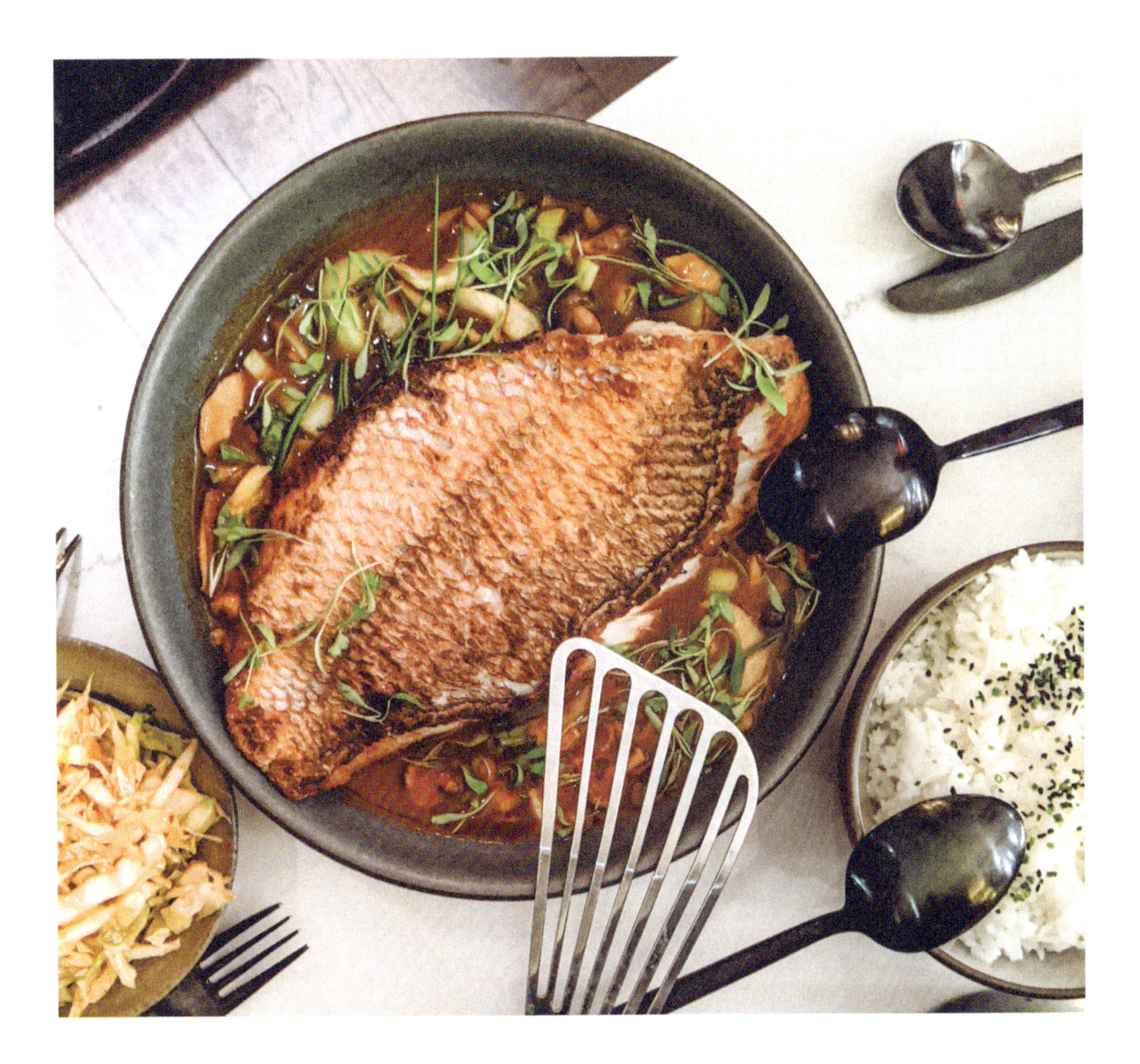

Cheater's Diet (by Paul Rivas)

Premise of the Diet: Eat a Mediterranean-style diet during the week, "cheat" during the weekend, and lose weight, because cheating strengthens our motivation to eat well the rest of the week.

Claims of the Diet: Purposely blowing it on weekends cranks up the metabolism, reversing the metabolic slowdown that happens when calories are restricted during the week.

Diet Description: Monday through Friday, fruits and vegetables should make up half the plate, while one-quarter is lean protein and one-quarter is whole grains. Be sure to have at least 3 servings of fruit per day and 4 servings of vegetables. Sugar, bread, white rice, potatoes, saturated fats, most fried foods, and alcohol are off-limits until the weekend. On Saturday and Sunday, add an extra 10 calories per day for every pound of weight.

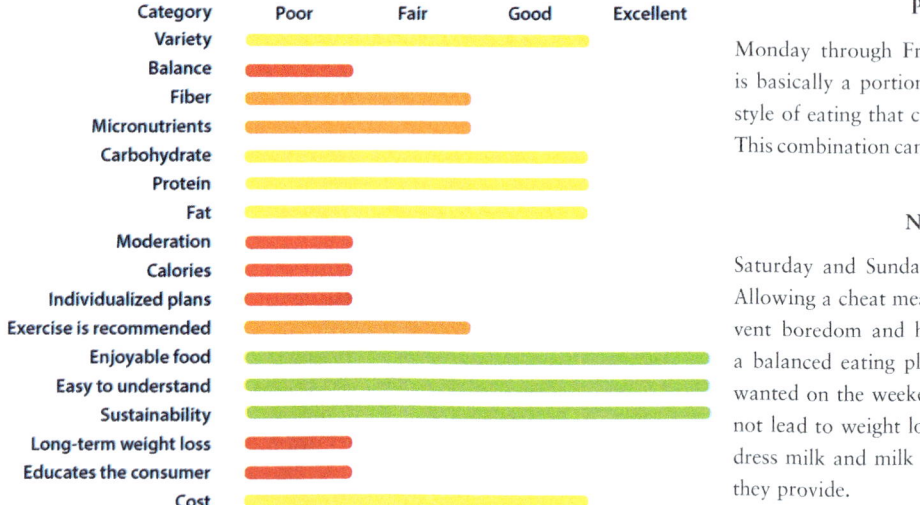

Category	Poor	Fair	Good	Excellent
Variety			Good	
Balance	Poor			
Fiber		Fair		
Micronutrients		Fair		
Carbohydrate			Good	
Protein			Good	
Fat			Good	
Moderation	Poor			
Calories	Poor			
Individualized plans	Poor			
Exercise is recommended		Fair		
Enjoyable food				Excellent
Easy to understand				Excellent
Sustainability				Excellent
Long-term weight loss	Poor			
Educates the consumer	Poor			
Cost			Good	

Positives

Monday through Friday meals are healthy. It is basically a portion-controlled Mediterranean style of eating that considers calorie restriction. This combination can lead to healthy weight loss.

Negatives

Saturday and Sunday eating is out of control. Allowing a cheat meal once in a while may prevent boredom and help us continue to follow a balanced eating plan, but eating whatever is wanted on the weekend is a bad habit and will not lead to weight loss. Doesn't adequately address milk and milk products and the nutrients they provide.

The hook/catch or brilliant selling point: Eat what we want, don't exercise, and still lose weight. This is exactly what most people want to hear. Finally!

Truths/Myths

- Myth - Cheating on weekends will rev up our metabolism. p. 65

- Truth - It is not wise to over-indulge on weekly basis, it will only serve to cause weight gain.

Final decision: Thumbs down

How to improve this diet: Continue the meal plan for 7 days a week and if the urge for a cheat comes, have a taste of it but don't overindulge. Work into the mindset that we need a lifestyle of healthy eating where we occasionally veer off course, knowing the more often we do, the slower our weight loss will be. Engage in aerobic exercise at least 150 minutes a week. No need for the recommended supplements.

Clean and Lean Diet: 30 Days, 30 Foods, A New You

Premise of the Diet: Intermittent fasting and 30 natural foods consumed for 30 days will set the foundation for adopting a new healthier lifestyle.

Claims of the Diet: Will inspire creativity in cooking and assembling meals.

Diet Description: Involves preparing by choosing an intermittent fasting schedule. Eating 3 meals and 3 snacks. Provides a list of items to be avoided, including MSG, white flour, alcohol, fried foods, soda, and foods with added sugar. Provides a list of 30 recommended foods to be combined and consumed in meals and snacks. The diet allows the dieter to alter that list based on personal preferences, as long as the new additions are natural and not processed with artificial ingredients.

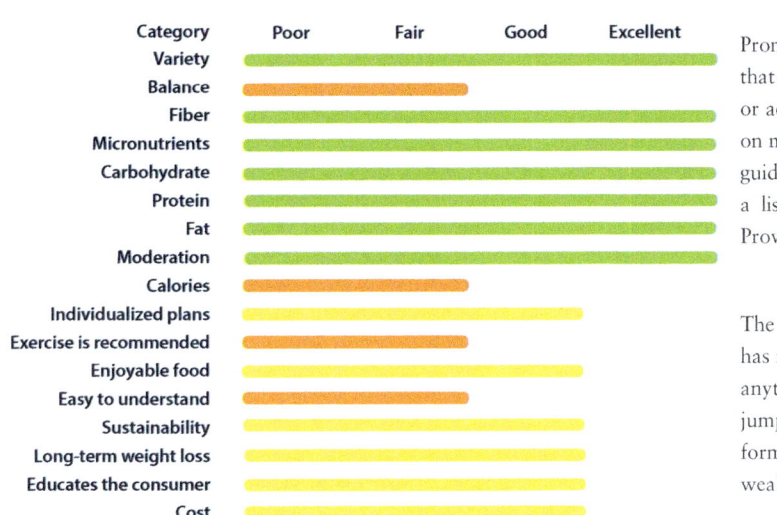

Category	Rating
Variety	Excellent
Balance	Fair
Fiber	Excellent
Micronutrients	Excellent
Carbohydrate	Excellent
Protein	Excellent
Fat	Excellent
Moderation	Excellent
Calories	Fair
Individualized plans	Good
Exercise is recommended	Fair
Enjoyable food	Good
Easy to understand	Fair
Sustainability	Good
Long-term weight loss	Good
Educates the consumer	Good
Cost	Good

Positives

Promotes natural whole foods. Promotes exercise that can be individualized by beginner, intermediate or advanced exercisers. Provides recipes. Focuses on making sustainable lifestyle changes. Provides guidelines for choosing healthy foods. Provides a list of spices to be incorporated into meals. Provides nutritional facts about various nutrients.

Negatives

The recommendation for intermittent fasting has no integrity. In other words, it means nearly anything and therefore means nothing. It merely jumps on the most recent bandwagon. The informational support for intermittent fasting is weak.

The hook/catch or brilliant selling point: Author has written many successful diet books.

Truths/Myths

- **Myth** - Intermittent fasting is a good way to lose weight. 🔍 p. 81

- **Truth** - This diet offers so many variations of intermittent fasting, the question must be asked: What is the point? Some approaches are what many people do anyway.

- **Truth** - Long periods of fasting can decrease the metabolic rate, making fat loss more difficult.

Final decision: Thumbs up (without intermittent fasting) 👍

How to improve this diet: Include a variety of the whole, natural foods eaten in moderation. Don't bother incorporating the intermittent fasting time frames.

Cookie Diet

Premise of the Diet: Snacking throughout the day on low-calorie cookies made with a secret "hunger-controlling" formula keeps us from feeling hungry.

Claims of the Diet: Lose 10 to 15 pounds per month, without feeling hunger.

Diet Description: In place of breakfast and lunch, eat 1-2 "hunger controlling" cookies, every 2 hours every day, for a total of 9 cookies a day. Have a 500- to 700-calorie dinner consisting of lean meat and salad/vegetables. Do this indefinitely.

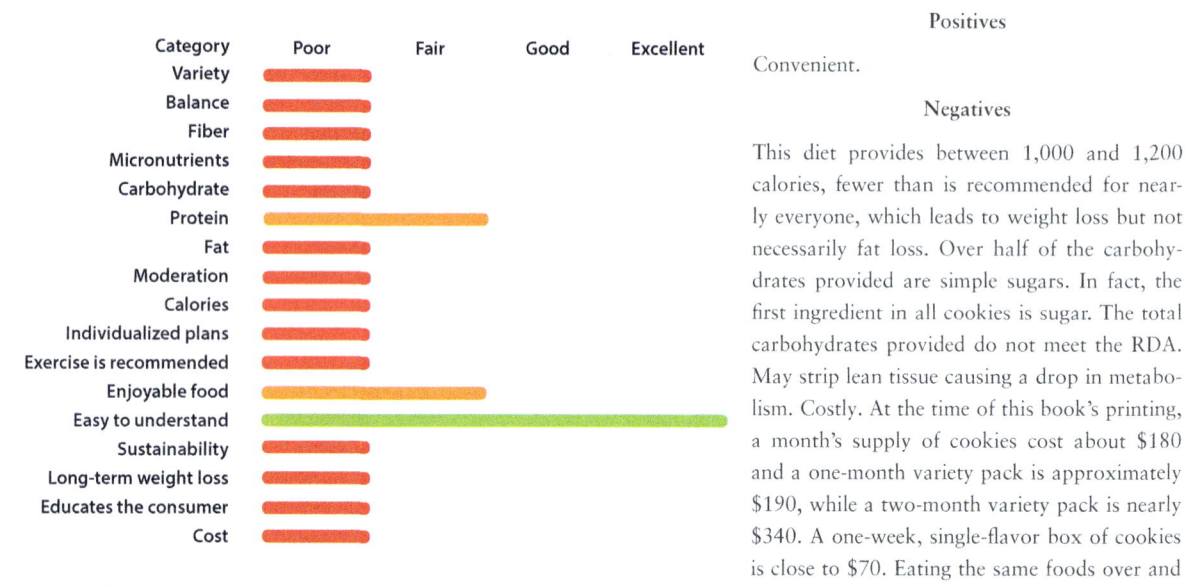

Category	Poor	Fair	Good	Excellent
Variety	■			
Balance	■			
Fiber	■			
Micronutrients	■			
Carbohydrate	■			
Protein		■		
Fat	■			
Moderation	■			
Calories	■			
Individualized plans	■			
Exercise is recommended	■			
Enjoyable food		■		
Easy to understand				■
Sustainability	■			
Long-term weight loss	■			
Educates the consumer	■			
Cost	■			

Positives

Convenient.

Negatives

This diet provides between 1,000 and 1,200 calories, fewer than is recommended for nearly everyone, which leads to weight loss but not necessarily fat loss. Over half of the carbohydrates provided are simple sugars. In fact, the first ingredient in all cookies is sugar. The total carbohydrates provided do not meet the RDA. May strip lean tissue causing a drop in metabolism. Costly. At the time of this book's printing, a month's supply of cookies cost about $180 and a one-month variety pack is approximately $190, while a two-month variety pack is nearly $340. A one-week, single-flavor box of cookies is close to $70. Eating the same foods over and over gets boring and monotonous for most of us. Furthermore, while other diets fortify their packaged foods with vitamins and minerals, this diet does not.

The hook/catch or brilliant selling point: Eating "hunger-controlling cookies" helps us lose weight. Our dream comes true!

Truths/Myths

- *Myth* - Eating "hunger-controlling cookies" can help us lose weight. 🔍 p. 17

- *Truth* - Burning more calories than we consume is how we lose weight. In fact, following this diet will not result in sustainable fat loss and may ultimately result in a lower metabolic rate and more body fat.

Final decision: Thumbs down 👎

How to improve this diet: Can't be improved.

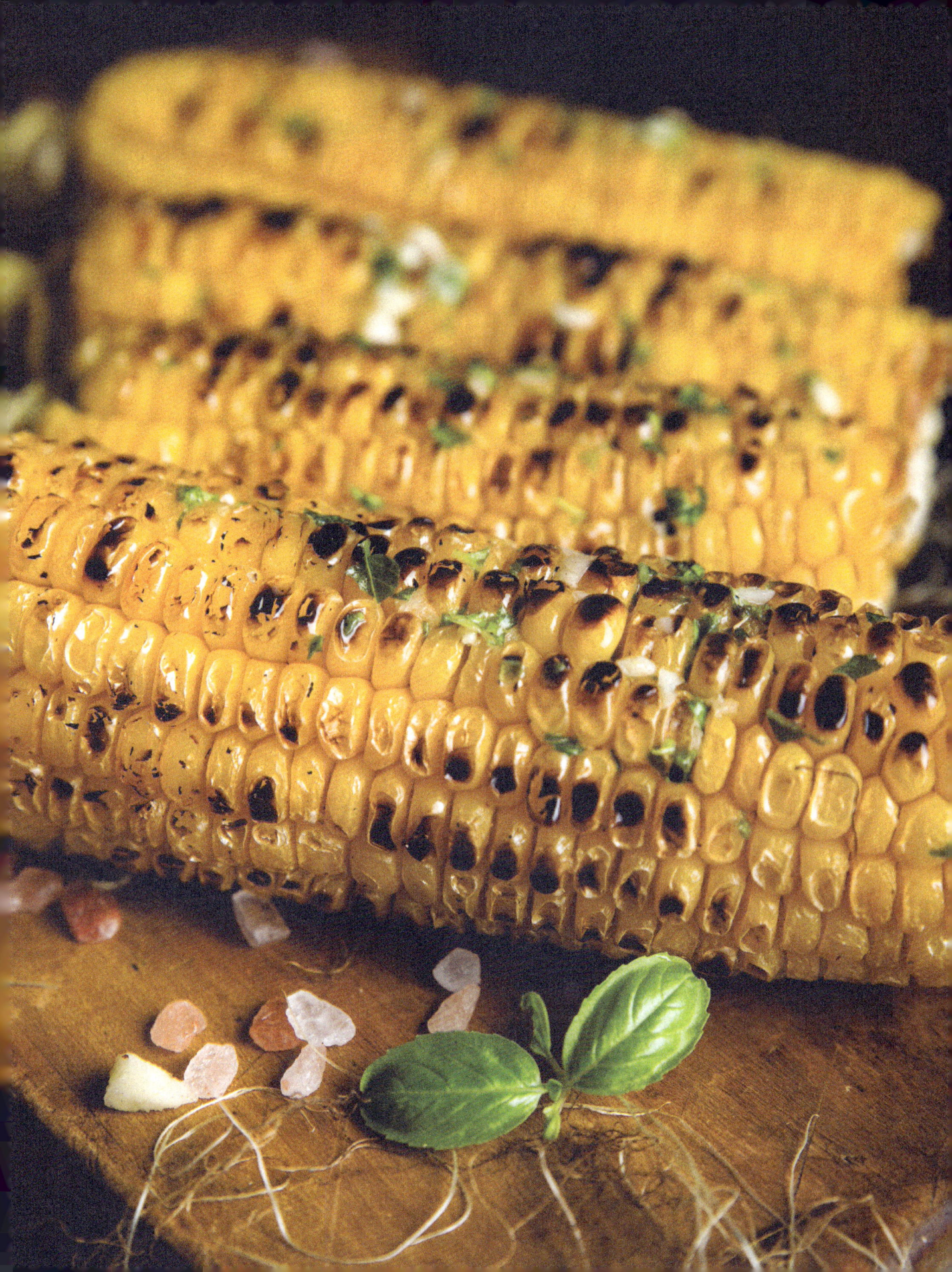

Cruise Control Diet

Premise of the Diet: A whole-foods method of weight loss.

Claims of the Diet: Speedy, long-lasting weight loss.

Diet Description: Based on four rules: 1) Eat natural foods, which will help the body burn fat. 2) Avoid processed and packaged foods because they cause the body to store fat. 3) Sweets are allowed from time to time to avoid feelings of restriction. 4) Do not count calories, keep food journals, or attempt to monitor portion controls. Choose an 8-hour window that's convenient to eat meals and snacks each day. During that window, consume 2 meals and 2 snacks that emphasize protein, non-starchy veggies, and healthy fat. A couple of servings of healthy carb-rich foods or wine is also allowed. The other 16 hours (the "burn zone"), consume any treat that gets almost 100% of its calories from fat.

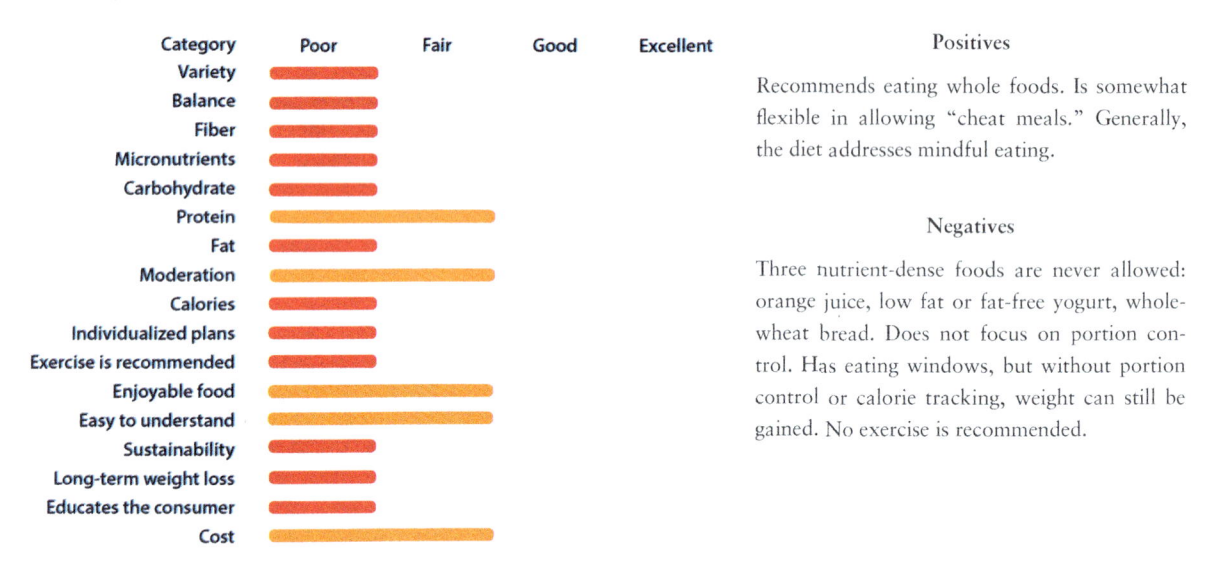

Category	Poor	Fair	Good	Excellent
Variety	■			
Balance	■			
Fiber	■			
Micronutrients	■			
Carbohydrate	■			
Protein		■		
Fat	■			
Moderation		■		
Calories	■			
Individualized plans	■			
Exercise is recommended	■			
Enjoyable food		■		
Easy to understand		■		
Sustainability	■			
Long-term weight loss	■			
Educates the consumer	■			
Cost		■		

Positives

Recommends eating whole foods. Is somewhat flexible in allowing "cheat meals." Generally, the diet addresses mindful eating.

Negatives

Three nutrient-dense foods are never allowed: orange juice, low fat or fat-free yogurt, whole-wheat bread. Does not focus on portion control. Has eating windows, but without portion control or calorie tracking, weight can still be gained. No exercise is recommended.

The hook/catch or brilliant selling point: Brilliant marketing of sensational claims.

Truths/Myths

- **Myth** - Bringing insulin down means weight comes down automatically. 🔍 p. 73

- **Truth** - Bringing insulin down means there will be fewer spikes in blood glucose, which would naturally mean there is less glucose to convert to glycogen and fat. However, for weight to be lost, total number of calories must also be controlled.

- **Myth** - Constant overloading on carbohydrates and protein foods causes body systems to malfunction, ending up with chronically elevated insulin that locks us into burning sugar instead of fat. The body then sends most blood sugar directly to fat cells.

- **Truth** - Rising blood glucose is the major cause of rising insulin, which locks us into storing calories, not the burning of calories. The burning of fat is influenced by low levels of insulin. Low levels of insulin automatically mean high levels of glucagon. This myth is suggesting that an overload of carbohydrates and protein creates insulin resistance. Research shows that insulin resistance is more related to excess body fat.

- **Truth** - Constant overloading of any form of calories (carbohydrates, proteins or fats) causes excess body fat which is associated with insulin resistance. As body fat accumulates in tissues other than adipose cells, those tissues (like skeletal muscle) become insulin resistant and don't respond well to insulin's cue to move glucose from the blood to tissues for storage. As a result, blood glucose levels are not reduced, which in turn causes the pancreas to make more insulin. Many risk factors are associated with insulin resistance, including obesity, an inactive lifestyle, gestational diabetes, polycystic ovary syndrome, family history of diabetes, and smoking, to name a few.

• Myth - This diet is better than keto at unleashing the metabolism because keto diets eliminate carbohydrates to slash insulin, which is too extreme for a lot of people. This diet allows for a gentle lowering of insulin and dips into ketosis where fat is being burned. (The burn zone) 🔍 p. 84

• Truth - The above myth twists the facts. Ketosis doesn't occur at the same time as insulin secretion. Ketosis is a process that normally occurs between meals, when glucagon is secreted from the pancreas instead of insulin. This diet is just suggesting that the dieter eat healthy by including a normal amount of carbohydrates in their diet which will control insulin to normal levels. The keto diet reduces carbs so low that glucagon is secreted instead of insulin and ketosis is occurring continuously, after meals and between meals. Including carbohydrates above those recommended in the ketogenic diets will not allow ketosis to occur except between meals when insulin levels are low and glucagon is in control. In other words, this diet doesn't put the body into ketosis any more than occurs normally between meals. The ketogenic diet is, in fact, too extreme and many dieters either can't get into ketosis or can't sustain deep ketosis. One has to remain in a fasting state for more than a few hours in order to burn mostly fat. But the best way to burn fat for weight loss is by monitoring calorie intake and regularly exercising at a moderate or high intensity.

• Myth - After the "burn zone," the "boost zone" is entered, during which traditional meals and snacks are eaten that include plenty of metabolism-boosting protein, vegetables, and moderate amounts of healthy carbs during that chosen 8-hour window. Some insulin will be produced, but not enough to slow your progress.

• Truth - Ketosis occurs when glucagon is secreted by the pancreas instead of insulin. A moderate amount of vegetables and healthy carbohydrates will not keep someone in ketosis because it will result in insulin secretion instead of glucagon. Therefore, the process of ketosis will have to slow down. Adding carbohydrates back after placing the body in a carb-starved state, could increase the storage of those carbohydrates as fat since the body will be planning for another period of starvation.

Final decision: Thumbs down 👎

How to improve this diet: Can't be improved.

DASH Diet Weight-Loss Solution
(aka Dietary Approaches to Stop Hypertension)

Premise of the Diet: Good for people with metabolic syndrome, high blood pressure, prediabetes, or diabetes, and post-menopausal women who have gained weight around the midriff.

Claims of the Diet: Lowers cholesterol and blood pressure without medication while improving metabolism, lowering body fat, and improving strength and cardiovascular fitness. Reduces body's demand for insulin and reduces midsection fat.

Diet Description: Specific calorie requirements must be determined using the recommended food groups, including grains or grain products, vegetables, fruits, low-fat dairy, meat, poultry, or fish, fats and oils, and nuts, seeds, or dry beans. Sweets and added sugars are limited. The plan defines the serving sizes of each. The sample plans are provided by the National Heart Lung and Blood Institute (NHLBI). Requires meal planning. Provides 28 days of meal plans, 45+ recipes, and lifestyle plan to lose weight, lower blood pressure, lower cholesterol and triglycerides.

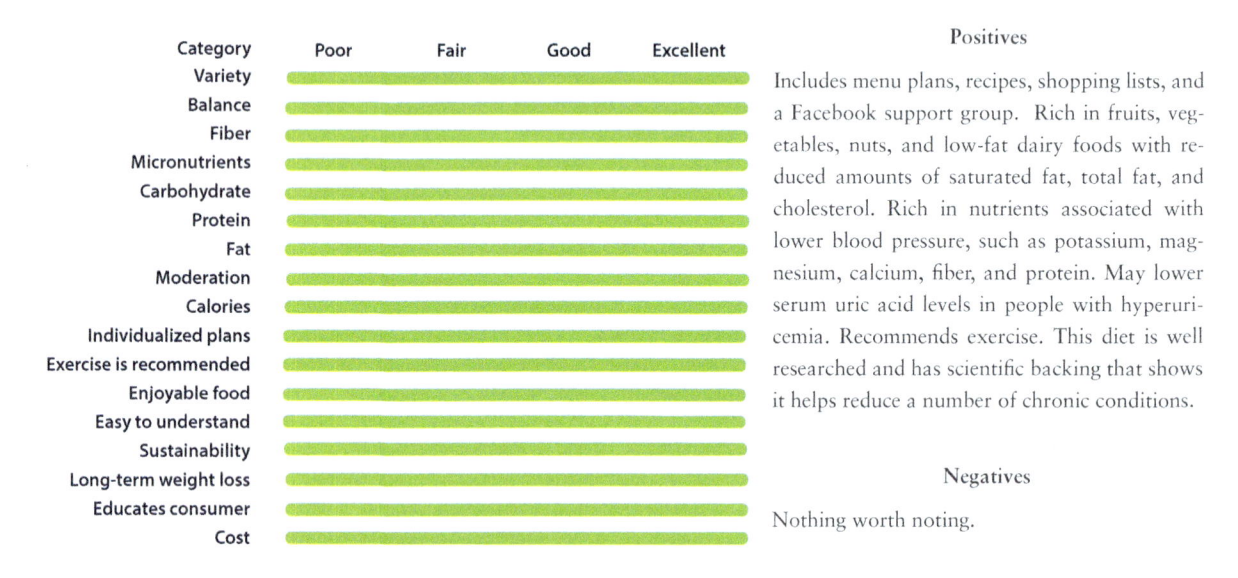

Category	Poor	Fair	Good	Excellent
Variety				✓
Balance				✓
Fiber				✓
Micronutrients				✓
Carbohydrate				✓
Protein				✓
Fat				✓
Moderation				✓
Calories				✓
Individualized plans				✓
Exercise is recommended				✓
Enjoyable food				✓
Easy to understand				✓
Sustainability				✓
Long-term weight loss				✓
Educates consumer				✓
Cost				✓

Positives

Includes menu plans, recipes, shopping lists, and a Facebook support group. Rich in fruits, vegetables, nuts, and low-fat dairy foods with reduced amounts of saturated fat, total fat, and cholesterol. Rich in nutrients associated with lower blood pressure, such as potassium, magnesium, calcium, fiber, and protein. May lower serum uric acid levels in people with hyperuricemia. Recommends exercise. This diet is well researched and has scientific backing that shows it helps reduce a number of chronic conditions.

Negatives

Nothing worth noting.

The hook/catch or brilliant selling point: Combines the healthy DASH diet with weight loss strategies and suggestions.

Truths/Myths: None worth noting.

Final decision: Thumbs up 👍

How to improve this diet: Nothing worth noting.

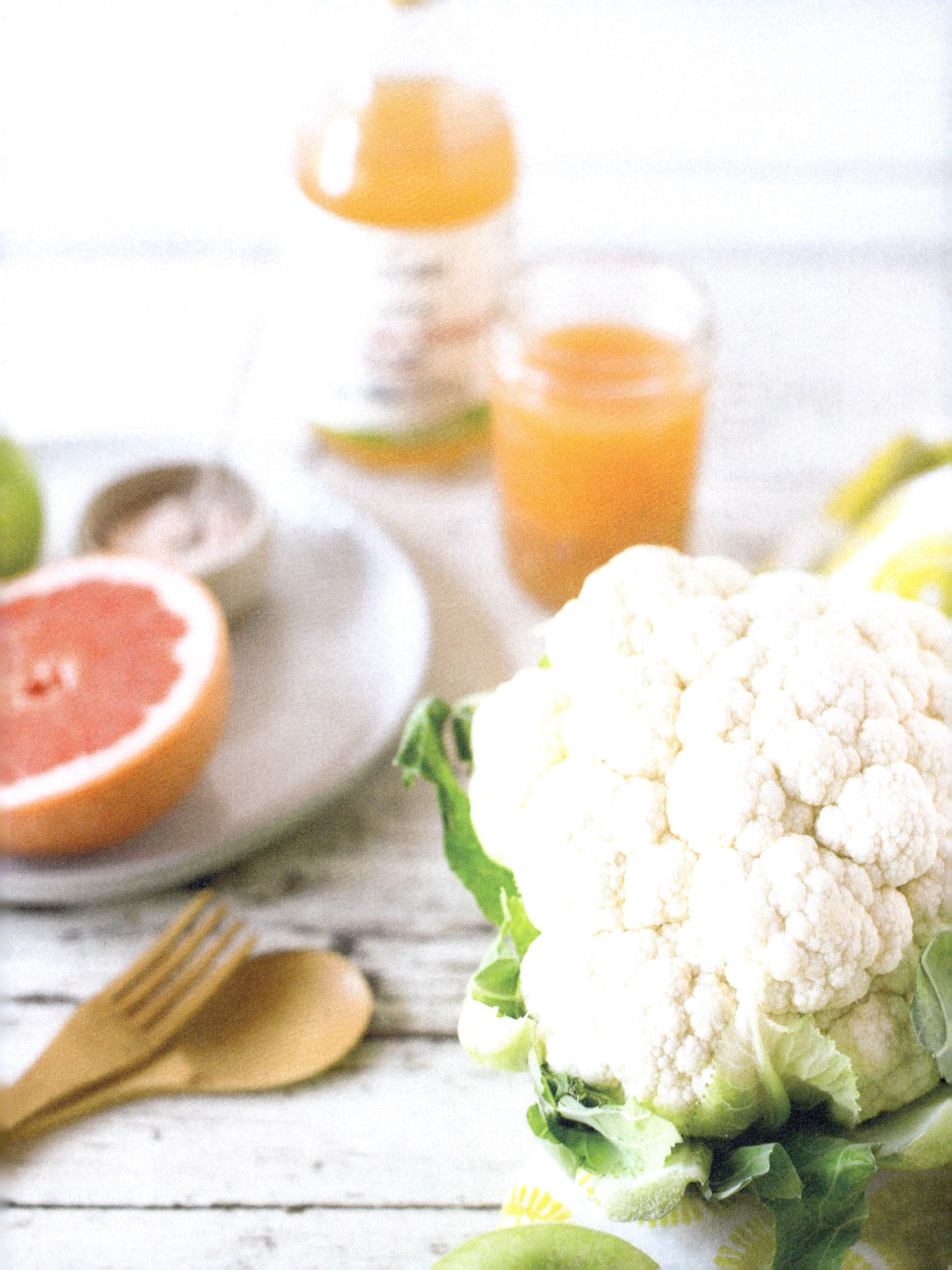

Diet Solution (aka The Beyond Diet)

Premise of the Diet: The Diet Solution program is a holistic diet and lifestyle approach that combines specific foods that match our specific metabolic type. There are three metabolic diet types: protein, carb, or mixed. Eliminating foods that don't suit a particular metabolic type will promote weight loss.

Claims of the Diet: Answering the program's questionnaire (which asks questions about dieting history, motivation level, eating habits, reactions toward dieting, response to hunger and cravings, and reasons for overeating) can determine our metabolic type.

Diet Description: Answer program questionnaire, calculate calorie goal, and follow the 6-week meal plan, customizing it by adding more protein or carbs to satisfy the determined metabolic type. Limits food intake to whole, natural, organic foods, mostly healthy meats, fish, vegetables, seeds, nuts, and raw high-fiber fruits.

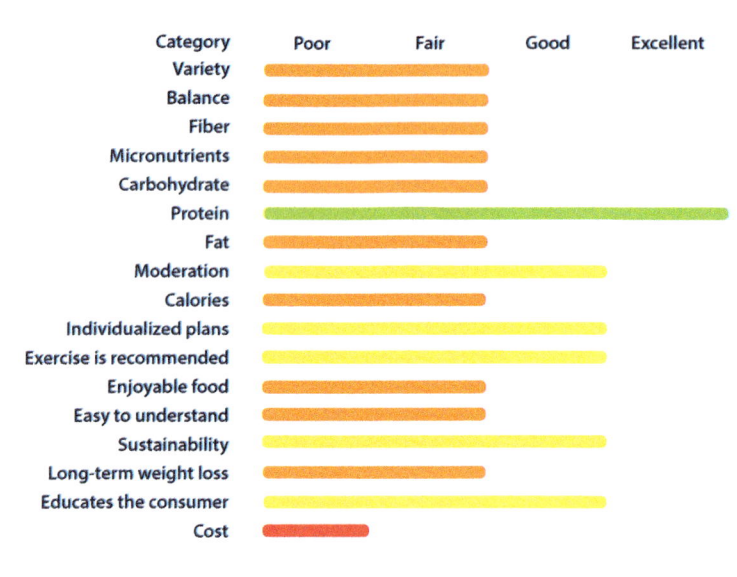

Category	Poor	Fair	Good	Excellent
Variety	■			
Balance	■			
Fiber	■			
Micronutrients	■			
Carbohydrate	■			
Protein				■
Fat	■			
Moderation		■		
Calories	■			
Individualized plans		■		
Exercise is recommended		■		
Enjoyable food	■			
Easy to understand	■			
Sustainability		■		
Long-term weight loss	■			
Educates the consumer		■		
Cost	■			

Positives

Not a quick-fix diet. Recommends losing 1 to 2 pounds per week. Encourages keeping a food journal to record daily intake. Regardless of the metabolic type determined, this plan encourages eating 3 meals and 2 snacks. Requires no calorie counting. Weight loss may occur due to a lower intake of calories from consuming plenty of lean protein and adequate fiber. Educates about the dangers of hydrogenated fats. Encourages rethinking the concept of snacks as junk food to choosing nutritious alternatives such as raw nuts, boiled eggs, and fruits or vegetables. Emphasizes foods high in the heart-healthy Omega-3 fats, encourages the intake of fresh fruit and vegetables. Provided meal plans can be adjusted to suit individual needs. Teaches about portion sizes. Encourages drinking water.

Negatives

Restrictive. Expensive. Can be deficient in calcium. For many, it will be hard to follow long term. Raw, organic eggs and unpasteurized dairy can be a health hazard. These are not recommended for consumption. The entire premise of this diet is not grounded in science.

The hook/catch or brilliant selling point: Cleverly capitalizes on the mass push for low carbs or low-fat diets by reasoning that if we don't experience success on one, it is because we are not eating right for our particular metabolic type.

Truths/Myths

- **Myth** - Everyone fits into three metabolic diet types. 🔍 p. 65

- **Truth** - Everyone needs to eat the right balance of carbs, protein, and fat at meals. 🔍 p. 41

- **Myth** - A questionnaire based mostly on emotions and psychological concepts can determine our body's physiology.

- **Truth** - Only lab values and anthropometrics (height, weight, waist circumference and calculations) could come close to determining our actual metabolism.

- Myth - Organic foods foster weight loss.

- Truth - A calorie deficit fosters weight loss.

- Myth - Foods containing ingredients that can't be pronounced are "toxins."

- Truth - Ingredients that are difficult to pronounce are just that, difficult to pronounce. For example, ascorbic acid and alpha-tocopherol are the scientific terms for vitamin C and vitamin E.

- Truth - Consuming fewer processed foods is recommended.

- Myth - Natural foods have a rigid definition and are limited to organic whole foods.

- Truth - There is no set definition for a natural food. Standard definitions for some terms have been established by the FDA. For example, the word "Fresh" is defined by the FDA as "never been frozen or heated and contains no preservatives." Healthy foods can still be frozen, canned or packaged.

- Truth - Motivation and staying positive while dieting is helpful.

Final decision: This was a tough one, because most recommendations are viable. However, not all recommendations are safe, and it is not based on science. Thumbs down. 👎

How to improve this diet: Loosen rigid definitions. Do not eat raw eggs or unpasteurized dairy products. We should all eat the right balance of carbs, protein, and fat at meals.

Diet-to-Go

Premise of the Diet: A chef prepares and portions meals, so all the work is already done.

Claims of the Diet: No matter what your weight-loss and healthy living goals, Diet-to-Go can help you achieve them. This approach will save you time and you will eat better.

Diet Description: Chef-prepared healthy meals delivered weekly. Choose from four menus: 1) Balanced menu, 2) Balanced Diabetic menu, 3) Keto-carb30 menu, or 4) Vegetarian. Can choose to receive two meals a day (lunch and dinner) for 5 days a week ($12.70 per meal totaling $127 per week plus shipping) up to three meals a day for 7 days ($8.90 per meal totaling $187 per week plus shipping). The Keto-carb30 menu runs slightly higher for $10.14 per meal totaling $212.99 per week plus shipping.

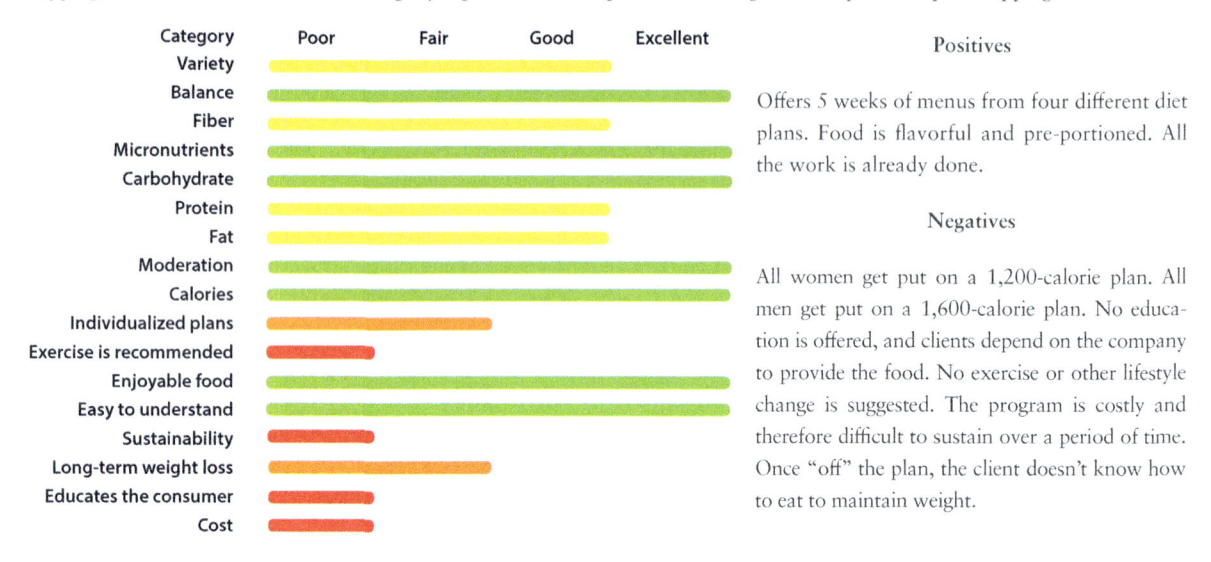

Category	Rating
Variety	Fair
Balance	Excellent
Fiber	Fair
Micronutrients	Excellent
Carbohydrate	Excellent
Protein	Fair
Fat	Fair
Moderation	Excellent
Calories	Excellent
Individualized plans	Poor–Fair
Exercise is recommended	Poor
Enjoyable food	Excellent
Easy to understand	Excellent
Sustainability	Poor
Long-term weight loss	Poor–Fair
Educates the consumer	Poor
Cost	Poor

Positives

Offers 5 weeks of menus from four different diet plans. Food is flavorful and pre-portioned. All the work is already done.

Negatives

All women get put on a 1,200-calorie plan. All men get put on a 1,600-calorie plan. No education is offered, and clients depend on the company to provide the food. No exercise or other lifestyle change is suggested. The program is costly and therefore difficult to sustain over a period of time. Once "off" the plan, the client doesn't know how to eat to maintain weight.

The hook/catch or brilliant selling point: Easy.

Truths/Myths

- Myth - All women should try to lose weight by consuming 1,200-calorie diets, and all men should consume no more than 1,600 calories when trying to lose weight.

- Truth - People are unique individuals with different food preferences and calorie requirements. Losing weight too quickly can harm one's metabolism, making it difficult to lose weight later. p. 13, 21

Final decision: Thumbs down

How to improve this diet: Follow a balanced eating plan that offers the required number of calories needed to lose weight. Make necessary lifestyle changes, including incorporating regular exercise.

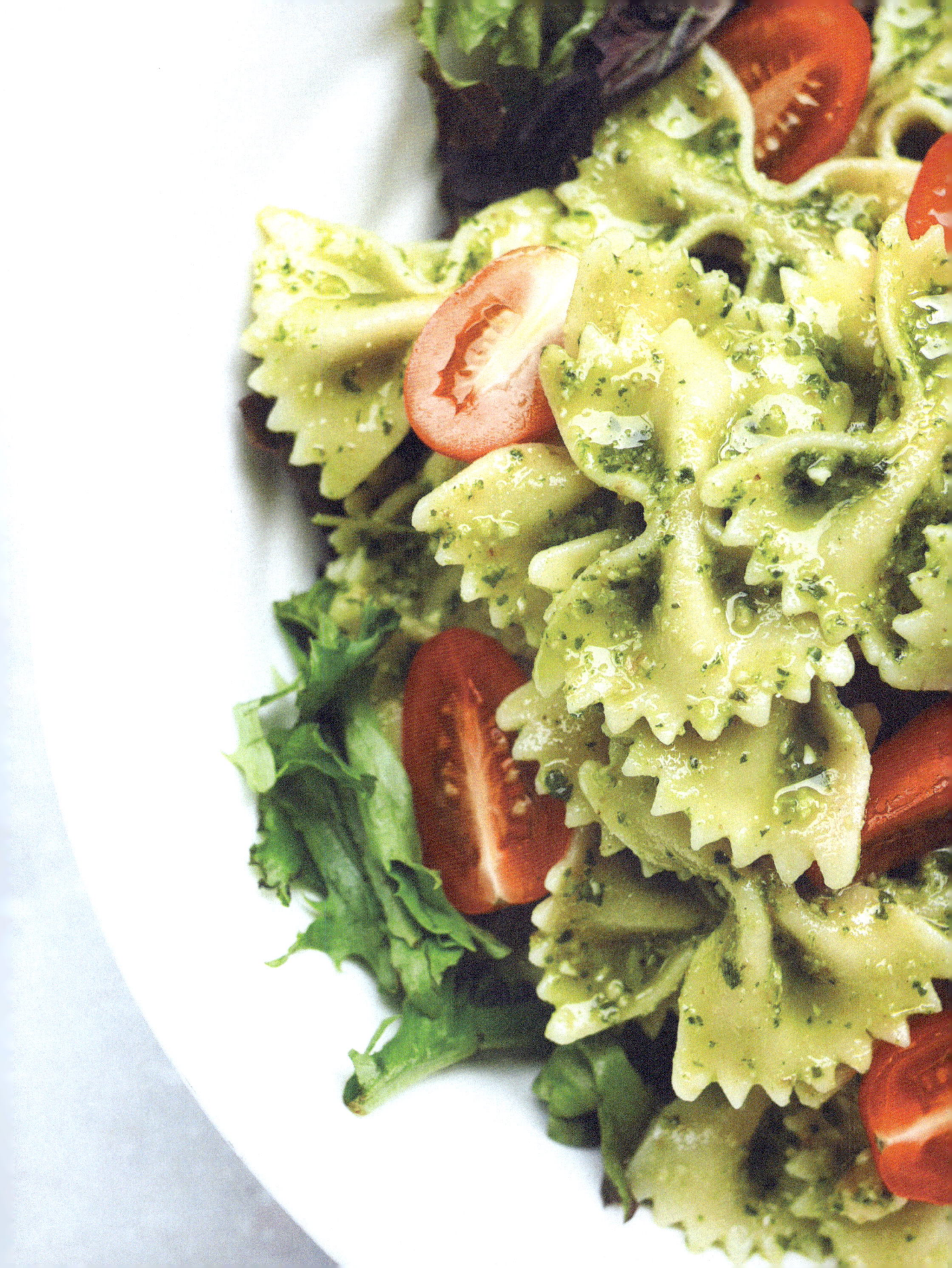

Dr. Andrew Weil Diet

Premise of the Diet: An anti-inflammatory diet that curbs inflammation and helps with weight loss.

Claims of the Diet: Will decrease inflammation.

Diet Description: Complex carbohydrates make up 40% to 50% of daily calories. Healthy fats make up 30% of your daily calories, while protein accounts for 20% to 30% of daily calories. Except for fish, some cheeses and yogurt, animal protein is limited. Processed foods are not allowed. Tea is preferred to coffee. One or two glasses of red wine daily is acceptable, as is plain dark chocolate in moderation if the cocoa content is at least 70%.

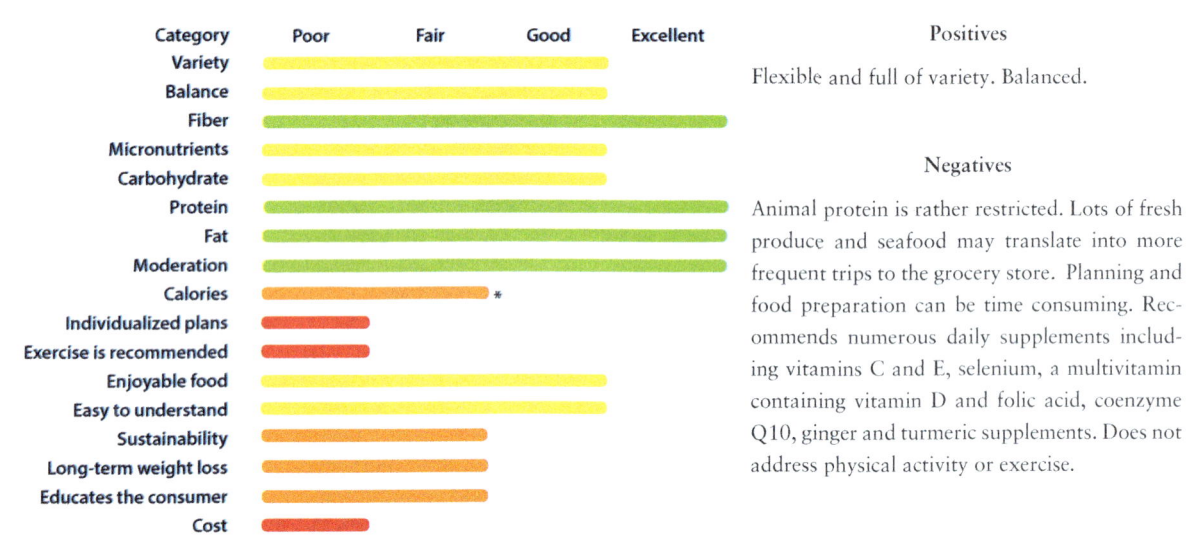

Category	Poor	Fair	Good	Excellent
Variety			██████	
Balance			██████	
Fiber				████████
Micronutrients			██████	
Carbohydrate			██████	
Protein				████████
Fat				████████
Moderation				████████
Calories			██*	
Individualized plans	██			
Exercise is recommended	██			
Enjoyable food			██████	
Easy to understand			██████	
Sustainability		████		
Long-term weight loss		████		
Educates the consumer		████		
Cost	██			

Positives

Flexible and full of variety. Balanced.

Negatives

Animal protein is rather restricted. Lots of fresh produce and seafood may translate into more frequent trips to the grocery store. Planning and food preparation can be time consuming. Recommends numerous daily supplements including vitamins C and E, selenium, a multivitamin containing vitamin D and folic acid, coenzyme Q10, ginger and turmeric supplements. Does not address physical activity or exercise.

*Gives the range needed for most adults, 2,000-3,000 calories per day, but does not address calories in relation to weight loss.

The hook/catch or brilliant selling point: Decrease inflammation and lose weight in the process.

Truths/Myths

- **Myth** - This is a weight-loss diet.

- **Truth** - This is an anti-inflammatory diet, but some weight may be lost due to following a healthy eating plan. Since being overweight is also associated with inflammation, it is logical that losing excess weight may help decrease inflammation in the body.

- **Myth** - All the supplements are necessary in the diet. 🔍 p. 99

- **Truth** - It is wiser to consume these nutrients in the form of food.

Final decision: Thumbs down 👎

How to improve this diet: Follow this plan, making sure the calorie amount consumed is less than expended to ensure weight loss. Do not purchase all the supplements but instead make wise, nutrient-dense choices.

Dr. Phil's Ultimate Weight Solution
(aka Dr. Phil's 20/20 Ultimate Weight Solution)

Premise of the Diet: Using psychology can help change the way we approach food, as well as our relationship with food as it relates to weight control.

Claims of the Diet: Ends the dieting frustration and provides the tools for life-changing weight loss.

Diet Description: This diet is divided into four phases: 1. The five-day boost: eat only the 20 foods listed in the guideline. 2. Five-day sustain: add foods outside the original 20, but all meals and snacks must have at least two of the original 20/20 foods. 3. 20-day sustain: more foods are allowed. Eat 4 meals, 4 hours apart for 20 days. Allows for two splurges that do not exceed 100 calories each week. 4. Management Phase: continue eating healthy foods from previous phases. If your goal is not reached by the end of Phase 3, repeat the first three phases until goal is reached.

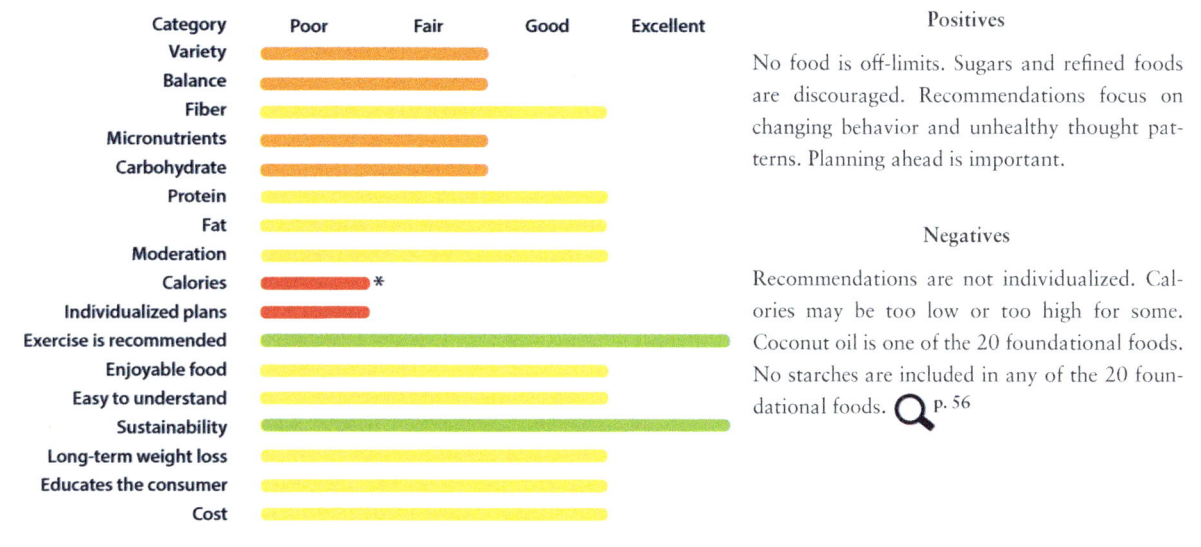

Category	Poor	Fair	Good	Excellent
Variety		Fair		
Balance		Fair		
Fiber			Good	
Micronutrients		Fair		
Carbohydrate		Fair		
Protein			Good	
Fat			Good	
Moderation			Good	
Calories	Poor*			
Individualized plans	Poor			
Exercise is recommended				Excellent
Enjoyable food			Good	
Easy to understand			Good	
Sustainability				Excellent
Long-term weight loss			Good	
Educates the consumer			Good	
Cost			Good	

Positives

No food is off-limits. Sugars and refined foods are discouraged. Recommendations focus on changing behavior and unhealthy thought patterns. Planning ahead is important.

Negatives

Recommendations are not individualized. Calories may be too low or too high for some. Coconut oil is one of the 20 foundational foods. No starches are included in any of the 20 foundational foods. 🔍 p. 56

*Calorie levels are not clearly addressed.

The hook/catch or brilliant selling point: Rides the coattails of TV celebrity and former psychologist Dr. Phil McGraw.

Truths/Myths

- Myth - A healthy relationship with food is sufficient for weight loss. 🔍 p. 1

- Truth - Improving our relationship with food can help us lose weight, but we need to have a balanced diet and consume a variety of healthy foods in moderation. Calories do count. 🔍 p. 21

Final decision: Thumbs down 👎

How to improve this diet: Consume a variety of interesting, nutrient-dense foods for all meals and snacks. Incorporate more complex carbohydrates. Keep calorie level near our BMR and increase/keep exercise level up to burn more calories than are being consumed.

Dukan Diet

Premise of the Diet: Eating protein is the key to weight loss.

Claims of the Diet: Lose up to 10 pounds the first week, then lose 2 to 4 pounds a week after that, all without being hungry.

Diet Description: Four phases with many do's and don'ts.

1. Attack Phase (1-7 days) – Eat all the pure protein we want, plus 1.5 tablespoons of oat bran.

2. Cruise Phase (1-12 months) – Add selected vegetables on selected days, plus 2 tablespoons of oat bran.

3. Consolidation Phase (5 days for every pound lost in early phases) – Unlimited lean protein and vegetables, plus 2.5 tablespoons of oat bran. Add more foods, such as cheese and bread.

4. Permanent Stabilization (indefinite) – Can eat nearly anything we want, plus 3 tablespoons oat bran.

Category	Poor	Fair	Good	Excellent
Variety	■			
Balance	■			
Fiber	■			
Micronutrients	■			
Carbohydrate	■			
Protein	■			
Fat	■			
Moderation	■			
Calories	■			
Individualized plans	■			
Exercise is recommended			■	
Enjoyable food	■			
Easy to understand	■			
Sustainability	■			
Long-term weight loss	■			
Educates the consumer	■			
Cost	■			

Positives

Provides many guidelines which tell us exactly what to do – this can be a good thing for those of us who do not want to think or learn. Promotes lower-fat proteins and oat bran to get fiber. Limits alcohol and sugar. Recommends exercise and water.

Negatives

Promotes more than the government's recommendation for protein, which may bring about health concerns. Complicated. Eliminates many healthy foods. Restricts both carbs and fat. Consuming 1.5–2 tablespoons of oat bran contain less than 5 grams of fiber, so it doesn't provide many health benefits. May feel too tired or exhausted to maintain exercise.

The hook/catch or brilliant selling point: If protein is good, more is even better.

Truths/Myths

- **Myth** - It is healthy and desirable to lose up to 10 pounds in a week. 🔍 p. 16

- **Truth** - Since water loss is part of the first stage of weight loss, it is therefore included in this number. Water must always be replaced.

- **Myth** - Eating only protein is what helps us lose those 10 pounds the first week. 🔍 p. 73

- **Truth** - When carbohydrates are eliminated from the diet, the body will use up stored glycogen in the body. Glycogen stores water with it, so when we burn up those last stores of glycogen in the body, the body also loses that accompanying water. 🔍 p. 15, 75

- **Myth** - It is safe to eliminate carbohydrates and fats from the diet in lieu of consuming more protein. 🔍 p. 40

- **Truth** - Both carbohydrates and fats provide essential health benefits.

Final decision: Thumbs down 👎

How to improve this diet: Can't be improved.

Eat Clean Diet

Premise of the Diet: Eating whole, nutrient-dense, well-sourced, and properly prepared foods leads to good health and our best appearance.

Claims of the Diet: Lose 3 pounds a week without being hungry. Stay healthy, have more energy. Eyes will look bright and alert. Teeth and gums will be healthier and skin will glow.

Diet Description: A balanced diet that focuses on whole grains at every meal, fruits, vegetables, 2-3 servings of healthy fats, and lean protein while encouraging portion control in 6 small meals a day. Drink 2 to 3 liters of water daily. Doesn't ban any food groups.

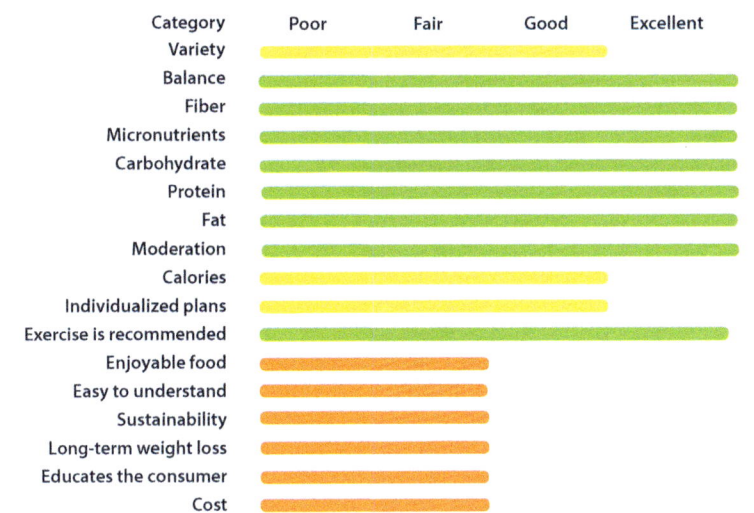

Category	Poor	Fair	Good	Excellent
Variety			Good	
Balance				Excellent
Fiber				Excellent
Micronutrients				Excellent
Carbohydrate				Excellent
Protein				Excellent
Fat				Excellent
Moderation				Excellent
Calories			Good	
Individualized plans			Good	
Exercise is recommended				Excellent
Enjoyable food		Fair		
Easy to understand		Fair		
Sustainability		Fair		
Long-term weight loss		Fair		
Educates the consumer		Fair		
Cost		Fair		

Positives

Provides flexible diet plans that range from 1,200 to 1,800 calories, which, may be on the lower end of calories needed to sustain energy, satisfy hunger, and help weight loss. Allows for a weekly cheat meal or treat, which may remove guilt and allow for continuation on the plan. Encourages learning where local foods come from and encourages developing relationships with local farmers to increase the likelihood of getting the freshest, in-season foods available. Encourages eating nutrient-dense foods and preparing meals at home.

Negatives

Recommends supplements. Suggests disputed medical treatments. Nutrition advice is not based on scientific evidence. Restrictive with lots of rules, which may make this diet difficult to follow for a long time. Difficult for those of us who want more flexibility.

The hook/catch or brilliant selling point: Rev up the metabolism, burn more fat faster, and never go hungry.

Truths/Myths

- **Myth** - We can eat more and weigh less.

- **Truth** - We can't eat more of everything /anything and expect to lose weight. Calories do matter. 🔍 p. 21

- **Myth** - Need to avoid "Chemically-charged foods."

- **Truth** - "Chemically-charged foods" do not exist. This is jargon used to sell. 🔍 p. 10

- **Myth** - Need to completely cut out saturated fats.

- **Truth** - Current recommendations are to eat 7-10% of total calories from saturated fat. Being too strict without a basis for it increases the likelihood of discouragement and failure.

- **Myth** - This diet can be a natural detox.

- **Truth** - Foods don't detoxify the body, the liver does. This is jargon used to sell.

Final decision: Thumbs up 👍

How to improve this diet: Be sure to consume sufficient calories. Do not take the supplements.

Eat More, Weigh Less Diet

Premise of the Diet: Encourages healthy lifestyle changes that accompany a healthy body weight.

Claims of the Diet: Many health benefits accompany a vegetarian diet.

Diet Description: A low-fat vegetarian diet that recommends consuming less than 10 percent fat, no cholesterol and as much fruit, vegetables, and legumes as desired. Allows moderate amounts of low-fat dairy but no meats, oils, nuts, alcohol, and anything containing sugar.

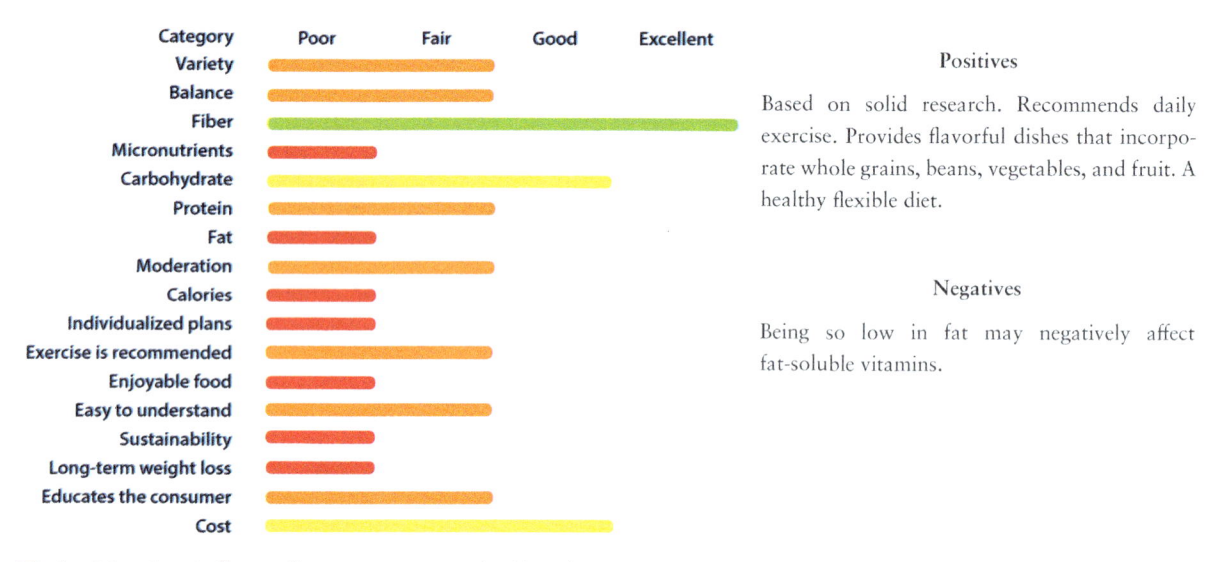

Category	Rating
Variety	Fair
Balance	Fair
Fiber	Excellent
Micronutrients	Poor
Carbohydrate	Good
Protein	Fair
Fat	Poor
Moderation	Fair
Calories	Poor
Individualized plans	Poor
Exercise is recommended	Fair
Enjoyable food	Poor
Easy to understand	Fair
Sustainability	Poor
Long-term weight loss	Poor
Educates the consumer	Fair
Cost	Good

Positives

Based on solid research. Recommends daily exercise. Provides flavorful dishes that incorporate whole grains, beans, vegetables, and fruit. A healthy flexible diet.

Negatives

Being so low in fat may negatively affect fat-soluble vitamins.

The hook/catch or brilliant selling point: Improves health and promotes weight loss.

Truths/Myths

- Truths - Consuming low-calorie foods that provide a large volume with a lot of water and fiber can increase the sense of fullness.

- Myths - No false claims made

Final decision: Thumbs up 👍

How to improve this diet: Occasionally add reasonable portions of lean meat for those who otherwise would have difficulty sustaining this diet.

Eat Right for Your Type Diet

Premise of the Diet: Eat a diet based on your blood type: O, A, B, or AB

Claims of the Diet: Foods eaten react chemically with blood types.

Diet Description: Type O blood: A high-protein diet with lots of lean meat, poultry, fish, and vegetables is recommended while being light on grains, beans, and dairy. These individuals suffer with GI problems.

Type A blood: A meat-less diet that is heavy on fruits and vegetables, beans, legumes, and whole grains. These individuals have a sensitive immune system.

Type B blood: Allows for green vegetables, eggs, certain meats, and low-fat dairy. Must avoid corn, chicken, wheat, buckwheat, lentils, tomatoes, peanuts, and sesame seeds.

Type AB blood: Focus on tofu, seafood, dairy, and green vegetables. Avoid caffeine, alcohol, and smoked or cured meats. These individuals tend to have low stomach acid.

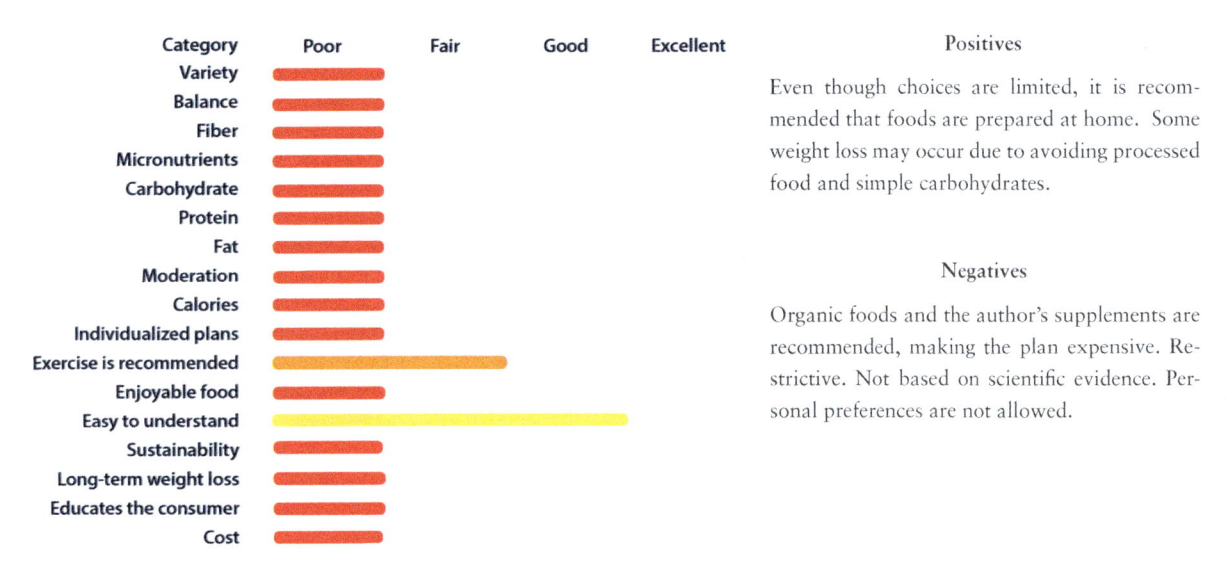

Category	Poor	Fair	Good	Excellent
Variety	■			
Balance	■			
Fiber	■			
Micronutrients	■			
Carbohydrate	■			
Protein	■			
Fat	■			
Moderation	■			
Calories	■			
Individualized plans	■			
Exercise is recommended		■		
Enjoyable food	■			
Easy to understand			■	
Sustainability	■			
Long-term weight loss	■			
Educates the consumer	■			
Cost	■			

Positives

Even though choices are limited, it is recommended that foods are prepared at home. Some weight loss may occur due to avoiding processed food and simple carbohydrates.

Negatives

Organic foods and the author's supplements are recommended, making the plan expensive. Restrictive. Not based on scientific evidence. Personal preferences are not allowed.

The hook/catch or brilliant selling point: Crazy, weird ideas get a lot of attention.

Truths/Myths

- Myth - The entire premise of the diet. 🔍 p. 13

- Truth - I have found no evidence to support any benefits based on blood type diets. There is no proven connection between blood type and digestion.

Final decision: Thumbs down 👎

How to improve this diet: Can't be improved.

Eat This, Not That Diet

Premise of the Diet: Consume fewer calories than the amount expended daily by swapping higher-calorie foods with items that are lower in fat and calories.

Claims of the Diet: Lose 10-30+ pounds.

Diet Description: Swap higher-calorie foods with items that are lower in fat and calories.

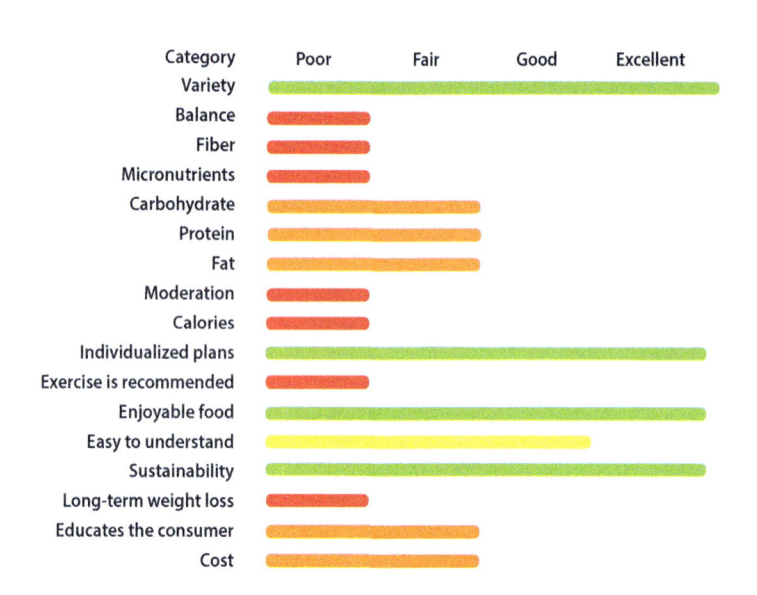

Category	Rating
Variety	Excellent
Balance	Poor
Fiber	Poor
Micronutrients	Poor
Carbohydrate	Fair
Protein	Fair
Fat	Fair
Moderation	Poor
Calories	Poor
Individualized plans	Excellent
Exercise is recommended	Poor
Enjoyable food	Excellent
Easy to understand	Good
Sustainability	Excellent
Long-term weight loss	Poor
Educates the consumer	Fair
Cost	Fair

Positives

Can help with making smarter choices for those who eat out often. Could be useful for those who don't want to go on a weight-loss diet but are trying to make healthier choices. No special rules to follow. Looking up "swaps" at restaurants is not difficult. Provides an easy-to-follow list of approved foods.

Negatives

This is more of a calorie-counter's guide that can assist in making wiser choices, than a diet to follow. Not everything on the "eat this" list is healthy. Not a nutritionally-balanced diet plan. Weight will not be lost unless total calories consumed are fewer than the number of calories expended.

The hook/catch or brilliant selling point: Swap to a healthier lifestyle.

Truths/Myths

- **Myth** - A revolutionary weight-loss plan exists that allows meals at Burger King, McDonald's, Dunkin' Donuts, Olive Garden, and ordering takeout pizza, ice cream and indulging in comfort foods whenever desired and still promotes weight loss.

- **Truth** - Calories consumed must be less than calories expended in order to lose body fat.   p. 21

Final decision: Thumbs down

How to improve this diet: Limit its use to the occasional eating out episode.

Eat to Live Diet (aka Nutritarian Diet)

Premise of the Diet: Eating foods high in nutrients and low in calories allows eating more and feeling fuller longer.

Claims of the Diet: Lose 20 pounds in 6 weeks, slows aging, increases lifespan, and helps prevent chronic illnesses.

Diet Description: A 6-week plan that limits carbs, sugar, oil, meat, and dairy while increasing whole fruits, vegetables, beans, and legumes. In essence, this is a plant based, low-salt, gluten free, low-fat plan. Recommended food group percentages include 30-60% coming from vegetables, with at least half of vegetables being raw, 10-40% from fruits—which translates to at least 3–5 servings of fresh fruit daily, and at least ½ cup of beans and legumes daily, which converts to 10-40% of total calories. At least one ounce of nuts, seeds, or avocados should be consumed, which translates to 10–40% of total calories. Consumption of whole grains and potatoes should not exceed 20% of total calories. Non-factory-farmed animal products, such as meat, dairy and eggs should comprise less than 10% of intake. Minimally-processed foods are allowed, but they should not exceed 10% of total calories.

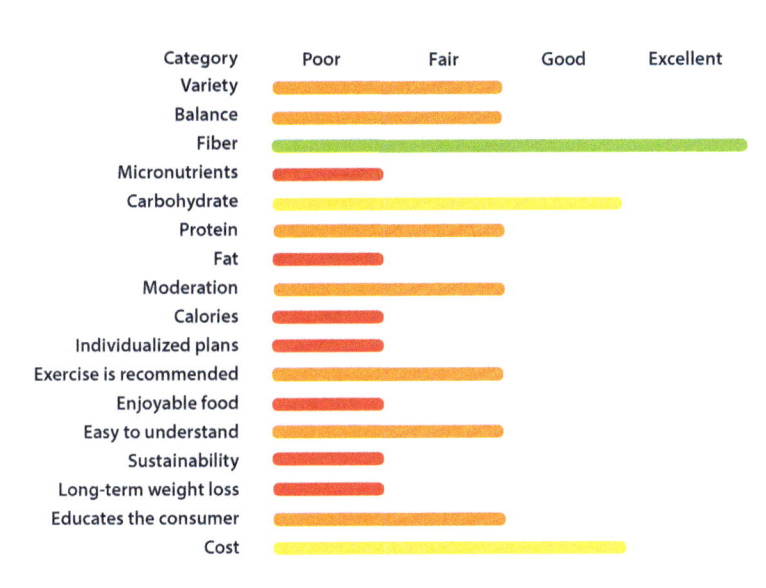

Category	Rating
Variety	Fair
Balance	Fair
Fiber	Excellent
Micronutrients	Poor
Carbohydrate	Good
Protein	Fair
Fat	Poor
Moderation	Fair
Calories	Poor
Individualized plans	Poor
Exercise is recommended	Fair
Enjoyable food	Poor
Easy to understand	Fair
Sustainability	Poor
Long-term weight loss	Poor
Educates the consumer	Fair
Cost	Good

Positives

High in fiber. Perfect for vegans and those who enjoy large volumes of fresh produce. Designed to be nutrient-dense. Minimizes processed foods.

Negatives

Eliminates dairy products, animal products, snacking between meals, and oils. Is extremely restrictive; very low in calories, fat, and sodium (fewer than 1,000 mg per day), which may make it difficult to maintain. Although not too low in protein, it does eliminate animal protein. Many do not have access to non-factory-farmed animal products. Because of the increased risk of nutrient deficiencies, supplements may be necessary, including a multivitamin containing B12, iodine, zinc, and vitamin D.

The hook/catch or brilliant selling point: Promises impressive weight loss and other health benefits.

Truths/Myths

- Myth - It is healthy to lose 20 pounds in 6 weeks. p. 16

- Truth - While plant-based diets naturally restrict calorie intake by limiting calorie-rich foods, they can be healthy if required supplements are consumed to replace missing nutrients. Losing 20 pounds in 6 weeks far exceeds the recommended rate of weight loss, which generally translates into loss of lean tissue and water. Research suggests severe calorie restriction can slow metabolism, strip lean tissue, promote hunger and increase the risk of regaining the weight lost. p. 84

- Myth - This is a healthy approach to weight loss.

- Truth - Weight will most likely be lost on this plan but the chance of being able to sustain the plan long term is low.

Final decision: Thumbs down

How to improve this diet: Incorporate modest amounts of lean meat and dairy.

Eat What You Love, Love What You Eat Diet

Premise of the Diet: It is possible to lose weight and enjoy foods if we eat mindfully.

Claims of the Diet: This is a mindful eating program that helps heal one's relationship with food.

Diet Description: Before eating, it is important to identify what we are feeling. We need to ask ourselves if we are hungry or feeling another emotion like anger, loneliness, or boredom. It is also important to notice when we are no longer hungry but full. Guidelines are also given for different food groups:

1. Produce: choose colorful, high-fiber fruits and vegetables.

2. Grains: half of the servings should be whole grains.

3. Dairy: choose low-fat or nonfat products.

4. Protein: choose lean cuts of meat and poultry, while seafood should be consumed at least twice a week.

5. Sweets: cake and other sugary treats are allowed in moderation. Alcohol is allowed in moderation.

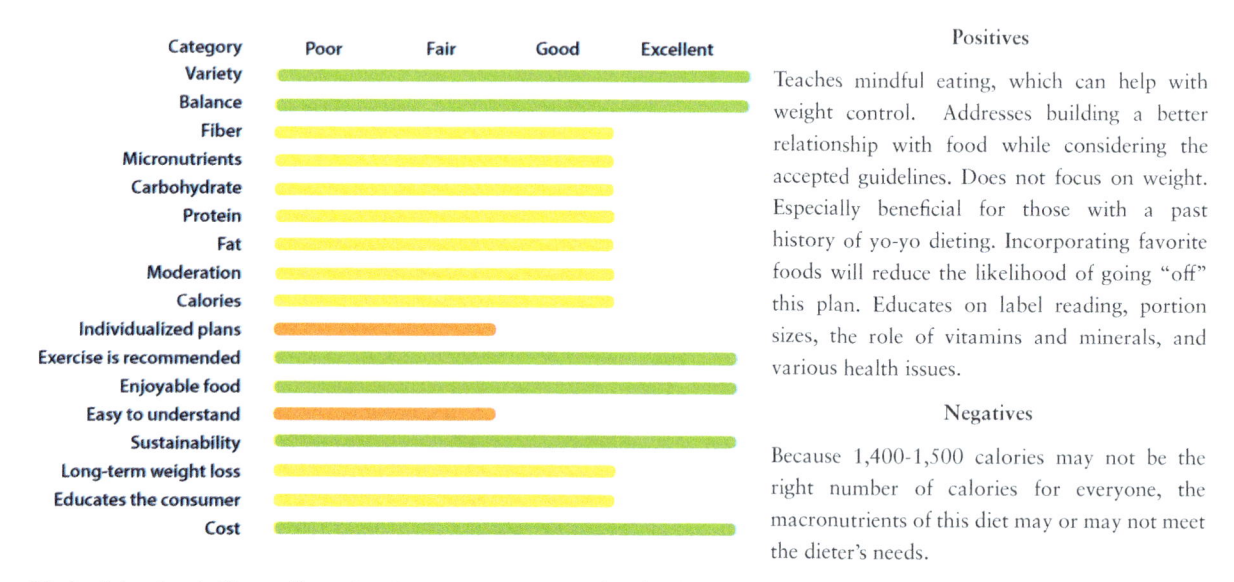

Category	Poor	Fair	Good	Excellent
Variety				Excellent
Balance				Excellent
Fiber			Good	
Micronutrients			Good	
Carbohydrate			Good	
Protein			Good	
Fat			Good	
Moderation			Good	
Calories			Good	
Individualized plans		Fair		
Exercise is recommended				Excellent
Enjoyable food				Excellent
Easy to understand		Fair		
Sustainability				Excellent
Long-term weight loss			Good	
Educates the consumer			Good	
Cost				Excellent

Positives

Teaches mindful eating, which can help with weight control. Addresses building a better relationship with food while considering the accepted guidelines. Does not focus on weight. Especially beneficial for those with a past history of yo-yo dieting. Incorporating favorite foods will reduce the likelihood of going "off" this plan. Educates on label reading, portion sizes, the role of vitamins and minerals, and various health issues.

Negatives

Because 1,400-1,500 calories may not be the right number of calories for everyone, the macronutrients of this diet may or may not meet the dieter's needs.

The hook/catch or brilliant selling point: Everyone wants to eat what they love! No deprivation on this diet.

Truths/Myths

- Myth - None worth noting

- Truth - Mindful eating is important for weight loss and weight maintenance.

Final decision: Thumbs up 👍

How to improve this diet: Since calories do matter, they need to be considered and adjusted based on each person's needs in order for slow, sustainable weight loss to occur.

Eco Atkins Diet

Premise of the Diet: High-protein, vegetarian diet

Claims of the Diet: Provides new advice and insights into doing the Atkins Diet correctly.

Diet Description: Instead of the rich animal fats suggested in the original Atkins diet, healthy fats, such as canola oil, olive oil, avocado, and nuts, soy foods, beans, and seeds are recommended. About 31% of the calories come from plant proteins, 43% from vegetable oils, and 26% from carbs. Carbs are provided mostly from fruits, vegetables, and cereals, but not enriched white bread, rice, potatoes, or baked goods.

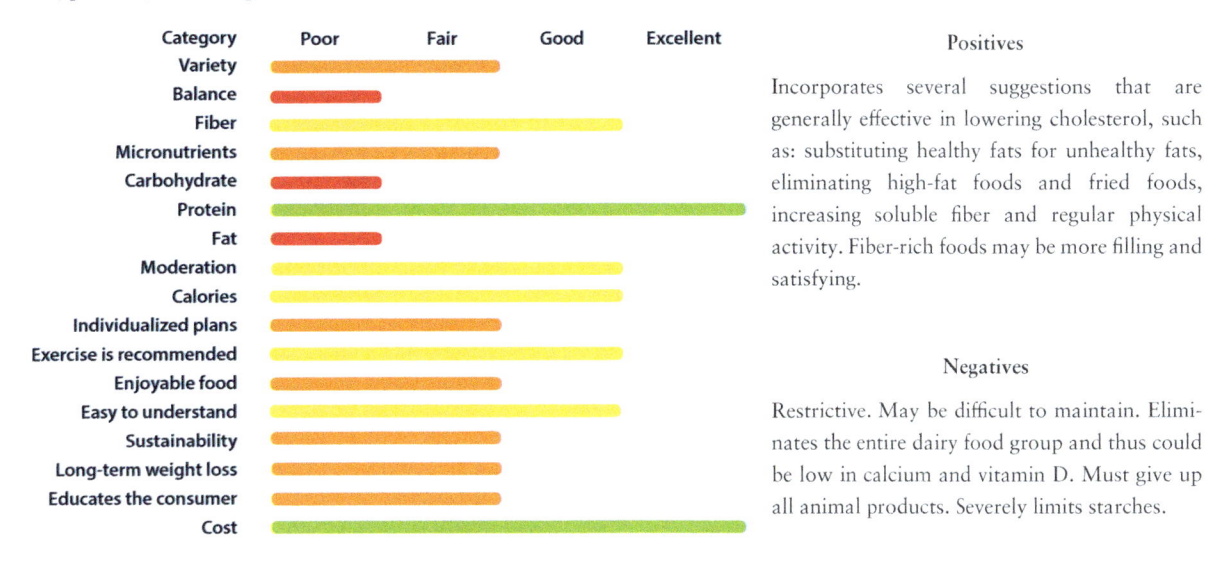

Category	Poor	Fair	Good	Excellent
Variety		██		
Balance	█			
Fiber		███		
Micronutrients		██		
Carbohydrate	█			
Protein				████
Fat	█			
Moderation		███		
Calories		███		
Individualized plans		██		
Exercise is recommended		███		
Enjoyable food		██		
Easy to understand		███		
Sustainability		██		
Long-term weight loss		██		
Educates the consumer		██		
Cost				████

Positives

Incorporates several suggestions that are generally effective in lowering cholesterol, such as: substituting healthy fats for unhealthy fats, eliminating high-fat foods and fried foods, increasing soluble fiber and regular physical activity. Fiber-rich foods may be more filling and satisfying.

Negatives

Restrictive. May be difficult to maintain. Eliminates the entire dairy food group and thus could be low in calcium and vitamin D. Must give up all animal products. Severely limits starches.

The hook/catch or brilliant selling point: Changes one of the major glaring criticisms of the original Atkins diet: lots of unhealthy fats.

Truths/Myths

- Myth - Substituting healthy fats for saturated fats is sufficient and makes up for not consuming all food groups. 🔍 p. 16

- Truth - Eating a variety of foods from all food groups is important for health and the sustainability of consist healthy eating.

Final decision: Thumbs down 👎

How to improve this diet: In moderation, include foods in the starch and dairy groups.

Engine 2 Diet

Premise of the Diet: Vegan Lifestyle

Claims of the Diet: This plan could help save your life.

Diet Description: There are two 28-day plans.

1. The "Fire Cadet" gradually cuts out foods dubbed unhealthy, while at the same time adding nutritious foods.

    Week 1: Eliminates dairy, processed, and refined foods.

    Week 2: Eliminates many sources of protein, such as meat, chicken, eggs, and fish.

    Week 3: Eliminates added or extracted oils.

    Week 4: Accompanying the above eliminations, add more fruits, vegetables, whole grains, legumes, nuts, and seeds.

2. "Firefighter" is the more extreme version which follows week 4 for 4 weeks.

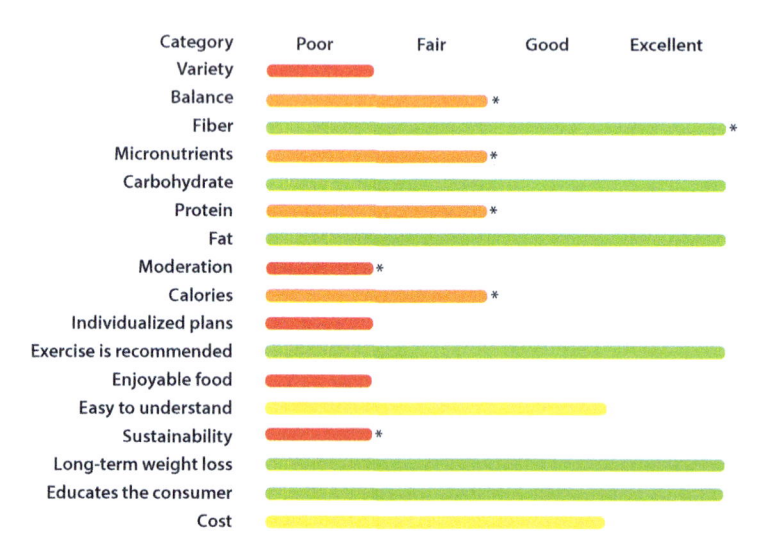

Category	Poor	Fair	Good	Excellent
Variety	■			
Balance		■*		
Fiber				■*
Micronutrients		■*		
Carbohydrate				■
Protein		■*		
Fat				■
Moderation	■*			
Calories		■*		
Individualized plans	■			
Exercise is recommended				■
Enjoyable food	■			
Easy to understand			■	
Sustainability	■*			
Long-term weight loss				■
Educates the consumer				■
Cost			■	

Positives

Emphasizes plant-based foods like vegetables, fruits, tofu, tempeh, soy yogurt, brown rice, hummus, herbs, and nut butters. Encourages giving up alcohol. Recommends exercising 5 days a week for 10 to 45 minutes. Provides educational workbooks, tools, seminars, podcasts, coaches, educational videos, small groups, recipes.

Negatives

Eliminates meat, dairy, cheese substitutes, oil, all processed grains, and most canned and packaged foods. Because so many foods and food groups are eliminated, supplements or fortified foods may be necessary. When packaged foods are eliminated, it can be difficult to consume fortified foods. Deficiencies in vitamin D, B12, and fish oils are likely. There is no real benefit for making this change for only 28 days; it would have to be continued.

*This plan requires much dedication and enthusiasm. It is a way of life that must be fully embraced. For those embracing it, making the switch, and learning how to fuel their body properly with allowable foods could bring about excellent health and weight loss. Without full dedication, adequate education and motivation to consume a variety of nutrient-dense, allowable foods, many deficiencies are possible.

The hook/catch or brilliant selling point: Go Plant Strong!

Truths/Myths

- Myth - None worth mentioning

- Truth - Many health benefits accompany a vegan and vegetarian diet.

- Truth - When food choices are nutrient-dense, weight loss can be expected.

- Truth - The author is a dedicated fitness enthusiast and spent a decade as one of the premier triathletes in the world.

Final decision: Thumbs down (for those who are not completely enthusiastic about this lifestyle)

How to improve this diet: Be sure to make protein a priority. Seek out plant sources of omega-3 fatty acids, such as chia and flaxseeds. Be sure to consume calcium and vitamin D-rich foods. Become educated about which foods provide various nutrients. In the absence of set calorie levels, monitor the consumption of starchy foods like pasta and rice carefully, as they can easily be overeaten and hinder weight loss.

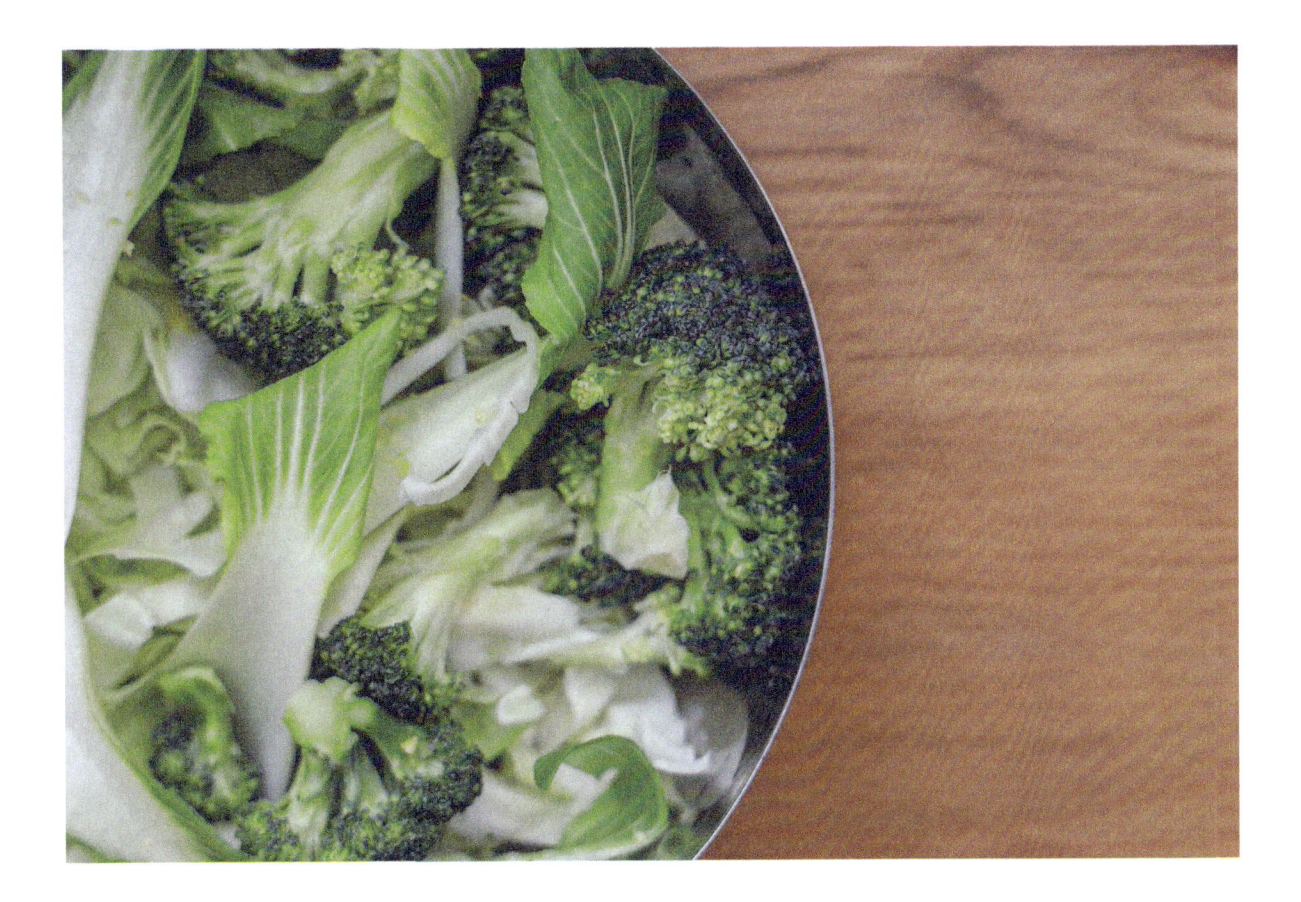

F-Factor Diet

Premise of the Diet: A diet high in fiber helps with weight loss and creates a feeling of fullness.

Claims of the Diet: Will rev-up metabolism so you can shed pounds and help achieve target weight. Will improve health and increase energy and even defy the aging processes, all while maintaining a normal lifestyle.

Diet Description: Recommends 3 meals and 1 snack a day, focusing on combining lean proteins with high-fiber complex carbohydrates. The four principles include eating carbohydrates, dining out, drinking alcohol, and working out less. Through several phases of the diet, net carbs are increased from 35 grams (3 carb servings) to 75 grams (6 carb servings) to about 125 grams (9 carb servings) or until the carb goal is reached. Thus, it provides general guidelines regarding what to eat but allows room for flexibility.

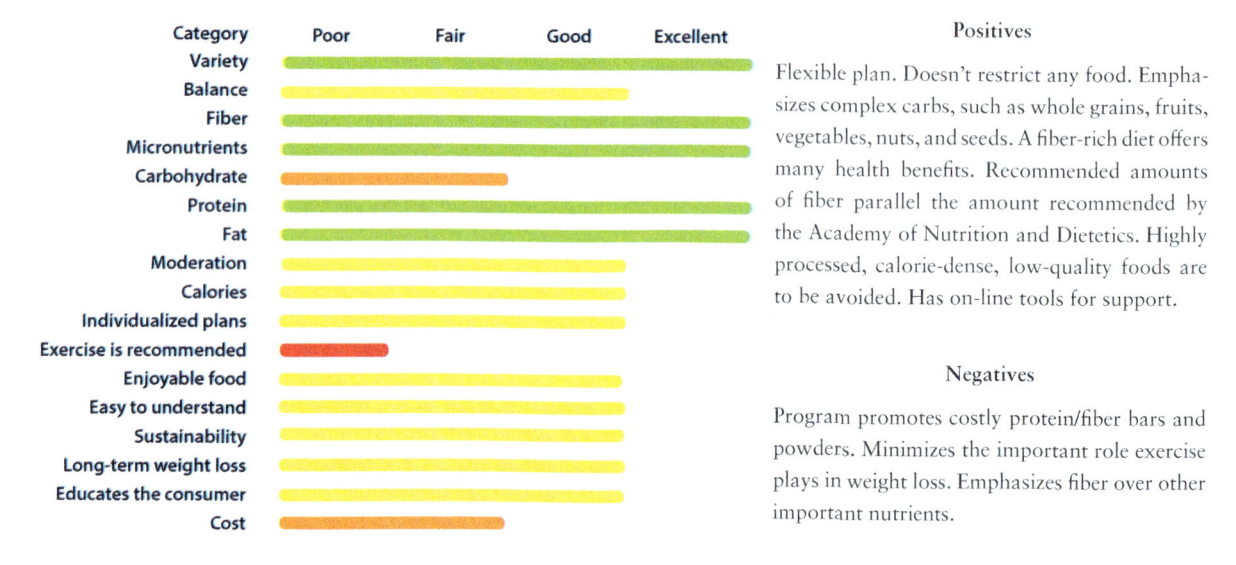

Category	Poor	Fair	Good	Excellent
Variety				●
Balance			●	
Fiber				●
Micronutrients				●
Carbohydrate		●		
Protein				●
Fat				●
Moderation			●	
Calories			●	
Individualized plans			●	
Exercise is recommended	●			
Enjoyable food			●	
Easy to understand			●	
Sustainability			●	
Long-term weight loss			●	
Educates the consumer			●	
Cost		●		

Positives

Flexible plan. Doesn't restrict any food. Emphasizes complex carbs, such as whole grains, fruits, vegetables, nuts, and seeds. A fiber-rich diet offers many health benefits. Recommended amounts of fiber parallel the amount recommended by the Academy of Nutrition and Dietetics. Highly processed, calorie-dense, low-quality foods are to be avoided. Has on-line tools for support.

Negatives

Program promotes costly protein/fiber bars and powders. Minimizes the important role exercise plays in weight loss. Emphasizes fiber over other important nutrients.

The hook/catch or brilliant selling point: In a culture where carbohydrates are demonized, this diet focuses on allowing carbohydrates.

Truths/Myths

- **Myth** - None worth noting.

- **Truth** - The Institute of Medicine suggests 45%-65% of calories should come from carbohydrates. Since 20-130 grams of carbohydrates are recommended in this diet, it is considered by most a low-carb diet. 🔍 p. 41

Final decision: Thumbs up 👍

How to improve this diet: Since eating large amounts of fiber at once can lead to bloating, cramping, gas, and diarrhea, increase fiber consumption slowly.

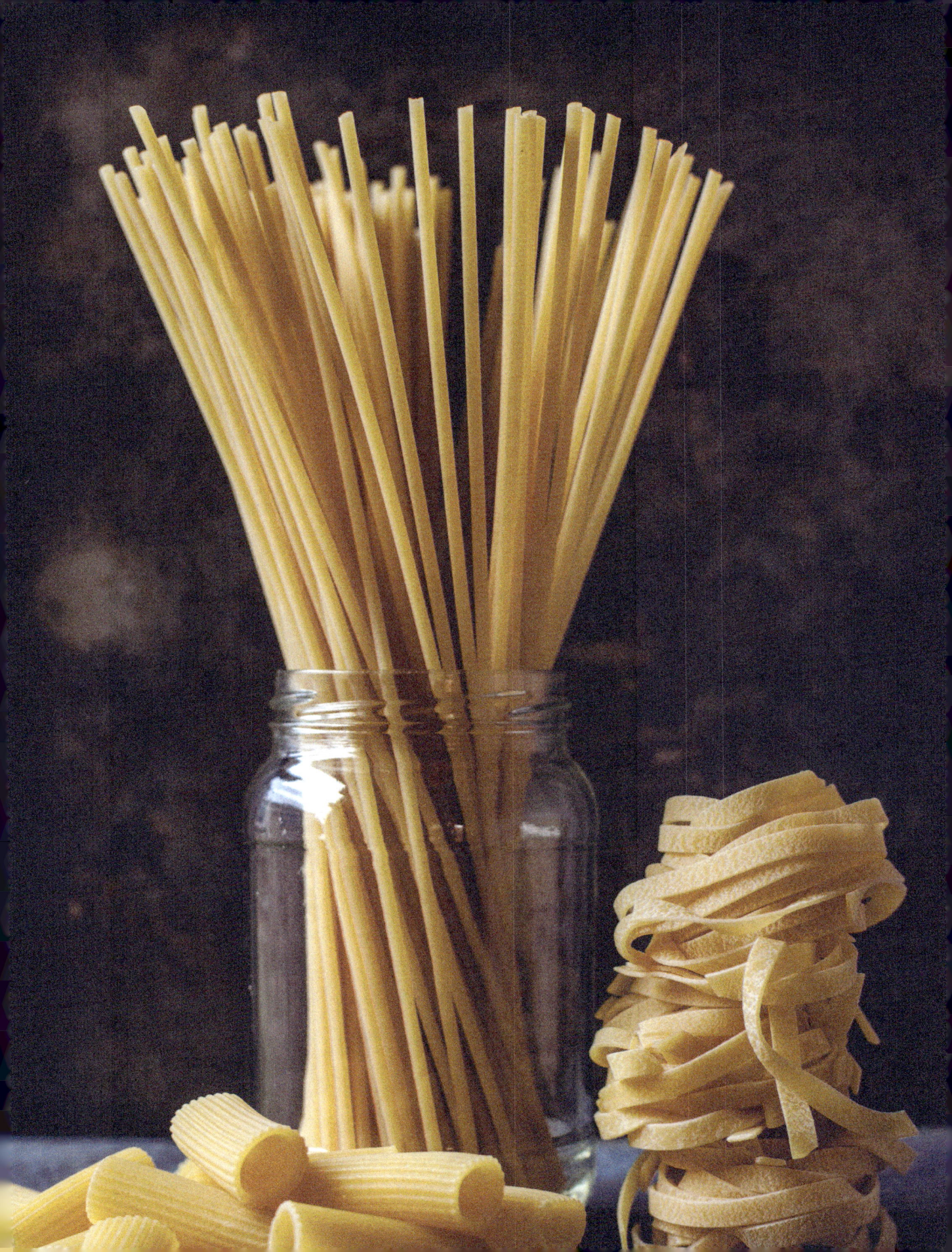

Fast Diet

Premise of the Diet: Restricts energy intake severely for 2 days a week, then recommends eating normally the rest of the week.

Claims of the Diet: Fasting from time to time is effective for weight loss.

Diet Description: Is basically the 5:2 intermittent diet. Eat normally for 5 days of the week and cut calories to about 25% of normal intake on 2 nonconsecutive days. Those calories should provide high-protein foods, aiming for about 50 grams.

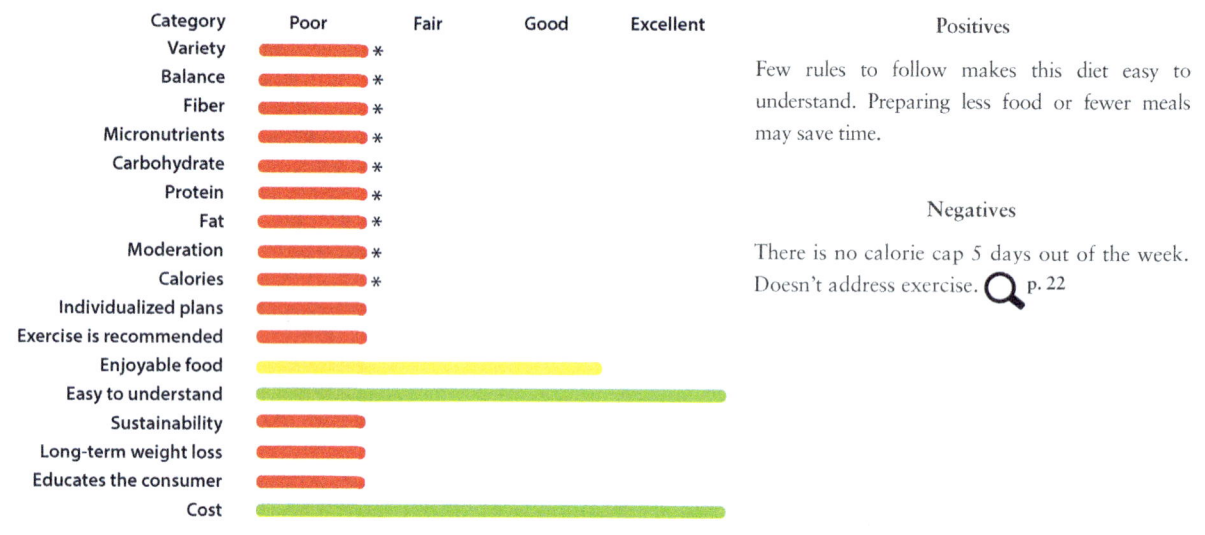

Category	Poor	Fair	Good	Excellent
Variety	*			
Balance	*			
Fiber	*			
Micronutrients	*			
Carbohydrate	*			
Protein	*			
Fat	*			
Moderation	*			
Calories	*			
Individualized plans	■			
Exercise is recommended	■			
Enjoyable food			■	
Easy to understand				■
Sustainability	■			
Long-term weight loss	■			
Educates the consumer	■			
Cost				■

Positives

Few rules to follow makes this diet easy to understand. Preparing less food or fewer meals may save time.

Negatives

There is no calorie cap 5 days out of the week. Doesn't address exercise. 🔍 p. 22

*Can vary depending on food choices. Little guidance is provided by the diet.

The hook/catch or brilliant selling point: We love the word FAST in relationship to dieting and losing weight.

Truths/Myths

• Myth - This type of fasting is a good approach to weight loss.

• Truth - This diet makes no changes in eating patterns for 5 out of the 7 days of the week. It is this eating pattern that puts on excess body fat. As soon as fasting is over, any weight lost will be regained unless long-term changes are made in eating habits.

• Truth - One of the downfalls of many diets is the hunger experienced while dieting. Being hungry decreases the likelihood of adherence. Long-term compliance is unlikely. 🔍 p. 76

• Truth - Wow! The fact that so many people are excluded from this diet suggests it may not be a healthy approach. Those excluded include: pregnant women, anyone underweight, or with a history of eating disorders or diabetes, kids, teens, frail seniors, or anyone who isn't feeling well or has a fever. With all these restrictions, careful promotion of a diet like this is prudent.

• Truth - Studies indicate there is weight regain once fasting is done.

• Truth - Short-term periods of rapid weight loss involve mostly a loss of water and glycogen, not fat. 🔍 p. 75

• Truth - Insufficient research is available to know how the human body's metabolism adapts or changes to repeated intermittent or alternate-day fasting.

• Truth - Insufficient research is available to known what the long-term health effects are of intermittent fasting.

- Truth - Depriving the body of food can lead to an unhealthy relationship with food, which can make weight loss more difficult.

- Truth - It can be difficult to exercise while fasting due to low energy. Intermittent fasting will not allow full replenishment of glycogen stores, because trying to refuel more than 2 hours after exercise misses the primary window of opportunity to replenish glycogen stores for future bouts of exercise.

- Truth - Exercise when fasting can result in stripping lean tissue. A net negative nitrogen balance will occur if the exerciser does not consume the necessary protein. Skeletal muscle protein degradation is elevated for 24-48 hours after exercise. Muscle net protein balance will remain negative without nutrient intake. If exercising during intermittent fasting, there is a decrease in circulating levels of amino acids, which can lead to an increase in muscle protein degradation, or an increase in amino acids released from muscles. This ultimately decreases metabolic rate, making it harder to lose weight.

- Truth - Some of the studies cited to support fasting monitor the metabolism of unhealthy subjects such as anorexics near death, use short time frames of intervention, and few subjects. None of these studies translate well to a healthy population trying to lose weight for the long haul.

Final decision: Thumbs down

How to improve this diet: Eat fewer calories than is expended daily. Choose a variety of whole, nutrient dense foods whose macronutrient distribution follow the recommended guidelines. Engage in regular exercise that involves cardiovascular and strength training most days of the week.

Fast Food Diet

Premise of the Diet: If we eat "right" 80% of the time, it's OK to splurge 20% of the time. It is possible to lose weight without giving up the drive-thru and without requiring a lot of cooking.

Claims of the Diet: If you want to lose weight, there is no need to stop visiting drive-up windows or to start cooking.

Diet Description: Consume fast foods in three meals and two snacks. Eliminates fried foods and sodas sweetened with high-fructose corn syrup. Offers suggestions for better substitutions and tips for cutting fat and calories while still enjoying a diet mainly from fast-food restaurants. Alcohol is allowed in moderation.

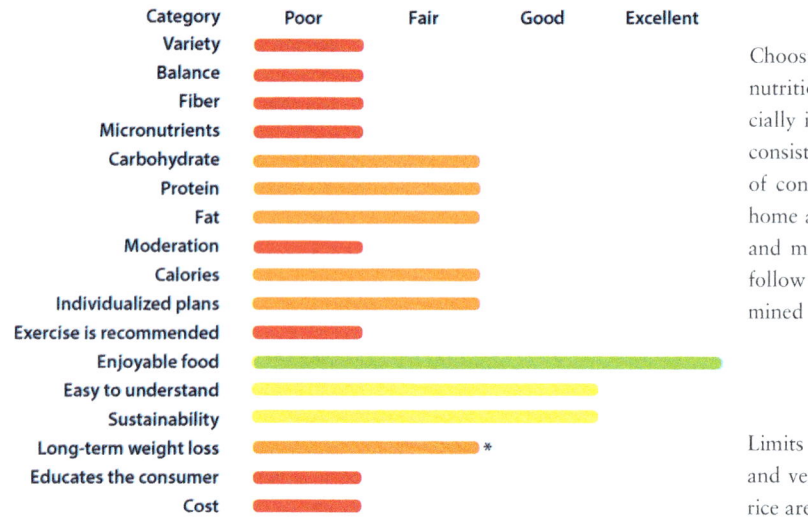

Category	Poor	Fair	Good	Excellent
Variety	■			
Balance	■			
Fiber	■			
Micronutrients	■			
Carbohydrate		■		
Protein		■		
Fat		■		
Moderation	■			
Calories		■		
Individualized plans		■		
Exercise is recommended	■			
Enjoyable food				■
Easy to understand			■	
Sustainability			■	
Long-term weight loss		■*		
Educates the consumer	■			
Cost	■			

Positives

Choosing items lower in calories and higher in nutrition is better when eating out. This is especially important for people who won't cook or consistently choose to eat out. Allows enjoyment of convenience foods. Can eat out or cook at home as much as desired, as long as the calorie and menu suggestions are adhered to. Easy to follow in that the portion size is already determined and there is no food preparation.

Negatives

Limits options, choices, and amounts of fruits and vegetables. Whole-grain breads and brown rice are not often offered. Fish choices are limited. Overall, healthy choices are narrow and restricted. Requires great self-control to order a healthy option (baked potato without sour cream) when the aroma of flavorful French fries is right there. It can be hard to stick to.

*Weight loss is more likely for individuals who are excessively overweight. Weight loss is less likely for individuals who only want to lose a few pounds.

The hook/catch or brilliant selling point: We all want to believe we can achieve weight loss and improved health while frequently dining out and maintaining busy lives that don't allow us to cook or prepare our own food.

Truths/Myths

- Myth - It is possible to eat healthy while eating every meal away from home.

- Truth - While some fast-food choices are healthier than others, it is unrealistic to regularly eat "healthy" or consistently eat meals at fast-food establishments and lose weight. 🔍 p. 3

- Myth - Making substitutions for favorite foods is satisfying and sustainable.

- Truth - Making substitutions for favorite foods are exactly that. The favorite food is not consumed. Although it sounds good "in words," the reality is a different flavor and level of satisfaction.

Final decision: Thumbs down 👎

How to improve this diet: Can't be improved.

Fast Metabolism Diet

Premise of the Diet: It is possible to speed up metabolism by eating certain foods in a particular order.

Claims of the Diet: Speeds up metabolism so 20 pounds can be lost in 28 days.

Diet Description: Three rotating and repeating phases that focus on distinct foods for a total of 4 weeks. Switching between the phases allows different systems and organs to rest and be restored.

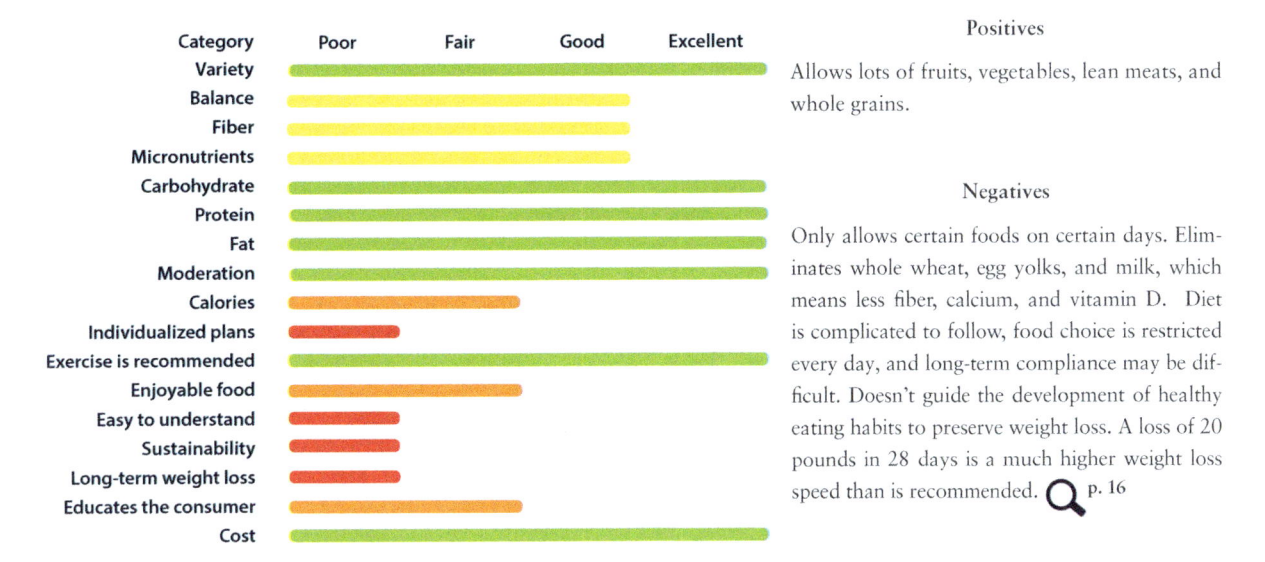

Category	Poor	Fair	Good	Excellent
Variety				████
Balance		██		
Fiber		██		
Micronutrients		██		
Carbohydrate				████
Protein				████
Fat				████
Moderation				████
Calories	██			
Individualized plans	█			
Exercise is recommended				████
Enjoyable food	██			
Easy to understand	█			
Sustainability	█			
Long-term weight loss	█			
Educates the consumer	██			
Cost				████

Positives

Allows lots of fruits, vegetables, lean meats, and whole grains.

Negatives

Only allows certain foods on certain days. Eliminates whole wheat, egg yolks, and milk, which means less fiber, calcium, and vitamin D. Diet is complicated to follow, food choice is restricted every day, and long-term compliance may be difficult. Doesn't guide the development of healthy eating habits to preserve weight loss. A loss of 20 pounds in 28 days is a much higher weight loss speed than is recommended. 🔍 p. 16

The hook/catch or brilliant selling point: Weight loss hasn't occurred or has been difficult because foods were not eaten in the right order.

Truths/Myths

- Myth - Metabolism can be manipulated by the food eaten. 🔍 p. 84

- Truth - While this is true to some extent, the work involved in manipulating food choices has such a small rate of metabolic return in comparison to the rather large impact on nutrients (or lack of) consumed. In addition, it is usually not sustainable. Confusion, poor health, or frustration often lead to "going off" the diet. It would be better to make healthy food choices long term. Given various life circumstances, this usually requires being flexible.

- Myth - Low-nutrient foods, plus too much stress, can slow the metabolism, resulting in weight gain.

- Truth - Calorie-dense foods or foods low in nutrients can often add excess calories, which causes weight gain. It doesn't really slow the metabolism. But, indeed, the end result is the same: weight gain. Stress does affect hormones and can have an impact on weight gain. 🔍 p. 16

- Truth - Weight loss is most likely possible on this diet, not because it speeds up metabolism or foods are eaten in the proper order, but because of calorie restriction.

Final decision: Thumbs down 👎

How to improve this diet: Don't worry about the difficult schedule and simply eat the various recommended foods (including wheat, eggs and dairy, if so desired) in moderation.

Faster Way to Fat Loss Program (FWTFL)

Premise of the Diet: A 6-week program that combines three dieting approaches simultaneously: intermittent fasting, macro counting, and carb cycling

Claims of the Diet: Intermittent fasting causes weight loss even when calories aren't restricted.

Diet Description: This $199, 6-week-long program includes a weight-loss coach, a weekly workout schedule, and a calorie/macro counting schedule to be tracked on the My Fitness Pal app. While days of the week can be shifted around to adapt to your personal schedule, it is recommended that Monday and Tuesday are Low Carb days where 50g of carbs or less are eaten. Wednesday, Thursday, and Saturday are Regular Calorie/Macro days. Friday and Sunday are Low Calorie/Macro days in which calories are reduced by 25%. The program also outlines how to apply at least a 12-hour fast daily (with the goal of working up to a 16-hour fast). This equates to eating only during an 8-hour window of time each day and fasting the remaining 16 hours. Monthly 24-hour fasts are to eventually be worked into the program. Specific workouts are provided that coordinate with calorie intake.

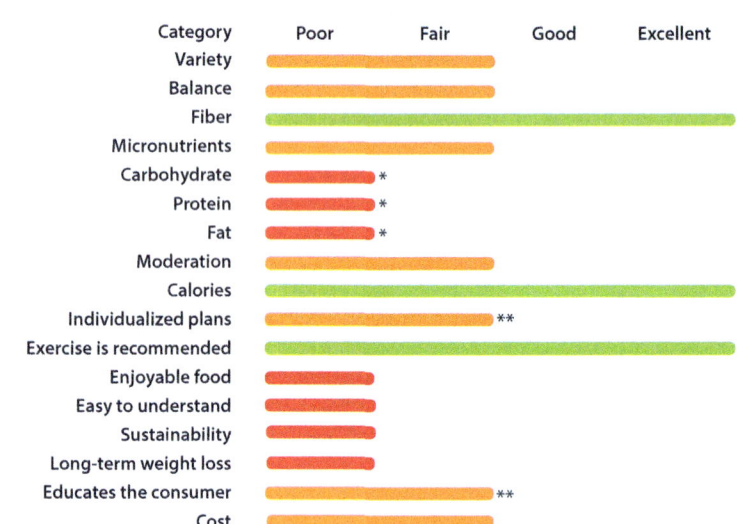

Category	Poor	Fair	Good	Excellent
Variety		Fair		
Balance		Fair		
Fiber				Excellent
Micronutrients		Fair		
Carbohydrate	Poor*			
Protein	Poor*			
Fat	Poor*			
Moderation		Fair		
Calories				Excellent
Individualized plans		Fair**		
Exercise is recommended				Excellent
Enjoyable food	Poor			
Easy to understand	Poor			
Sustainability	Poor			
Long-term weight loss	Poor			
Educates the consumer		Fair**		
Cost		Fair		

Positives

Promotes a variety of whole foods, offers a virtual coach to answer questions, can be customized for preferences and allergies. Offers a "prep week" to introduce the program, define terms, and familiarize new participants with concepts before starting the program. Can be tailored for men or women. Website offers a Frequently Asked Questions (FAQ) section. Highly processed foods are discouraged. Provides streamed videos for daily exercise. Incorporates high-intensity interval training, strength training for different muscle groups, and cardio.

Negatives

Coaches are program graduates who have paid between $3,000 and $5,000 to receive the program's non-accredited "coaching certification." In addition to helping people lose weight, coaches earn money for each client and new coach they recruit into the program. They are financially invested in the program as they build their business online. The program is intensely focused on eating habits and exercise, as it incorporates three different weight-loss approaches rolled into one program. Policy states that the program is suitable for breastfeeding women. Everyone is encouraged to avoid dairy and foods containing gluten.

*This score could be higher if weekly fasting didn't occur.

** This score could fall anywhere depending on the knowledge of the life coach and the accuracy of the advice given.

The hook/catch or brilliant selling point: Uses enticing buzz words from three different fad-diet approaches.

Truths/Myths

- Myth - Fasting helps the body detox naturally, and it is important to drink a lot of water so toxins can be flushed out. 🔍 p. 13

- Truth - One of the functions of the liver is to detoxify the body

- Myth - The body requires an occasional 24-hour fast to allow the digestive system complete rest and allow cellular repair. 🔍 p. 81

- Truth - Your body doesn't need rest from food for cellular repair.

194

- **Myth** - Pregnant and postpartum/breastfeeding women should go on a diet.

- **Truth** - Pregnant and postpartum/breastfeeding women shouldn't be dieting or actively attempting to lose weight during these times, as additional calories are needed for growth and milk production. Members of this population should not avoid gluten and dairy products unless they have sensitivities to them.

- **Myth** - People will lose weight on this program because it provides all the necessary approaches.

- **Truth** - People may lose weight on this program because they are eating fewer calories than they are expending.

- **Myth** - Intermittent fasting is necessary for weight loss. 🔍 p. 81

- **Truth** - While intermittent fasting can help dieters lose weight, it has not been proven to be more effective in long-term weight loss than general calorie restriction. However, fasting can lead to an unhealthy relationship with food.

- **Myth** - There are no dangers of combining three intense dieting approaches at once.

- **Truth** - In addition to being very restrictive, reducing "food and nutrition" to nothing but numbers can dissociate a dieter from internal cues. This heavy emphasis on counting may trigger at-risk dieters into disordered eating.

- **Myth** - Carb cycling is important for weight loss.

- **Truth** - There is no credible evidence in humans that supports carb cycling for weight loss or health. Carb cycling alternates carb intake on a daily, weekly or monthly basis.

- **Truth** - Intermittent fasting is associated with decreased insulin levels and it may decrease inflammation. It is currently unclear if the above changes are from the fasting or the resulting weight loss.

Final decision: Thumbs down 👎

How to improve this diet: Don't limit carbohydrates for 48 hours weekly without consulting a doctor, and don't fast for 24 hours each month.

Fat Smash Diet

Premise of the Diet: Was originally designed for celebrities trying to lose weight on the show "Celebrity Fit Club." Other than the first two phases of the diet, it is based on healthy principles.

Claims of the Diet: Will "rewire" the body and its relationship to food and physical activity. Detoxifies the body, promotes rapid weight loss, teaches sustainable weight-maintenance skills, reduces the risk of diet-related disease, leads to a healthier lifestyle. It is an alternative program for people wanting to lose weight in a short period of time.

Diet Description: This diet has four phases:

1. Detox: Start with a 9-day vegetarian "detox." Meat, fish, pasta, and alcohol are not allowed. Requires 30 minutes of aerobic exercise.

2. Foundation: Begin to allow meats, fish, healthy grains, fats, and some alcohol. Exercise is increased to 35 minutes, 5 times a week.

3. Construction: Lasts for 4 weeks. Add more variety to the diet while focusing on portion control. Exercise is increased to 45 minutes a day.

4. Temple: Continue adding more foods until all are allowed. Addresses slip-ups. Requires 60 minutes of moderate to intense exercise that can include weight training 5 times a week.

Category	Poor	Fair	Good	Excellent
Variety				●
Balance				●
Fiber				●
Micronutrients				●
Carbohydrate				●
Protein				●
Fat				●
Moderation				●
Calories			●	
Individualized plans		●		
Exercise is recommended		●		
Enjoyable food			●	
Easy to understand				●
Sustainability				●
Long-term weight loss				●
Educates the consumer				●
Cost				●

Positives

Last two phases adhere to dietary recommendations. Promotes a diet low in saturated fat, high in fruits and vegetables. Does not exclude food groups. Recommends eating throughout the day with no more than 3-4 hours between meals. Recommends eating no later than 1.5 hours before going to bed. Establishes a regular eating schedule. Allows for ready-made foods, though preparing at home is recommended. The last two phases allow for a slow, gradual, and consistent weight loss, which increases the likelihood of maintaining that loss.

Negatives

The first two phases do not adhere to recommendations from major health organizations and are very restrictive. Needs to address maintenance more thoroughly. The exercise recommendation is about twice the current recommendation, and thus may not be feasible for many dieters.

*Information provided is based on the final phase of the diet.

The hook/catch or brilliant selling point: Starting with very restricted eating makes us eager to eat anything, so healthy eating is seen as a treat to which we look forward.

Truths/Myths

- **Myth** - Detoxification is necessary.

- **Truth** - The liver detoxifies our bodies. We don't need to detox our bodies by choosing or eliminating certain foods. Therefore, the first two phases of this diet are unnecessary. 🔍 p. 16, 75

Final decision: Thumbs up on the last 2 phases 👍

How to improve this diet: Other than keeping the progression of exercise, eliminate the first two phases of the diet.

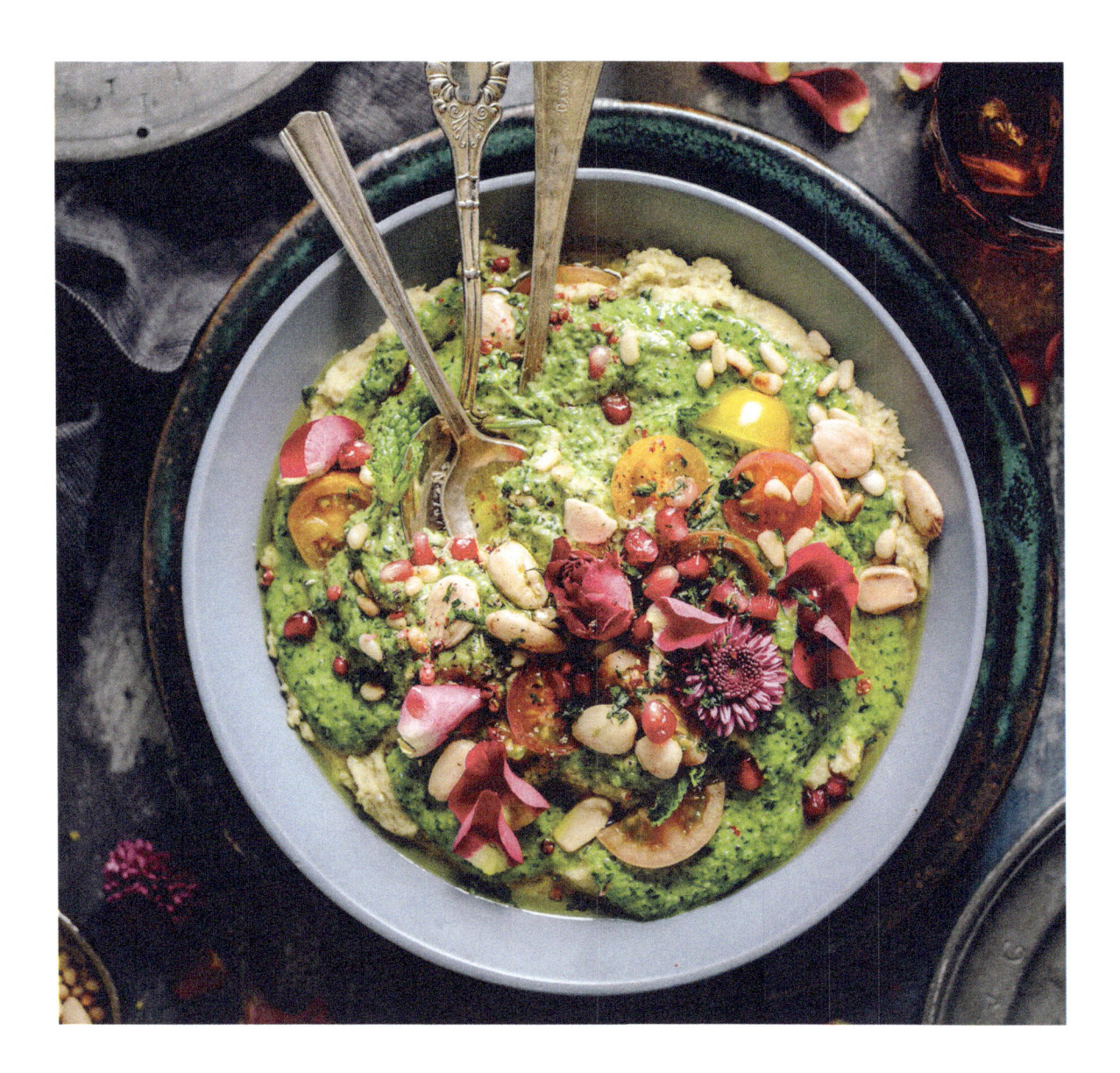

5 Factor Diet

Premise of the Diet: If you can count to five, you have an idea of the plan's basic principles. This diet plan has helped shape some of the hottest bodies.

Claims of the Diet: Promises that eating a balanced meal 5 times a day will keep blood sugar stable, which will improve mood and energy.

Diet Description: Five meals a day, each consisting of five elements: lean protein, low-to-moderate glycemic complex carbohydrate, fiber, healthy fat, and sugar-free fluids. Includes one "cheat day" per week.

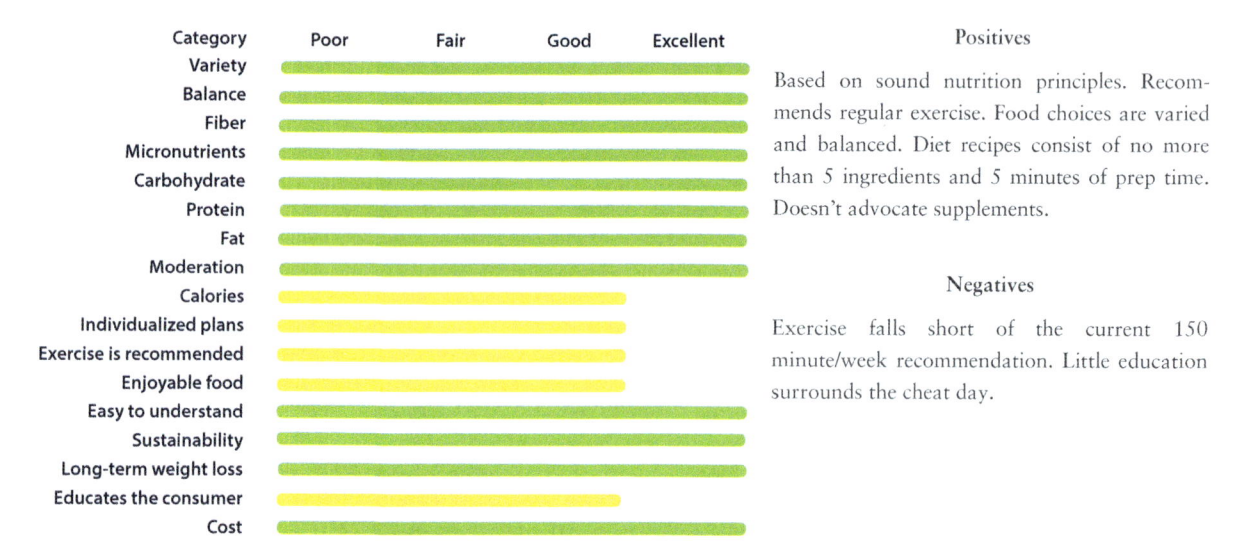

Category	Poor	Fair	Good	Excellent
Variety				█
Balance				█
Fiber				█
Micronutrients				█
Carbohydrate				█
Protein				█
Fat				█
Moderation				█
Calories			█	
Individualized plans			█	
Exercise is recommended			█	
Enjoyable food			█	
Easy to understand				█
Sustainability				█
Long-term weight loss				█
Educates the consumer			█	
Cost				█

Positives

Based on sound nutrition principles. Recommends regular exercise. Food choices are varied and balanced. Diet recipes consist of no more than 5 ingredients and 5 minutes of prep time. Doesn't advocate supplements.

Negatives

Exercise falls short of the current 150 minute/week recommendation. Little education surrounds the cheat day.

The hook/catch or brilliant selling point: Catchy title. Celebrity endorsements. Sound nutrition recommendations.

Truths/Myths: None worth noting

Final decision: Thumbs up 👍

How to improve this diet: Increase exercise to 150 minutes/week and incorporate weight-bearing exercises. Learn how to incorporate "junk" foods into an overall healthy eating plan for the cheat day. Additional flavorful herbs, spices and low-calorie vegetables could be incorporated into the easy recipes provided for more interest and excitement.

Flat Belly Diet*

Premise of the Diet: No clear basis, simply incorporates monounsaturated fats into each meal.

Claims of the Diet: Eat fat and lose weight. In 32 days, you can lose 15 pounds and drop belly fat.

Diet Description: Starts with 4 days of consuming 1,200 calories each day with no added salt and no processed foods or gas-producing foods like beans, cabbage or broccoli, and no carbs like pasta, bananas, or breads. Also requires drinking 2 liters of "Sassy Water," which is water mixed with ginger root, cucumber, lemon, and mint leaves. After that, a Mediterranean-style diet is eaten for 4 weeks, consisting of 4 meals of 400 calories per meal for a total of 1,600 calories per day. Go no longer than 4 hours between eating. Eat monounsaturated fats at every meal.

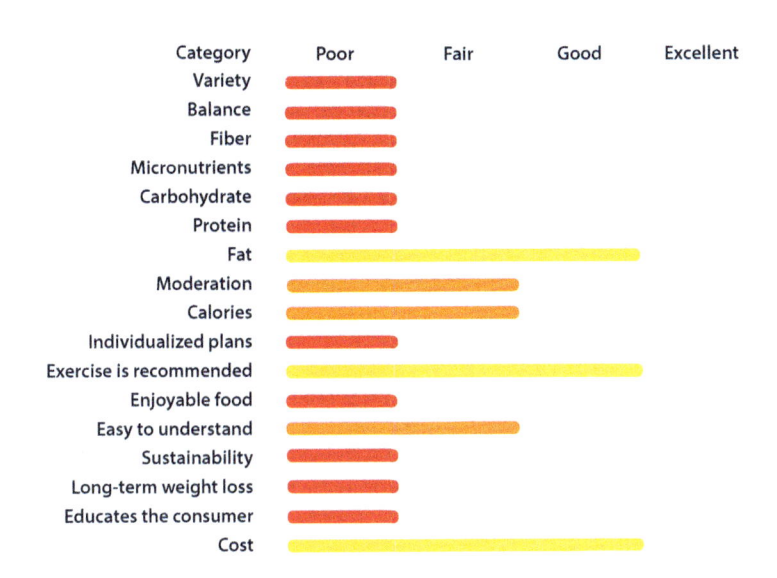

Category	Poor	Fair	Good	Excellent
Variety	▬			
Balance	▬			
Fiber	▬			
Micronutrients	▬			
Carbohydrate	▬			
Protein	▬			
Fat				▬▬▬▬
Moderation		▬▬		
Calories		▬▬		
Individualized plans	▬			
Exercise is recommended			▬▬▬	
Enjoyable food	▬			
Easy to understand		▬▬		
Sustainability	▬			
Long-term weight loss	▬			
Educates the consumer	▬			
Cost			▬▬▬	

Positives

Recommends consuming monounsaturated fats in place of saturated fats. Ultimately ends with a Mediterranean diet, a heart-healthy eating plan that's been shown to help people lose weight. Might lose weight because of limited total calories.

Negatives

The first 4 days are very restrictive and are unnecessary. It cuts out fibrous foods, which should be promoted because they can be helpful in weight loss and can help add the feeling of fullness. Not flexible with the calorie level. Purchase of a monthly membership would increase the cost.

*These scores are based on the first 4 days of the Flat Belly Diet. If starting and following a Mediterranean Diet, the scores would be excellent and the recommendation would be thumbs up, because it would in essence then be the Mediterranean Diet.

The hook/catch or brilliant selling point: Touts a silver bullet: "Sassy Water" and Fast Weight Loss.

Truths/Myths

- **Myth** - Belly fat can be targeted and lost by eating monounsaturated fats. 🔍 p. 56, 63

- **Truth** - There is nothing magical about the monounsaturated fats that lead to a flat belly.

- **Myth** - Sassy Water is essential to kick-start weight loss. 🔍 p. 13

- **Truth** - Sassy Water is not necessary. Any diet that cuts calories can lead to weight loss.

Final decision: Thumbs down 👎

How to improve this diet: Skip the first 4 days of the diet, avoid the "Sassy Water" and adopt the Mediterranean Diet long term.

Flavor Point Diet

Premise of the Diet: Limiting flavors helps us better recognize the sensation of fullness.

Claims of the Diet: Promises 9-16 pounds lost in 6 weeks.

Diet Description: Three meals and two snacks daily, plus an optional dessert that all total 1,200-1,500 calories a day. Provides Flavor Point guidelines. Has 3 phases that follow a "flavor theme" and suggests sticking with the same flavors will train the brain to turn off the hunger switch. In other words, we reach the Flavor Point faster if we eat the same flavor over and over during the day.

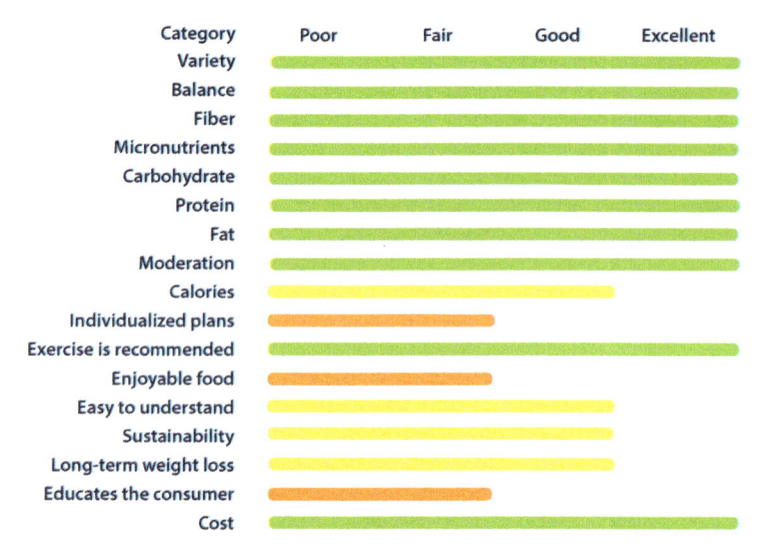

Category	Poor	Fair	Good	Excellent
Variety				●
Balance				●
Fiber				●
Micronutrients				●
Carbohydrate				●
Protein				●
Fat				●
Moderation				●
Calories			●	
Individualized plans		●		
Exercise is recommended				●
Enjoyable food		●		
Easy to understand			●	
Sustainability			●	
Long-term weight loss			●	
Educates the consumer		●		
Cost				●

Positives

Encourages reading food labels. Allows alcoholic beverages in moderation. Low in saturated fat and high in fiber. Focuses on fruits, vegetables, and whole grains, making it good for many health conditions, like high cholesterol, high blood pressure, and heart disease. Recommends fresh and whole foods. Doesn't eliminate any particular flavor or food.

Negatives

Flavor themes may take some time to get accustomed to and be tedious. Requires time cooking and preparing food. Some food items may not be easily obtained. Plan starts out restrictive and rigid. Doesn't adequately address eating out.

The hook/catch or brilliant selling point: Focuses on one thing; narrow and simple.

Truths/Myths: None worth mentioning.

Final decision: Thumbs up 👍

How to improve this diet: No suggestions.

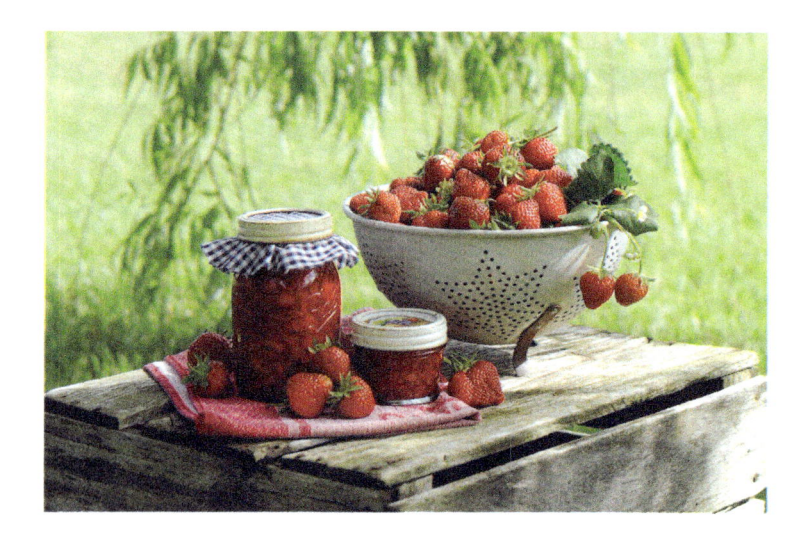

Flexitarian Diet

Premise of the Diet: A flexible vegetarian diet that encourages mostly plant-based foods but allows meat and other animal products.

Claims of the Diet: Eat a healthy diet that minimizes meat without excluding it altogether.

Diet Description: No specific guidelines or calorie levels. Based on fruits, vegetables, legumes, whole grains, and protein from plants. Incorporates meat and animal products from time to time. Recommends avoiding processed foods and limiting added sugars in favor of foods in their most natural form.

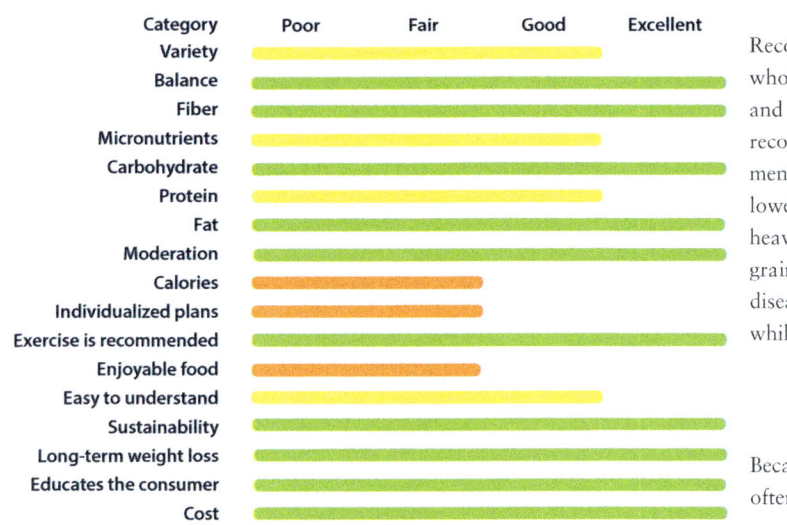

Category	Poor	Fair	Good	Excellent
Variety			Good	
Balance				Excellent
Fiber				Excellent
Micronutrients			Good	
Carbohydrate				Excellent
Protein			Good	
Fat				Excellent
Moderation				Excellent
Calories		Fair		
Individualized plans		Fair		
Exercise is recommended				Excellent
Enjoyable food		Fair		
Easy to understand			Good	
Sustainability				Excellent
Long-term weight loss				Excellent
Educates the consumer				Excellent
Cost				Excellent

Positives

Recommends mostly fruits, vegetables, legumes, whole grains while minimizing processed foods and sugar. Decreases meat consumption while recommending plant-based proteins. Recommends nutrient-dense foods that are naturally lower in calories and high in antioxidants. The heavy emphasis on vegetables, legumes, whole grains, and fruits may lower the risk of heart disease, blood pressure, cancer, and diabetes, all while promoting fat loss.

Negatives

Because vitamin B12, zinc, iron, and calcium are often found in animal products, special attention must be given to them to avoid deficiency.

p. 47, 29

The hook/catch or brilliant selling point: Catchy name deems further investigation.

Truths/Myths

- Truths - No claims made that need explaining.
- Myths - No false claims made.

Final decision: Thumbs up 👍

How to improve this diet: Be sure to consume good sources of vitamin C to help absorb the iron found in legumes, whole grains, nuts and seeds. Eat plant-based sources of calcium such as kale, chard and sesame seeds.

Four Day Diet

Premise of the Diet: It is important to vary diet and physical activity every 4 days.

Claims of the Diet: Varying diet and physical activity every 4 days increases weight loss.

Diet Description: Recommends keeping a record of food and exercise for 10 days prior to starting the diet. Discusses personal challenges with a self-evaluation. Requires that a weight-loss goal be determined. Has seven phases or modules, each lasting 4 days. Most modules do not have to be followed in order. The seven modules are low in calories. Foods are chosen from a food list. Less may be eaten, but not more than is indicated.

- Module 1 Induction: Eating mostly fruits, vegetables, beans, and legumes.
- Module 2 Transition: Start reintroducing all food groups.
- Module 3 Protein Stretch: Increase protein consumption.
- Module 4 Smooth: Can cheat.
- Module 5 Push: 4 days of limited calories and an hour of cardio each day.
- Module 6 Pace: Basic steady exercise and balanced eating.
- Module 7 Vigorous: (The most strict) - 4 days of vegetables and fruit, with lots of cardio.

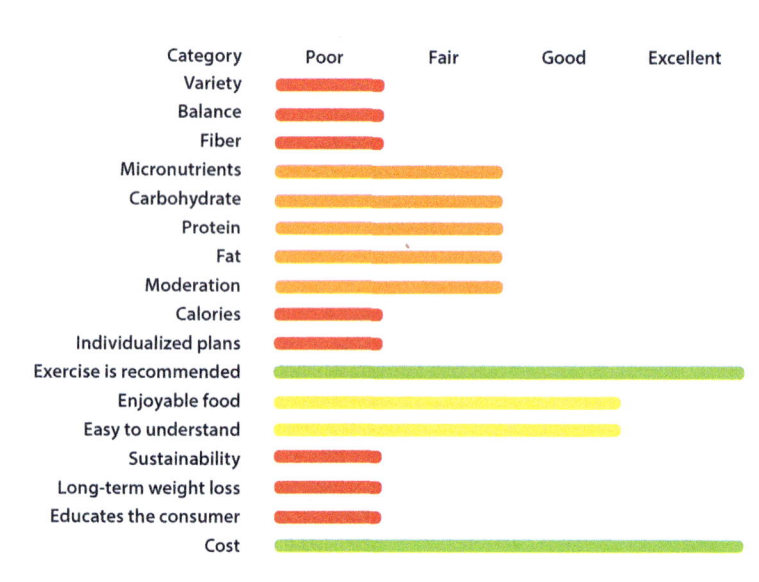

Category	Poor	Fair	Good	Excellent
Variety	■			
Balance	■			
Fiber	■			
Micronutrients		■		
Carbohydrate		■		
Protein		■		
Fat		■		
Moderation		■		
Calories	■			
Individualized plans	■			
Exercise is recommended				■
Enjoyable food			■	
Easy to understand			■	
Sustainability	■			
Long-term weight loss	■			
Educates the consumer	■			
Cost				■

Positives

Each phase has a different focus with lots of food choices, minimizing the likelihood of getting bored. Generally, eliminates high-fat, high-carb foods. The book recommends meals for each specific day.

Negatives

Requires determination and willpower to make it through some of these modules. Choices and amounts are limited. Food prep and the exercise requires significant time and can be challenging. Includes nutritious foods, but may be too low in calories, vitamin D, calcium, whole grains, and dairy products. May not provide sufficient calories for the intense cardio it requires. During the most vigorous phase of exercise, only fruits and vegetables are consumed. p. 35

The hook/catch or brilliant selling point: Magic formula is revealed for fast weight loss.

Truths/Myths

- **Myth** - 4-day blocks of alternating restrictions works best for weight loss. p. 81

- **Truth** - No research supports this. Any number of days when calorie consumption is less than calories expended will help with weight loss. Nothing magical about 4-day blocks of time.

Final decision: Thumbs down

How to improve this diet: Eat a moderate, balanced diet daily and exercise regularly.

French Women Don't Get Fat Diet: The Secret of Eating for Pleasure

Premise of the Diet: Unlocks the "French paradox"— secrets of how French women enjoy food while staying slim and healthy.

Claims of the Diet: Provides a positive way to stay trim.

Diet Description: Keep a record for 3 weeks of what is eaten. Note which foods should be added or subtracted. For 2 days, eat only leek soup and water. Eat a wide variety of fresh, seasonal ingredients. Use plenty of seasonings and herbs. Eat two servings of yogurt daily. No liquor, but wine and champagne are allowed in moderation. Sweets are OK in small amounts.

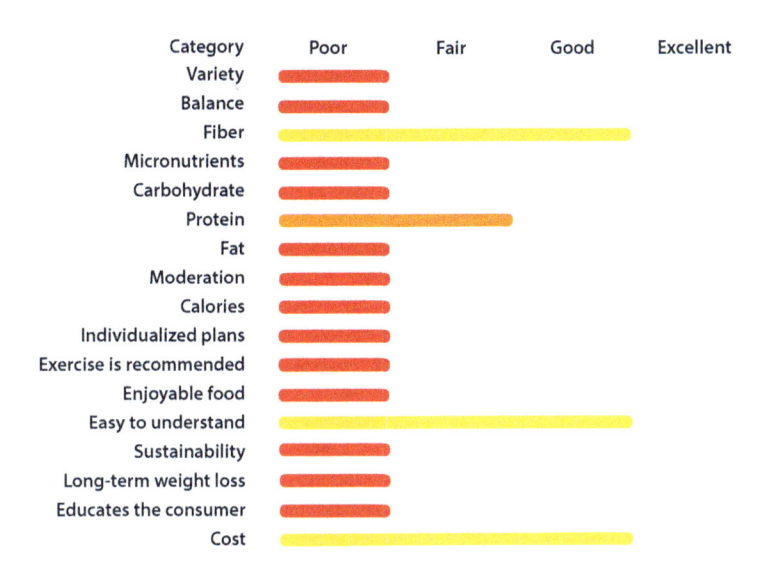

Category	Poor	Fair	Good	Excellent
Variety	■			
Balance	■			
Fiber			■	
Micronutrients	■			
Carbohydrate	■			
Protein	■	■		
Fat	■			
Moderation	■			
Calories	■			
Individualized plans	■			
Exercise is recommended	■			
Enjoyable food	■			
Easy to understand			■	
Sustainability	■			
Long-term weight loss	■			
Educates the consumer	■			
Cost			■	

Positives

Recommends nutrient-dense foods in small portions, values quality over quantity in food choices, every bite should be savored and enjoyed, recommends walking and weight training regularly and eating 3 meals a day at regular times. Recommends keeping good posture. No foods are forbidden. Allows for foods like chocolate, wine, and cheese in moderation. Recommends eating slowly. Educates on how to get the most from the dining experience.

Negatives

While no food is off-limits, there is not a strict meal plan accounting for calorie amounts, which does matter for weight loss.

*This ranking excludes the leek soup day.

The hook/catch or brilliant selling point: Catchy title describes the romantic culture and how beautiful women in France keep their figures.

Truths/Myths

- Myth - Leek soup has "magical qualities" that promote weight loss. 🔍 p. 13

- Truth - No need for leek soup. It is just soup.

Final decision: Thumbs up for the concept, it is a great idea. However, too many areas are not adequately addressed, so it ultimately gets a thumbs down. 👎

How to improve this diet: Skip the leek soup stage and jump right into eating well. Find out how many calories are needed and stay within that range.

Fruit Flush Diet

Premise of the Diet: Eating fruit will cleanse the GI system and put it into fat-burn mode and help you overcome food addictions.

Claims of the Diet: Lose 9 pounds in 3 days.

Diet Description: Three-day detox session involving: 12 glasses of bottled or filtered water each day, protein supplement drinks, any type of fresh fruit, a salad in the evening (no starchy vegetables), no exercise, and no other drinks but water.

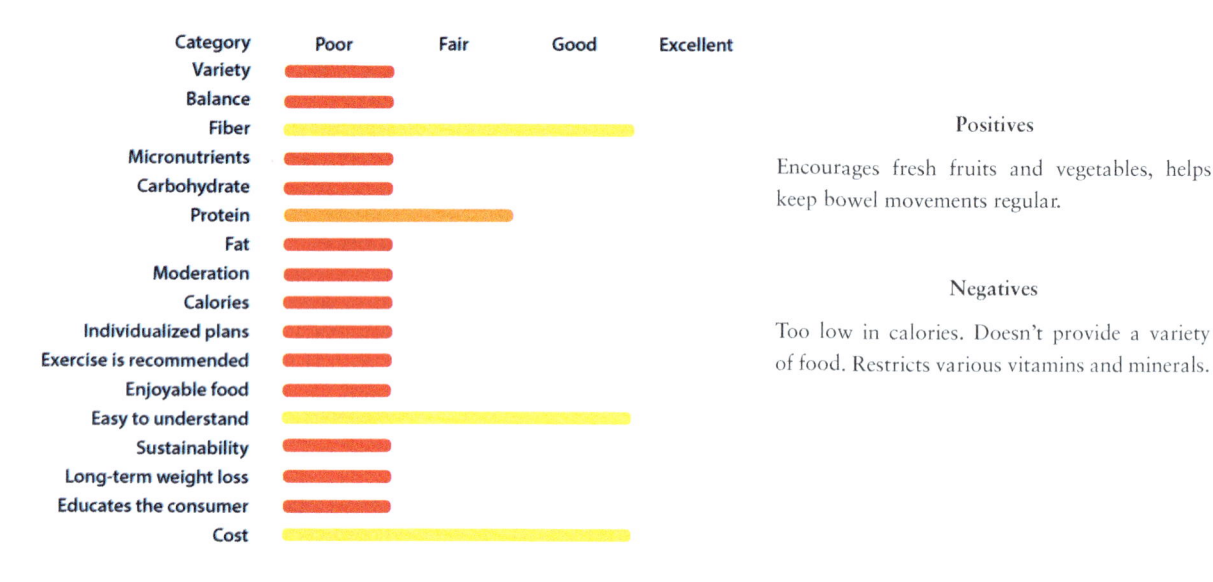

Category	Rating
Variety	Poor
Balance	Poor
Fiber	Good
Micronutrients	Poor
Carbohydrate	Poor
Protein	Fair
Fat	Poor
Moderation	Poor
Calories	Poor
Individualized plans	Poor
Exercise is recommended	Poor
Enjoyable food	Poor
Easy to understand	Good
Sustainability	Poor
Long-term weight loss	Poor
Educates the consumer	Poor
Cost	Good

Positives

Encourages fresh fruits and vegetables, helps keep bowel movements regular.

Negatives

Too low in calories. Doesn't provide a variety of food. Restricts various vitamins and minerals.

The hook/catch or brilliant selling point: Fast, easy weight loss

Truths/Myths

- *Myth* - Our digestive system needs a break.

- *Truth* - No healthy, functioning system in the body needs a break, and this includes the GI system.

- *Myth* - A low-calorie, fiber-rich fruit diet is needed to cleanse our GI system.

- *Truth* - Fiber-rich foods are recommended in the diet. Fiber reduces the likelihood of constipation and keeps the GI tract healthy. The only thing that really "cleans" the GI tract is a colonoscopy prep, but it would be unwise and unhealthy to frequently engage in a colonoscopy prep-like cleanse, as it would have a negative impact on the gut microbiome.

- *Myth* - A low-calorie, fiber-rich fruit diet will put a body into fat-burning mode. 🔍 p. 72

- *Truth* - Only exercise can make the body burn calories and put the body into a fat-burning mode.

- *Myth* - This diet will detoxify the body. 🔍 p. 13

- *Truth* - Our liver detoxifies our body. Specific foods or even combinations of different foods can't detoxify.

Final decision: Thumbs down 👎

How to improve this diet: Can't be improved.

FullBar Diet

Premise of the Diet: Mimics the surgical approach of physically making a smaller stomach, ultimately leading to weight loss.

Claims of the Diet: The 150- to 180-calorie FullBar swells up in the belly, creating the feeling of fullness before meals so less is eaten at the meal.

Diet Description: Eat a FullBar, a pre-meal snack made of high-fiber grains, 30 minutes before the two largest meals of the day, along with 8 ounces of water. Each bar contains 1 to 4.5 grams of fat, 4 to 5 grams of fiber, and 5 to 7 grams of protein.

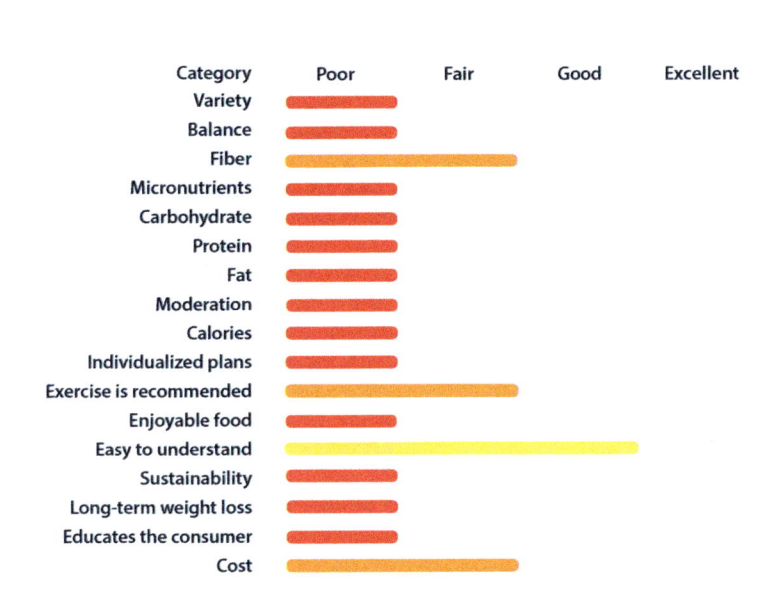

Category	Poor	Fair	Good	Excellent
Variety	●			
Balance	●			
Fiber		●		
Micronutrients	●			
Carbohydrate	●			
Protein	●			
Fat	●			
Moderation	●			
Calories	●			
Individualized plans	●			
Exercise is recommended		●		
Enjoyable food	●			
Easy to understand			●	
Sustainability	●			
Long-term weight loss	●			
Educates the consumer	●			
Cost		●		

Positives

Bars do not contain any chemical appetite suppressers. "Taking the edge off" hunger before a meal should help in controlling amount of food eaten. This is technically not a weight loss diet. It requires consuming a bar before meals. It would still be important to listen to hunger cues and eat the proper number of calories in order to lose weight. 🔍 p. 13

Negatives

Is based on the assumption that the foods eaten at meals will be nutrient-dense, healthy choices, and that the total calories consumed will be less than expended. While "taking the edge off" hunger before a meal should help in controlling the amount of food eaten, it has no influence on food choices. Weight could be gained on this diet.

The hook/catch or brilliant selling point: Takes the guesswork and control out of the hands of the consumer.

Truths/Myths

- **Myth** - None worth noting.

- **Truth** - Drinking water before a meal may help some feel fuller, leading to eating less at the meal.

Final decision: Thumbs down 👎

How to improve this diet: Be empowered by learning how to create flavorful, high-fiber, nutrient-dense snacks equaling the same number of calories as the bars to eat 30 minutes before meals. Be sure to eat nutrient-dense, low-calorie meals. Exercise regularly.

Gene Smart Diet

Premise of the Diet: Our genes are mismatched with today's lifestyles and methods of dieting.

Claims of the Diet: In order to get our genes back in sync, we need to reduce calories, eat more fiber, increase antioxidant intake from fruits and vegetables, consume omega-3 fatty acids, and exercise more.

Diet Description: Day 1 consists of a celery soup fast. Days 2–21 are the "Adaptive phase," during which dieters consume 1,600 calories daily. Days 22–35 are the "Preconditioning phase," when dieters consume 1,800 calories a day. In the "Optimal Maintenance phase," dieters consume 2,000 calories a day. These meals focus on the four principles:

1. Increasing polyphenols
2. Adding omega-3 fattyacids
3. Increasing fiber
4. Reducing calories

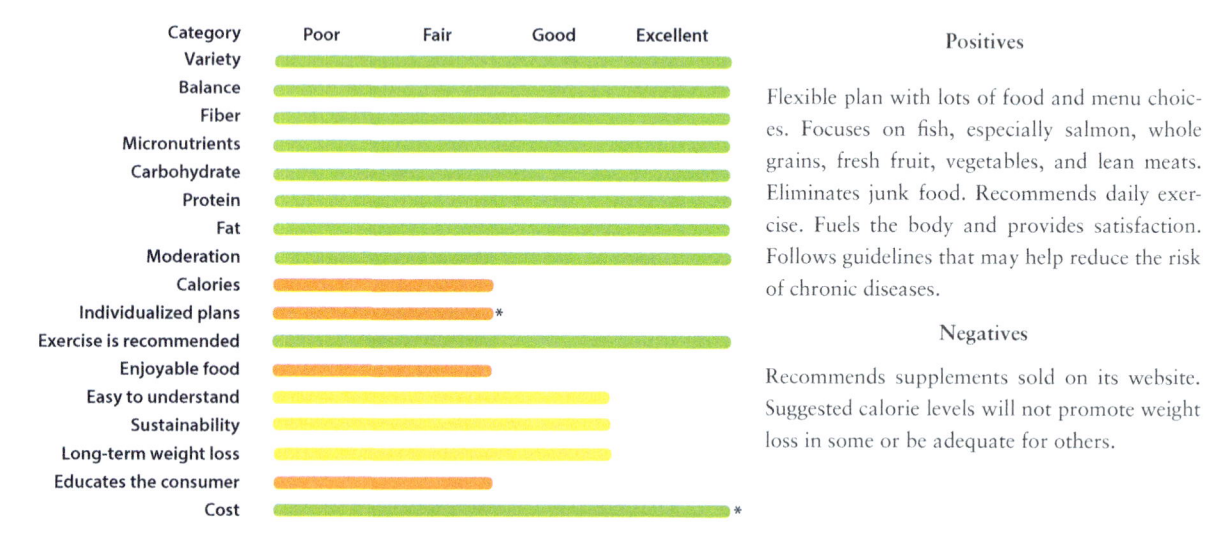

Category	Poor	Fair	Good	Excellent
Variety				●
Balance				●
Fiber				●
Micronutrients				●
Carbohydrate				●
Protein				●
Fat				●
Moderation				●
Calories		●		
Individualized plans		●*		
Exercise is recommended				●
Enjoyable food		●		
Easy to understand			●	
Sustainability			●	
Long-term weight loss			●	
Educates the consumer		●		
Cost				●*

Positives

Flexible plan with lots of food and menu choices. Focuses on fish, especially salmon, whole grains, fresh fruit, vegetables, and lean meats. Eliminates junk food. Recommends daily exercise. Fuels the body and provides satisfaction. Follows guidelines that may help reduce the risk of chronic diseases.

Negatives

Recommends supplements sold on its website. Suggested calorie levels will not promote weight loss in some or be adequate for others.

*Excludes the celery soup fast.
**Cost would rank poorly if all supplements were consumed.

The hook/catch or brilliant selling point: The magic bullet has been found – it's the perfect individualized diet!

Truths/Myths

- **Myth** - We know enough about the human genome to make specific diet recommendations for each of the specific genes. 🔍 p. 66

- **Truth** - We still have much to learn about the interaction between different foods and different genes. To date, the traditional Mediterranean Diet's influence on genes has been studied more than any other diet. The Mediterranean Diet appears to exert beneficial effects on risk factors for stroke, improved lipid profile, and even emotional eating.

- **Truth** - The idea behind this diet is very complex. The complexity of relationships among foods, nutrients, and genes is immense, and the field is still in the infancy stage. For example, the SLC19A3 gene provides instructions for making a protein that serves to transport the vitamin thiamine. This transporter is needed to move thiamine into cells so it can be used by the body, where it is needed for proper functioning of the nervous system and the breakdown of sugars and protein. But at least seven mutations in the SLC19A3 gene have been identified. People with biotin-thiamine-responsive basal ganglia disease experience recurrent episodes of neurological problems, including brain dysfunction. SLC19A3 gene mutations likely result in impairment of the protein that transports thiamine into cells, but the relationship between specific brain abnormalities and the abnormal thiamine transporter is unknown. 🔍 p. 15

• Truth - Obesity is a multifaceted disease. More than just genes impact obesity. Both environmental and biological factors contribute. Research demonstrates that the dramatic rise in the prevalence of obesity is primarily due to environmental factors, specifically the abundant consumption of energy-dense foods and little physical activity.

• Truth - In the years to come, we will undoubtedly see more about the effectiveness of personalized nutrition and the mechanisms in epigenetic inheritance. 🔍 p. 78

• Truth - Most likely weight can be lost on this diet, but it is probably due to consuming a low calorie level, not because genes were changed.

Final decision: Thumbs up 👍

How to improve this diet: Skip the celery soup fast and dive right into following a diet that is high in whole grains, fresh fruit, vegetables, healthy fats, and lean meats that corresponds to required caloric needs. Exercisenomics indicates regular exercise is important.

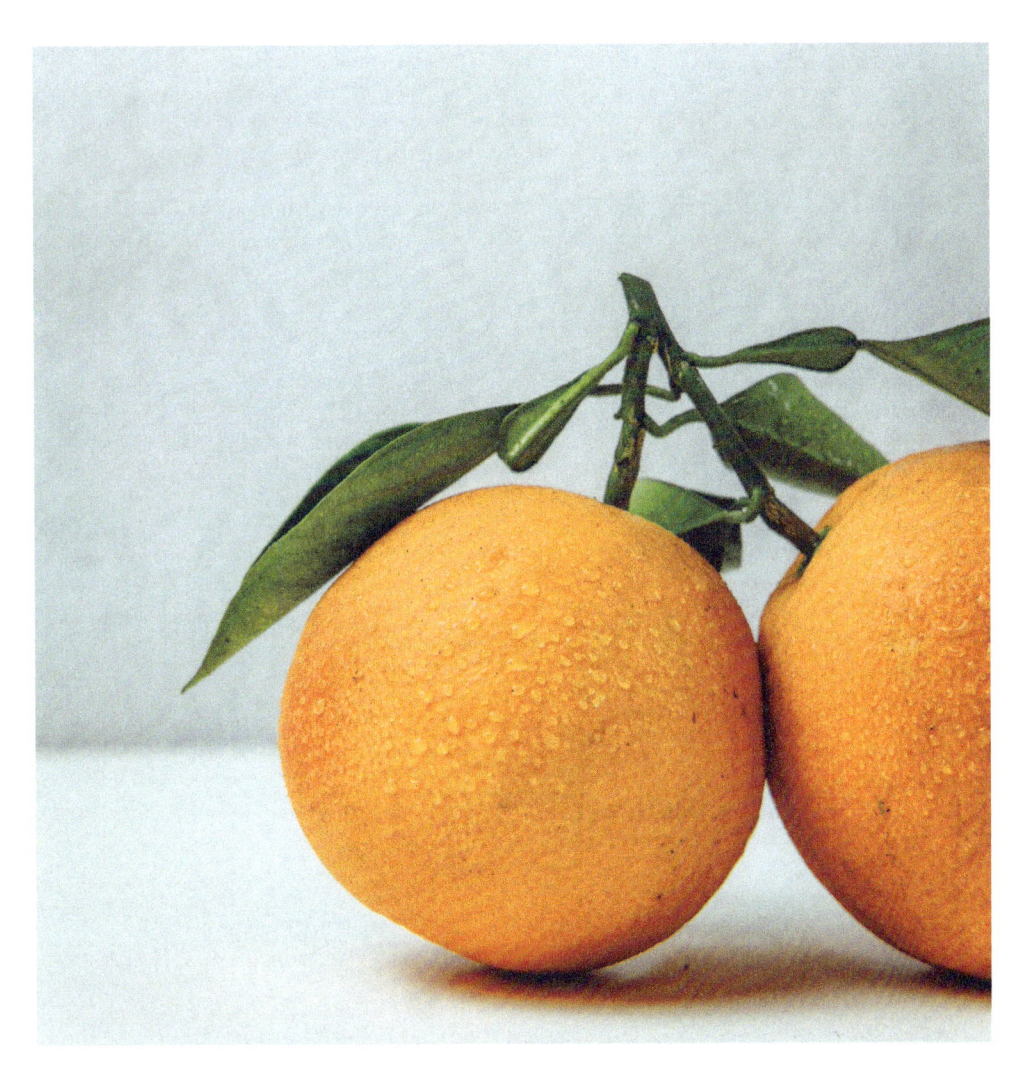

Genotype Diet

Premise of the Diet: Eat to fuel ancestral genetic type.

Claims of the Diet: Will change genetic destiny to enable living the longest, fullest, and healthiest life possible.

Diet Description: Six genotypes with their own evolutionary story are created for this diet.

GenoType 1 - The Hunter is tall, thin, and intense, with an overabundance of adrenaline and a fierce, nervous energy that winds down with age. Vulnerable to systemic burnout when overstressed, the Hunter's modern challenge is to conserve energy for the long haul.

GenoType 2 - The Gatherer is full-figured, even when not overweight. Struggles with body image in a culture where thin is "in." An unsuccessful crash dieter with a host of metabolic challenges. Becomes a glowing example of health when properly nourished.

GenoType 3 - The Teacher is strong, sinewy, and stable, with great chemical synchronicity and stamina. Built for longevity given the right diet and lifestyle. This is the genotype of balance with a tremendous capacity for growth and fulfillment.

GenoType 4 - The Explorer is muscular and adventurous, and a biological problem solver, with an ability to adapt to environmental changes. Possesses a better than average capacity for gene repair. Is vulnerable to hormonal imbalances and chemical sensitivities, but can overcome with a balanced diet and lifestyle.

GenoType 5 - The Warrior is long, lean, and healthy in youth. Is subject to a bodily rebellion in midlife. Can overcome quick-aging metabolic genes and experience a second, "silver" age of health with the optimal diet and lifestyle.

GenoType 6 - The Nomad is all about extremes with a high sensitivity to environmental conditions like changes in altitude and barometric pressure. Is vulnerable to neuromuscular and immune problems. But has little trouble controlling caloric intake and adapting to changes of aging.

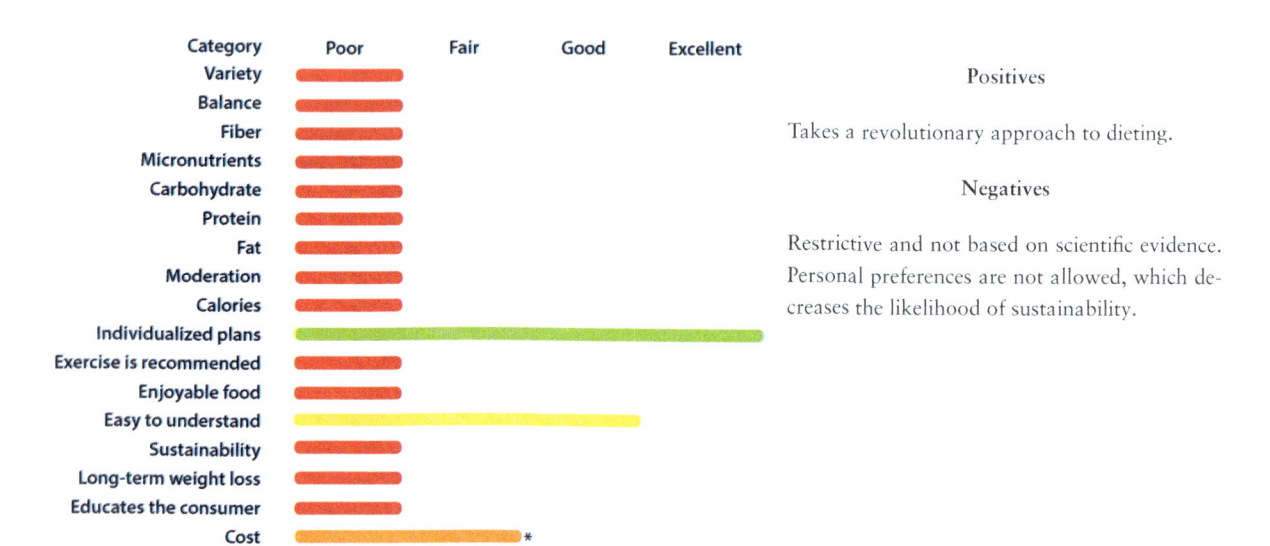

Category	Rating
Variety	Poor
Balance	Poor
Fiber	Poor
Micronutrients	Poor
Carbohydrate	Poor
Protein	Poor
Fat	Poor
Moderation	Poor
Calories	Poor
Individualized plans	Excellent
Exercise is recommended	Poor
Enjoyable food	Poor
Easy to understand	Good
Sustainability	Poor
Long-term weight loss	Poor
Educates the consumer	Poor
Cost	Fair*

Positives

Takes a revolutionary approach to dieting.

Negatives

Restrictive and not based on scientific evidence. Personal preferences are not allowed, which decreases the likelihood of sustainability.

*Depends on which category a person falls into and whether they purchase supplements.

The hook/catch or brilliant selling point: Uses individual differences with claims about genetic backing to fuel the body and optimize genetic programing.

Truths/Myths

- Myth - Addresses the effect of epigenetics on an individual's health.

- Truth - Epigenetics is the study of changes in gene expression that occur without altering DNA sequence. While there is evidence for epigenetics, we are not yet at the point of classifying people and certainly not at the point of making specific, clear, and confident meal recommendations.

- Myth - Groundbreaking research has been conducted that identifies six unique genetic types, and these specific GenoTypes represent the identified and known survival strategy. 🔍 p. 13

- Truth - While dieters may identify their specific GenoType using the book's rationale, by identifying family history, blood type, fingerprint analysis, leg length measurements, and dental characteristics, it is impossible at this point in time to determine one's own genetic identity. It took decades of highly skilled geneticists throughout the world to even identify the genes and determine their sequence through the Human Genome Project. Additionally, the Human Genome Project sequenced the genomes of brewers' yeast, the roundworm, the fruit fly, and mice. Studying similarities and differences between human and nonhuman genes, researchers hope to discover the functions of particular genes. Moreover, some research suggests that how a person eats may actually influence the health of children and grandchildren based on genes being altered. While this area of science is exciting and is being worked on…we have not arrived. There is much we don't yet know about this area. What we do know is depicted in the current recommendations.

- Myth - This diet has precisely determined how we can alter our genetic destiny by turning on the good genes while silencing the bad ones so health risks, weight, and life span can all be improved. The GenoType Diet reveals previously hidden genetic strengths and weaknesses and provides a precise diet and lifestyle plan for every individual.

- Truth - It has been determined that environmental factors, including diet and lifestyle, influence how genes are expressed; however, we are not yet able to make complete, firm recommendations for all foods or for all people.

- Truth - Obesity is multifaceted and results from the interplay of both environmental and biological factors. The dramatic rise in the prevalence of obesity is primarily due to the increased consumption of energy-dense foods and reduced physical activity, both of which are environmental factors.

- Truth - Most obesity genes remain to be identified.

- Truth - It is worth noting that the creator of this diet also created the "Eat Right for Your Type Diet" and sells many supplements for personal financial gain. 🔍 p. 99

Final decision: Thumbs down 👎

How to improve this diet: Can't be improved

Gluten Free Diet (aka G-free diet)

Premise of the Diet: Celiac disease is an autoimmune disorder in which gluten triggers immune system activity that damages the lining of the small intestine. If not properly managed, over time the damage prevents absorption of nutrients from food.

Claims of the Diet: Eating gluten-free is critical for managing symptoms of celiac disease and other medical conditions associated with gluten, such as gluten ataxia and non-celiac gluten sensitivity.

Diet Description: Do not eat foods with the protein gluten. Gluten is found in wheat, barley, rye, and a cross between wheat and rye called triticale, and in some cases, oats. Oats are naturally gluten-free but may be contaminated during manufacturing with wheat, barley, or rye products. May eat: Amaranth, arrowroot, buckwheat, corn and cornmeal, flax, hominy, millet, quinoa, rice, sorghum, soy, tapioca, and gluten-free flours such as rice, soy, corn, potato, and bean. Label reading is important. Foods that are labeled gluten-free must have less than 20 ppm of gluten, according to the Food and Drug Administration.

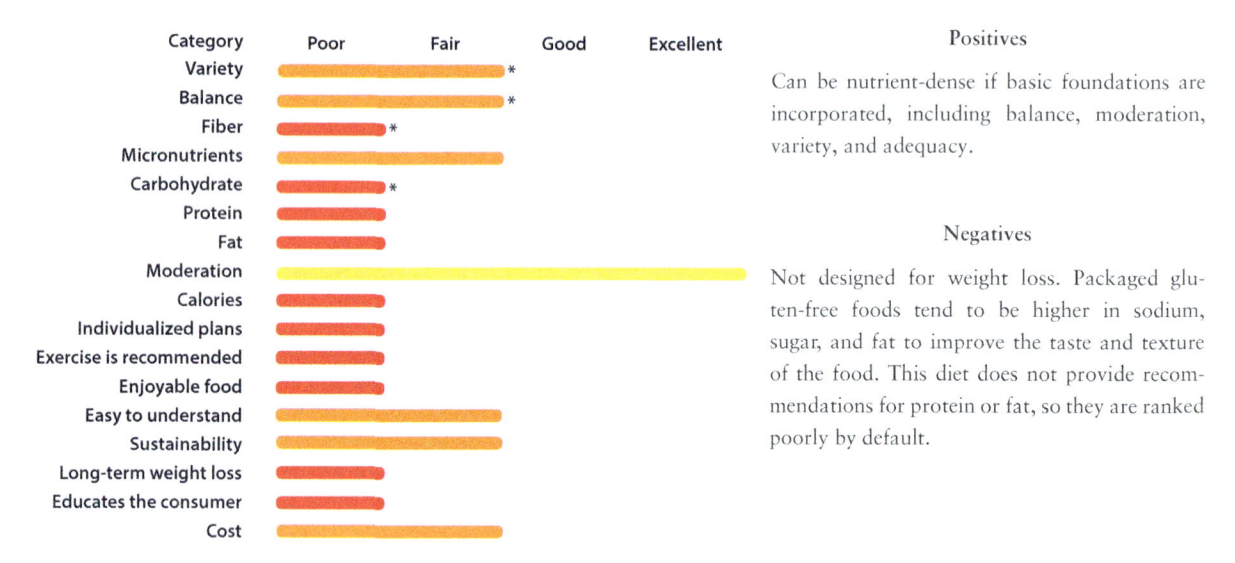

Category	Poor	Fair	Good	Excellent
Variety		*		
Balance		*		
Fiber	*			
Micronutrients				
Carbohydrate	*			
Protein				
Fat				
Moderation				
Calories				
Individualized plans				
Exercise is recommended				
Enjoyable food				
Easy to understand				
Sustainability				
Long-term weight loss				
Educates the consumer				
Cost				

Positives

Can be nutrient-dense if basic foundations are incorporated, including balance, moderation, variety, and adequacy.

Negatives

Not designed for weight loss. Packaged gluten-free foods tend to be higher in sodium, sugar, and fat to improve the taste and texture of the food. This diet does not provide recommendations for protein or fat, so they are ranked poorly by default.

*Most people who follow a gluten-free diet tend to reduce their carbohydrate intake, particularly from grains. This will lead to a reduction in fiber intake, an increase in risk for micronutrient deficiencies and a carbohydrate intake likely less than the AMDR. It is possible to have a well-balanced, gluten-free diet that includes high-fiber grains; however, because few gluten-free grains are enriched, those following a normal carbohydrate-level gluten-free diet may still be at risk for riboflavin, folate and iron deficiencies.

The hook/catch or brilliant selling point: Media hype: this is not a weight loss or a fat-loss diet.

Truths/Myths

- Myth - This is a diet to follow in order to lose weight.

- Truth - This is not a weight-loss diet.

Final decision: Thumbs down

How to improve this diet: Follow a diet designed to lose body fat.

Glycemic Index Diet

Premise of the Diet: A diet designed to help diabetics control blood sugar levels will also help others lose excess weight.

Claims of the Diet: It's the easiest, most satisfying eating plan possible.

Diet Description: The glycemic index scores foods from 0 to 100 based on how much they raise blood sugar levels. High-GI foods score 70 or higher and are considered bad. These include foods like white rice, white bread, white bagels, white potatoes, crackers, and sugar-sweetened beverages. Medium-GI foods score 56 to 69. Sweet potatoes, corn, brown rice, couscous, spaghetti, ice cream, raisins, and grapes fall into this category. Low-GI foods score 55 and below and are considered good. These include foods like barley, soy products, grainy breads, lentils, oatmeal, peanuts, peas, carrots, hummus, and skim milk. Eat more foods in the low-GI category and fewer in the high-GI group.

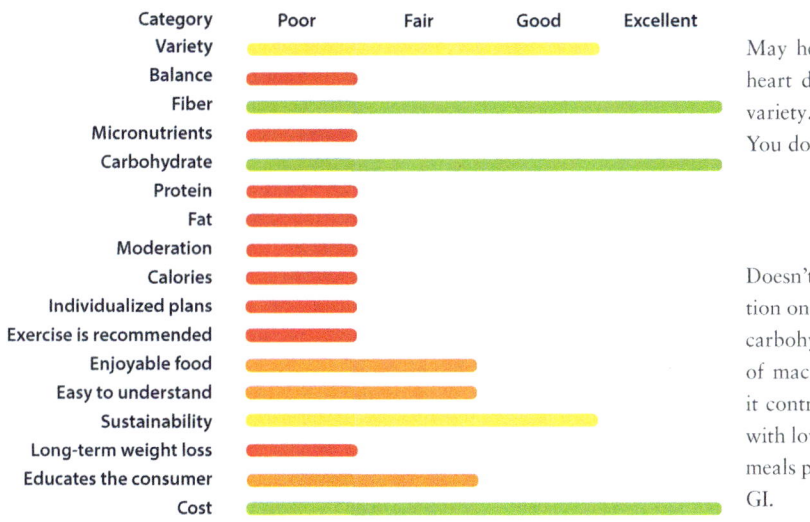

Category	Poor	Fair	Good	Excellent
Variety			Good	
Balance	Poor			
Fiber				Excellent
Micronutrients	Poor			
Carbohydrate				Excellent
Protein	Poor			
Fat	Poor			
Moderation	Poor			
Calories	Poor			
Individualized plans	Poor			
Exercise is recommended	Poor			
Enjoyable food		Fair		
Easy to understand		Fair		
Sustainability			Good	
Long-term weight loss	Poor			
Educates the consumer		Fair		
Cost				Excellent

Positives

May help prevent conditions like diabetes and heart disease. No calorie counting. Allows for variety. You also don't need to cut out all carbs. You do need to be selective about your carbs.

Negatives

Doesn't offer advice, suggestions, or information on non-carb foods, or calories. In addition, carbohydrates make up the largest percentage of macronutrients in a balanced diet. To limit contributions of carbohydrates to only those with low GI is challenging considering that most meals provide a mixture of both high GI and low GI.

The hook/catch or brilliant selling point: The glycemic index is a breakthrough nutritional discovery that helps us identify the speed at which the body digests food and the impact a particular food has on weight.

Truths/Myths

- **Myth** - Following this diet will promote weight loss.

- **Truth** - Portion sizes matter, and while this diet may be a useful guide in planning a diet that helps control blood sugar levels, it does not provide guidelines for overall healthful eating or calorie control.

Final decision: Thumbs down

How to improve this diet: Choose mostly low GI foods when making carbohydrate choices, choose lean meats, healthy fats, make ½ the plate fruits and vegetables, choose low-fat dairy, exercise regularly and make sure calorie intake is lower than calories expended.

GOLO Diet

Premise of the Diet: Manage insulin levels through a calorie-controlled, low-glycemic diet and exercise.

Claims of the Diet: Eat more food and lose more weight while feeling fuller longer. Will help restore hormonal balance and repair metabolism while removing hunger or cravings.

Diet Description: There is a 30-, 60-, or 90-day GOLO Rescue Program. The GOLO Metabolic Fuel Matrix allows choices for each meal from four "fuel groups": proteins, carbs, vegetables, and fats. Allows 1 to 2 servings of each fuel group per meal and 3 meals per day. Avoid processed foods, fatty red meats, processed sugar and sugar-laden beverages, artificial sweeteners, and dairy.

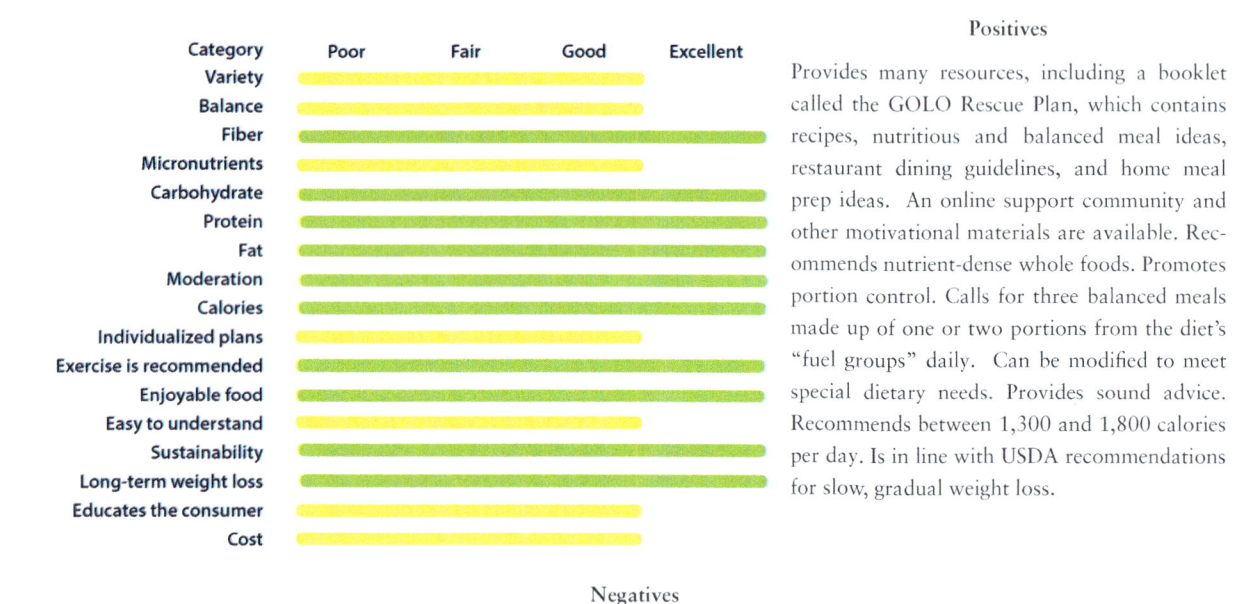

Category	Poor	Fair	Good	Excellent
Variety			Good	
Balance			Good	
Fiber				Excellent
Micronutrients			Good	
Carbohydrate				Excellent
Protein				Excellent
Fat				Excellent
Moderation				Excellent
Calories				Excellent
Individualized plans			Good	
Exercise is recommended				Excellent
Enjoyable food				Excellent
Easy to understand			Good	
Sustainability				Excellent
Long-term weight loss				Excellent
Educates the consumer			Good	
Cost		Fair		

Positives

Provides many resources, including a booklet called the GOLO Rescue Plan, which contains recipes, nutritious and balanced meal ideas, restaurant dining guidelines, and home meal prep ideas. An online support community and other motivational materials are available. Recommends nutrient-dense whole foods. Promotes portion control. Calls for three balanced meals made up of one or two portions from the diet's "fuel groups" daily. Can be modified to meet special dietary needs. Provides sound advice. Recommends between 1,300 and 1,800 calories per day. Is in line with USDA recommendations for slow, gradual weight loss.

Negatives

Encourages the GOLO Release supplement. The supplement is the cornerstone of the diet and, according to the company, is what makes the program different than others on the market. Consists of magnesium, zinc and chromium and some herbs.

The hook/catch or brilliant selling point: According to Google rankings, this was the most searched diet in 2016.

Truths/Myths:

- *Myth* - The GOLO Release supplement is necessary. p. 99

- *Truth* - Consuming a well-balanced diet full of variety should supply all nutrients in the supplement in adequate amounts.

Final decision: Thumbs up. 👍

How to improve this diet: Add milk to make the diet more nutritionally adequate and don't bother taking the supplement.

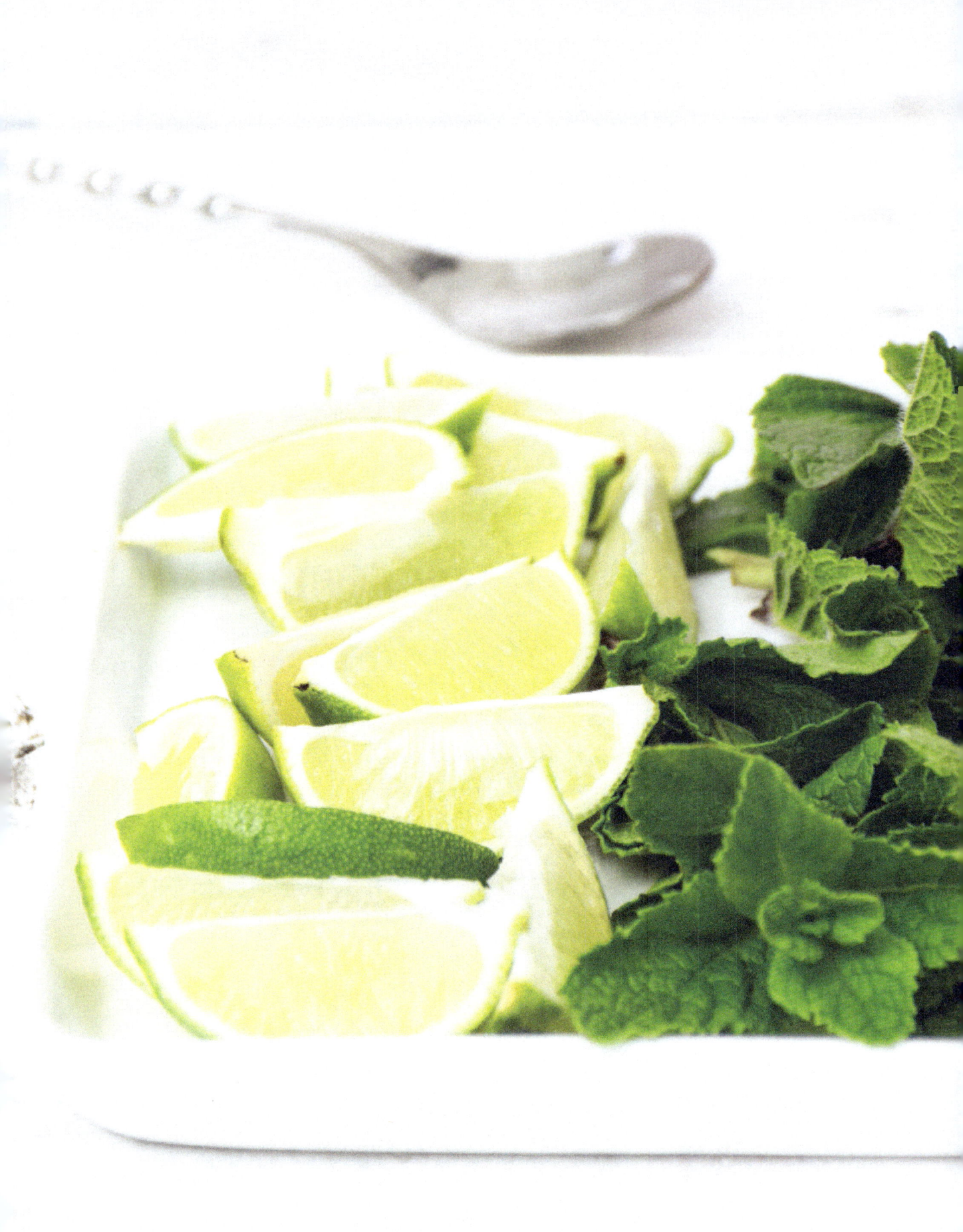

Good Calories–Bad Calories

Premise of the Diet: Poor science has led to faulty beliefs about the relationship between diet, obesity, and other chronic health conditions.

Claims of the Diet: The best diet is one with lots of protein and fat and little carbohydrates.

Diet Description: Eat lots of protein and animal fat.

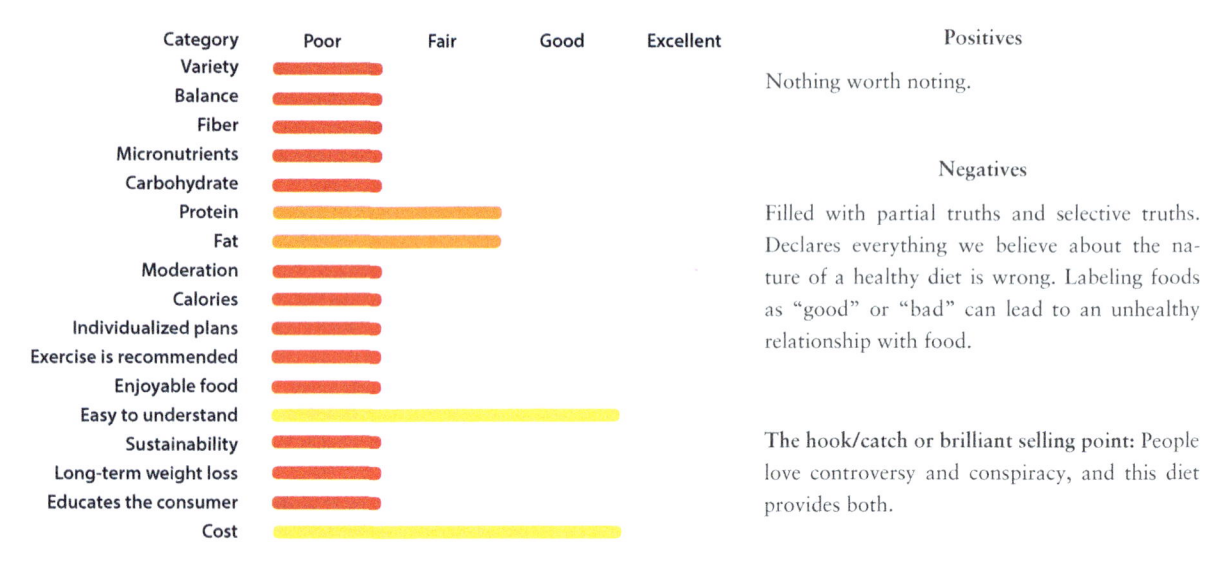

Category	Poor	Fair	Good	Excellent
Variety	■			
Balance	■			
Fiber	■			
Micronutrients	■			
Carbohydrate	■			
Protein		■		
Fat		■		
Moderation	■			
Calories	■			
Individualized plans	■			
Exercise is recommended	■			
Enjoyable food	■			
Easy to understand			■	
Sustainability	■			
Long-term weight loss	■			
Educates the consumer	■			
Cost			■	

Positives

Nothing worth noting.

Negatives

Filled with partial truths and selective truths. Declares everything we believe about the nature of a healthy diet is wrong. Labeling foods as "good" or "bad" can lead to an unhealthy relationship with food.

The hook/catch or brilliant selling point: People love controversy and conspiracy, and this diet provides both.

Truths/Myths

- *Myth* - It is a myth that dietary fat and heart disease, salt and high blood pressure and dietary fiber and cancer are connected.

- *Truth* - Much research supports the associations between the above nutrients and the corresponding chronic diseases.

- *Myth* - People store excess body fat because carbohydrates drive up the insulin level in the blood, which in turn encourages fat to be stored. 🔍 p. 73

- *Truth* - Calories can only be stored as body fat if they are not burned for energy. Excess calories can come from protein and fat just as easily as carbohydrates.

- *Myth* - A calorie of fat is much less fattening than a calorie of sugar. 🔍 p. 55

- *Truth* - A gram of fat contributes 9 calories per gram while a gram of sugar provides 4 calories per gram. The body has the ability to efficiently store fat calories as body fat, while it is slightly less efficient at storing calories from carbohydrates as body fat.

- *Myth* - Saturated fats, especially those coming from animal sources, are good for health.

- *Truth* - Many studies do not support this. Current dietary recommendations do not support this notion.

- *Myth* - Obesity is a result of carbohydrates.

- *Truth* - This is not true. Obesity is a complex chronic condition that has many contributing factors.

- Myth - Consuming excess calories does not create body fat. 🔍 p. 21

- Truth - Consumed excess calories (more than expended) are stored as body fat.

- Myth - Carbohydrates are addictive and those who have tried to break their addiction crave them just like alcoholics crave a drink.

- Truth - Researchers debate whether or not the term addiction can be applied to a nutrient that is vital to life.

Final decision: Thumbs down 👎

How to improve this diet: Can't be improved.

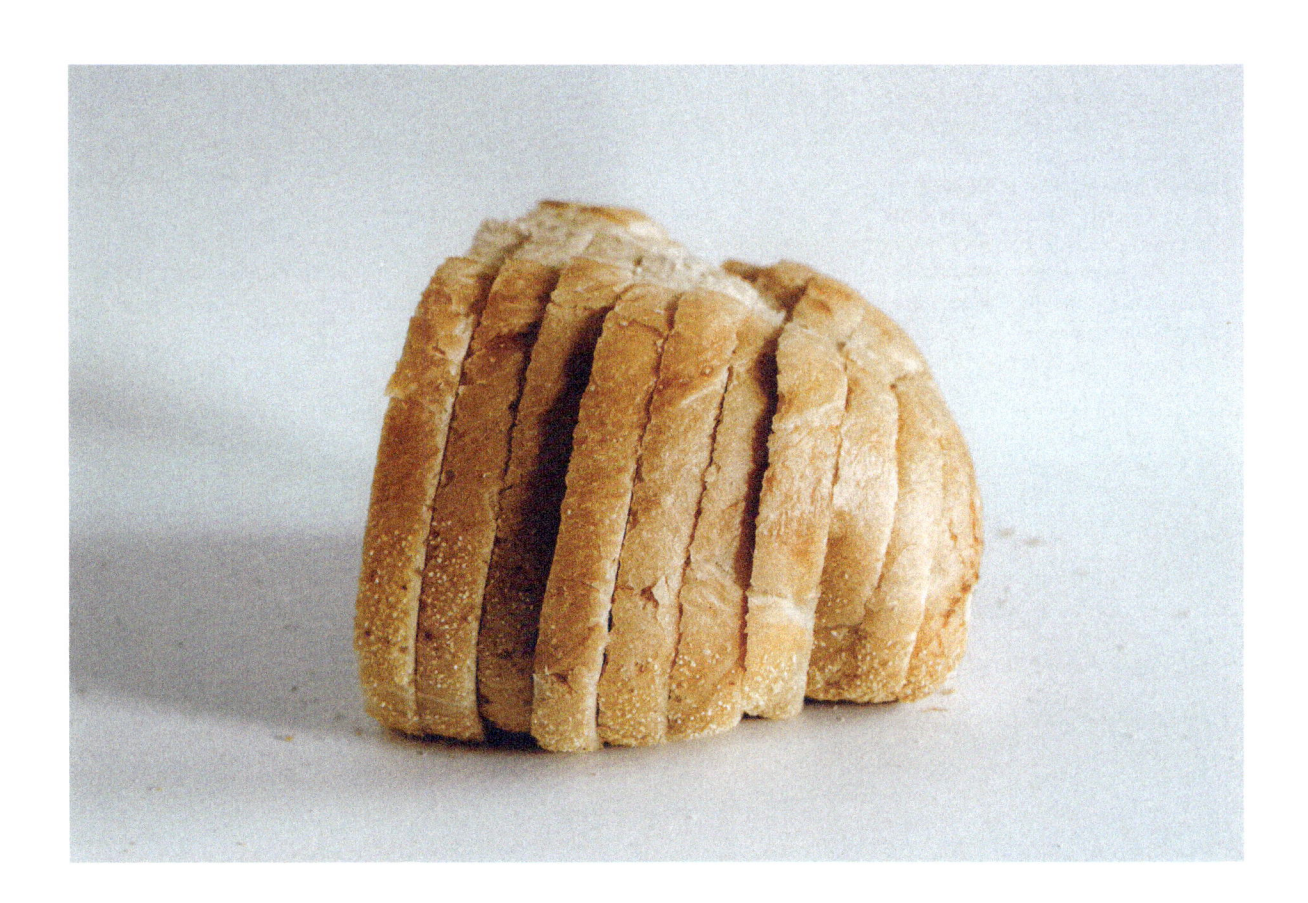

Grapefruit Diet

Premise of the Diet: Grapefruit has fat-burning enzymes.

Claims of the Diet: Promises 10 pounds can be lost in 12 days.

Diet Description: Many versions exist, but most promote a 10- to 12-day plan of 800-1,000 calories, no extremely hot or extremely cold foods, nothing prepared in aluminum pans, and grapefruit at every meal.

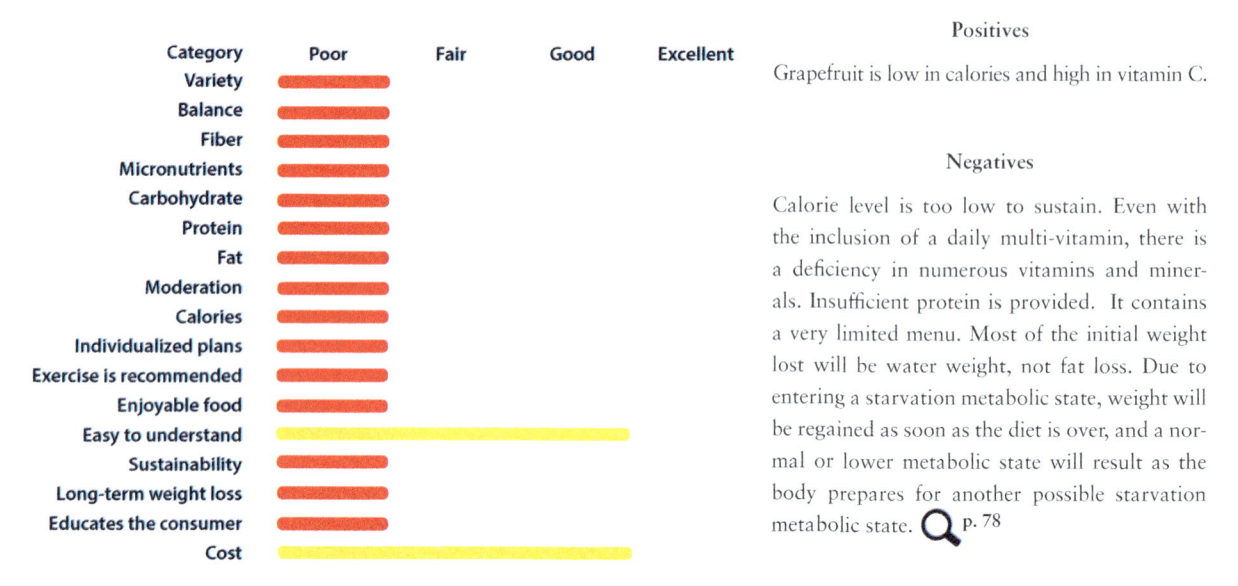

Category	Poor	Fair	Good	Excellent
Variety	■			
Balance	■			
Fiber	■			
Micronutrients	■			
Carbohydrate	■			
Protein	■			
Fat	■			
Moderation	■			
Calories	■			
Individualized plans	■			
Exercise is recommended	■			
Enjoyable food	■			
Easy to understand			■	
Sustainability	■			
Long-term weight loss	■			
Educates the consumer	■			
Cost			■	

Positives

Grapefruit is low in calories and high in vitamin C.

Negatives

Calorie level is too low to sustain. Even with the inclusion of a daily multi-vitamin, there is a deficiency in numerous vitamins and minerals. Insufficient protein is provided. It contains a very limited menu. Most of the initial weight lost will be water weight, not fat loss. Due to entering a starvation metabolic state, weight will be regained as soon as the diet is over, and a normal or lower metabolic state will result as the body prepares for another possible starvation metabolic state. p. 78

The hook/catch or brilliant selling point: Most people are looking for something natural that burns fat without exercising.

Truths/Myths

- Myth - Enzymes in grapefruit burn fat.

- Truth - Enzymes in grapefruit do not burn fat. If research were to show that they can burn fat, the amount burned would have to exceed the calories consumed in order for the diet to work.

Final decision: Thumbs down

How to improve this diet: Can't be improved.

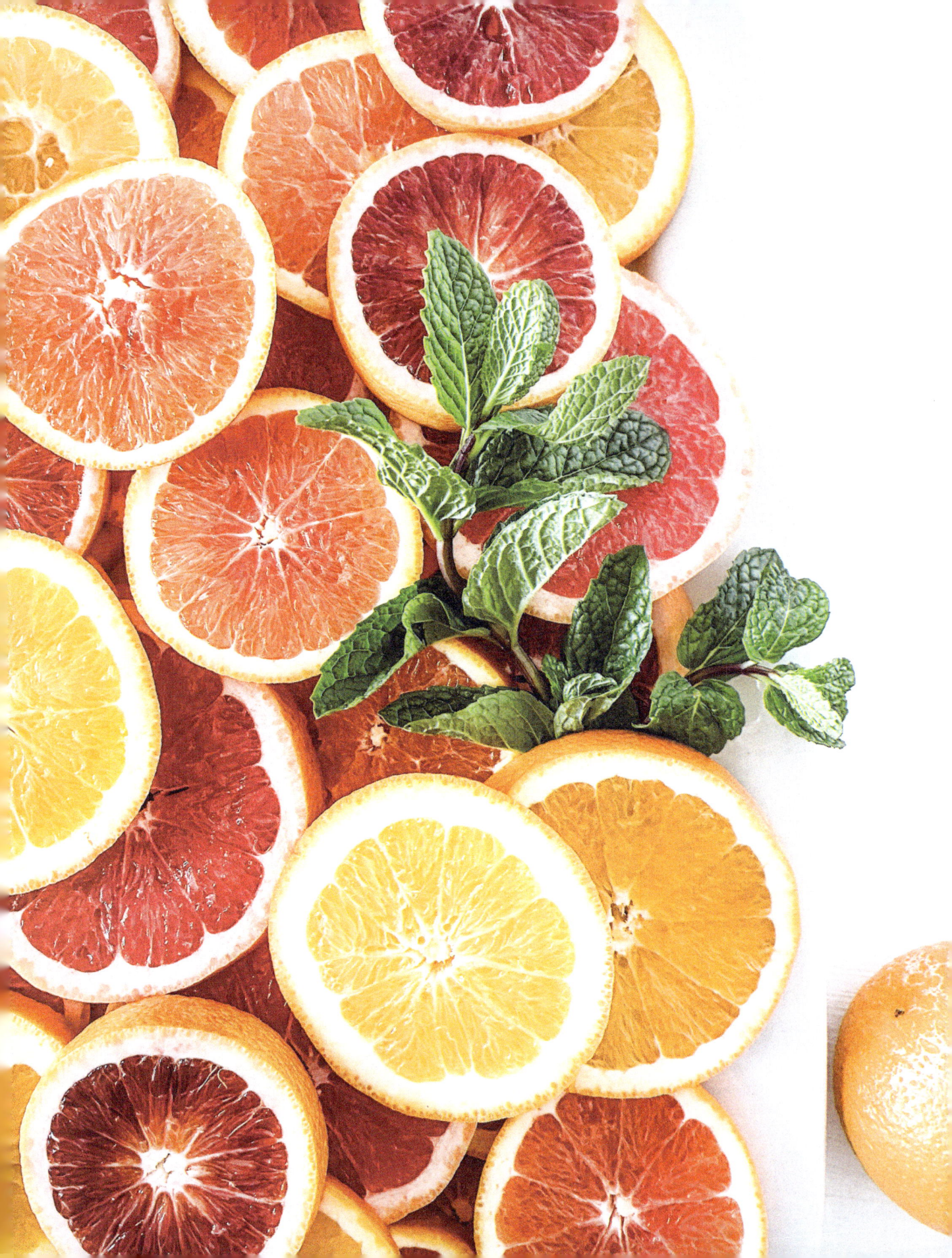

Hallelujah Diet

Premise of the Diet: Replaces the Standard American Diet (SAD) foods with plant-based foods that nourish our bodies so we can reclaim our natural self-healing power.

Claims of the Diet: Has everything you need to thrive in healthy eating. Biblically based.

Diet Description: Consists of 4 Steps.

Step 1: Consume raw vegetables, fruits, nuts, and seeds.

Step 2: Eliminate toxic foods like white flour and sugar.

Step 3: Consume BarleyMax and vegetable juice.

Step 4: Take their supplements.

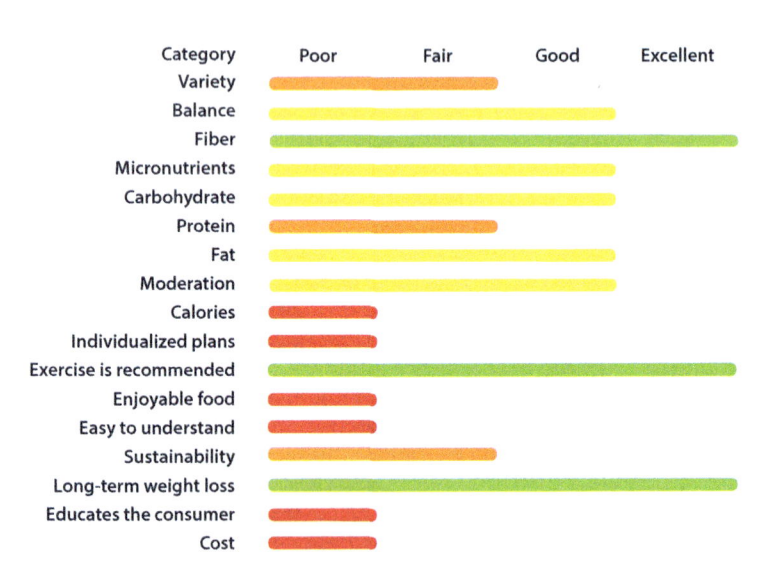

Category	Rating
Variety	Poor–Fair
Balance	Fair–Good
Fiber	Excellent
Micronutrients	Fair–Good
Carbohydrate	Fair–Good
Protein	Poor–Fair
Fat	Fair–Good
Moderation	Fair–Good
Calories	Poor
Individualized plans	Poor
Exercise is recommended	Excellent
Enjoyable food	Poor
Easy to understand	Poor
Sustainability	Poor–Fair
Long-term weight loss	Excellent
Educates the consumer	Poor
Cost	Poor

Positives

Requires minimal cooking. Is low in saturated fat, added sugars, and sodium. May be good for people with chronic diseases, such as hypertension, diabetes, heart disease, or high cholesterol.

Negatives

Requires a lot of prep work and planning for juicing. Supplements costing nearly $2,000/year are encouraged to be taken at specific times throughout the day to make up for the low levels of iron, zinc, omega-3 fatty acids, vitamin B12, vitamin D, and calcium that more than likely are insufficiently provided by the diet alone. This is nearly an additional $167 per month on top of a regular grocery bill. May be challenging to stick with long term, due to the many restrictions.

The hook/catch or brilliant selling point: It is empowering to think that it is possible to reclaim our natural self-healing power.

Truths/Myths

- **Myth** - Since meat, dairy, white flour, sugar products, and refined salt are manufactured with additives, preservatives, and artificial ingredients, they are bad and should be eliminated.

- **Truth** - Containing additives and preservatives does not automatically make foods bad. Some foods are fortified and enriched with vitamins and minerals which are considered additives.

- **Myth** - Even if your digestive system is healthy, you can only absorb a portion of the nutrients in fruits and vegetables. Juicing with BarleyMax allows you to gain maximum nutrition naturally.

- **Truth** - It is true that only about 40-90% of the vitamins we consume are bioavailable, meaning that 40-90% of all the vitamins we consume can be used by our bodies. However, vitamins in animal products are better absorbed than those coming from plant sources. But research also shows nutrients in whole foods have a more positive influence on health than nutrients consumed in a supplement.

• Myth - No matter what kind of diet you follow, there are likely gaps in your nutrition and therefore supplements should be taken.

• Truth - Eating a well-balanced diet that provides a variety of foods in moderation should provide adequate nutrients. However, eliminating entire food groups (like meats and dairy) will also eliminate many nutrients. Nutrients are better absorbed and have greater health benefits when we consume them in whole foods rather than pill or powder form.

• Myth - Meat can "get trapped" in our system, delay elimination, and cause toxicity and illness.

• Truth - Meat is broken down by stomach acid and digestive enzymes. In the small intestine, proteins are broken down into amino acids, which are absorbed into the blood, while fats are broken down into fatty acids and absorbed.

• Myth - Eating raw foods is the best way to get nutrients, restore damaged cells, and have long-lasting health.

• Truth - Vitamins are rather delicate and can be destroyed by light, heat, oxygen, water, pH, and the passing of time. Eating raw does eliminate destruction done by heat. However, if raw food is too unfamiliar or un-flavorful and thus not eaten, it will supply no nutrients.

Final decision: Thumbs down

How to improve this diet: Eating raw vegetables is fine, as long as vegetables are eaten. But for people who don't like raw vegetables, cooking them is better than not eating them at all. Make ½ the plate fruits and vegetables and consume lean protein and complex carbohydrates and healthy fats.

The hCG Diet
(Human Chorionic Gonadotropin, a hormone present at high levels in early pregnancy)

Premise of the Diet: The Human Chorionic Gonadotropin (hCG) hormone, which is present in high levels in early pregnancy, boosts metabolism.

Claims of the Diet: Boosts in metabolism result in large amounts of fat loss (1-2 pounds/day). Won't feel hungry.

Diet Description: Combines the Human Chorionic Gonadotropin hormone with a 500 calorie a day diet. It is illegal to sell products claiming to contain hCG as an over the counter (OTC) drug product. Yet hCG products can still be found in various forms including oral drops, pellets, and sprays through websites and retail stores. The FDA has called this diet dangerous, illegal, and fraudulent.

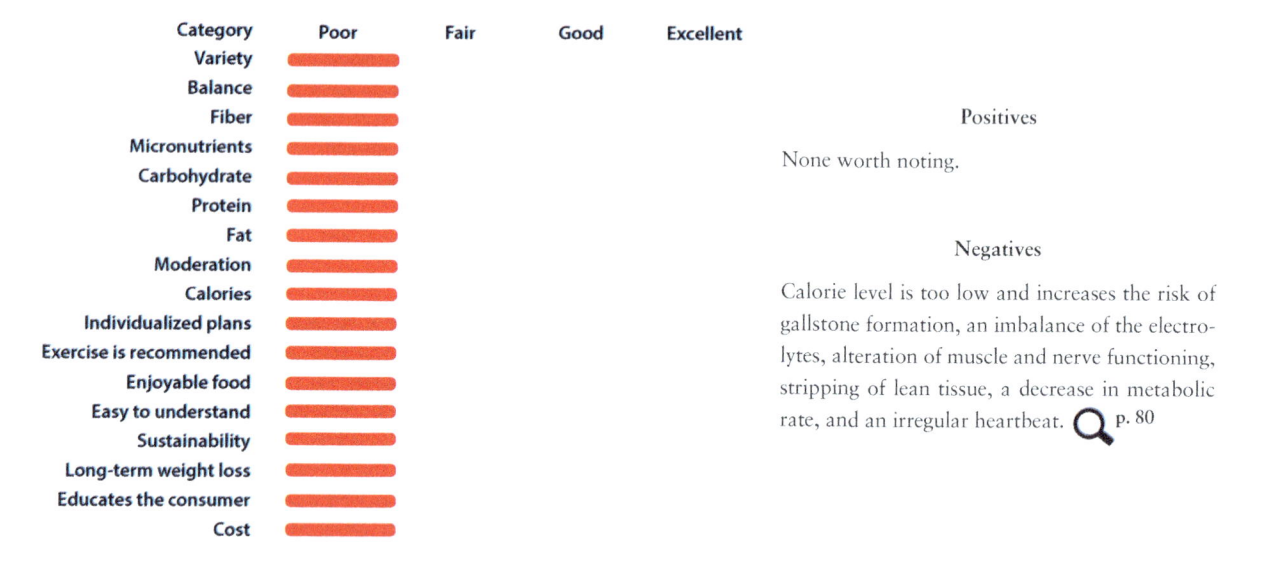

Category	Poor	Fair	Good	Excellent
Variety	■			
Balance	■			
Fiber	■			
Micronutrients	■			
Carbohydrate	■			
Protein	■			
Fat	■			
Moderation	■			
Calories	■			
Individualized plans	■			
Exercise is recommended	■			
Enjoyable food	■			
Easy to understand	■			
Sustainability	■			
Long-term weight loss	■			
Educates the consumer	■			
Cost	■			

Positives

None worth noting.

Negatives

Calorie level is too low and increases the risk of gallstone formation, an imbalance of the electrolytes, alteration of muscle and nerve functioning, stripping of lean tissue, a decrease in metabolic rate, and an irregular heartbeat. 🔍 p. 80

The hook/catch or brilliant selling point: Fast weight loss

Truths/Myths

- **Myth** - This diet boosts metabolism. 🔍 p. 13

- **Truth** - Any weight loss achieved while being on the hCG diet is due to low calorie intake alone. hCG does not boost metabolism or help in weight loss.

- **Truth** - hCG is approved by the FDA as a prescription drug for the treatment of female infertility. It is not approved for weight loss.

Final decision: Thumbs down 👎

How to improve this diet: Can't be improved

High School Reunion Diet

Premise of the Diet: Eat well to lose weight

Claims of the Diet: You will look great and lose weight within 30 days.

Diet Description: Meals and snacks consist of vegetables, legumes, fruit, fish and lean meats, low-fat dairy, and whole grains. Avoids processed foods.

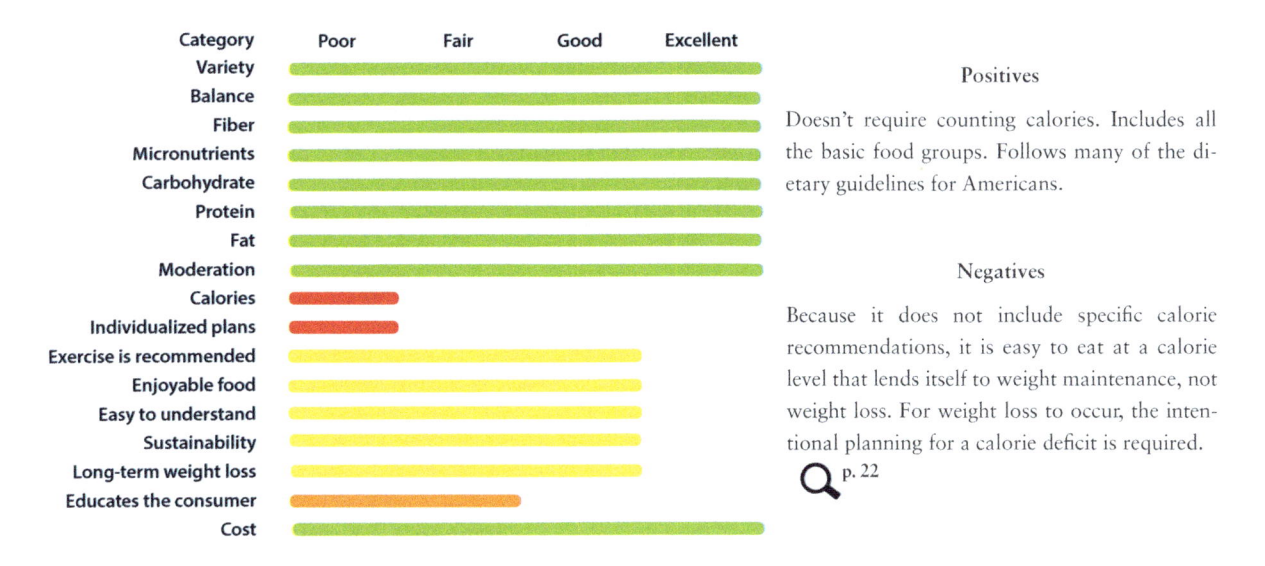

Category	Poor	Fair	Good	Excellent
Variety				■
Balance				■
Fiber				■
Micronutrients				■
Carbohydrate				■
Protein				■
Fat				■
Moderation				■
Calories	■			
Individualized plans	■			
Exercise is recommended			■	
Enjoyable food			■	
Easy to understand			■	
Sustainability			■	
Long-term weight loss			■	
Educates the consumer		■		
Cost				■

Positives

Doesn't require counting calories. Includes all the basic food groups. Follows many of the dietary guidelines for Americans.

Negatives

Because it does not include specific calorie recommendations, it is easy to eat at a calorie level that lends itself to weight maintenance, not weight loss. For weight loss to occur, the intentional planning for a calorie deficit is required.

🔍 p. 22

The hook/catch or brilliant selling point: Catches the attention of those with a specific goal in mind.

Truths/Myths: Nothing worth noting

Final decision: Thumbs up 👍

How to improve this diet: Be sure to consume fewer calories than expended.

Hormone Diet (aka Hormone Reset Diet)

Premise of the Diet: Hormonal imbalances and fluctuations contribute to excess body fat.

Claims of the Diet: Lose up to 15 pounds in 21 days and sync hormones to promote an overall healthier body.

Diet Description: A three-step, 6-week process starts with a 2-week "detox," eliminating caffeine, alcohol, sugar, dairy, gluten-containing grains, artificial sweeteners, and most oils. It then adopts a "Glyci-Med" diet, which is a mix of foods low on the glycemic index and a traditional Mediterranean diet, while taking supplements such as multivitamins, omega-3 fatty acids, calcium, vitamin D, and magnesium. Eat every 3-4 hours. Make healthy food choices 80% of the time. Includes one to two "cheat meals" a week. Use pH strips and ketone strips to test body's pH. Get blood, urine, or saliva tests to check hormone levels.

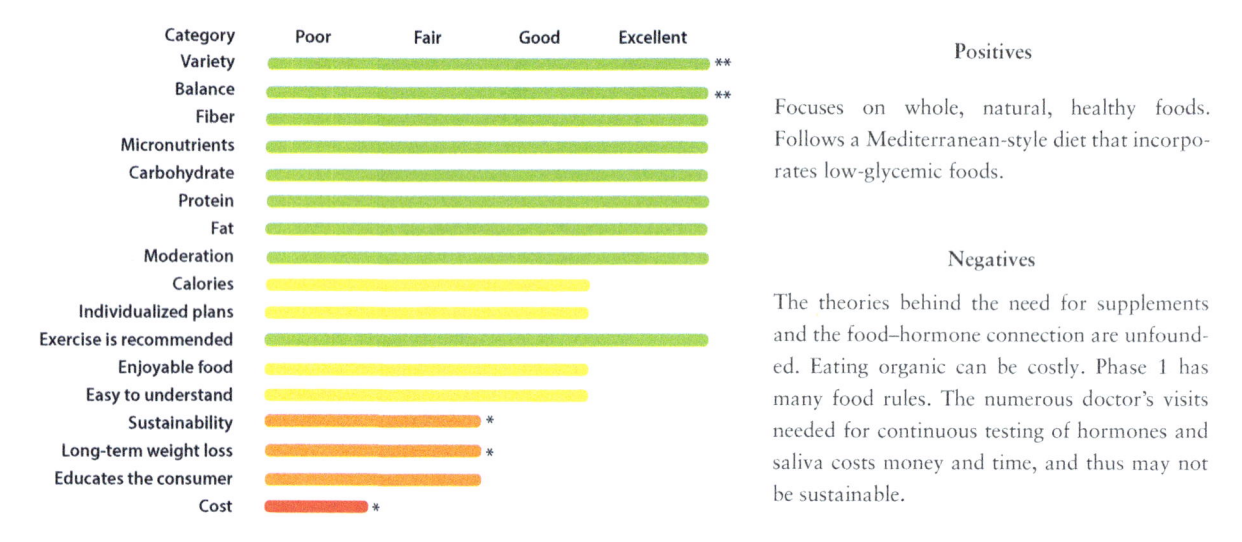

Category	Poor	Fair	Good	Excellent
Variety				✓ **
Balance				✓ **
Fiber				✓
Micronutrients				✓
Carbohydrate				✓
Protein				✓
Fat				✓
Moderation				✓
Calories			✓	
Individualized plans			✓	
Exercise is recommended				✓
Enjoyable food			✓	
Easy to understand			✓	
Sustainability		✓ *		
Long-term weight loss		✓ *		
Educates the consumer		✓		
Cost	✓ *			

Positives

Focuses on whole, natural, healthy foods. Follows a Mediterranean-style diet that incorporates low-glycemic foods.

Negatives

The theories behind the need for supplements and the food–hormone connection are unfounded. Eating organic can be costly. Phase 1 has many food rules. The numerous doctor's visits needed for continuous testing of hormones and saliva costs money and time, and thus may not be sustainable.

*These are lower due to continuous lab work and doctor's appointments.

** These are rated as excellent as long the detox period is not done. The detox period eliminates dairy.

The hook/catch or brilliant selling point: Most people know hormones are powerful.

Truths/Myths

- *Myth* - It is healthy to lose 15 pounds in 21 days.

- *Truth* - If 15 pounds is lost in 21 days, it will not be fat weight. 🔍 p. 14

- *Myth* - Hormones are directly affected by the foods consumed.

- *Truth* - Hormones are affected by many things. Saying certain foods are "hormone hindering" is not true.

Final decision: Thumbs up only if lab work and detox are not done. 👍

How to improve this diet: Do not engage in the detox portion of the diet. No need for all the blood tests. Make sure the calories consumed are less than the calories expended. 🔍 p. 13

Instinct Diet (aka the "i" Diet)

Premise of the Diet: Food and eating habits must be aligned with our hard-wired neurobiology.

Claims of the Diet: Lose an average of 30 pounds over 6 months. Will retrain our brain.

Diet Description: The diet is divided into 2 stages. The first stage lasts 2 weeks and eliminates refined carbohydrates and alcohol. The later stages adds "free choices" that send the brain messages that say "satisfied." Based on 5 universal food instincts that control our eating behavior and our weight: hunger, availability, variety, calorie density and familiarity.

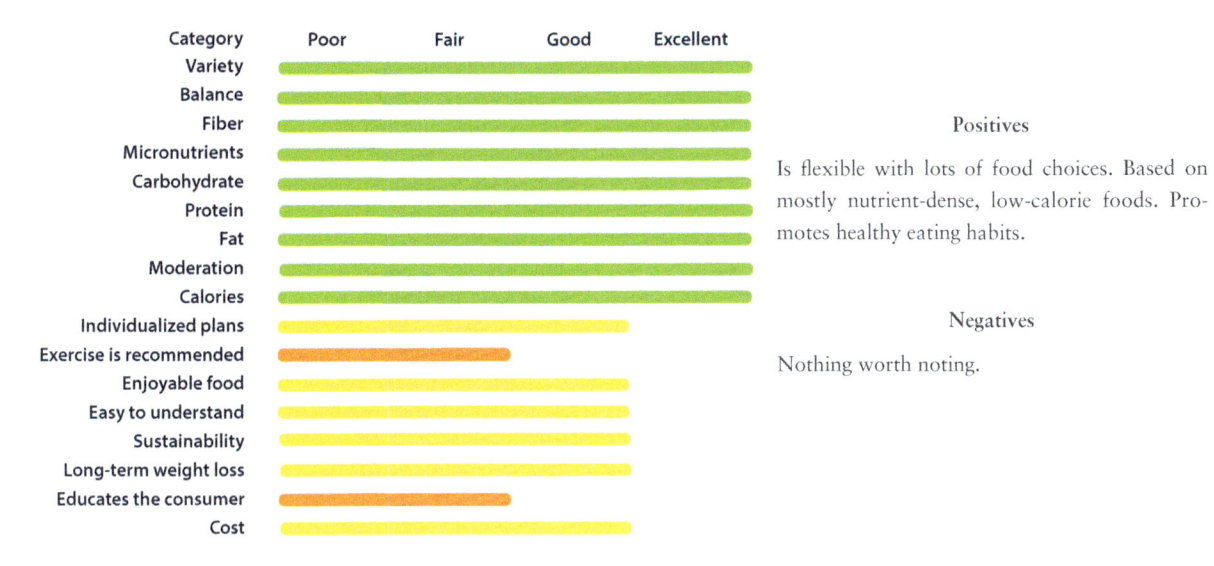

Category	Poor	Fair	Good	Excellent
Variety				████
Balance				████
Fiber				████
Micronutrients				████
Carbohydrate				████
Protein				████
Fat				████
Moderation				████
Calories				████
Individualized plans			████	
Exercise is recommended	████			
Enjoyable food			████	
Easy to understand			████	
Sustainability			████	
Long-term weight loss			████	
Educates the consumer	████			
Cost			████	

Positives

Is flexible with lots of food choices. Based on mostly nutrient-dense, low-calorie foods. Promotes healthy eating habits.

Negatives

Nothing worth noting.

The hook/catch or brilliant selling point: Past difficulties in weight loss may be attributed to not eating the right food for our hard-wiring. This diet can help overcome this obstacle.

Truths/Myths

- Myth - None worth noting.

- Truth - We need to satisfy hunger in order to sustain a weight-loss diet over time.

- Truth - We want to eat more when more food is available for the taking.

- Truth - We are attracted to a variety of foods and eat more when presented with more choices.

- Truth - We enjoy calorie-dense foods, as they are often loaded with flavor.

- Truth - Familiar foods feel safe, and thus, we are often drawn to them.

Final decision: Thumbs up 👍

How to improve this diet: Be sure the calories consumed are less than the calories expended.

Intermittent Fasting
(aka One Meal a Day Plan, OMAD)

Premise of the Diet: An eating pattern that cycles between periods of fasting and eating.

Claims of the Diet: Lose weight.

Diet Description: Varies. May involve daily 16-hour fasts or fasting for 24 hours, twice per week. May involve eating 1 hour per day and fasting the other 23 hours. Recommends eating the one meal within the same 4-hour window each day. Meal can consist of whatever is desired but is limited to 800-1,000 calories.

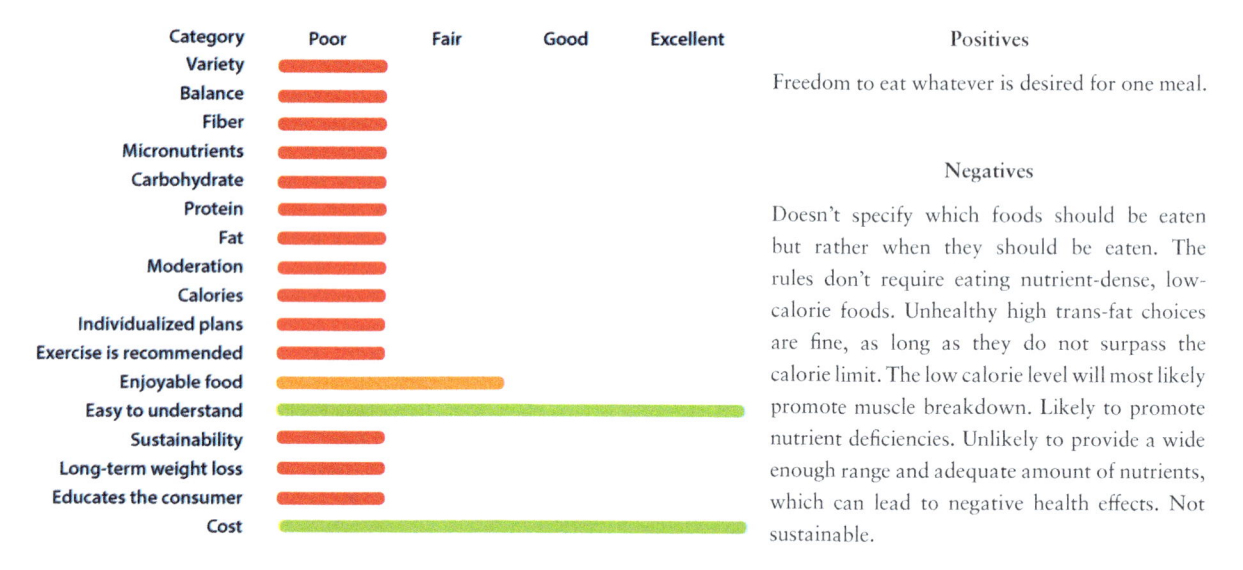

Category	Poor	Fair	Good	Excellent
Variety	■			
Balance	■			
Fiber	■			
Micronutrients	■			
Carbohydrate	■			
Protein	■			
Fat	■			
Moderation	■			
Calories	■			
Individualized plans	■			
Exercise is recommended	■			
Enjoyable food		■		
Easy to understand				■
Sustainability	■			
Long-term weight loss	■			
Educates the consumer	■			
Cost				■

Positives
Freedom to eat whatever is desired for one meal.

Negatives
Doesn't specify which foods should be eaten but rather when they should be eaten. The rules don't require eating nutrient-dense, low-calorie foods. Unhealthy high trans-fat choices are fine, as long as they do not surpass the calorie limit. The low calorie level will most likely promote muscle breakdown. Likely to promote nutrient deficiencies. Unlikely to provide a wide enough range and adequate amount of nutrients, which can lead to negative health effects. Not sustainable.

The hook/catch or brilliant selling point: Suffering and starving is the silver bullet that is equated with the freedom to eat anything.

Truths/Myths

- **Myth** - Fasting is a good way to lose weight.

- **Truth** - A daily 23-hour fast is likely to create an unhealthy relationship with food, which can lead to isolation and decrease overall social health.

- **Truth** - One of the downfalls of many diets is we get hungry while dieting. Being hungry decreases the likelihood of adherence. Long-term compliance is unlikely.

- **Truth** - Fasting does not provide a wide enough range or adequate amount of nutrients, which can lead to nutrient deficiencies.

- **Truth** - Long periods of fasting can decrease the metabolic rate, making fat loss more difficult.

- **Truth** - The metabolic benefits of fasting have not been proven superior to those of continuous energy restriction.

- **Truth** - Properly-controlled and powered studies of different types of fasting regimen interventions in humans are lacking.

- **Truth** - It is not yet known whether long-term intermittent fasting is safe or effective.

- Myth - Our digestive system needs a break from food processing.

- Truth - No organ or system in the body takes a break. Our heart, our lungs, and our liver never take a break.

Final decision: Thumbs down

How to improve this diet: Can't be improved. We need to eat more frequently to prevent nutrient deficiencies, feel satisfied, maintain our metabolic rate and safeguard a healthy relationship with food.

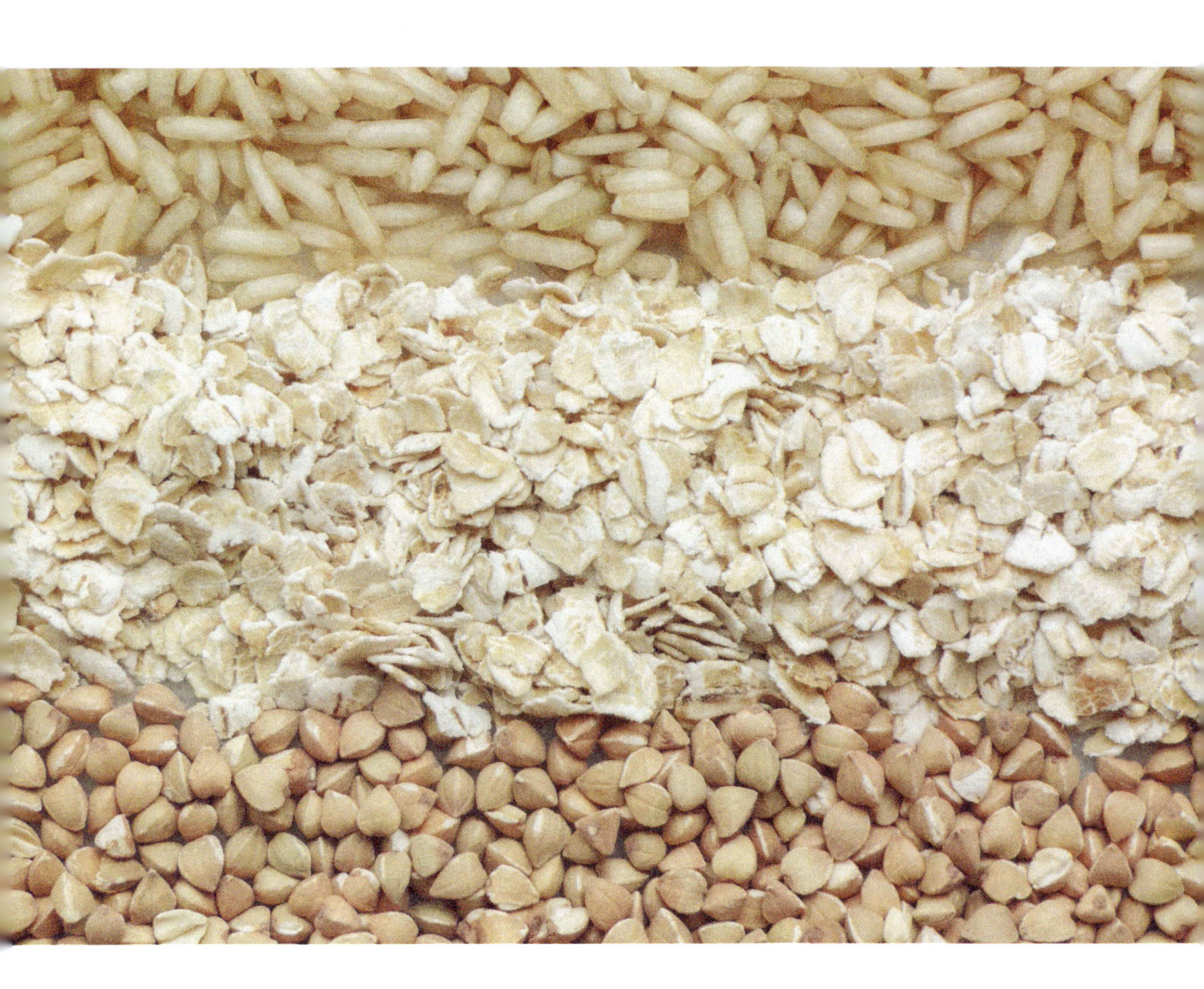

Jenny Craig Diet

Premise of the Diet: Everything needed to succeed is provided, including food, online/phone and center consultants, weekly personal coaching sessions, access to premium menus, and full access to digital tools.

Claims of the Diet: Lose up to 16 pounds in the first 4 weeks without changing your day-to-day eating habits.

Diet Description: Eat prepackaged Jenny Craig chef-crafted food items 6 times a day, consuming about 1,200 calories. Start eating a few meals made at home when you reach half of your goal. Once target weight is reached, spend 4 weeks transitioning to home-cooked meals.

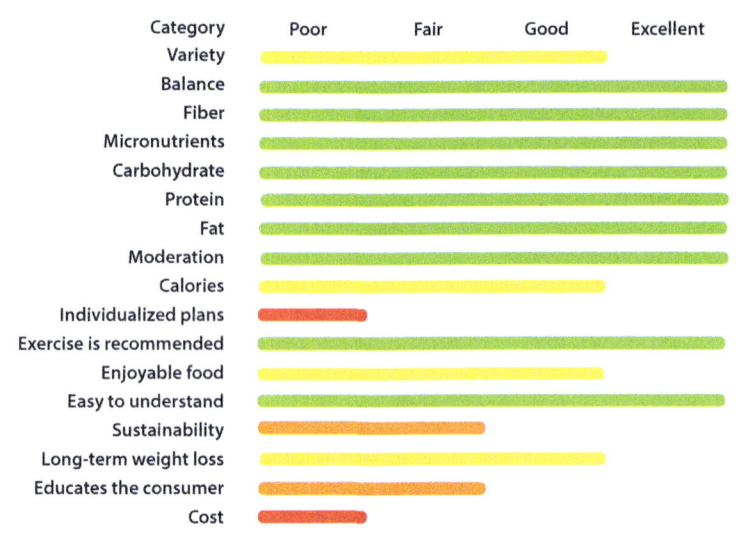

Category	Rating
Variety	Fair/Good
Balance	Excellent
Fiber	Excellent
Micronutrients	Excellent
Carbohydrate	Excellent
Protein	Excellent
Fat	Excellent
Moderation	Excellent
Calories	Good
Individualized plans	Poor
Exercise is recommended	Excellent
Enjoyable food	Good
Easy to understand	Excellent
Sustainability	Poor/Fair
Long-term weight loss	Good
Educates the consumer	Poor/Fair
Cost	Poor

Positives

Focuses on low-fat foods, water, fiber, protein, and non-starchy vegetables. Recommends 30 minutes or more of moderate activity at least 5 days a week. There is research to show that it works. It meets most of the U.S. Department of Agriculture's Dietary Guidelines for Americans, including fiber, potassium, and calcium. Provides support systems to answer questions. Allows for occasional splurges, like alcoholic beverages. No food is completely off-limits.

Negatives

Costly; according to their website the average cost of food is $15- $26 daily, which can limit sustainability. Relies on their purchased foods, which can cause isolation from others at mealtime. Consumption is limited to purchased food items. Providing everything without necessary education and learning how to eat limits a person's success in various unpredictable life situations.

The hook/catch or brilliant selling point: We give everything needed for success.

Truths/Myths

- Myths - None worth noting

- Truths - Relying on prepackaged foods can develop dependence on those meals and the system. Successful transitioning off the system is critical to long-term success. Thus, being educated and confident in how to do this is imperative.

Final decision: Thumbs up for those who can afford the program and who are willing to put special effort into transitioning off the prepackaged foods. 👍

How to improve this diet: None worth noting

Keto Cycle Diet

Premise of the Diet: The Keto Cycle meal plan is a fat-rich (70–80% of total daily calories), low-carb eating plan.

Claims of the Diet: It takes proficiency to create meal plans that guarantee substantial weight-loss results, and we've already done that for you!

Diet Description: A variation of the ketogenic diet involving a standard ketogenic diet (under 50g of carbohydrates a day) for 5–6 days a week, followed by 1–2 days of higher carb consumption, referred to as "refeeding days"; these are intended to replenish glycogen stores. Approximately 65–90% of total calories should come from healthy fats, while 10–30% of calories should come from protein. Various subscription lengths are available. Offers the Keto Diet Plan, App, and Keto Bars.

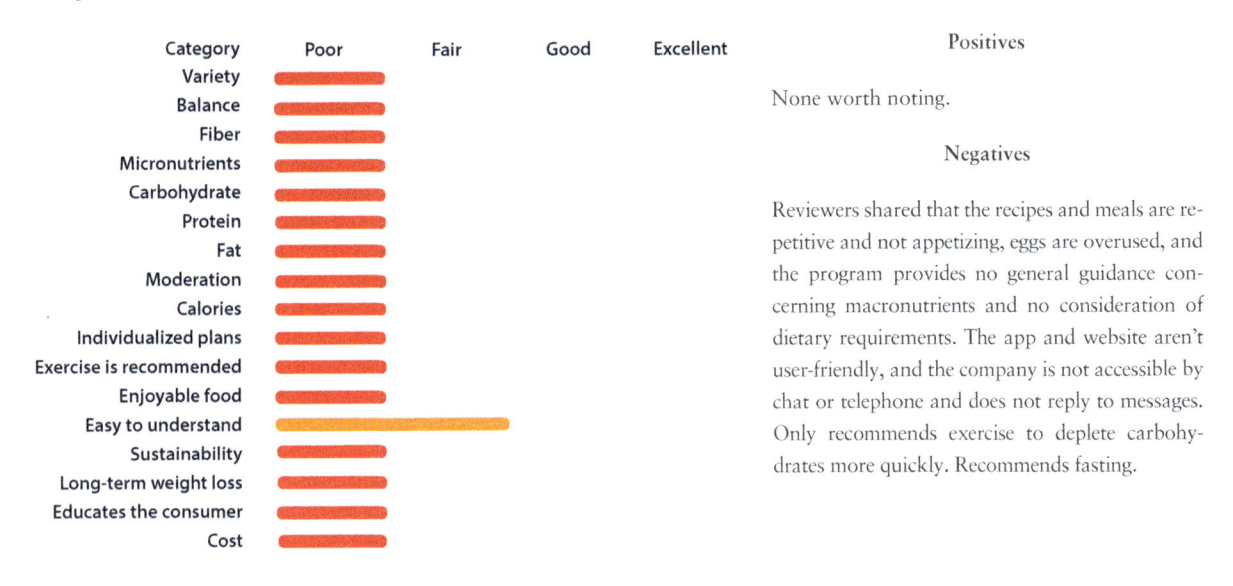

Category	Poor	Fair	Good	Excellent
Variety	●			
Balance	●			
Fiber	●			
Micronutrients	●			
Carbohydrate	●			
Protein	●			
Fat	●			
Moderation	●			
Calories	●			
Individualized plans	●			
Exercise is recommended	●			
Enjoyable food	●			
Easy to understand		●		
Sustainability	●			
Long-term weight loss	●			
Educates the consumer	●			
Cost	●			

Positives

None worth noting.

Negatives

Reviewers shared that the recipes and meals are repetitive and not appetizing, eggs are overused, and the program provides no general guidance concerning macronutrients and no consideration of dietary requirements. The app and website aren't user-friendly, and the company is not accessible by chat or telephone and does not reply to messages. Only recommends exercise to deplete carbohydrates more quickly. Recommends fasting.

The hook/catch or brilliant selling point: Title includes popular, enticing words.

Truths/Myths

- Myth - During the cyclical ketogenic diet, switching out of ketosis during refeeding days allows the dieter to reap the benefits of carb consumption for a temporary period.

- Truth - It is unhealthy to switch in and out of ketosis rapidly. 🔍 p. 85

- Myth - This diet is the same as a carbohydrate cycling diet.

- Truth - While both the keto cycling diet and the carbohydrate cycling diet include reducing carbohydrates on some days (typically 4–6 days) and consuming higher carbs on other days (typically 1–3 days), ketosis is not usually reached on carb cycling diets.

Final decision: Thumbs down 👎

How to improve this diet: Can't be improved.

Keto Diet Hypnosis

Premise of the Diet: Rewire your brain.

Claims of the Diet: This is a smooth and powerful manner to lose weight.

Diet Description: This diet provides an overview of a keto diet (see Keto Diet description). But this diet acknowledges that the keto diet can be overwhelming and challenging and thus provides hypnosis techniques to help increase the adherence. Discusses topics such as making eating a pleasurable experience, dealing with cravings, letting go of old patterns and behaviors, mentally rehearsing outcomes, and integrating activities for well-being.

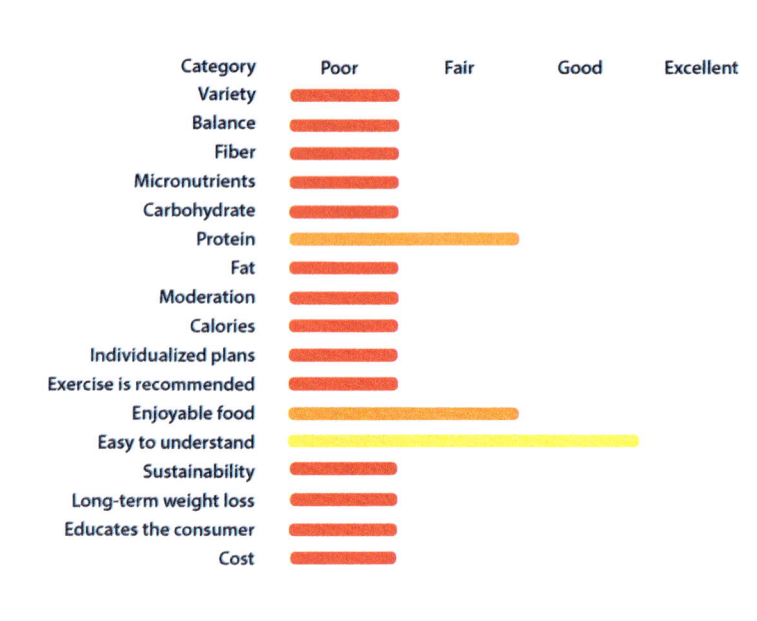

Category	Poor	Fair	Good	Excellent
Variety	■			
Balance	■			
Fiber	■			
Micronutrients	■			
Carbohydrate	■			
Protein		■		
Fat	■			
Moderation	■			
Calories	■			
Individualized plans	■			
Exercise is recommended	■			
Enjoyable food		■		
Easy to understand			■	
Sustainability	■			
Long-term weight loss	■			
Educates the consumer	■			
Cost	■			

Positives

Attempts to re-educate the subconscious about meals and discusses sensible eating habits and attitudes about weight. Seeks to exchange the style of thought that initially led to unhealthy and unhelpful behaviors. Recommends keeping a food-mood journal. Addresses emotional and habitual eating. Creating new strategies is also addressed.

Negatives

There is no calorie restriction. Carbohydrates, which are restricted on this diet, are a large source of daily fiber. Many people experience "keto flu" their first week on the diet, which leaves them feeling fatigue, brain fog, nausea, headaches, and muscle cramps. Protein sources come from both lean protein foods and foods high in saturated fat.

The hook/catch or brilliant selling point: A solution for staying on this very difficult diet is offered.

Truths/Myths

- Myth - One of the diets that can do you no wrong is the ketogenic diet.

- Truth - There are many deficiencies in the keto diet.

- Myth - Hypnosis is a proven treatment for obesity.

- Truth - Although there is some evidence that hypnosis may have a beneficial role in the treatment of obesity, most studies are lacking details and follow-up. More extensive, well-designed research studies need to be conducted in order to establish the best methods, most effective approaches, and the extent of its usefulness.

- Myth - Hypnosis and mindfulness are ancient strategies that in recent years have garnered renewed interest, due to the variety of therapeutic applications and the flexibility of use, which also includes self-administration.

- Truth - Mindfulness and hypnosis do not share the same definition, suggesting that the name of this diet is misleading and in fact may be nothing more than self-administered, mindful-eating self-talk.

- Myth - Burning ketones instead of other fuels is the ideal way to lose weight.

• Truth - In order to get the body to burn ketones we must deprive ourselves of carbohydrates, eating fewer than 20–50 grams per day. It typically takes a few days to reach a state of ketosis, during which time a "keto flu" may be experienced. Eating too much protein can also interfere with ketosis. But eating too little protein can cause the body to strip its own lean tissue, which is not helpful for people trying to lose weight.

• Myth - Keto diets are great for athletes and body builders. 🔍 p. 48

• Truth - Since this diet requires such a high percentage of calories coming from fat (75%–90%) and such a low percentage from carbohydrates (less than 5%), very little room is left for protein, which is essential for maintaining muscle mass. Moreover, decades of research indicate that carbohydrates are the body's preferred source of fuel, which is essential for physically active individuals.

• Myth - So many people are on this diet; therefore it must be safe and effective.

• Truth - Many people are on this diet, but that does not mean it is safe or effective over the long term. This diet is seen and heard about everywhere, and nearly all of us have heard anecdotal reports of lots of weight loss. We do not yet have enough information to know the long-term effects. What we do know is that eating any restrictive diet is difficult to sustain. Once "off" the diet, most people will return to their normal way of eating, and the weight lost will likely be regained. 🔍 p. 13

• Myth - The keto diet is safe, healthy, and nutritionally balanced. 🔍 p. 39

• Truth - Whole grain and unrefined carbohydrates lower the risk of stroke, dementia, and certain cancers. This diet removes those protective foods. Not eating a wide variety of vegetables, fruits, and grains puts us at risk for deficiencies in several micronutrients, including selenium, magnesium, phosphorus, and vitamins B and C. Because so much fat is consumed and needs to be metabolized, the diet could make existing liver conditions worse. The low intake of carbohydrates can cause confusion, irritability, and mood swings. Constipation may result due to consuming low amounts of fibrous foods like grains and legumes.

• Truth - Due to the high saturated-fat content, the American Heart Association cautions against this diet, indicating it can be hard on the heart, kidneys, and bones. 🔍 p. 56

• Truth - Due to the lack of carbohydrates, the body mobilizes its stored carbohydrates, in the form of glycogen, from the liver and muscle tissues. In this process water is lost; thus, much of the rapid weight loss in the beginning is water weight. 🔍 p. 15

• Truth - For the most part, not all types of this diet have been studied. Overall, only the standard and high-protein types have been examined to any degree.

Final decision: Thumbs down 👎

How to improve this diet: If you are set on hypnotherapy, set your sights on a well-balanced, healthful eating plan that can be sustained and allows for a safe, gradual weight loss of ½–2 pounds a week.

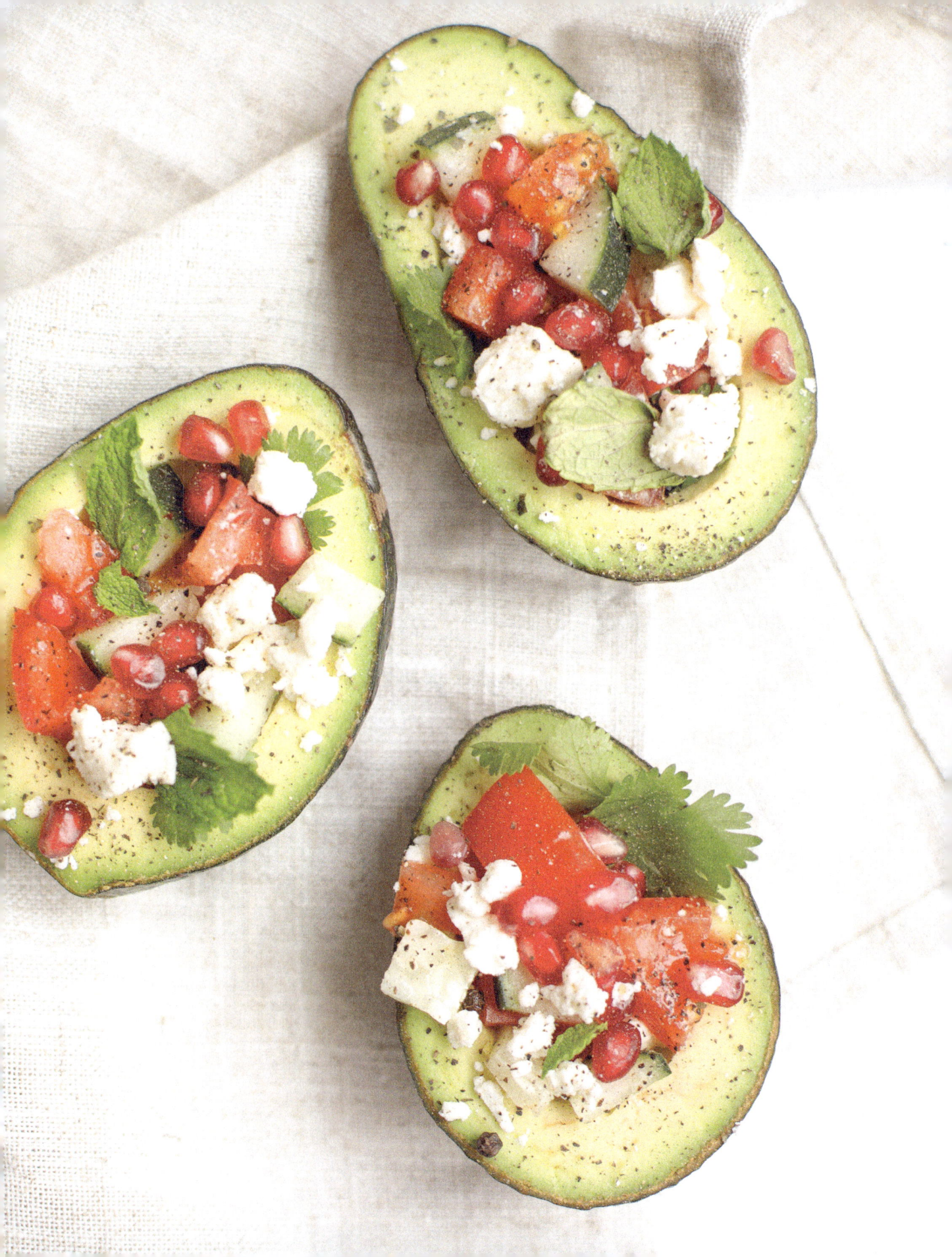

Keto Fast

Premise of the Diet: Reach ketosis faster through intermittent fasting.

Claims of the Diet: Burns more fat than the Keto Diet alone. Produces quick weight loss and provides a person with more energy.

Diet Description: Eat mostly high-fat foods within certain allotted time frames.

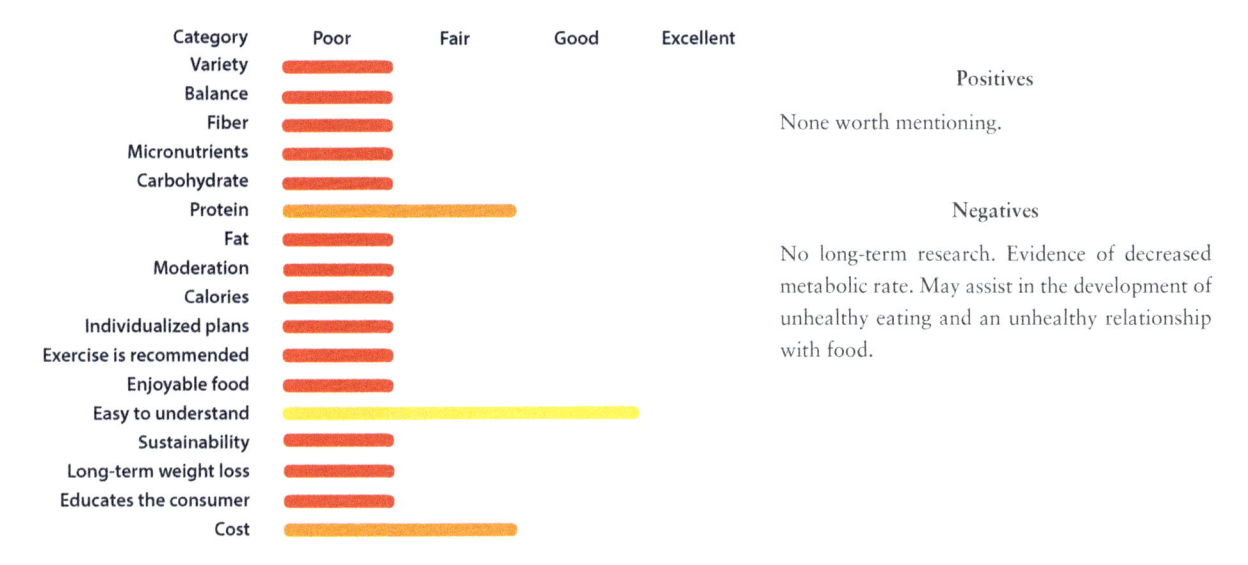

Category	Poor	Fair	Good	Excellent
Variety	■			
Balance	■			
Fiber	■			
Micronutrients	■			
Carbohydrate	■			
Protein		■		
Fat	■			
Moderation	■			
Calories	■			
Individualized plans	■			
Exercise is recommended	■			
Enjoyable food	■			
Easy to understand			■	
Sustainability	■			
Long-term weight loss	■			
Educates the consumer	■			
Cost		■		

Positives

None worth mentioning.

Negatives

No long-term research. Evidence of decreased metabolic rate. May assist in the development of unhealthy eating and an unhealthy relationship with food.

The hook/catch or brilliant selling point: Combines two popular fad diets for twice the power.

Truths/Myths

- **Myth** - Intermittent fasting preserves muscle mass during weight loss and improves energy levels, which may be helpful for keto dieters attempting to improve athletic performance and lose body fat. 🔍 p. 75

- **Truth** - Studies show lean body mass is lost during the caloric restriction of intermittent fasting. To avoid lean body mass loss, it is recommended for dieters to increase protein intake to around 2.3 g/kg of body weight or to supplement with branched-chain amino acids that maintain lean mass while promoting the loss of fat mass. Increasing dietary protein while engaging in calorie restriction means insufficient amounts of other macronutrients are consumed. Moreover, studies show this approach has led to micronutrient and vitamin intake below RDAs, which can negatively impact health, exercise performance and metabolic rate. 🔍 p. 29

- **Myth** - Intermittent fasting can reduce hunger and promote feelings of fullness, which may aid in weight loss. 🔍 p. 81

- **Truth** - Most studies on this topic are short term, as it is difficult to sustain.

Final decision: Thumbs down 👎

How to improve this diet: Cannot be improved.

Ketogenic Diet

Premise of the Diet: Classic keto diets include mostly fat (75-90% of calories), relatively low levels of protein (5-20% of calories), and very low levels of carbohydrates (less than 5% of calories). May also be calorie-restricted.

Claims of the Diet: A far superior diet where weight can be lost without counting calories or tracking food intake. Eat all the fat you want.

Diet Description: There are several versions of the ketogenic diet.

Standard ketogenic diet: Very low-carb (5%), moderate-protein (20%), and high-fat diet (75%).

Cyclical ketogenic diet: Primarily used by bodybuilders or athletes. Involves periods of higher carb re-feed days. For example: 5 ketogenic days, followed by 2 high-carb days.

Targeted ketogenic diet: Primarily used by bodybuilders and athletes. Allows additional carbs for workouts.

High-protein ketogenic diet: Very low-carb (5%), moderate-protein (35%), and high-fat diet (60%).

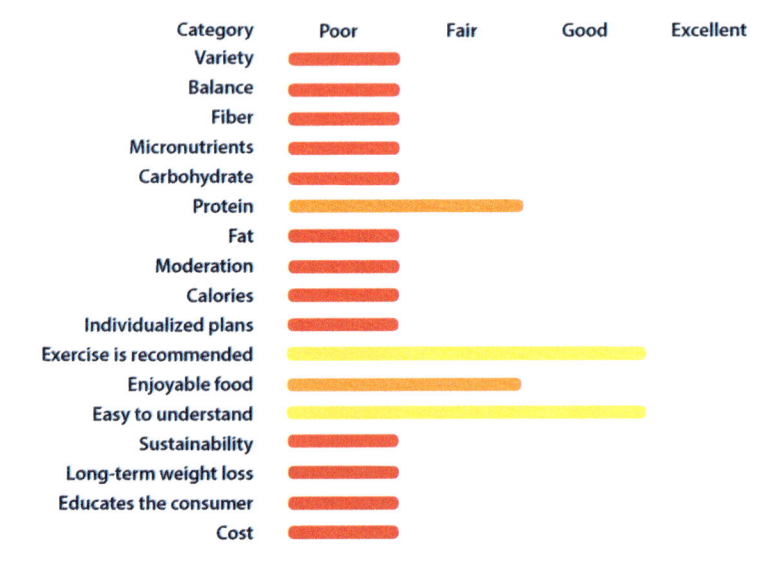

Category	Poor	Fair	Good	Excellent
Variety	▬			
Balance	▬			
Fiber	▬			
Micronutrients	▬			
Carbohydrate	▬			
Protein		▬		
Fat	▬			
Moderation	▬			
Calories	▬			
Individualized plans	▬			
Exercise is recommended			▬	
Enjoyable food		▬		
Easy to understand			▬	
Sustainability	▬			
Long-term weight loss	▬			
Educates the consumer	▬			
Cost	▬			

Positives

While this diet might not provide health benefits for an otherwise healthy person, under close doctor supervision, it may be beneficial for type 2 diabetics because of reducing carbohydrate consumption, which reduces the need for insulin to be secreted. May feel fuller for a longer period of time. Some healthy unsaturated fats like almonds, walnuts, seeds, avocados, tofu, and olive oil are allowed.

Negatives

Keeping the body in a constant state of ketosis requires strict dietary adherence. Cheating or sneaking just a few carbohydrates can be enough to disrupt this constant state of ketosis and results in the storage of fat, rather than the burning of fat. There is no calorie restriction. Carbohydrates, which are restricted on this diet, are a large source of daily fiber. Weight loss may be short-lived, because the diet is difficult to stick with long term, so the likelihood of returning to old eating habits is great. Many experience "keto flu" their first week on the diet, which leaves them experiencing fatigue, brain fog, nausea, headaches, and muscle cramps. Protein sources come from both lean protein foods and foods high in saturated fat. 🔍 p. 21

The hook/catch or brilliant selling point: It is a weight-loss wonder. Let's have everyone do it!

Truths/Myths

- **Myth** - Because there is solid evidence showing a ketogenic diet is beneficial in reducing seizures in children, these neuroprotective effects must be beneficial for other brain disorders like Parkinson's, Alzheimer's, multiple sclerosis, and autism.

- **Truth** - Robust evidence shows ketogenic diets reduce seizures in children, sometimes as well as medication; but there is little evidence suggesting ketosis should be used to treat these other conditions in humans. In fact, because it is not easy to get an adult body into deep ketosis, which is necessary to have an impact on epilepsy, health care providers in general do not attempt or recommend this approach except in the case of Type 2 (T2D) diabetes. In the case of T2D, close monitoring of patients for potential problems and to ensure they are actually staying in ketosis is required. Because staying in true, deep ketosis is especially challenging for adults, the medical diet is used to treat children and infants with epilepsy. In many instances, dieters trying this diet for weight loss often are not even in ketosis. If they are in ketosis, they are not in deep ketosis, which has problems of its own.

- **Myth** - It is a weight-loss wonder.

- **Truth** - It is actually a medical diet that comes with serious risks when not under a doctor's supervision. It is not the type of diet with which to leisurely experiment. It is used to help reduce seizures in children with epilepsy. In a manner of speaking, only short-term results have been studied. We still need long-term studies, as we do not know much about the long-term effects, possibly because it's difficult to stick with long term and thus most can't eat this way for a long time. If this diet can't be sustained for a long time, lost weight will be regained; much evidence indicates it is unhealthy to engage in practices that result in "yo-yo dieting" or rapid weight-loss fluctuation, as they are associated with increased mortality. 🔍 p. 84

- **Truth** - Weight loss is the primary reason many people go on the ketogenic diet.

- **Myth** - Burning ketones instead of other fuels is the ideal way to lose weight.

- **Truth** - In order to get the body to burn ketones, we must deprive ourselves of carbohydrates, fewer than 20 to 50 grams per day. It typically takes a few days to reach a state of ketosis, during which time a "keto flu" may be experienced. Eating too much protein can also interfere with the use of ketone bodies for energy, but eating too little protein can cause the body to strip its own lean tissue, which is not helpful for people trying to lose weight.

- **Myth** - Keto diets are great for athletes and bodybuilders.

- **Truth** - Since this diet requires such a high percent of calories coming from fat (75%-90%) and such a low percent from carbohydrates (less than 5%), very little room is left for protein, which is essential for maintaining muscle mass. Moreover, decades of research indicate carbohydrates are the preferred source of fuel, which is essential for physically active individuals. 🔍 p. 48

- **Myth** - So many people are on this diet that it must be safe and effective.

- **Truth** - Many people are on this diet, but that does not mean it is safe or effective long term. This diet is seen and heard about everywhere, and nearly all of us have heard anecdotal reports of lots of weight loss. We do not yet have enough information to know the long-term effects. What we do know is any diet that severely restricts or eliminates food groups is difficult to sustain. Once "off" the diet, most will return to their normal way of eating and the weight lost will likely be regained. 🔍 p. 13

- **Myth** - The keto diet is safe, healthy, and nutritionally balanced.

- **Truth** - Whole grain and unrefined carbohydrates lower the risk of stroke, dementia, and certain cancers. This diet removes those protective foods. It's high in saturated fat. Not eating a wide variety of vegetables, fruits, and grains puts us at risk for deficiencies in several micronutrients, including selenium, magnesium, phosphorus, and vitamins B and C. Because so much fat is consumed and needs to be metabolized, the diet could make existing liver conditions worse. The low intake of carbohydrates can cause confusion, irritability, and mood swings. Constipation may result, due to consuming low amounts of fibrous foods like grains and legumes.

- **Truth** - Due to the high saturated fat content, the American Heart Association cautions against this diet, indicating it can be hard on the heart, kidneys and bones. 🔍 p. 56

- **Truth** - Due to the lack of carbohydrates, the body depletes its stored carbohydrates, glycogen, from the liver and muscle tissues. In this process, water is lost; thus, much of the rapid weight loss in the beginning is water weight.

- Truth - For the most part, not all types of this diet have been studied. Overall, only the standard and high-protein types have been examined to any degree.

- Truth - Under close physician supervision, at least in the short term, ketogenic diets have been shown to improve blood sugar levels in people with type 2 diabetes.

- Truth - There is no long-term research analyzing this diet's effects over time on diabetes and high cholesterol.

- Truth - Some researchers are concerned that once someone has reached their goal weight and gotten a taste preference for foods with no carbs in them, it might be hard to keep calorie levels high enough to maintain that target weight because of being satisfied with fewer calories.

- Myth - Insulin is a fat-storage hormone. 🔍 p. 73

- Truth - Insulin helps glucose exit blood and enter tissues. It also helps fatty acids and amino acids enter tissues. Insulin's primary function is to transport glucose out of blood and into tissues to be either burned as fuel or stored as glycogen for later use. A secondary function is to transport fatty acids into tissues to be burned for fuel in the muscle or stored as triglycerides in the liver for later use; and a third function of insulin is to take amino acids out of circulating blood and get them into tissues so they can be synthesized into new proteins, converted into new compounds, burned for energy, converted to triglycerides, and stored for later use. Just because it transports glucose doesn't mean it is the fat-storage hormone. Insulin secretion is stimulated by glucose, but its role is to metabolize all excess calories. It promotes more fuel storage than any other hormone. It promotes more growth than estrogen, testosterone, or growth hormones. Any amount of circulating insulin doesn't mean it increases the risk of fat storage. A physiologically normal amount of insulin is required for life. Excess insulin increases risk for chronic diseases, such as type 2 diabetes.

- Myth - Eating carbohydrates spikes blood insulin levels.

- Truth - It is important to discuss what type of carbohydrate is being consumed. The amount of glucose in blood is a reflection of dietary carbohydrate and dietary fat consumed. Excess body fat can lead to insulin resistance. Blood glucose profile is determined by how much fat is eaten and secondarily by the amount of carbs eaten. Carbohydrate tolerance or the ability to eat carbohydrates may increase when a low-fat, plant-based diet of whole foods is consumed. This type of diet can result in increased insulin sensitivity and can decrease insulin resistance.

- Myth - Diabetes is a state of carbohydrate toxicity and insulin resistance is a state of carbohydrate intolerance. Insulin resistance is caused by insulin itself, which is triggered by eating carbohydrates.

- Truth - Diabetes is the accumulation of glucose in the blood. In type 1 diabetes (T1D), the pancreas does not produce sufficient insulin to signal the muscles, adipose, and liver to remove glucose from the blood and store it as glycogen (made and stored in muscle and liver) or fat (made in adipose and liver and stored in adipose). In type 2 diabetes (T2D), the pancreas secretes insulin but the target tissues (muscle, adipose, and liver) become resistant to the insulin signal. T2D is very complex, but evidence shows that accumulation of fat in tissues other than adipose (ectopic "fat") can cause those tissues to become resistant to the insulin signal. In both T1D and T2D, an inability to lower glucose from the blood produces many forms of tissue damage.

- Myth - Carbohydrates cause diabetes.

- Truth - Carbs are not the primary cause of diabetes. Dietary fat provides more than two times the number of calories per gram that carbohydrates provide (9 vs 4). Thus, it is often excess dietary fat that causes weight gain. Insulin receptors are surrounded by all this stored fat, so when insulin comes along to let more glucose in to be stored, the body rejects the additional glucose stating, "we already have so much fat here... wait till this fat is burned up and gone, in the meantime you – glucose – stay in the blood." Dysfunctional insulin receptors in muscles and the liver can't accept glucose, so the glucose is trapped in blood. Insulin resistance is a state of carbohydrate intolerance first created by the consumption of excess dietary fat, resulting in an increased need for oral medication or insulin to help insulin get out of blood and into tissues.

• Myth - Amino acids and fatty acids are essential nutrients in the diet, but carbohydrates are not because the body can make them.

• Truth - In a fed metabolic state, skeletal muscle and heart can use glucose, amino acids, and fatty acids for fuel, while the brain, kidneys, and other tissues use glucose. Muscle and liver store excess glucose as glycogen, and adipose and the liver make fat from excess glucose, amino acids, and fat, and it is stored in the adipose. In a fasted metabolic state, skeletal muscle uses its own protein, stored glycogen, fat from adipose, and ketone bodies from the liver for energy. Furthermore, in the fasted metabolic state, the brain cannot use amino acids or fatty acids for fuel. The brain can use ketone bodies but prefers glucose, yet it doesn't have the stores of glucose, like skeletal muscle. So, when carbohydrates are limited, the liver makes ketone bodies from adipose-released fatty acids and glucose from its glycogen stores, and glucose from amino acids. The glucose and ketones are used by the brain for fuel in the fasted metabolic state. So, as you can see, carbohydrates are essential. If we do not consume carbohydrates, the liver will make the essential carbohydrates needed for tissues, like the brain, that need it for energy. Even though fats are available for energy, without dietary or stored carbohydrates, which is the case in the Keto Diet, skeletal muscle must rely on its own protein (lean tissue) as it uses the fat for energy. In other words, even though the liver is producing glucose, the amount of glucose it produces is insufficient to supply the skeletal muscle and the rest of body without stripping lean tissue. 🔍 p. 73

• Myth - There are no negative consequences that result from Ketogenic Diets.

• Truth - Research has shown that the keto diet can lead to diarrhea, nausea, constipation, vomiting, acid reflux, hair loss, kidney stones, muscle cramps or weakness, hypoglycemia, low platelet count, impaired cognition, inability to concentrate, impaired mood, disordered mineral metabolism, stunted growth in children, increased risks for bone fractures, osteopenia and osteoporosis, increased bruising, acute pancreatitis, hyperlipidemia, high cholesterol, insulin resistance, elevated cortisol, heart arrhythmia, myocardial infarction (heart attacks), amenorrhea (lack of menstrual cycle), and increased risk of premature death. In its totality, people on a low-carbohydrate diet can die sooner and suffer from more disease in the long run. It results in many health conditions that have been associated with a shortened life.

• Myth - Low-carbohydrate diets are high-protein diets.

• Truth - The proportion of calories from protein in low-carbohydrate diets remains in the AMDR for percent of calories from protein. Carbohydrates tend to be exchanged for fat in low-carbohydrate diets. High-fat diets may increase risk of CVD and diabetes mortality, especially if those fats come from animal sources. In essence, a low-carbohydrate diet based on animal sources is associated with higher mortality, while a vegetable-based low-carbohydrate diet seemed to lower CVD mortality rates.

• Myth - Low-carbohydrate diets are effective for weight loss. 🔍 p. 15

• Truth - While some studies have demonstrated weight loss with a low carbohydrate diet, they tend to be conducted over short periods of time and with a small number of subjects; therefore, they fail to document the long-term effects

Final decision: Thumbs down 👎

How to improve this diet: Eat a balanced, unprocessed diet, with adequate, colorful fruits and vegetables, lean meats, fish, whole grains, nuts, seeds, olive oil, and lots of water. Be sure to consume a calorie amount that allows for weight loss.

The Kind Diet

Premise of the Diet: Vegan

Claims of the Diet: Going vegan will improve health.

Diet Description: Contains 3 phases of veganism:

1. Flirting: A gradual transition away from animal-based foods

2. Going Vegan: Committing to a vegan lifestyle

3. Superhero: Eating unprocessed vegetables, fruit, nuts, and sweets. Limit nightshade vegetables (such as potatoes, tomatoes, and eggplants).

Cannot consume white sugar, honey, or organic evaporated cane syrup. Allows brown rice syrup, barley malt, maple syrup, agave, molasses, and fruit.

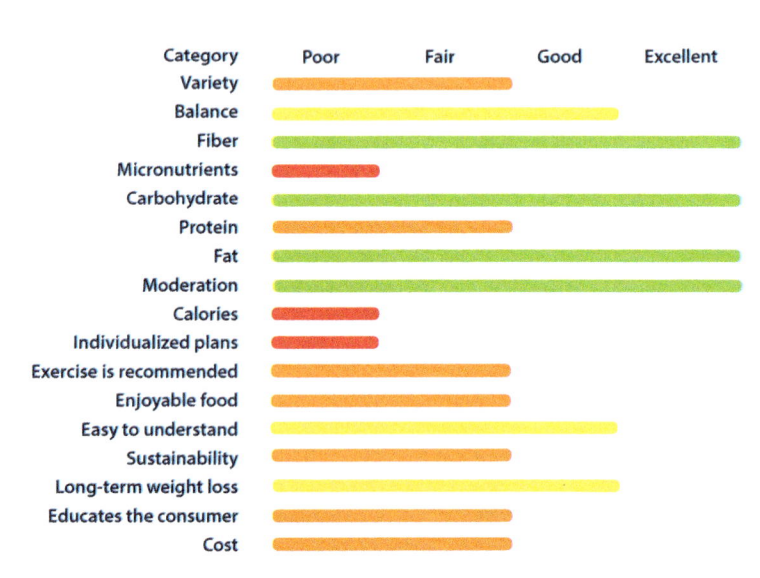

Category	Poor	Fair	Good	Excellent
Variety		■		
Balance			■	
Fiber				■
Micronutrients	■			
Carbohydrate				■
Protein		■		
Fat				■
Moderation				■
Calories	■			
Individualized plans	■			
Exercise is recommended		■		
Enjoyable food		■		
Easy to understand			■	
Sustainability		■		
Long-term weight loss			■	
Educates the consumer		■		
Cost		■		

Positives

This diet is really a vegan how-to cookbook more than a weight-loss diet, but if followed, most would probably lose weight. Discusses cooking methods, as well as foods to choose when traveling. Recommends eating whole grains, beans, and vegetables, especially choosing locally and in-season varieties. May help prevent heart disease, diabetes, and high cholesterol.

Negatives

Without careful selection, it may become deficient in calcium, iron, vitamin B12, vitamin D, and folate. Very restrictive. May be difficult to adhere to long term. Strict adherence may increase food costs. Nightshades, meats, and dairy are restricted. 🔍 p. 29

The hook/catch or brilliant selling point: Uses the fame of actress and animal lover Alicia Silverstone

Truths/Myths

- Myth - None worth noting.

- Truth - A vegan diet can be healthy, though you'll need to make sure all your nutritional needs are met.

Final decision: Thumbs down 👎

How to improve this diet: For sustainability, you may need to lighten up on the restrictions.

LA Weight Loss Diet
(LA Weight Loss Centers are franchised centers.)

Premise of the Diet: Balanced eating and lifestyle changes with support.

Claims of the Diet: Has helped millions of people to achieve their goal.

Diet Description: Clients fill out detailed questionnaires providing information on their eating habits and emotional attachment to food. Counselors interview clients and prescribe a plan that is laid out in portions, not calories. Menu plans range from 1,200 calories to 2,400 calories. Includes 3-4 phases. Some plans recommend an initial 2-day cleanse, which can increase the program from 3 to 4 phases. Most programs recommend seeing the counselor three times a week for guidance, support, education, coaching, and monitoring weight and food choices during the second phase. After achieving the goal weight, phase 3 is a 6-week stabilization period where calories are slowly increased. It includes meeting with a counselor 2 times a week. The last phase is maintenance and recommends a weekly check-in with a counselor for a year. Sodium is restricted to 2,100 milligrams daily. Caffeine is allowed. One alcoholic beverage is allowed 3 times a week.

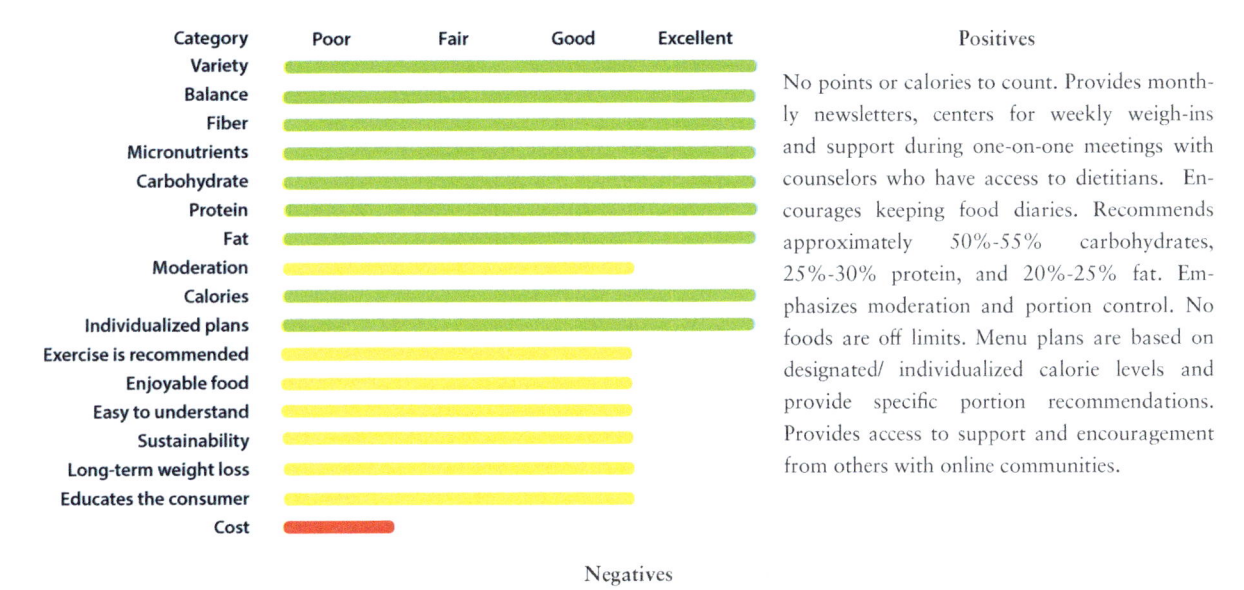

Category	Poor	Fair	Good	Excellent
Variety				✓
Balance				✓
Fiber				✓
Micronutrients				✓
Carbohydrate				✓
Protein				✓
Fat				✓
Moderation			✓	
Calories				✓
Individualized plans				✓
Exercise is recommended			✓	
Enjoyable food			✓	
Easy to understand			✓	
Sustainability			✓	
Long-term weight loss			✓	
Educates the consumer			✓	
Cost	✓			

Positives

No points or calories to count. Provides monthly newsletters, centers for weekly weigh-ins and support during one-on-one meetings with counselors who have access to dietitians. Encourages keeping food diaries. Recommends approximately 50%-55% carbohydrates, 25%-30% protein, and 20%-25% fat. Emphasizes moderation and portion control. No foods are off limits. Menu plans are based on designated/ individualized calorie levels and provide specific portion recommendations. Provides access to support and encouragement from others with online communities.

Negatives

Promises fast, easy weight loss. Includes and sells nutritional supplements, bars, juices, and snacks that are sold exclusively at centers and are available only to clients. Counselors are not dietitians and earn commission on products they sell. Rather strict. There is little room for splurges, cheating, or special occasions. 🔍 p. 99

The hook/catch or brilliant selling point: Flashy name associated with fame and popularity.

Truths/Myths

- Myth - None worth noting

- Truth - Balanced, slow weight loss increases the likelihood of keeping weight off.

Final decision: Thumbs up 👍

How to improve this diet: Follow meal and exercise lifestyle and behavior changes, but you should avoid bars and supplements; they are not needed. Skip the 2-day cleanse. Make sure all expenses associated with the program are received in writing prior to starting.

Lemonade Diet (aka the Master Cleanse)

Premise of the Diet: Fast weight loss while detoxifying the body.

Claims of the Diet: Will drop pounds, "detox" the digestive system, increase energy and happiness, improve health, and curb cravings for unhealthy food.

Diet Description: A liquid-only diet consisting of a lemonade drink (fresh-squeezed lemon juice, pure maple syrup, cayenne pepper, and water), a salt-water drink, and herbal laxative tea for 10 days.

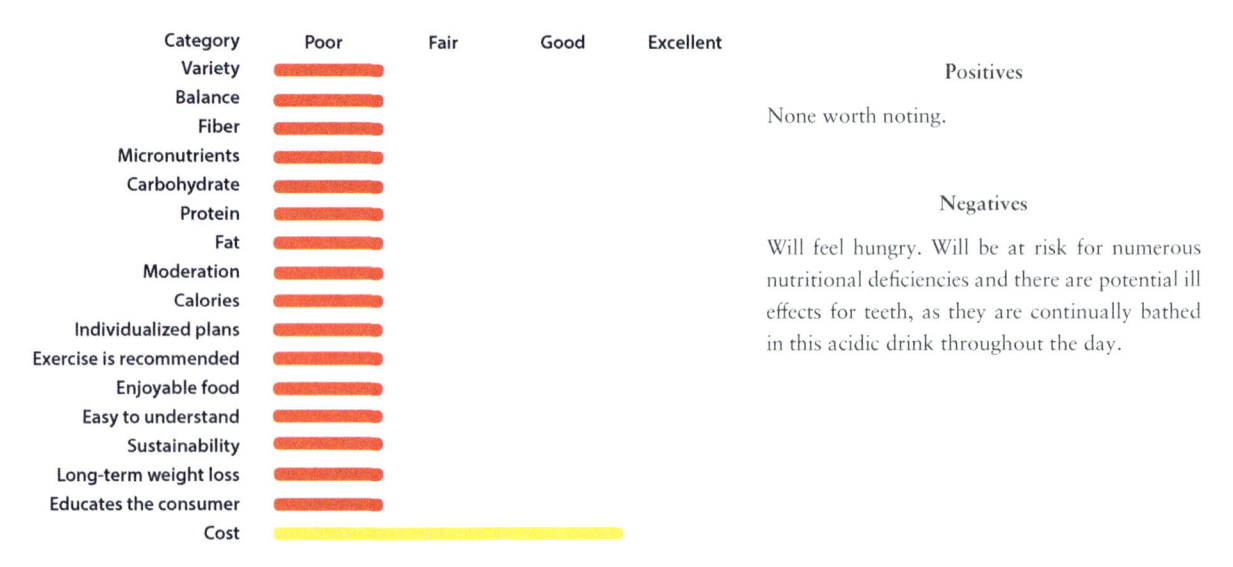

Category	Poor	Fair	Good	Excellent
Variety	■			
Balance	■			
Fiber	■			
Micronutrients	■			
Carbohydrate	■			
Protein	■			
Fat	■			
Moderation	■			
Calories	■			
Individualized plans	■			
Exercise is recommended	■			
Enjoyable food	■			
Easy to understand	■			
Sustainability	■			
Long-term weight loss	■			
Educates the consumer	■			
Cost			■	

Positives

None worth noting.

Negatives

Will feel hungry. Will be at risk for numerous nutritional deficiencies and there are potential ill effects for teeth, as they are continually bathed in this acidic drink throughout the day.

The hook/catch or brilliant selling point: Fast weight loss while detoxifying the body.

Truths/Myths

- **Myth** - Will detox the body.

- **Truth** - Although no evidence is provided, because the liver detoxes the body, the theory is that fat-soluble toxins stored in adipose tissue would be released and cycled through the liver; however, the body is constantly recycling fatty acids in the adipose tissue.

- **Myth** - Claims "detox symptoms" like cravings, tiredness, boredom, and headaches may be experienced. 🔍 p. 13

- **Truth** - Cravings, tiredness, boredom, and headaches are symptoms of starvation, not detoxification.

- **Myth** - Will lose weight.

- **Truth** - Consuming very few calories will cause weight loss. However, the loss will include muscle, bone, and water, not necessarily fat. Any lost weight will likely be regained right back. This is an unhealthy way to temporarily lose weight. 🔍 p. 78

Final decision: Thumbs down 👎

How to improve this diet: Can't be improved.

Living Low Carb Diet

Premise of the Diet: Low-carb diet plan.

Claims of the Diet: Will cause weight loss by reducing the amount of carbohydrates consumed.

Diet Description: Limits carbs to 0 - 30 grams a day. Going lower helps you to lose more weight. Avoid white foods like potatoes, white rice, white breads, and flour. Consume half a gram of protein for every pound of ideal weight. Make sure protein is part of every meal. Drink 8 to 12 eight-ounce glasses of water daily. Eat whole organic foods. Include healthy fats, such as olive oil and avocados.

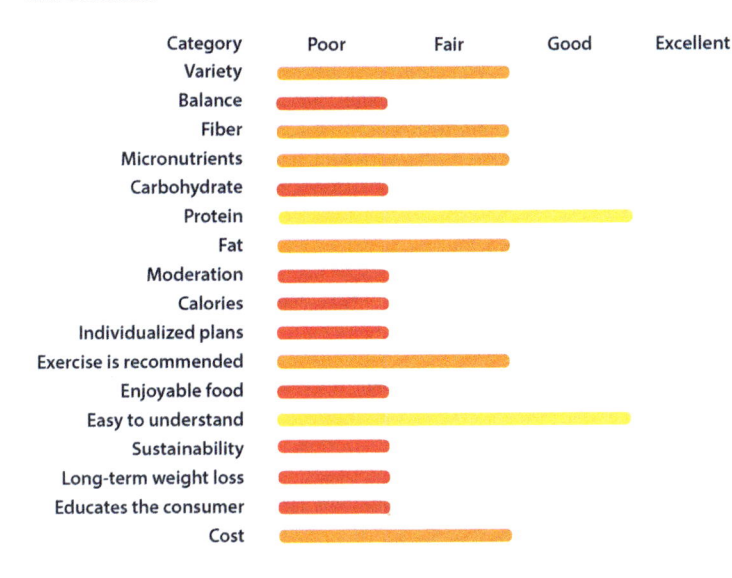

Category	Rating
Variety	Fair
Balance	Poor
Fiber	Fair
Micronutrients	Fair
Carbohydrate	Poor
Protein	Good
Fat	Fair
Moderation	Poor
Calories	Poor
Individualized plans	Poor
Exercise is recommended	Fair
Enjoyable food	Poor
Easy to understand	Good
Sustainability	Poor
Long-term weight loss	Poor
Educates the consumer	Poor
Cost	Fair

Positives

May help create a feeling of fullness.

Negatives

May be more challenging if living with people who are not on the same plan. Can lead to an increase in ketones or ketosis, bad breath, gout, and constipation. Limiting the amount of fruits and whole grains eaten can lead to deficiencies in vitamins, minerals, and fiber.

The hook/catch or brilliant selling point: Jumps on the "Low Carb" Craze.

Truths/Myths

- Myth - Eating low carb helps with weight loss.

- Truth - To keep the weight off, you will need to make other lifestyle changes.

- Truth - While many overeat processed grains, the solution is not eliminating them from the diet. The solution is eating complex carbohydrates in moderation. 🔍 p. 41

- Myth - Being in ketosis is ideal for people wanting to lose weight. 🔍 p. 86

- Truth - When in ketosis, the metabolism slows and lean tissue and minerals may be lost.

Final decision: Thumbs down 👎

How to improve this diet: Include at least 130 grams of complex carbohydrates a day.

Macrobiotic Diet

Premise of the Diet: Combines the concepts of Buddhism and certain dietary principles. Aims to balance spiritual and physical wellness while avoiding "toxins" that come from eating dairy products, meats, and oily foods.

Claims of the Diet: Can prevent and cure diseases, including cancer.

Diet Description: Whole grains, vegetables, and beans are staples. Excludes potatoes, tomatoes, eggplant, peppers, asparagus, spinach, beets, zucchini, and avocados and non-locally grown fruit. Recommends consuming locally grown produce. Recommends cooking with pots, pans, and utensils made only from glass, wood, stainless steel, ceramic, and enamel. Doesn't use microwaves or electricity for food preparation. Little to no meat, dairy, eggs, and poultry is consumed. Does allow fish. Forty to 60% of diet should be organically grown whole grains. Twenty to 30% of diet should come from locally grown vegetables. Five percent to 10% should come from beans and bean products and sea vegetables, like seaweed. Only drink when feeling thirsty. Chew each mouthful of food at least 50 times. Eat two to three times a day. Stop before feeling full. Rice syrup is the only recommended sweetener and should be used sparingly. Consuming foods in the form of soup is recommended.

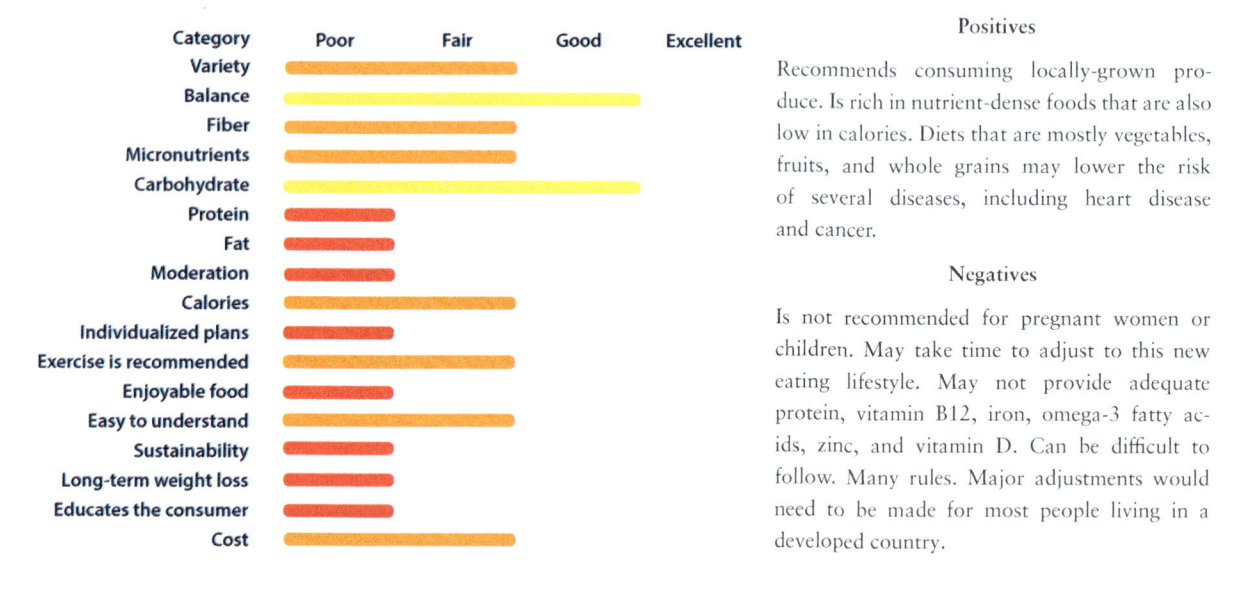

Category	Poor	Fair	Good	Excellent
Variety	▬			
Balance			▬	
Fiber	▬			
Micronutrients	▬			
Carbohydrate			▬	
Protein	▬			
Fat	▬			
Moderation	▬			
Calories	▬			
Individualized plans	▬			
Exercise is recommended	▬			
Enjoyable food	▬			
Easy to understand		▬		
Sustainability	▬			
Long-term weight loss	▬			
Educates the consumer	▬			
Cost		▬		

Positives

Recommends consuming locally-grown produce. Is rich in nutrient-dense foods that are also low in calories. Diets that are mostly vegetables, fruits, and whole grains may lower the risk of several diseases, including heart disease and cancer.

Negatives

Is not recommended for pregnant women or children. May take time to adjust to this new eating lifestyle. May not provide adequate protein, vitamin B12, iron, omega-3 fatty acids, zinc, and vitamin D. Can be difficult to follow. Many rules. Major adjustments would need to be made for most people living in a developed country.

The hook/catch or brilliant selling point: A unique combination of spirituality and diet.

Truths/Myths

- Myth - It is important to avoid anything spicy, dairy, eggs, meat, and nightshade vegetables, coffee, fruit juice, and too much water.

- Truth - Except for those who are allergic to nightshades and lactose intolerant, research does not show that consuming the above food items in moderation contributes to being unbalanced or the development of diseases. 🔍 p. 29

- Truth - A plant-based, low-fat, high-fiber diet lowers the risk of heart disease and some cancers.

- Truth - Soups can retain nutrients in the broth during the cooking process.

Final decision: Thumbs down. 👎

How to improve this diet: Since dairy is eliminated, be sure to include non-dairy foods fortified with calcium and vitamin D, such as soy and almond milk.

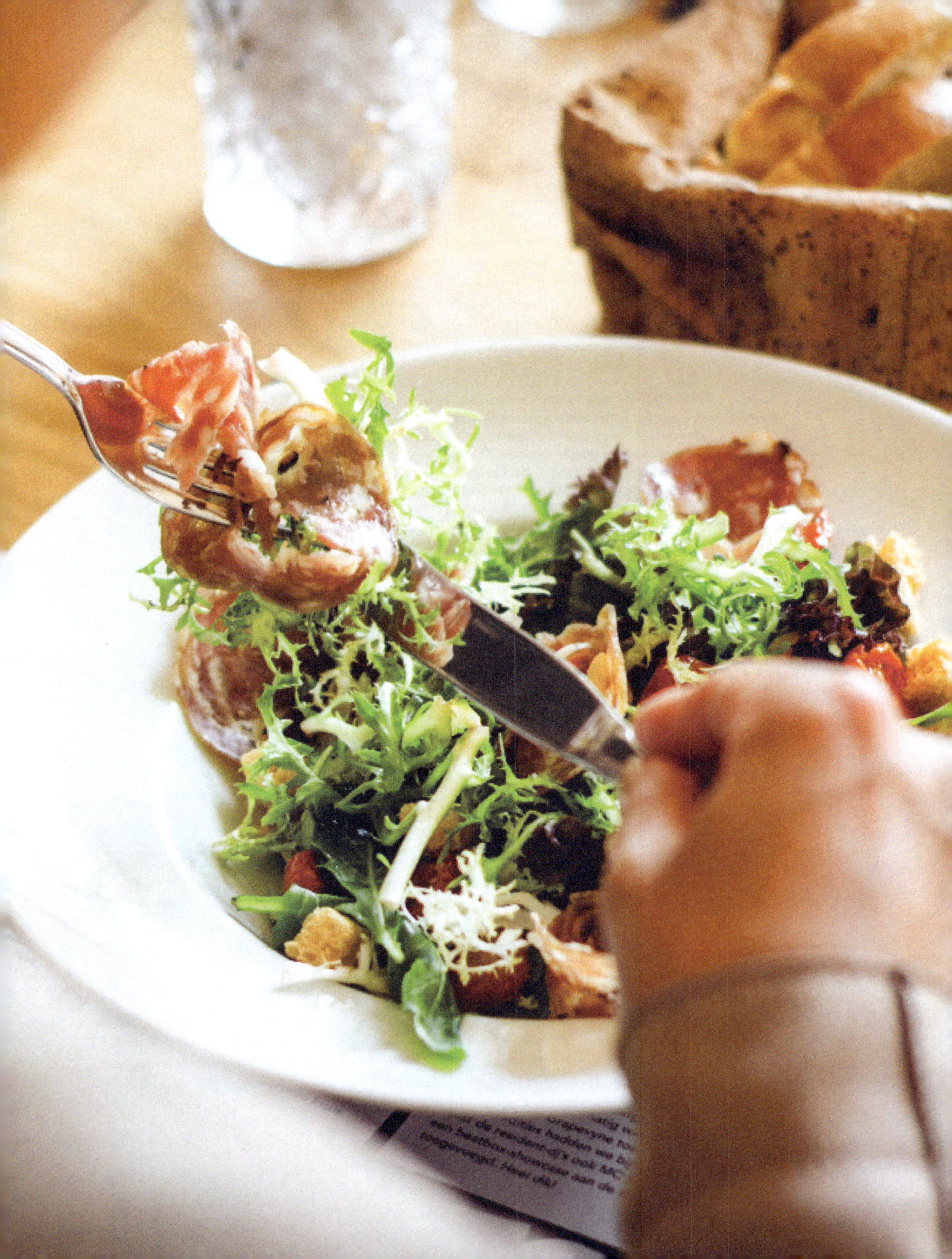

The Maker's Diet

Premise of the Diet: Eat what Jesus ate.

Claims of the Diet: A health plan that is biblically based and scientifically proven, resulting in 10-15 pounds lost in the first 40 days.

Diet Description: This is more than a diet. It involves hygiene in the form of hand washing before meals. It recommends beginning and ending each day with a prayer for healing and/or thanks. Reducing toxins is a key component. It suggests avoiding water and toothpaste if it has been treated with fluoride. Do not get cavities filled with mercury. Avoid overexposure to electromagnetic fields such as excess X-rays and cell phones. Pertaining to food, it provides a 40-day guide built on principles first described in the Bible. All foods must be whole, organic, and consumed unprocessed, unrefined, and untreated with pesticides or hormones. Eventually includes red meat and some saturated fats. Starches and sugars are allowed in their natural, unrefined form. Natural fats found in fish, cod liver oil, butters, cheeses, milk, and creams are allowed. Includes weekly partial fast days in each phase of the diet.

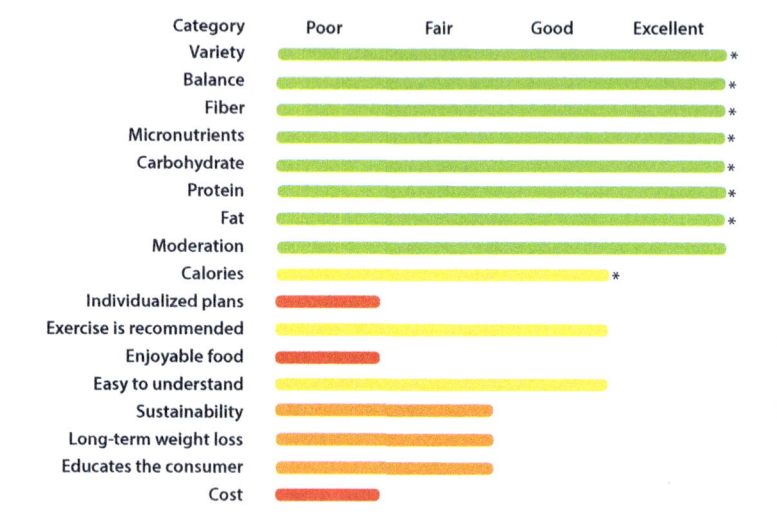

Category	Poor	Fair	Good	Excellent
Variety				Excellent*
Balance				Excellent*
Fiber				Excellent*
Micronutrients				Excellent*
Carbohydrate				Excellent*
Protein				Excellent*
Fat				Excellent*
Moderation				Excellent
Calories			Good*	
Individualized plans	Poor			
Exercise is recommended		Fair		
Enjoyable food	Poor			
Easy to understand		Fair		
Sustainability		Fair		
Long-term weight loss		Fair		
Educates the consumer		Fair		
Cost	Poor			

Positives

Involves some kosher practices and holistic living habits that may assist a strict Orthodox Jewish population.

Negatives

Very restrictive on the kinds of foods allowed. Indicates that numerous cleansing agents and supplements are essential. Includes saturated fat and extra-virgin coconut oil. 🔍 p. 55

*Ratings exclude the partial-day fasts.

The hook/catch or brilliant selling point: This groundbreaking diet uses a holistic approach to health, leading the follower on a life-changing journey.

Truths/Myths

- **Myth** - Organic is better than other produce.

- **Truth** - Organic produce, on the whole, is not better than other produce. But in all cases, it is more expensive, which can prohibit and limit its purchase and ultimately hinder one's ability to continue on this diet. It is better to consume non-organic produce than no produce if the budget doesn't allow for the former.

- **Myth** - "Organic" and "natural" items should be preferred.

- **Truth** - Not everything natural is safe. Natural toxins are chemicals naturally produced by living organisms. While the terms "Organic" and "Natural" sound healthy and desirable, there are many natural items (poisons and carcinogens) that are dangerous to humans, including the botulinum family of neurotoxins, yet some are used in the cosmetic industry (including in botox). Other toxins include glycoalkaloids plant toxins found in potatoes and aflatoxin, found in the edible portion of nuts. However, the amount of these are monitored in the food industry to ensure they do not reach high enough levels in our food supply to cause harm.

- Myth - Fluoride is a toxin.

- Truth - Fluoride is a trace mineral required for health. Fluoride is the safe ion form of the poisonous gas fluorine. It is found naturally in plants and animals. It is added to the water supply in many municipalities to assist community members with oral health. Once fluoride is absorbed, it is taken up by bones and developing teeth. One of the best-known functions of fluoride is its role in maintaining healthy teeth and hardening enamel, the outer portion of teeth. Fluoride from food, beverages, and dental products such as toothpaste can repair enamel that has started to erode. Fluoride also helps maintain strong bones by stimulating osteoblasts. In general, osteoblasts are cells that secrete materials that make up the matrix for bone formation. In combination with calcium and vitamin D, fluoride may increase bone mineral density, which helps in the reduction of osteoporosis. It is an essential nutrient needed by the body. Like any nutrient, too much or too little can be harmful.

- Myth - Cavities filled with mercury are dangerous.

- Truth - Mercury is not an essential nutrient. It is not needed by the body. It is a naturally occurring element found in air, water, and soil. It exists in various forms: elemental (or metallic); inorganic (exposure through various occupations); and organic (e.g., methylmercury, which can be consumed in the diet.) The forms of mercury differ in their degree of toxicity. Exposure may cause serious health effects for many parts of the body, including nerves, immune system, kidneys, eyes, lungs and skin. It can also threaten the development of children in utero and early life. Exposure to methylmercury (an organic compound) can occur when fish and shellfish are eaten. All humans are exposed to some level of mercury, as it occurs naturally in the earth's crust and is released into the environment. Dental amalgam fillings contain mercury and other metals. Although some people have allergic reactions to amalgam fillings, most scientific studies have found no relationship between this type of filling and symptoms of mercury poisoning in any age group.

- Truth - Overexposure to X-rays can be harmful. That is why physicians weigh the risks and benefits of using this imaging technology before subjecting patients to it.

- Truth - Prayer and a spiritual component have been found important in both research and in wellness fields.

- Truth - Hygiene in the form of hand washing before meals is important in reducing germs on the hands so they are not consumed with food.

Final decision: Thumbs down

How to improve this diet: Do not take the supplements or cleansing agents. They are not necessary. In order to achieve weight loss, be sure to consume fewer calories than are expended. Eat lots of fruits and vegetables, even if they are not organic.

Martha's Vineyard Diet Detox

Premise of the Diet: Bodies can be cleaned out and this helps with weight loss.

Claims of the Diet: Will lose a pound a day and rid the body of toxins.

Diet Description: There are three main principles: rest, reduce, and rebuild. In addition to traditional water enemas on most days, organic coffee enemas are required once a week, along with drinking 40-48 ounces of water, 32-40 ounces of herbal tea, 16 ounces of vegetable-based soup, and 32 ounces of either a green drink made from vegetables or a berry drink.

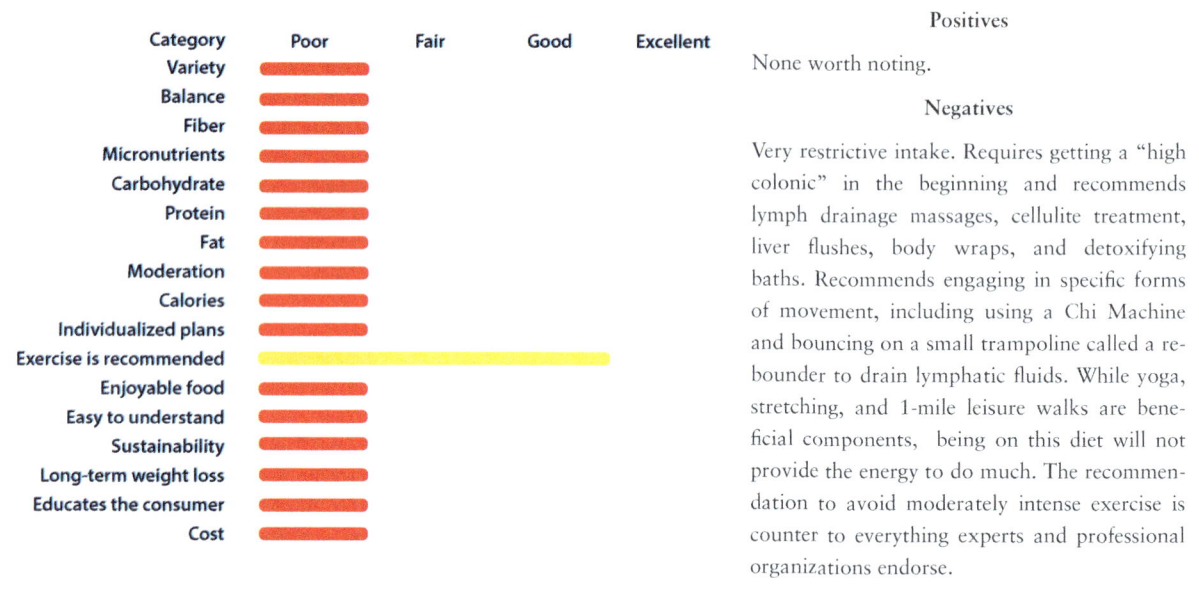

Category	Poor	Fair	Good	Excellent
Variety	■			
Balance	■			
Fiber	■			
Micronutrients	■			
Carbohydrate	■			
Protein	■			
Fat	■			
Moderation	■			
Calories	■			
Individualized plans	■			
Exercise is recommended		■		
Enjoyable food	■			
Easy to understand	■			
Sustainability	■			
Long-term weight loss	■			
Educates the consumer	■			
Cost	■			

Positives

None worth noting.

Negatives

Very restrictive intake. Requires getting a "high colonic" in the beginning and recommends lymph drainage massages, cellulite treatment, liver flushes, body wraps, and detoxifying baths. Recommends engaging in specific forms of movement, including using a Chi Machine and bouncing on a small trampoline called a rebounder to drain lymphatic fluids. While yoga, stretching, and 1-mile leisure walks are beneficial components, being on this diet will not provide the energy to do much. The recommendation to avoid moderately intense exercise is counter to everything experts and professional organizations endorse.

The hook/catch or brilliant selling point: Includes the name of an affluent summer colony that is home to celebrities.

Truths/Myths

- **Myth** - Lymph drainage massages and using a Chi Machine are helpful in weight loss.

- **Truth** - Lymph fluid buildup (lymphedema) results from a blockage in the lymphatic system, preventing lymph fluid from draining. Ultimately, the fluid can build up and cause swelling. Its most common cause is damage to or removal of lymph nodes. This is often part of cancer treatments, not patients trying to lose weight.

- **Myth** - It is important to take enzyme capsules, herbal cleansing formulas and/or enemas for health and weight loss.

- **Truth** - The liver and kidneys rid the body of toxins and wastes. A colonic, also known as colonic irrigation or colon hydrotherapy, streams gallons of water into the body through a tube inserted into the rectum. This can flush out beneficial bacteria in the colon, leaving the body in a worsened condition. 🔍 p. 85

- **Myth** - Bouncing on a small trampoline called a rebounder to drain lymphatic fluids is necessary for weight loss and health.

- **Truth** - There are no known health benefits to this approach to losing weight. There are no known health benefits to using these recommended supplements, products or techniques. In fact, any weight lost with this approach will most likely not be fat. Moreover lost weight will most likely be regained when the diet is over. A safer, cheaper, and less punishing path to weight loss and good health should be sought.

Final decision: Thumbs down 👎

How to improve this diet: Can't be improved.

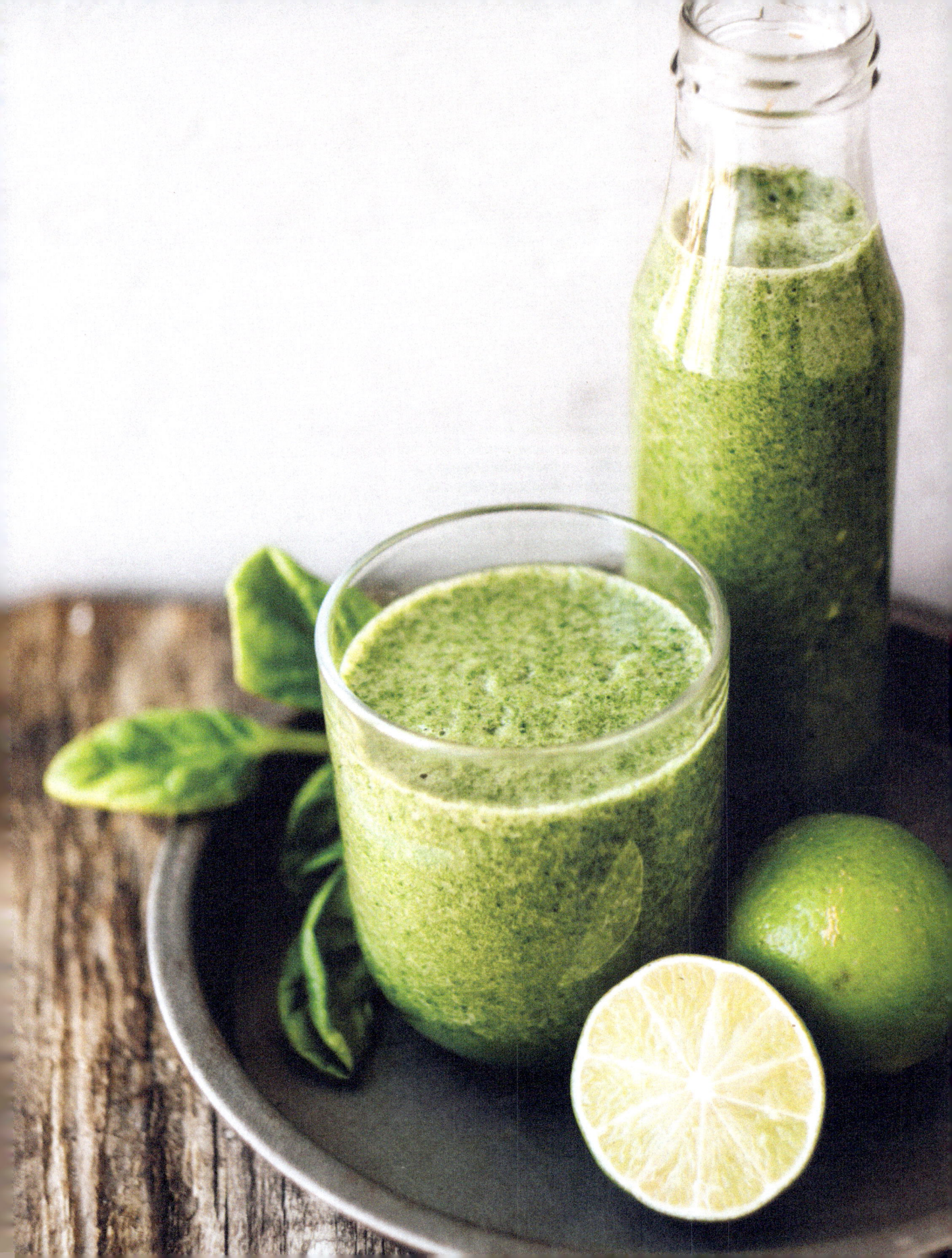

Master Your Metabolism Diet

Premise of the Diet: When hormones get out of balance, your health suffers, and the body has difficulty managing weight.

Claims of the Diet: Manipulates timing, quantities, and combinations of foods in order to make metabolism burn fat.

Diet Description: Swap "anti-nutrients" such as added fats, sugars, and chemical additives with organic and natural foods, in three phases. During the first phase, stop consuming foods containing hydrogenated fats, refined grains, high-fructose corn syrup, glutamates, artificial sweeteners, preservatives, and colors. Minimize consumption of starchy veggies, tropical dried and canned fruits, soy, alcohol, full-fat dairy, fatty meats, canned foods, and caffeine. In the second phase, consume 10 "power nutrient" food groups, including: legumes, peas and beans, alliums like onions and leeks, berries, meat and eggs, a variety of fruits and vegetables, nuts and seeds, organic low-fat dairy, and whole grains. The last phase involves eating every 4 hours, never skipping breakfast, eating until full, and not eating after 9 p.m. Fats, carbohydrates, and proteins are eaten in every meal and snack.

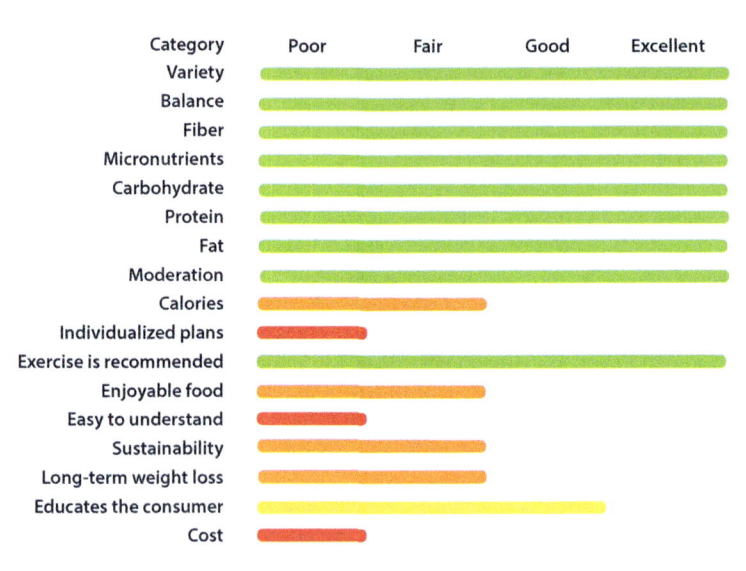

Category	Poor	Fair	Good	Excellent
Variety				■
Balance				■
Fiber				■
Micronutrients				■
Carbohydrate				■
Protein				■
Fat				■
Moderation				■
Calories		■		
Individualized plans	■			
Exercise is recommended				■
Enjoyable food		■		
Easy to understand	■			
Sustainability		■		
Long-term weight loss		■		
Educates the consumer			■	
Cost	■			

Positives

Addresses attitude and emotional triggers. Is well-balanced and healthy. Discusses how various glands including the thyroid, adrenal, and pituitary glands, and various hormones including insulin, thyroid hormones, estrogen and progesterone, testosterone, and leptin, may factor into weight management. Sample diets may help to improve the diet. Provides smart strategies for eating out, quick and easy recipes, shopping lists, and online shopping resources.

Negatives

Throwing out all plastics, bleached paper products, and other "toxic" household goods can be costly and wasteful. Calorie level may be low for certain people, especially heavy exercisers. Some may find the science in this diet overwhelming or confusing if they have not previously had some anatomy/physiology education.

The hook/catch or brilliant selling point: The author, Jillian Michaels, is well known as the tough-as-nails trainer on TV's "The Biggest Loser."

Truths/Myths

- **Myth** - Fat-burning genes can be spoken to by nutrients.

- **Truth** - Nutrients control hormone secretions, which control metabolism. For example, excess glucose (nutrient) controls insulin secretion (hormone), which controls the storage of the excess glucose (calories). Control of fat-burning enzymes is not well established.

- **Myth** - It is possible to rebalance energy and hormones for effortless weight loss.

- **Truth** - Weight loss is rarely effortless. Weight loss can be achieved by burning more calories than consumed.

- Myth - Environmental toxins cause weight gain.

- Truth - It is not scientifically accepted or established that environmental toxins inhibit weight loss.

Final decision: Thumbs down

How to improve this diet: While eating a combination of fats, carbs, and protein every 4 hours, never skipping breakfast, eating until full, and not eating after 9 p.m. are good ideas, loosen up some of the many restrictions and be sure to consume enough calories to continue routine exercise.

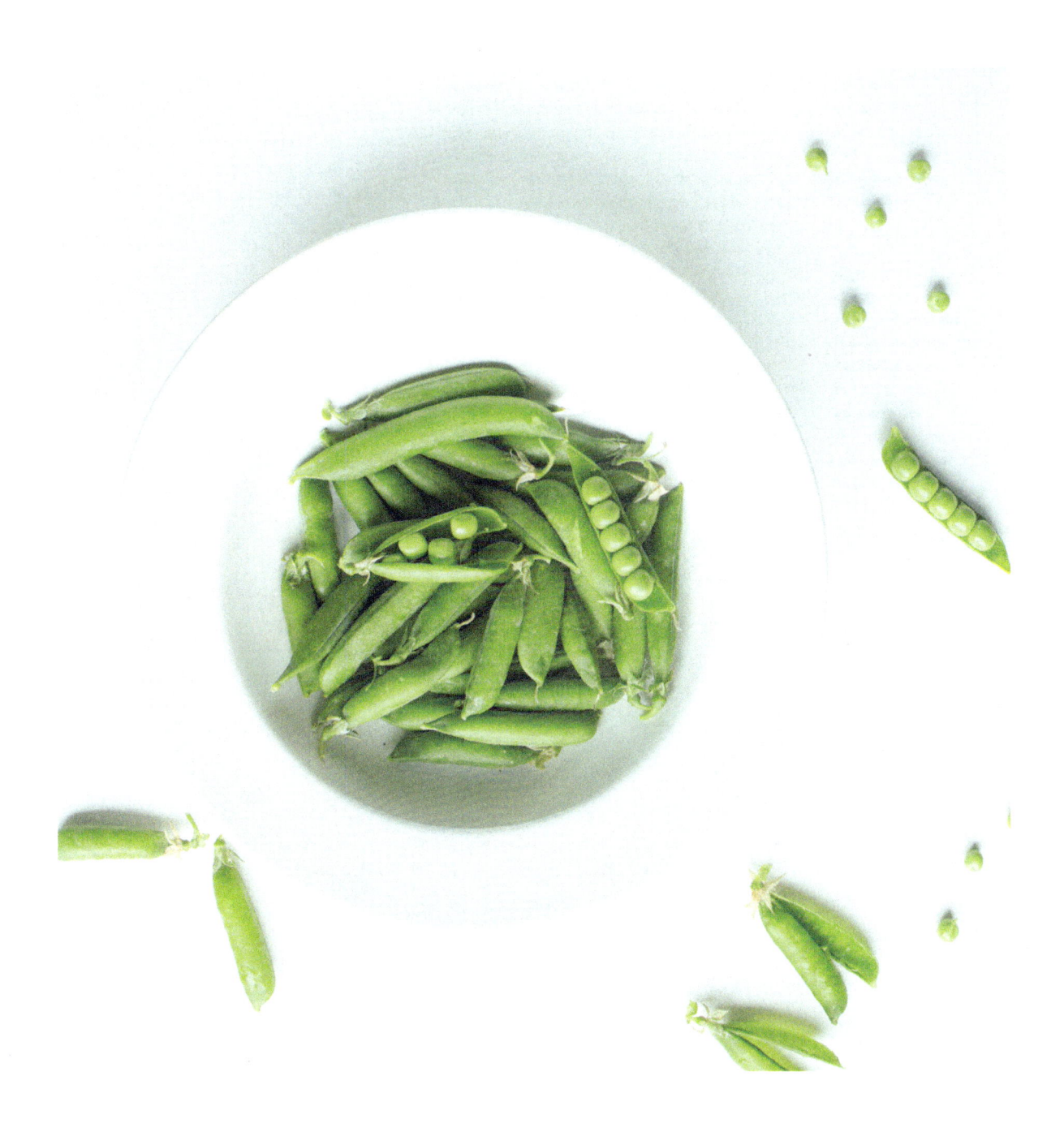

Mayo Clinic Diet

Premise of the Diet: By adopting and sustaining healthy habits long term, the goal weight can be maintained for life.

Claims of the Diet: Lose 1 to 2 pounds each week until goal weight is reached.

Diet Description: Two phases: 1. Lose It! Two-week phase designed to jump-start weight loss. May lose up to 6 to 10 pounds. Focuses on lifestyle habits associated with weight. Add five healthy habits, break five unhealthy habits, and adopt five bonus healthy habits. 2. Live It! Teaches healthy food choices, portion control, and taking a lifelong approach to diet and health to help maintain goal weight permanently.

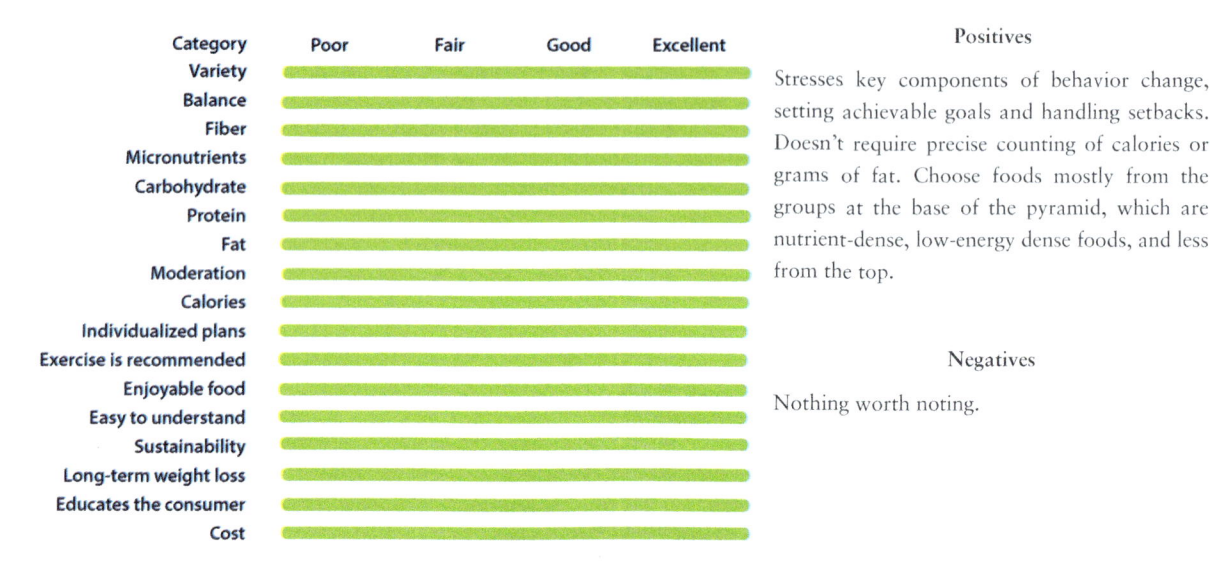

Category	Poor	Fair	Good	Excellent
Variety				✓
Balance				✓
Fiber				✓
Micronutrients				✓
Carbohydrate				✓
Protein				✓
Fat				✓
Moderation				✓
Calories				✓
Individualized plans				✓
Exercise is recommended				✓
Enjoyable food				✓
Easy to understand				✓
Sustainability				✓
Long-term weight loss				✓
Educates the consumer				✓
Cost				✓

Positives

Stresses key components of behavior change, setting achievable goals and handling setbacks. Doesn't require precise counting of calories or grams of fat. Choose foods mostly from the groups at the base of the pyramid, which are nutrient-dense, low-energy dense foods, and less from the top.

Negatives

Nothing worth noting.

The hook/catch or brilliant selling point: A diet from one of the most reputable clinics in the nation.

Truths/Myths:

- **Myth** - Nothing worth noting.

- **Truth** - The Mayo Clinic Diet was created by a team of weight-loss experts at Mayo Clinic and is designed for long-term weight management through reshaping lifestyles, adopting healthy new habits, and breaking unhealthy old habits. It focuses on generous amounts of healthy foods that contain a smaller number of calories so they can be eaten in a large volume, which helps avoid hunger.

Final decision: Thumbs up 👍

How to improve this diet: Nothing worth noting. But it is important to note that the first stage of any weight loss is water loss. Thus, do not be disappointed if "weight loss" slows after the initial Lose it phase. In fact, a slowdown is good and to be expected.

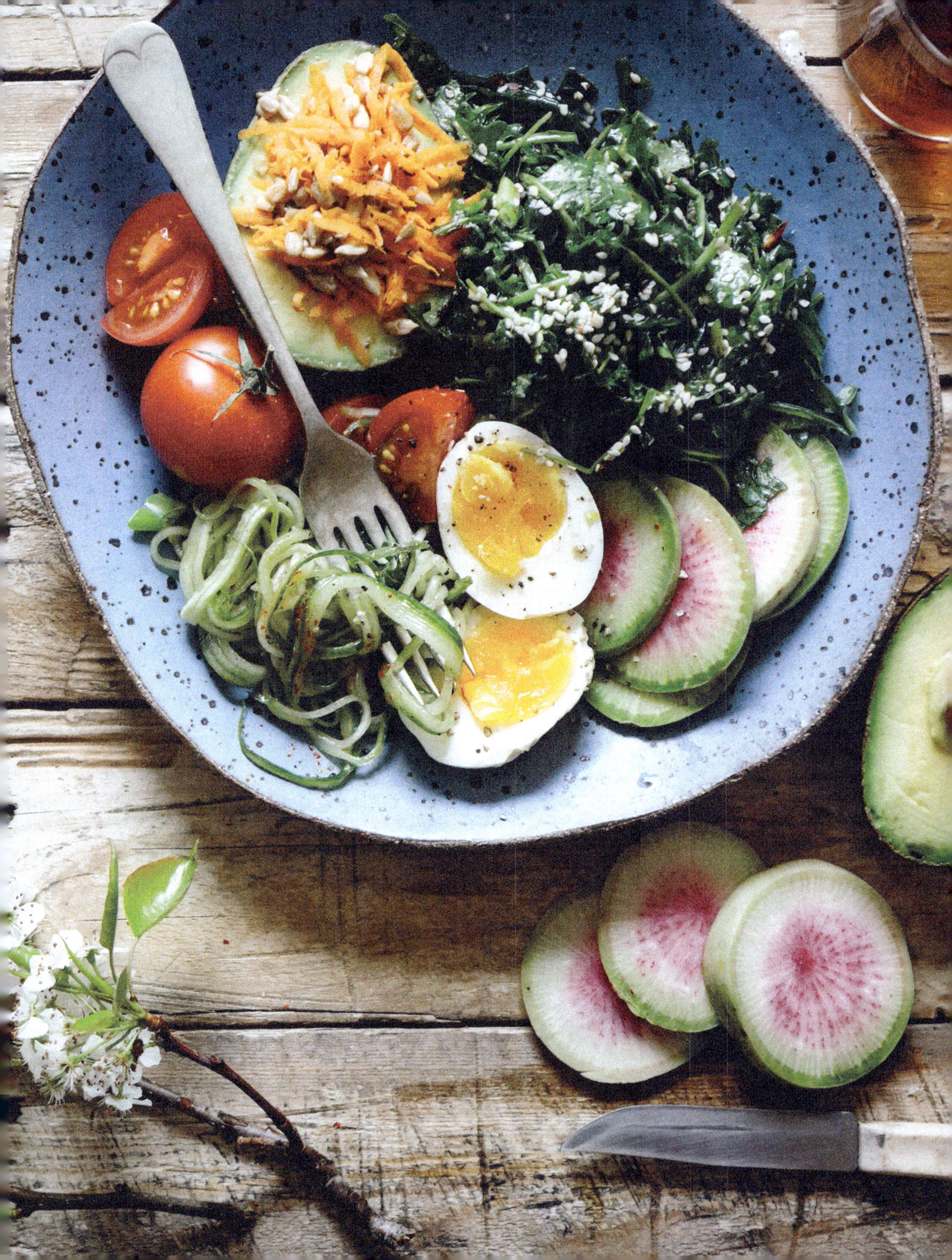

Medifast Diet

Premise of the Diet: No work or thinking on your part.

Claims of the Diet: Eat six meals a day and still lose weight.

Diet Description: Different calorie-restricted plans are offered.

1. Medifast GO! This is for busy people who need an easy-to-follow, rapid weight-loss program. Provides 800 to 1,000 calories a day.

2. Medifast Achieve provides a steady, gradual weight loss.

3. Thrive Healthy Living Plan is designed for healthy weight maintenance.

All programs are based on buying the company's specific products.

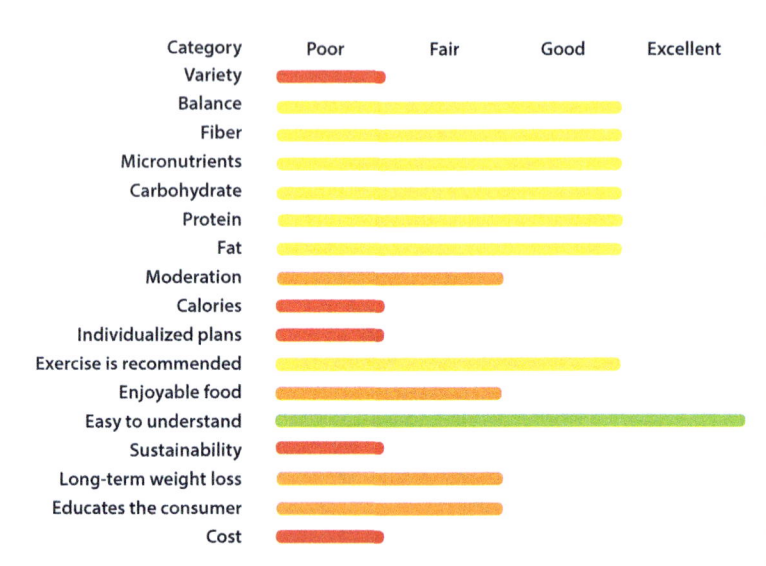

Category	Poor	Fair	Good	Excellent
Variety	■			
Balance		■■■		
Fiber		■■■		
Micronutrients		■■■		
Carbohydrate		■■■		
Protein		■■■		
Fat		■■■		
Moderation	■■			
Calories	■			
Individualized plans	■			
Exercise is recommended		■■■		
Enjoyable food	■■			
Easy to understand				■■■■
Sustainability	■			
Long-term weight loss	■■			
Educates the consumer	■■			
Cost	■			

Positives

Meals provide 5-7 ounces of lean protein, 3 servings of vegetables, and up to 2 servings of healthy fats. Replacement meals are enriched with nutrients in an attempt to offset nutrient deficiencies that can accompany very low-calorie diets and the fact that the program cuts out certain food groups, including dairy. Because meals are nutritionally based on a similar design, they are easily interchangeable with one another. There is some research to show meal replacement diets can be safe and help weight loss.

Negatives

In order to keep weight off, lifestyle changes must be made. If lifestyle changes are not made, those 65+ meal replacement foods are the only food choices for life. Making these lifestyle changes may make sticking with the program a challenge. While weight loss will mostly occur due to severe calorie restriction with the Medifast GO approach, this approach will most likely be tough to stick with and the weight loss may not be fat. Moreover, the low calorie level may make exercise, which is essential for weight loss, health, and weight maintenance, a challenge. It can be difficult to ensure all nutrients in adequate amounts are consumed on such a low-calorie diet and when entire food groups are eliminated. Eating different foods from those around us can create a situation of isolation and awkwardness. Foods are pricy.

The hook/catch or brilliant selling point: It's easy. Physicians developed this weight-loss program with fortified foods for nutritional adequacy.

Truths/Myths:

- **Myth** - Consuming meal replacements is an easy and good weight loss approach. 🔍 p. 13

- **Truth** - Becoming dependent on someone else to put nutritious meals in front of us makes us dependent on the provider. It is much wiser to become educated on how to prepare our own healthy foods. Preparing our own foods allows us to eat with others and greatly expands our food choices and flavors, all of which increases our likelihood of maintaining weight after extra weight is lost.

- Myth - The optimal fat-burning state can be achieved with a total daily carbohydrate intake of approximately 80–85 grams.
- Truth - The RDA for carbohydrates is 130 grams of carbohydrates in order to provide glucose to the brain and central nervous system. People's needs vary.

p. 39

Final decision: Thumbs down 👎

How to improve this diet: Because this is an extreme diet, be sure to talk with a physician before starting this meal replacement diet. For those on medication, stay in continuous communication with primary care providers while undertaking the program. It would be wiser to prepare our own meals in a healthful manner.

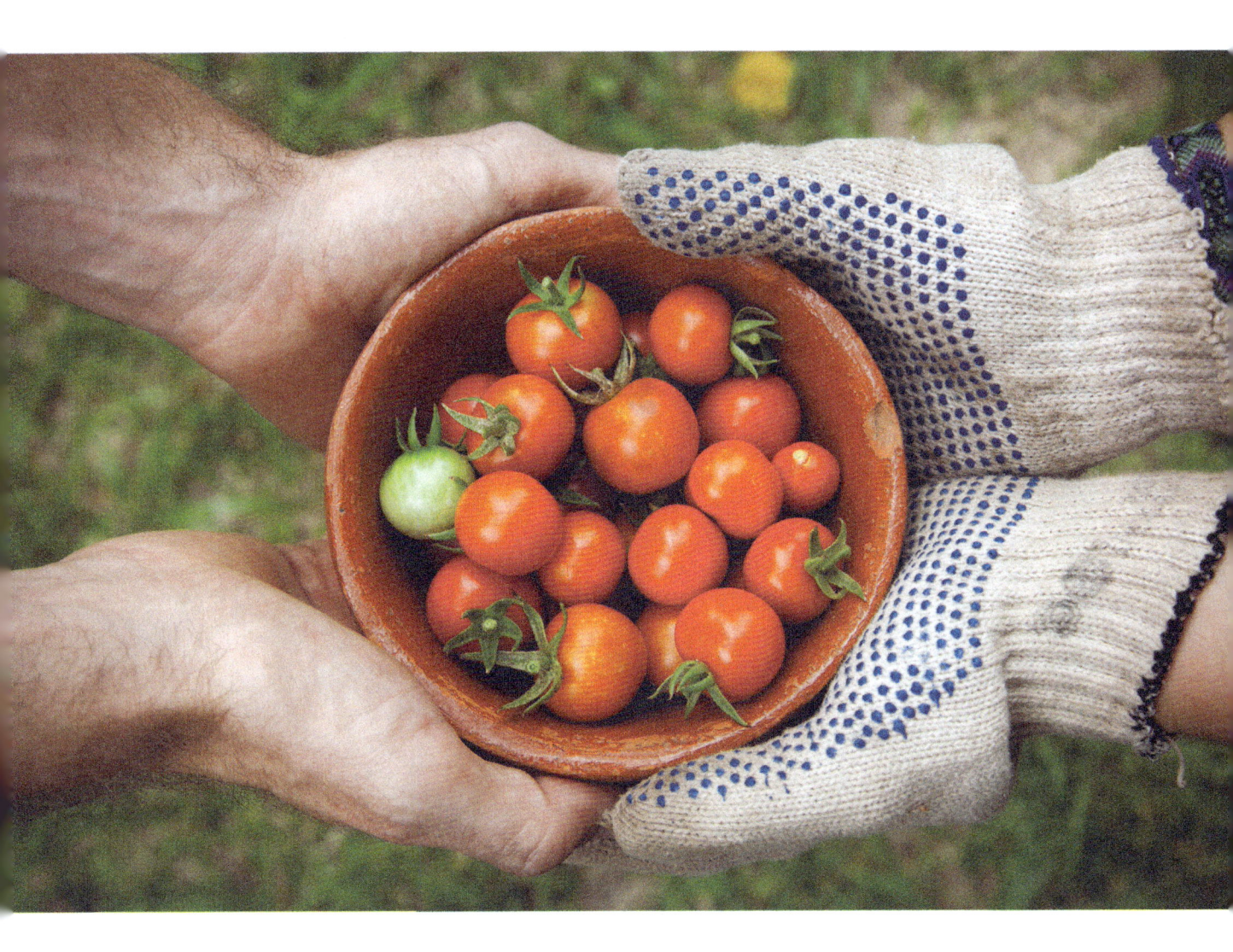

Mediterranean Diet

Premise of the Diet: Based on the traditional cuisine found in olive-growing regions bordering the Mediterranean Sea, where there are fewer deaths associated with cardiovascular diseases.

Claims of the Diet: A heart-healthy eating plan.

Diet Description: The foundation of the Mediterranean diet is plant-based. It includes daily consumption of vegetables, fruits, whole grains, and healthy fats, and weekly intakes of fish, poultry, beans, and eggs. It includes moderate amounts of dairy products and a limited amount of red meat. This plan involves making mealtimes social and enjoyable. May involve a glass of red wine and encourages physical activity.

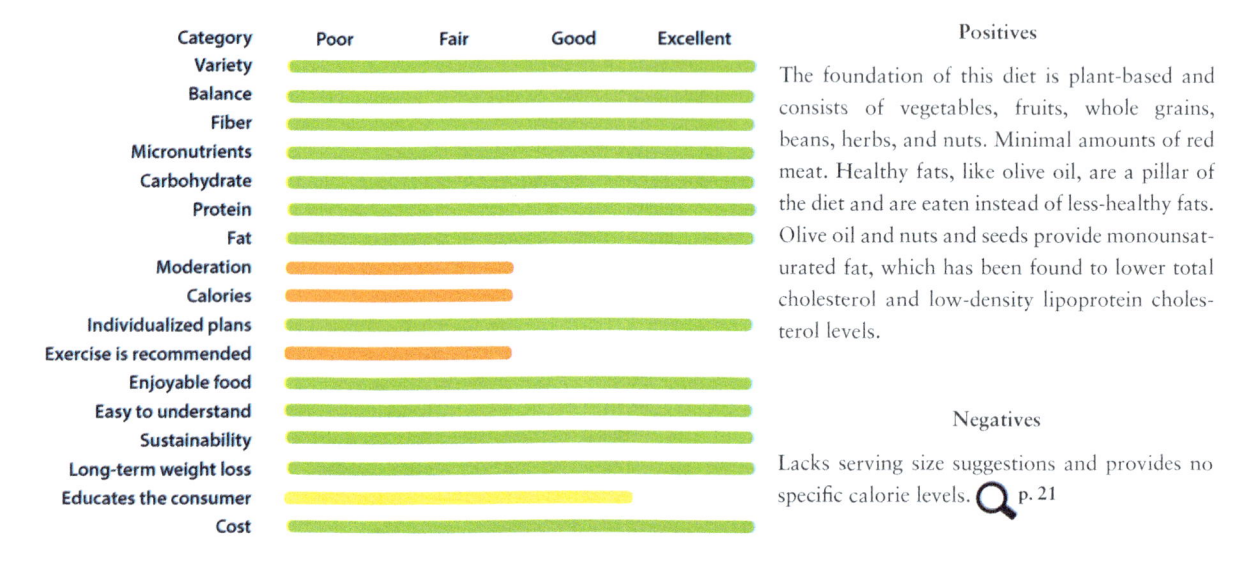

Category	Poor	Fair	Good	Excellent
Variety				✓
Balance				✓
Fiber				✓
Micronutrients				✓
Carbohydrate				✓
Protein				✓
Fat				✓
Moderation		✓		
Calories		✓		
Individualized plans				✓
Exercise is recommended		✓		
Enjoyable food				✓
Easy to understand				✓
Sustainability				✓
Long-term weight loss				✓
Educates the consumer			✓	
Cost				✓

Positives

The foundation of this diet is plant-based and consists of vegetables, fruits, whole grains, beans, herbs, and nuts. Minimal amounts of red meat. Healthy fats, like olive oil, are a pillar of the diet and are eaten instead of less-healthy fats. Olive oil and nuts and seeds provide monounsaturated fat, which has been found to lower total cholesterol and low-density lipoprotein cholesterol levels.

Negatives

Lacks serving size suggestions and provides no specific calorie levels. 🔍 p. 21

The hook/catch or brilliant selling point: Well-studied diet with a name that calls to mind beautiful beaches

Truths/Myths

- Myth - None worth noting
- Truth - Current studies support this diet's instrumental role in the prevention of cardiovascular disease.

Final decision: Thumbs up 👍

How to improve this diet: Be sure to consume fewer calories than are expended to achieve weight loss.

Morning Banana Diet (aka Asa-Banana Diet)

Premise of the Diet: A "stress-free" diet.

Claims of the Diet: Eating bananas in the morning will help you lose weight.

Diet Description: For breakfast, eat raw bananas (as many as you want) and drink room-temperature water. If still hungry, wait 15 to 30 minutes and you can eat something else that is < 200 calories. Eat a "normal" lunch and dinner. One afternoon snack is allowed, which is the only time sweets are allowed. Avoid dairy and ice cream. No desserts after meals. Go to bed before midnight.

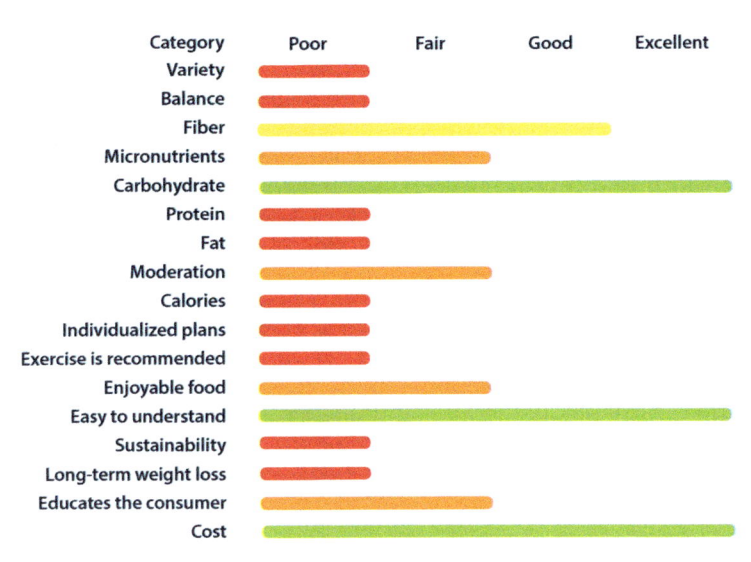

Category	Poor	Fair	Good	Excellent
Variety	■			
Balance	■			
Fiber		■		
Micronutrients	■			
Carbohydrate				■
Protein	■			
Fat	■			
Moderation		■		
Calories	■			
Individualized plans	■			
Exercise is recommended	■			
Enjoyable food		■		
Easy to understand				■
Sustainability	■			
Long-term weight loss	■			
Educates the consumer		■		
Cost				■

Positives

Teaches healthy techniques, such as to stop eating when 80% full, stresses the importance of a good night's sleep, encourages eating fruit, keeping a food journal, and becoming aware of hunger and fullness levels, which, if incorporated, increase the chance of long-term weight loss and improved health.

Negatives

Repetitive and may lead to monotony. Portion sizes are not adequately addressed. Does not require exercise. No clear parameters on lunch and dinner. While there are a number of success stories in Japan where the diet originated, lunch and dinner meals in other countries are different and therefore comparisons cannot be made.

🔍 p. 105

The hook/catch or brilliant selling point: So simple it sells

Truths/Myths

- **Myth** - Eating bananas in the morning (or at any time of the day) will help lose weight.

- **Truth** - There is nothing about bananas that specifically promotes weight loss. There is no scientific evidence that bananas will help with weight loss.

- **Truth** - While there is nothing specifically magical about not eating after 8 p.m., this behavior will likely cut out some extra calories, just as eating till 80% full will help.

- **Truth** - Studies show those getting 7 to 9 hours of sleep a night have lower weights. When tired, overeating unhealthy foods is more likely.

Final decision: Thumbs down 👎

How to improve this diet: Eat 3 balanced meals that, in total, have fewer calories than are expended.

Naturally Thin Diet

Premise of the Diet: Change your relationship with food. Eat well, but sparingly.

Claims of the Diet: Will show how to banish "Heavy Habits" and embrace "Thin Thoughts."

Diet Description: Provides 10 basic rules. Takes the view that a diet is like a "bank account." Balance all foods so as not to eat too much of any one item. Balance starches with proteins, and vegetables with sweets. Includes lots of vegetables, some whole grains, and lean protein. Recommends organic, locally grown vegetables, whole grains, and animal sources, while avoiding processed and packaged foods. Provides 10 basic rules revolving around eating in moderation, not denying self, and satisfying cravings.

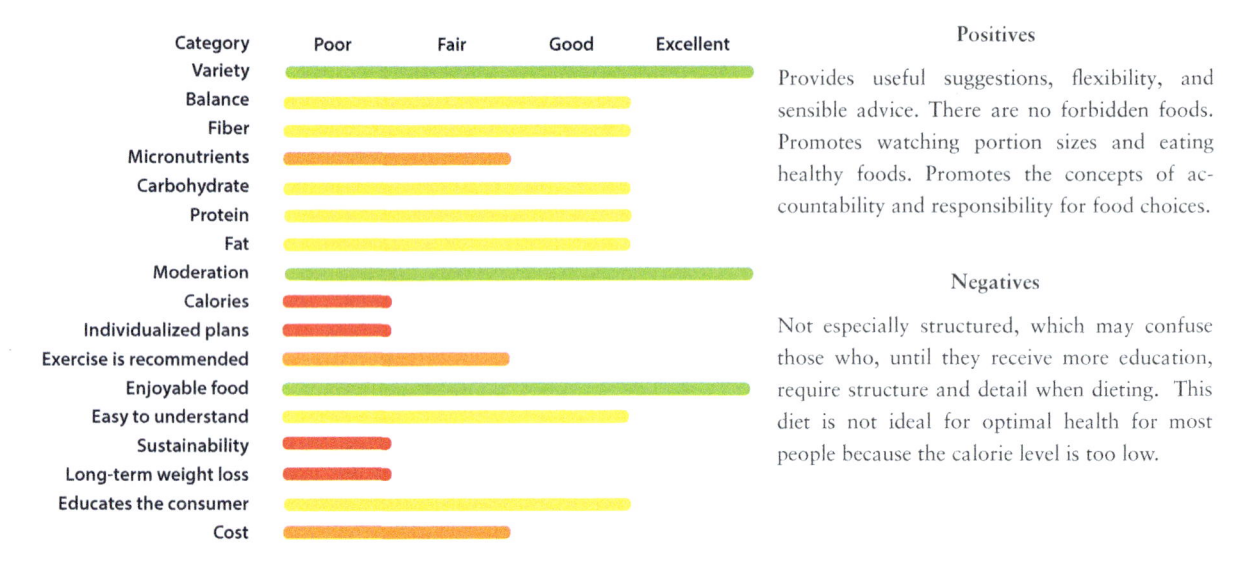

Category	Poor	Fair	Good	Excellent
Variety				●
Balance			●	
Fiber			●	
Micronutrients		●		
Carbohydrate			●	
Protein			●	
Fat			●	
Moderation				●
Calories	●			
Individualized plans	●			
Exercise is recommended		●		
Enjoyable food				●
Easy to understand			●	
Sustainability	●			
Long-term weight loss	●			
Educates the consumer			●	
Cost		●		

Positives

Provides useful suggestions, flexibility, and sensible advice. There are no forbidden foods. Promotes watching portion sizes and eating healthy foods. Promotes the concepts of accountability and responsibility for food choices.

Negatives

Not especially structured, which may confuse those who, until they receive more education, require structure and detail when dieting. This diet is not ideal for optimal health for most people because the calorie level is too low.

The hook/catch or brilliant selling point: The author, Bethenny Frankel, is one of reality TV's "Real Housewives of New York City."

Truths/Myths

- **Myth** - Healthy meal plans and calorie levels are offered.

- **Truth** - Strictly following the sample days would be too low in calories and nutrients provided. 🔍 p. 78, 21

Final decision: Thumbs down 👎

How to improve this diet: Follow many of the main premises, but be sure to fuel with adequate calories so the metabolic rate does not fall and nutrient deficiencies do not develop. Add a few servings of dairy and be sure to take a multi-vitamin. Do not skip meals or substitute alcoholic beverages for a meal.

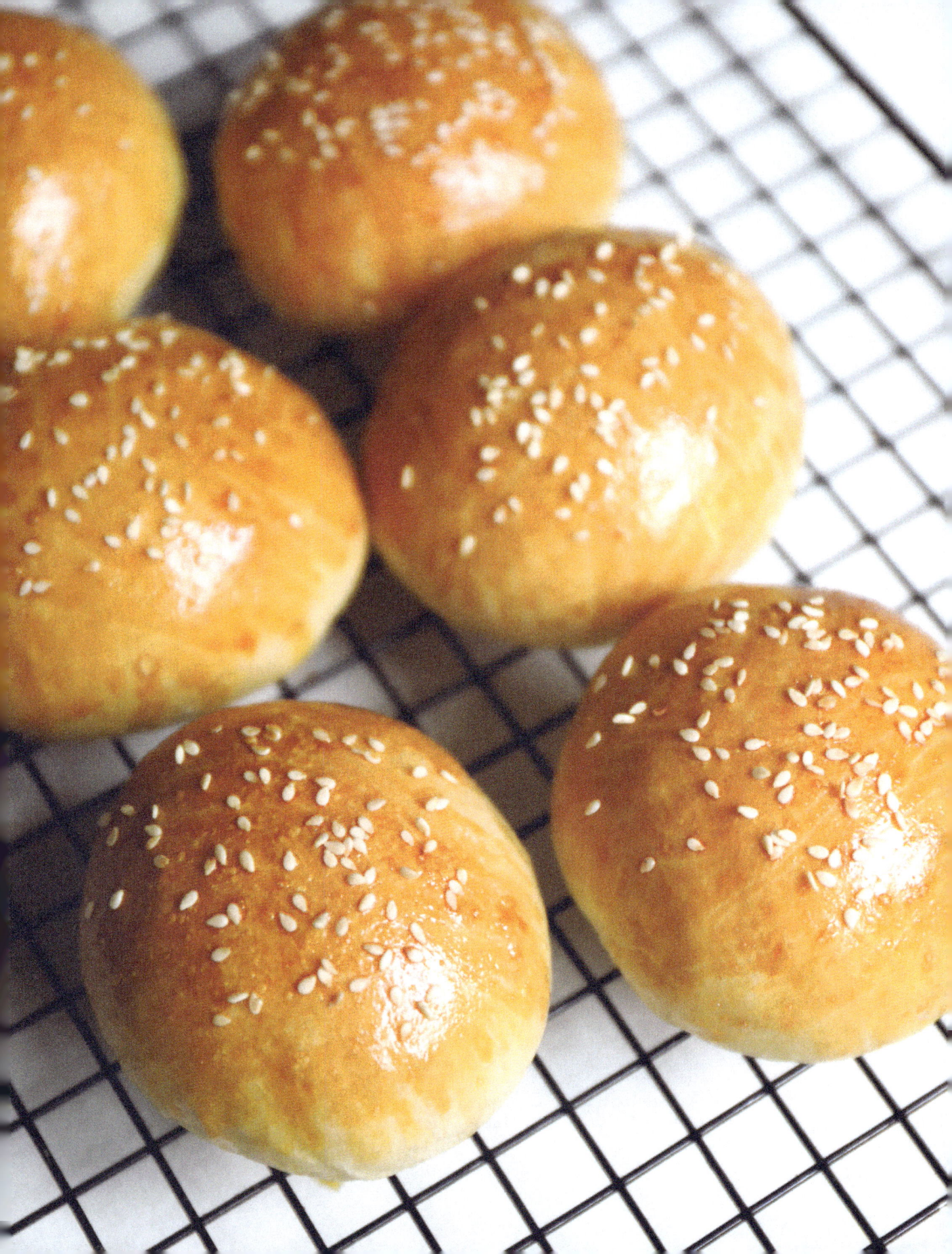

New Atkins For You Diet

Premise of the Diet: When there is too much sugar in the bloodstream, the body stores it as fat. A low-carb diet from the right sources of carbohydrates will help the body burn fat instead of sugar for fuel. It's a more realistic approach to the classic ketogenic diet.

Claims of the Diet: Expect to lose 1-2 lbs. per week. Will help improve health. Improves health markers for heart disease, insulin resistance, and diabetes. Will "flip the body's metabolic switch" from burning carbs to burning fat. Limits blood sugar and insulin spikes. The dieter will not experience hunger or cravings.

Diet Description: This diet is different from the old 20, 40, 100 Atkins diet in that it introduces the concept of "Net Carbs" (where fiber grams are subtracted from total carbohydrate grams) and the concept of Foundation Vegetables (12 to 15 grams of Net Carbs a day). It notes that fiber has been confirmed as having a minimal impact on blood sugar; as such, there is no need to limit your daily consumption of vegetables to 3 cups. Most people can consume up to 50 grams of carbohydrates and remain in ketosis.

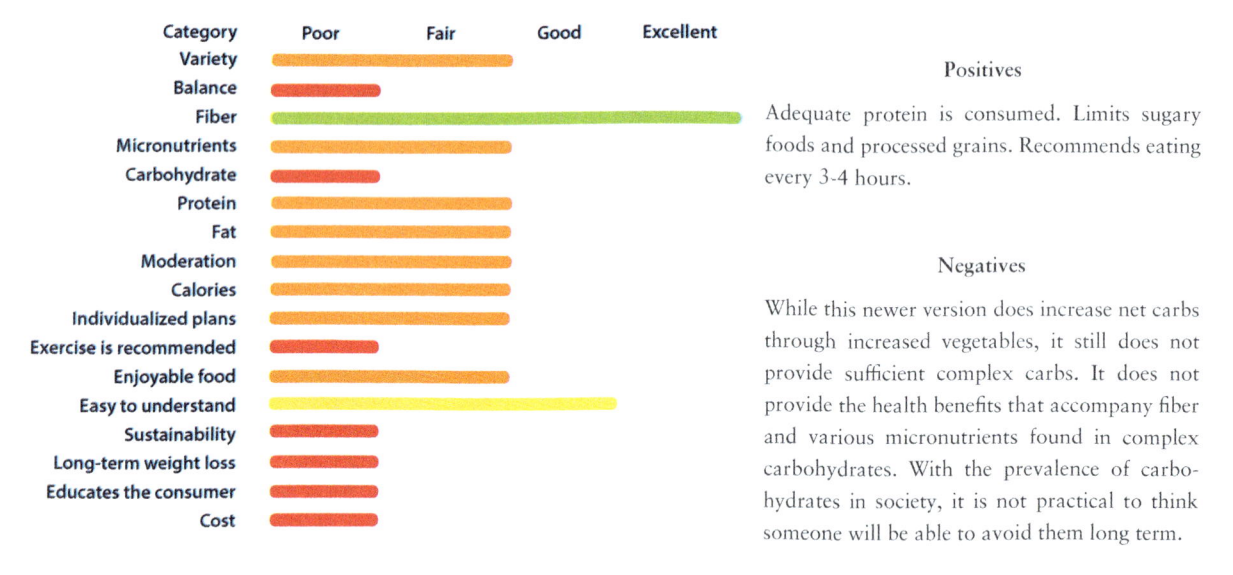

Category	Poor	Fair	Good	Excellent
Variety		Fair		
Balance	Poor			
Fiber				Excellent
Micronutrients		Fair		
Carbohydrate	Poor			
Protein		Fair		
Fat		Fair		
Moderation		Fair		
Calories		Fair		
Individualized plans		Fair		
Exercise is recommended	Poor			
Enjoyable food		Fair		
Easy to understand			Good	
Sustainability	Poor			
Long-term weight loss	Poor			
Educates the consumer	Poor			
Cost	Poor			

Positives

Adequate protein is consumed. Limits sugary foods and processed grains. Recommends eating every 3-4 hours.

Negatives

While this newer version does increase net carbs through increased vegetables, it still does not provide sufficient complex carbs. It does not provide the health benefits that accompany fiber and various micronutrients found in complex carbohydrates. With the prevalence of carbohydrates in society, it is not practical to think someone will be able to avoid them long term.

The hook/catch or brilliant selling point: It is easy to point the finger at one bad villain. Eliminate that one and we are home free!

Truths/Myths

- **Myth** - Carbs and weight loss are closely related. 🔍 p. 39, 15

- **Truth** - Actually, reducing calories and weight loss are closely related.

- **Myth** - Everyone's metabolism can use two different types of fuel for energy: either sugar (and carbs that are quickly turned into sugar by the body) or fat. But the type of fuel burned can have a huge difference in losing or maintaining weight. A typical diet reduces calories but is still high in carbohydrates (and thus sugar).

- **Truth** - Actually, everyone's metabolism can use varying components of carbohydrates, fats, proteins, and alcohol for fuel, depending on what is available and what the demands of the body are at any given moment. Carbs can turn into glucose quickly and are therefore a rather immediate source of fuel, while consumed fat and protein have to undergo more processes, but this is not bad. A combination of a variety of complex carbohydrates is recommended for a sustained feeling of satisfaction, and many health benefits accompany consuming complex carbohydrates. 🔍 p. 65

- **Myth** - Many people constantly cycle between sugar "highs" (where excess sugar is actually stored as fat in the body) and sugar "lows" (where you feel fatigued and ravenously hungry for more carbs and sugar).

• Truth - Candy bars and foods with simple sugars can cause an immediate rise in blood sugar and then a potential crash, depending on if any other food sources are consumed. Therefore, eating a candy bar or other sugary food (especially alone and with no other "healthy" food) is not recommended. The body can quickly turn consumed simple sugars into glucose (blood sugar). Fat and protein do have to go through more metabolic processes in order to be used as fuel.

• Myth - Limiting carbohydrates (sugar) means the body will burn fat, including body fat, for fuel.

• Truth - Limiting calories (regardless of their source) means the body may have to tap into body fat for fuel. Eating calories that provide carbs, proteins, and fats in recommended amounts and in sufficient amounts to meet BMR while exercising is the best way to burn body fat. Moreover, carbohydrates have a protein-spearing effect. In other words, carbohydrates are important for maintaining glycogen stores, which enable protein to be spared from being burned for fuel.

• Myth - Weight is lost, even when more calories are consumed.

• Truth - If more calories are consumed than the body burns, the body will store excess calories as fat. 🔍 p. 21

• Truth - Steady fueling also means more constant energy levels all day long, and many experience less hunger and cravings.

• Myth - There are no dangers associated with this style of eating.

• Truth - This type of diet should only be conducted under the close supervision of a physician. Attempting to try this diet without a physician's supervision can be dangerous.

Final decision: Thumbs down 👎

How to improve this diet: Add adequate carbohydrates in the form of complex carbohydrates. Carbohydrates should be at least 45-65% of all calories consumed. Continue to eat a variety of fruits, vegetables, and lean meats and consume no more than 35% of calories from fat sources.

New Beverly Hills Diet

Premise of the Diet: Digestive systems can be retrained by eating a fruit-based diet for 35 days, then adhering to strict rules about combining carbohydrates, fat, and protein.

Claims of the Diet: Will lose 10-15 pounds in 5 weeks, then will continue to lose weight.

Diet Description: There are four "conscious combining" principles:

1. Fruit must be eaten alone and should be eaten for breakfast. Wait an hour before eating different kinds of fruit.

2. Protein can be combined with fat, but not carbohydrates. Once protein is eaten, 80% of what is eaten the rest of the day should also be protein.

3. Carbohydrates can be combined with fat, but not protein.

4. Beer and spirits are considered carbohydrates. Red and white wine is considered fruit. Champagne is "neutral" and can be eaten with any type of food.

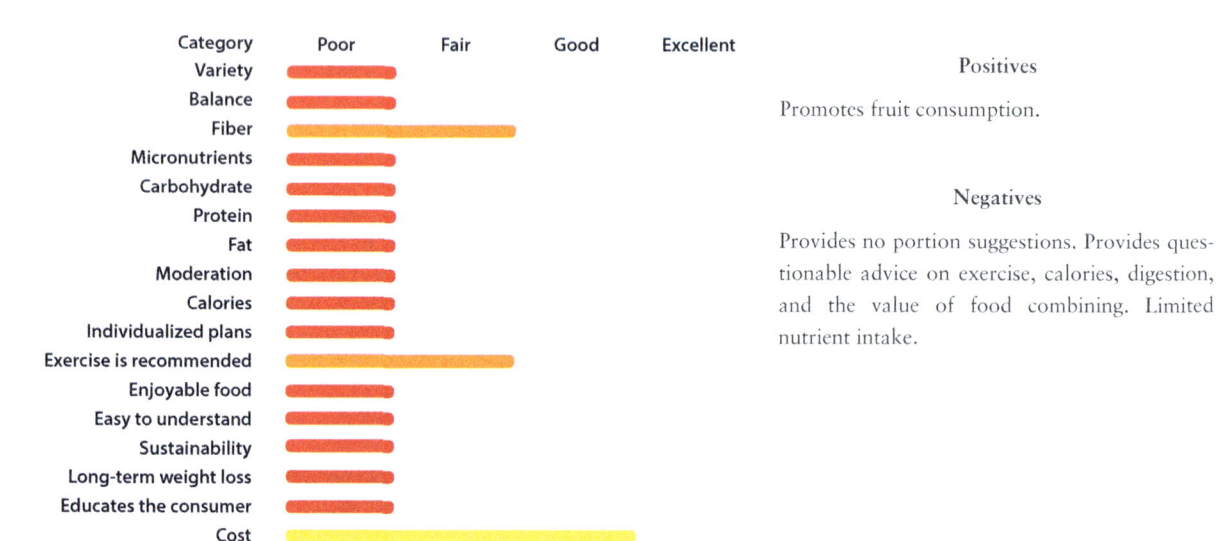

Category	Poor	Fair	Good	Excellent
Variety	▬			
Balance	▬			
Fiber		▬		
Micronutrients	▬			
Carbohydrate	▬			
Protein	▬			
Fat	▬			
Moderation	▬			
Calories	▬			
Individualized plans	▬			
Exercise is recommended		▬		
Enjoyable food	▬			
Easy to understand	▬			
Sustainability	▬			
Long-term weight loss	▬			
Educates the consumer	▬			
Cost				▬

Positives

Promotes fruit consumption.

Negatives

Provides no portion suggestions. Provides questionable advice on exercise, calories, digestion, and the value of food combining. Limited nutrient intake.

The hook/catch or brilliant selling point: Uses a flashy and popular location.

Truths/Myths

- **Myth** - Combining certain foods at meals will influence weight loss.

- **Truth** - Burning more calories than are consumed influences weight loss. 🔍 p. 13

Final decision: Thumbs down 👎

How to improve this diet: Can't be improved.

Noom

Premise of the Diet: A psychology-based diet and weight-loss program designed to help clients make healthy behavior changes surrounding diet and weight loss.

Claims of the Diet: The best diet is no diet at all.

Diet Description: Originally an app designed to track exercise and calorie intake, this program has grown to include psychology, behavior change, and support groups. Information to reframe thinking about food, weight, and overall life changes is presented. Price varies as it is based on personal goals. The recommended duration is based on how much weight loss is desired. The more months signed up for, the greater the monthly discount.

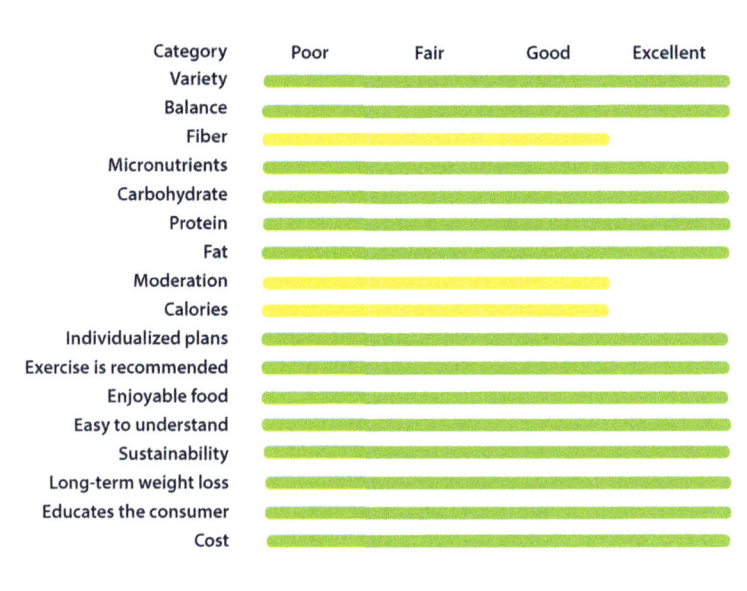

Category	Poor	Fair	Good	Excellent
Variety				✓
Balance				✓
Fiber			✓	
Micronutrients				✓
Carbohydrate				✓
Protein				✓
Fat				✓
Moderation			✓	
Calories			✓	
Individualized plans				✓
Exercise is recommended				✓
Enjoyable food				✓
Easy to understand				✓
Sustainability				✓
Long-term weight loss				✓
Educates the consumer				✓
Cost				✓

Positives

Takes numerous lifestyle factors into account, provides virtual support through coaches and peer groups, promotes lifestyle changes, includes all food groups, is easy to use, provides daily psychological articles, attempts to fit the program to the individual, and assigns a daily calorie budget, not a quick-fix approach. Dieters get to choose how much time they want to spend on lessons (5–16 minutes daily), which may help dieters become more self-aware of their relationship with food. Created by and provides a mobile health program recognized by the Centers for Disease Control (CDC) for delivering an evidence-based type-2 diabetes prevention program. Provides a step counter for those who keep their phone on them all day long. Uses a color-coded food system to help dieters prioritize food by caloric density. Offers a free one-week trial.

Negatives

Noom coaches are not dietitians. Requires food tracking and calorie counting. Program is calorie-based instead of nutrient-based which, for some, may promote behaviors that could be destructive such as calorie counting, food categorization, and preoccupation with weight from daily weigh-ins. May be difficult for those who struggle with freedom and too many choices, and feel they require that a specific meal plan be provided.

The hook/catch or brilliant selling point: Takes a psychological approach.

Truths/Myths

None worth noting.

Final decision: Thumbs up 👍

How to improve this diet: Those at risk for an eating disorder may be triggered by color-coding foods, and thus this program may best be avoided by those individuals.

NutriSystem Diet

Premise of the Diet: Meals are supplied, so there is no thinking or guessing.

Claims of the Diet: Lose up to 13 pounds and 7 inches overall in the first month.

Diet Description: Prepackaged meals and snacks are delivered and built around the glycemic index, which is a measure of how various carbs affect blood sugar. The program emphasizes "good" carbs that are digested slowly. About half of calories come from carbs, 25% from protein, and 25% from fat. Meals/plans are available for specific genders, vegetarians, diabetics, and can be customized for low sodium. Plans involve eating 5 to 6 times a day. The "core" 4-week plan generally costs $10-$11 a day. There is still a monthly grocery bill, as not all produce and meat/protein choices are provided. Therefore, costs will vary. Restaurant meals may count as one of the three "flex" meals allowed each week.

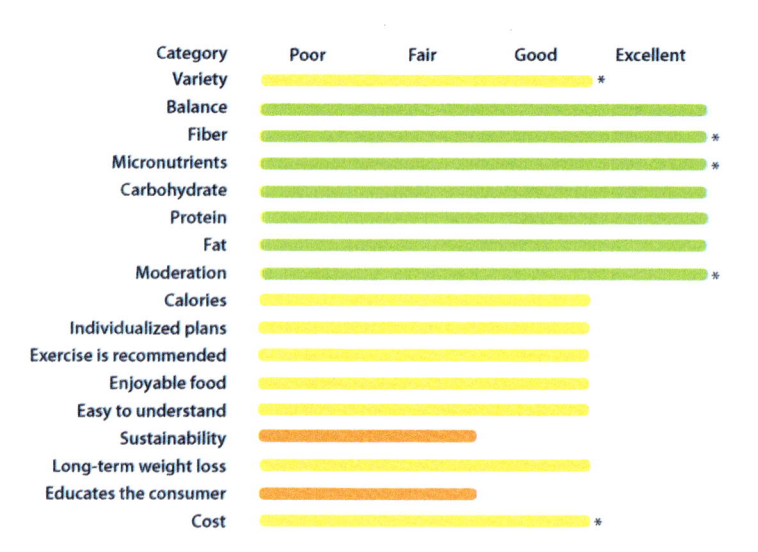

Category	Poor	Fair	Good	Excellent
Variety				*
Balance				
Fiber				*
Micronutrients				*
Carbohydrate				
Protein				
Fat				
Moderation				*
Calories				
Individualized plans				
Exercise is recommended				
Enjoyable food				
Easy to understand				
Sustainability				
Long-term weight loss				
Educates the consumer				
Cost				*

Positives

Provision of meals and meal-replacement products can promote weight loss and save time. No calorie counting. Pre-portioned food is delivered. Nearly all guess work is removed. Entrees, in general, will be smaller than some may be accustomed to, but the program requires frequent protein and fiber-rich produce, which can help reduce hunger. An "eating out guide," with recommendations categorized by cuisine, such as Italian or Mexican, is available. Suggestions are also made for diet-friendly foods at 30 popular nationwide chains. A number of member and company-generated recipes are available online for the transition period. Counselors are available 7 days a week by phone, chat or NuMi, the official NutriSystem tracking tool. Counselors are able to help clients wean off the program once goal weight is achieved. "NutriSystem Success" is a program that includes a portion-control container system to assist with making meals at home. Online resources are free.

Negatives

Diet may provide fewer calories than is generally recommended. While calorie level is designed for a loss of a pound or two each week, which is good, the "FreshStart" plan aims for women to lose up to 13 pounds and 7 inches in the first month, while men aim to lose 15 pounds and 7 inches. This rate of weight loss is not recommended. Becoming dependent on prepared foods may leave the user lost and uneducated on how to proceed once goal weight is reached. Eating prepacked foods can often isolate the dieter from friends and family during mealtimes. Consumption is mostly limited to purchased food items. Providing everything without education and learning how to eat limits a person's success in various unpredictable life situations. NutriSystem offers programs for teens ages 14 to 17.

*May vary depending on choices of prepackaged and grocery store items purchased.

The hook/catch or brilliant selling point: Ease of use, decreases the number of decisions to be made.

Truths/Myths

- **Myth** - Children ages 14 to 17 can benefit on their program.

- **Truth** - Children should not be put on a calorie-deficit program. Children need calories and nutrients to grow. If a child is overweight and should lose excess body fat, the recommended approach is to eat well-balanced, nutrient-dense meals and snacks at a calorie level that supports growth and increase exercise so they can grow into their weight.

- **Truth** - Relying on prepackaged foods can develop dependence on those meals and the system. Successful transitioning off the system is critical to long-term success. Thus, being educated and confident how to do this is imperative. This program allows for the consumer to shop for and choose certain foods, such as produce and meats, which provides practice for learning.

🔍 p. 16

Final decision: Thumbs up for adults who can afford the program and who are willing to put special effort into transitioning off the prepackaged foods. 👍

How to improve this diet: None worth noting.

The Obesity Code

Premise of the Diet: Intermittent fasting and eating whole, unprocessed foods help to balance hormones, which helps achieve long-term weight loss.

Claims of the Diet: Intermittent fasting allows the body to use its stored energy while insulin levels are low. Will reset and balance key hormones like insulin. The body exists only in two states: the fed state, when insulin levels are high; and the fasted state, when insulin levels are low. When insulin levels are high, fat is stored in the body.

Diet Description: Foods eaten include whole, unprocessed foods that trigger a minimal insulin response. The key, however, is when these foods are eaten. Incorporates short periods of intermittent fasting on a regular basis. There are many different types of fasts.

Short fasts are less than 24 hours.

- 16:8 – Eat all meals within 8 hours and fast for the remaining 16 hours. This pattern is usually practiced daily.

- 20:4 – All your meals are eaten within 4 hours and fast for the remaining 20 hours. In this pattern eat either one meal or two smaller meals during the feeding window.

Long fasts (more than 24 hours)

- 24-hour – Fast from dinner to dinner, or from lunch to lunch. This method allows eating once a day. Generally, this pattern is done two to three times a week.

- 5:2 – Usual eating for five days and fast for two days. Fast days usually consist of 500 calories each day.

- Alternate-day – Eat 500 calories every other day. Eat regularly on the alternate days.

The idea this diet proposes is that weight will be lost because insulin levels will lower during the fasting period.

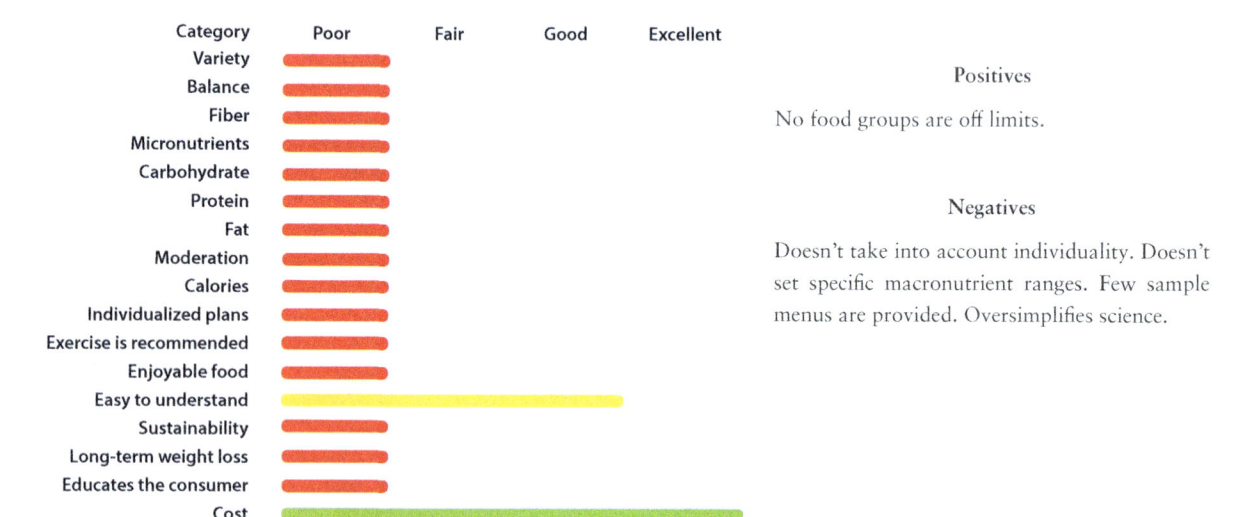

Category	Poor	Fair	Good	Excellent
Variety	▬			
Balance	▬			
Fiber	▬			
Micronutrients	▬			
Carbohydrate	▬			
Protein	▬			
Fat	▬			
Moderation	▬			
Calories	▬			
Individualized plans	▬			
Exercise is recommended	▬			
Enjoyable food	▬			
Easy to understand			▬	
Sustainability	▬			
Long-term weight loss	▬			
Educates the consumer	▬			
Cost				▬

Positives

No food groups are off limits.

Negatives

Doesn't take into account individuality. Doesn't set specific macronutrient ranges. Few sample menus are provided. Oversimplifies science.

The hook/catch or brilliant selling point: Unlocks the secret to weight loss.

Truths/Myths

• Myth - Weight gain and obesity in everyone are driven by hormones, and only by understanding the effects of insulin and insulin resistance can lasting weight loss be achieved.

• Truth - If hormonal imbalances are a problem, it is important to correct the imbalance. However, number of calories consumed also matters, and this diet doesn't consider individual causes for weight gain.

• Myth - Hormonal imbalances stem largely from food choices, frequent snacking, eating because it's mealtime not because of hunger, and consuming processed and refined foods with added carbohydrates, and added sugar. 🔍 p. 73

• Truth - Many things can cause hormonal imbalances. This diet does not take into account individuality.

• Myth - Fasting is a good approach for weight loss. 🔍 p. 78

• Truth - Studies indicate there is weight regain once fasting is done, especially if the fast moves the basal metabolic rate into a state of starvation.

• Truth - Short-term periods of rapid weight loss are mostly a loss of water and glycogen, not fat. 🔍 p. 15

• Truth - Insufficient research is available to conclusively show how each individual person's metabolism changes or adapts to repeated intermittent or alternate-day fasting.

• Truth - Insufficient research is available to know what the long-term health effects are of intermittent fasting.

• Truth - Depriving the body of food can lead to an unhealthy relationship with food and make weight loss more difficult. 🔍 p. 1

• Truth - It can be difficult to exercise while fasting due to low energy. Intermittent fasting will not allow full replenishment of glycogen stores, because trying to refuel more than 2 hours after exercise misses the primary window of opportunity to replenish glycogen stores for future bouts of exercise. 🔍 p. 105

• Truth - Exercise while fasting can result in stripping lean tissue. A net negative nitrogen balance will occur if the exerciser does not consume the necessary protein. Skeletal muscle protein degradation is elevated for 24-48 hours after exercise. Muscle net protein balance will remain negative without nutrient intake. If exercising during intermittent fasting, there is a decrease in circulating levels of amino acids, which can lead to an increase in muscle protein degradation, or an increase in amino acids released from muscles. This ultimately decreases metabolic rate, making it harder to lose weight.

• Truth - One study showed an increase in metabolic rate in healthy-weight subjects who did not eat for 4 days. However, the results of this study found that norepinephrine increased, with no change in insulin (the diet's named culprit). In other words, when food was not available, hormones adjusted, and this study found an increase in norepinephrine. Plasma glucose concentrations are increased by glucagon, epinephrine, norepinephrine but at the expense of lean tissue when the fast is longer than 72 hours. This time frame assumes glycogen stores are being completely restored between times of fasting. If glycogen stores are not completely restored, then lean tissue will be stripped earlier in the fast.

• Truth - Another study reported both lean and obese adults expended less energy during the morning when remaining in the fasted state than when consuming a breakfast.

• Myth - Much research supports the efficacy and safety of this type of diet.

• Truth - Much research done in this area has been conducted on near death anorexics, diabetics, children with epilepsy, rats, and penguins. Most people who undergo this diet do not fit into any of these categories.

• Myth - When insulin levels are low, the body switches to burning body fat. 🔍 p. 73

- Truth - This statement is only partially true. When insulin levels are low, glucagon levels are high, which means fat is released from body fat for fuel. However, this fat cannot be burned independent of carbohydrate or protein. Glucagon causes glucose to be released from glycogen stores in the liver and causes glucose to be made by the liver from lactate, glycerol, and select amino acids in the blood. This is done to maintain normal blood glucose levels for the brain, nervous system, and red blood cells. In addition, as glycogen stores are depleted in skeletal muscle, the muscle will use its own protein in order to burn fat for energy. This highlights that limiting protein and carbohydrates and focusing only on fat can lower the metabolism and make weight loss more difficult.

- Myth - All types of fasting are safe.

- Truth - Fasting for more than 14 days can lead to re-feeding syndrome, which involves a dangerous shift in fluids and electrolytes when food is re-introduced. 🔍 p. 79

Final decision: Thumbs down

How to improve this diet: Can't be improved.

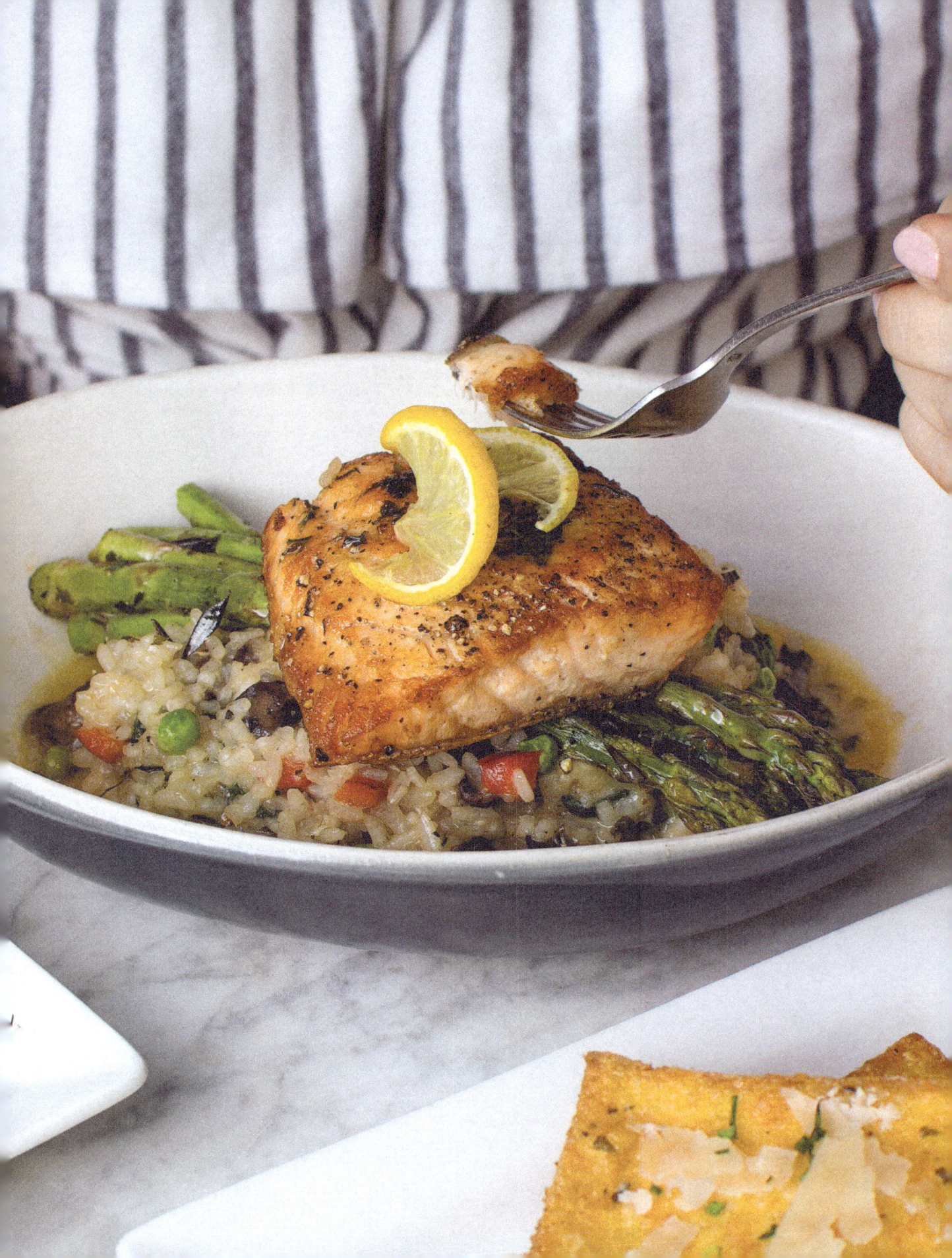

Omega-Z Diet

Premise of the Diet: Combines all the best weight-loss attributes and puts them in one diet. Provides simple dietary guidelines for optimal long-term weight loss.

Claims of the Diet: Teaches healthy eating and provides a researched rationale for healthy, sustainable weight loss.

Diet Description: Provides explanations while taking the dieter through a step-by-step process to determine their dietary needs and how to achieve healthy, sustainable weight loss.

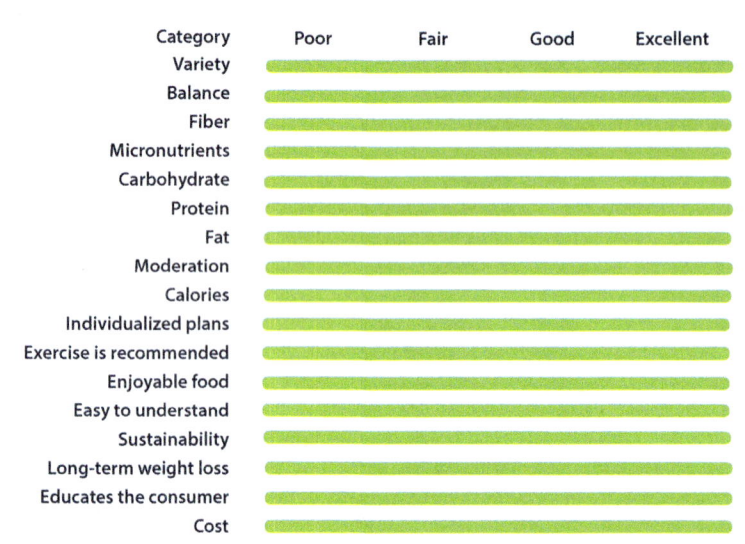

Category	Poor	Fair	Good	Excellent
Variety				✓
Balance				✓
Fiber				✓
Micronutrients				✓
Carbohydrate				✓
Protein				✓
Fat				✓
Moderation				✓
Calories				✓
Individualized plans				✓
Exercise is recommended				✓
Enjoyable food				✓
Easy to understand				✓
Sustainability				✓
Long-term weight loss				✓
Educates the consumer				✓
Cost				✓

Positives

Takes a holistic approach to creating a healthy lifestyle. Emphasizes fruits, vegetables, whole grains, and lean protein while minimizing fat, sugar, and fried foods. May help prevent some chronic conditions. Takes a healthful approach to weight loss. Emphasizes 150 minutes of exercise per week. Calls for cooking and eating a wide variety of foods. Based on solid research. Recommends keeping a food and physical activity record to help follow progress and identify problem areas. Is flexible and easy to modify to meet individual needs. Recommends nutrient-dense foods in small portions, no foods are forbidden. Recommends eating slowly. Educates people on how to get the most from the dining experience. Includes many helpful tips.

Negatives

None worth noting

The hook/catch or brilliant selling point: Combines the best attributes of the best weight loss diets.

Truths/Myths: None worth noting.

Final decision: Thumbs up 👍

How to improve this diet: None worth noting.

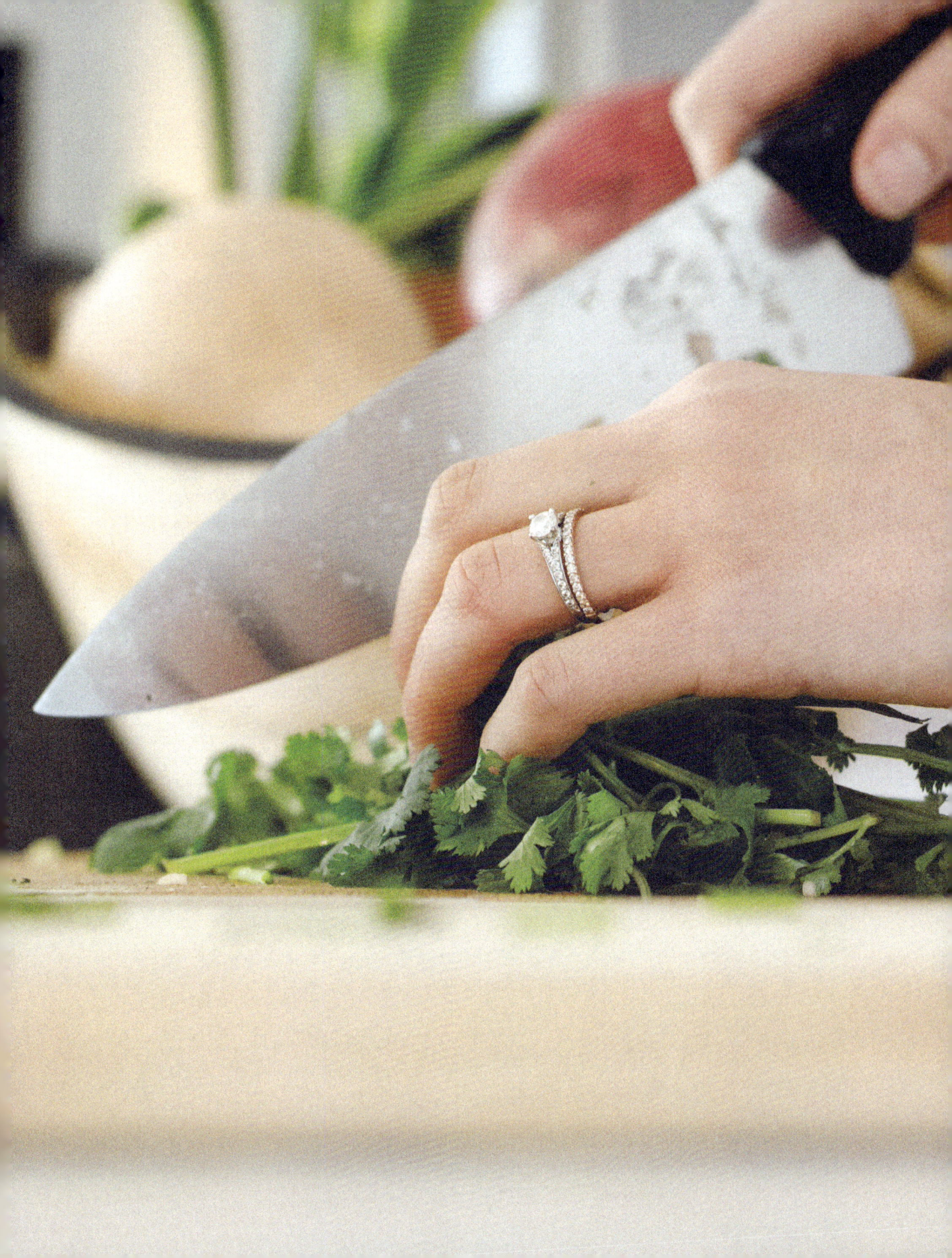

Optavia Diet

Premise of the Diet: Packaged bars, cookies, shakes, puddings, cereals, soups, and pastas that are reduced-carb, low-calorie, high in protein and probiotics.

Claims of the Diet: "No matter what you're facing, your Coach will be here to help steer you to success."

Diet Description: Includes two weight-loss programs and a weight-maintenance plan:

- Optimal Weight 5 & 1 Plan. Includes 5 Optavia Fuelings and 1 balanced Lean and Green meal daily. Provides 800–1,000 calories. Indicates 12 pounds can be lost over 12 weeks. You're meant to eat 1 meal every 2–3 hours and incorporate 30 minutes of moderate exercise most days of the week. One meal offers 5–7 ounces (145–200 grams) of cooked lean protein, 3 servings of non-starchy vegetables, and 2 servings of healthy fats. Provides no more than 100 grams of carbs per day.

- Optimal Weight 4 & 2 & 1 Plan. Provides more food flexibility and consists of 4 Optavia Fuelings, 2 Lean and Green meals, and 1 snack per day.

- Optimal Health 3 & 3 Plan. Consists of 3 Optavia Fuelings and 3 balanced Lean and Green meals per day for weight maintenance.

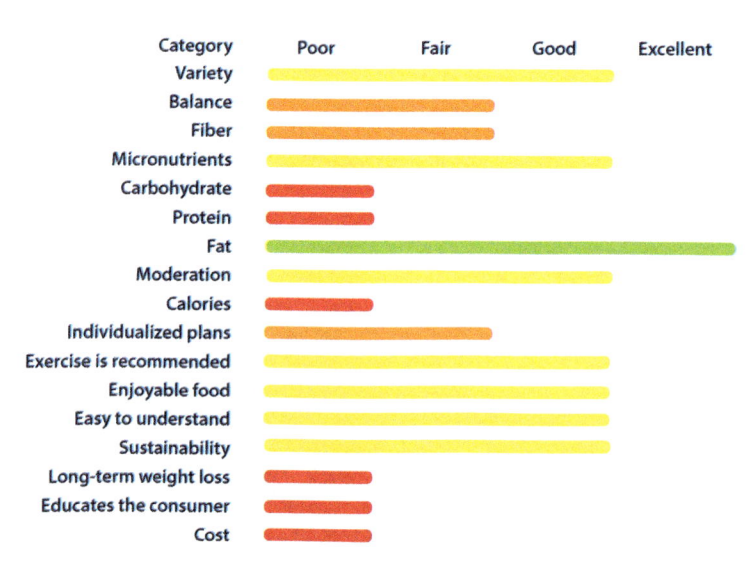

Category	Poor	Fair	Good	Excellent
Variety				Good
Balance		Fair		
Fiber		Fair		
Micronutrients				Good
Carbohydrate	Poor			
Protein	Poor			
Fat				Excellent
Moderation				Good
Calories	Poor			
Individualized plans		Fair		
Exercise is recommended				Good
Enjoyable food				Good
Easy to understand				Good
Sustainability				Good
Long-term weight loss	Poor			
Educates the consumer	Poor			
Cost	Poor			

Positives

Provides tools, including inspiring tips via text message, a dining-out guide, community forums, frequent support calls, and a meal and activity tracking app. Recommends meals be eaten every 2–3 hours and 30 minutes of moderate exercise most days of the week. Does not recommend skipping meals.

Negatives

Has limited food options and relies severely on prepackaged, heavily processed meals and snacks. Optavia coaches get paid on commission. The cost for one month's supply of Optavia Fuelings exceeds $400 on the 5&1 Plan, which substitutes for three to five daily meals depending on the plan. At 800-1,000 calories a day, the Optimal Weight 5 & 1 Plan is too low and unsafe for most people trying to lose weight. 🔍 p. 13

The hook/catch or brilliant selling point: Support and guidance increase chances for success – You will not be alone.

Truths/Myths

- Myth - None worth mentioning

- Truth - While support and guidance do increase chances for successful weight loss, it is difficult to determine the level of integrity coaches will have, since they are compensated based on orders placed by their personally-sponsored and supported Clients.

- Truth - Coaches are past clients who were successful with their weight loss; they are not required to be educated in a health or nutrition field.

Final decision: Thumbs down

How to improve this diet: Learn to portion real, whole foods. To avoid monotony, increase variety of meals allowed. Determine how many calories are needed for safe weight loss based on your individual requirements. Consume all macronutrients within the AMDR.

Park Avenue Diet

Premise of the Diet: A complete makeover. A lifetime of beauty and health.

Claims of the Diet: Will help people look and feel their best, lose weight, and attract the people and opportunities they desire.

Diet Description: A six-week program that addresses lifestyle components, including beauty, etiquette, poise, fitness, fashion weight, physique, hair, skin, clothing, self-confidence, and interpersonal skills. Phase 1 is a two-week self-discovery stage that teaches you how to apply each of the seven principles discussed in the book. Phase 2 is a week of "preparing for greatness" by practicing new skills. Phase 3, "making the A-list," unveils a "new you."

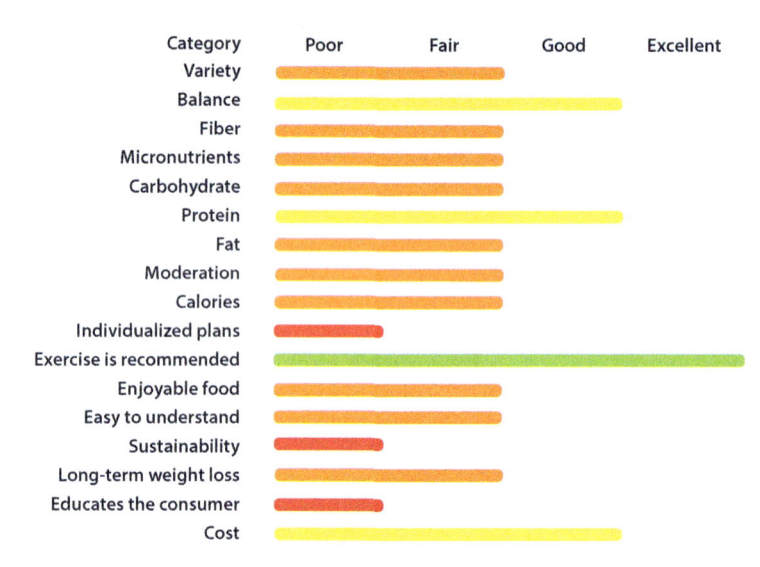

Category	Rating
Variety	Poor–Fair
Balance	Good
Fiber	Poor–Fair
Micronutrients	Poor–Fair
Carbohydrate	Poor–Fair
Protein	Good
Fat	Poor–Fair
Moderation	Poor–Fair
Calories	Poor–Fair
Individualized plans	Poor
Exercise is recommended	Excellent
Enjoyable food	Poor–Fair
Easy to understand	Poor–Fair
Sustainability	Poor
Long-term weight loss	Poor–Fair
Educates the consumer	Poor
Cost	Good

Positives

Includes lots of fruits, vegetables, lean meats, and seafood. Provides rather balanced menu plans and recipes. Recommended foods are readily available by most people. Exercises that increase in intensity and that can be done at home are outlined for 42 days.

Negatives

Low-calorie (1,250-1,350) restrictive diet. Not a healthy lifelong approach to weight loss. The calorie level is inadequate for many and may not adequately satisfy hunger. There is no guidance on exercise, calories, or alcohol. Dietary supplements are sold. While the book only briefly addresses weight maintenance, no particular plan is provided. Because of the limited amounts of whole grains and dairy, the suggested menus may be deficient in calcium, vitamin D, and potassium. 🔍 p. 22, 67, 39, 29

The hook/catch or brilliant selling point: Uses a popular location to grab attention, while addressing topics in addition to dietary intake.

Truths/Myths: None worth mentioning

Final decision: Thumbs down 👎

How to improve this diet: Determine how many calories are needed to maintain current weight, then subtract 500 calories from that total for a slow (1-2 pound a week) weight loss. Add low or non-fat dairy foods, along with whole grains, to this diet.

Perricone Diet

Premise of the Diet: Establish new dietary changes over time, leading to healthier long-term choices and lasting weight loss by eating anti-inflammatory foods rich in antioxidants and omega-3 fatty acids.

Claims of the Diet: Helps weight loss and keeps skin looking youthful.

Diet Description: A 28-day diet that begins with a restrictive 3-day diet. The 3-day diet features salmon, tofu, or poultry twice a day. After the initial 3 days, the food choices are less restrictive and are consumed in three meals and two snacks daily. Eliminates breads, cereals, crackers, fried foods, soft drinks, many processed foods, most snack foods, and desserts. Each meal includes lean protein, fruits and/or vegetables, and essential fatty acids from olive oil or nuts. Meals and snacks include a protein, which is eaten first. Allows for up to 2 ounces of antioxidant-rich dark chocolate a day.

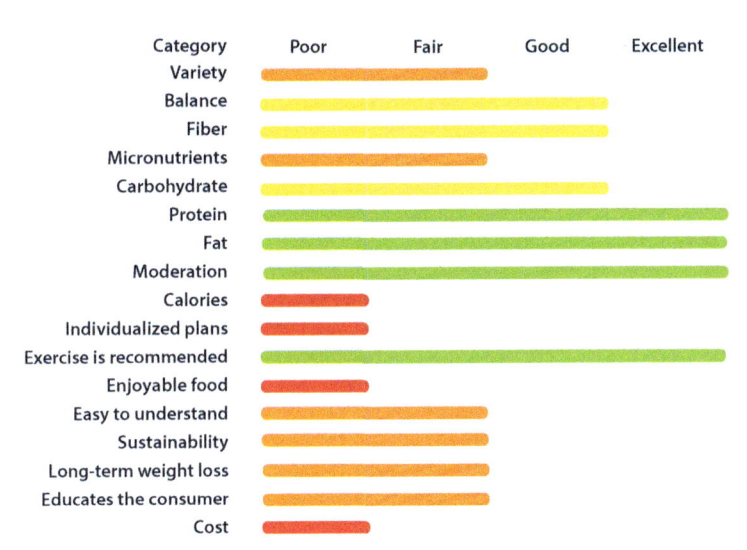

Category	Poor	Fair	Good	Excellent
Variety		■		
Balance			■	
Fiber			■	
Micronutrients		■		
Carbohydrate			■	
Protein				■
Fat				■
Moderation				■
Calories	■			
Individualized plans	■			
Exercise is recommended				■
Enjoyable food	■			
Easy to understand		■		
Sustainability		■		
Long-term weight loss		■		
Educates the consumer		■		
Cost	■			

Positives

High in salmon, fruit, and vegetables. Emphasizes fish as the "go-to" protein source, which is a major source of healthy fats, vitamin D, and selenium.

Negatives

Perricone's brand supplements are an important part of Perricone's plan. Requires 27 supplements a day. A packet of eight supplements, plus an extra omega-3 supplement, must be consumed an hour before every meal. A 30-day supply costs $150+. Supplements are at the heart of Dr. Perricone's philosophy on healthy aging and beautiful skin. The do-not-eat list is long and includes many foods.

The hook/catch or brilliant selling point: Written by respected physician, award-winning researcher, and bestselling author.

Truths/Myths

- Myth - It is important to avoid all foods associated with inflammation.

- Truth - A balance of food choices is important for weight loss. While constant consumption of many inflammation-inducing foods is unwise, eliminating all may not be realistic, leading to the inability to continue the diet. In biochemistry, eicosanoids are signaling molecules made by fatty acids. They exert complex control over many bodily systems, mainly in inflammation or immunity, and as messengers in the central nervous system. Eicosanoids help regulate blood clotting, blood pressure, immune function, and other body processes. The amount and balance of these fats in a diet will have an effect on cardiovascular disease, triglycerides, blood pressure and arthritis. The effect of an eicosanoid on these functions depends on the fatty acid from which it is made. p. 55

Final decision: Thumbs down

How to improve this diet: Don't purchase the supplements. Skip the very restrictive three-day diet and begin with the less restrictive 28-day diet. Mindfully consider the frequency of foods eaten on the "do not eat" list. Since weight loss comes down to how many calories are consumed versus how many are expended, be sure to consume approximately 500 calories a day less than are expended.

p. 99

Personality Type Diet

Premise of the Diet: Most diets fail because they do not address life patterns that can make us gain weight. This diet figures out our specific challenges to weight loss, then shows us how to overcome them.

Claims of the Diet: When patterns that keep people overweight are addressed, weight can be lost.

Diet Description: Answer 66 questions about personal habits and feelings toward eating patterns and exercise habits. A few categories include: "Mindless Muncher," "Nighttime Nibbler," "Hate-to-Move Struggler," "Persistent Procrastinator," or "No-Time-to-Exercise Protester." Based on categories, sensible advice and tips are offered. In general, the diet is based on low-fat foods while highlighting super foods such as fruits, vegetables, grains, nuts, seeds, dried beans, lentils, and soy products.

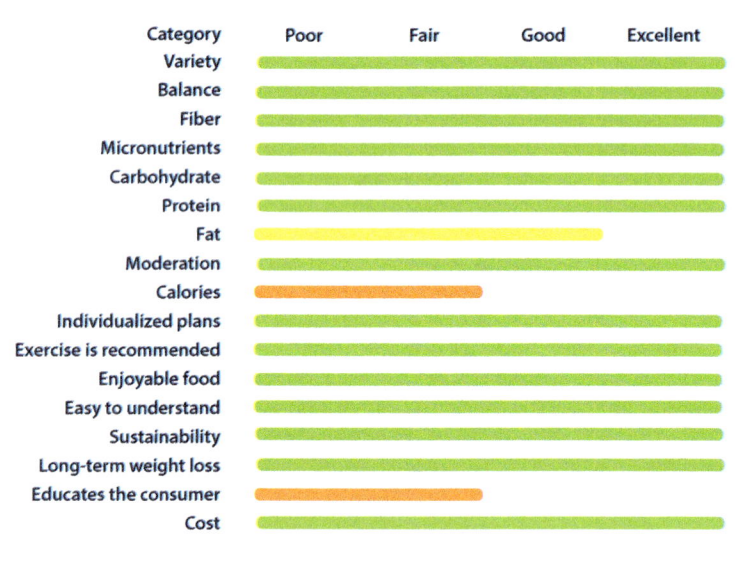

Category	Poor	Fair	Good	Excellent
Variety				●
Balance				●
Fiber				●
Micronutrients				●
Carbohydrate				●
Protein				●
Fat			●	
Moderation				●
Calories		●		
Individualized plans				●
Exercise is recommended				●
Enjoyable food				●
Easy to understand				●
Sustainability				●
Long-term weight loss				●
Educates the consumer		●		
Cost				●

Positives

No foods are forbidden. Everything is allowed in moderation. Gaining insight into eating and exercise habits as they relate to personality is helpful. The program is based on vegetarian, low-fat foods. It also highlights nutrient-dense foods, such as fruits, vegetables, and nuts. Is affordable and nonrestrictive and can be adapted to personal preferences. This plan is based on solid, evidence-supported principles of healthful eating and is designed to be sustained over time, which increases the likelihood of success.

Negatives

Does not provide much education to dieters. Calorie levels are not clearly addressed. In general, eating a vegetarian diet without proper planning can leave the dieter at risk of B12, calcium, zinc, and iron deficiencies.

The hook/catch or brilliant selling point: Information on personalities is always exciting and interesting.

Truths/Myths

- Truth - Understanding personality traits can help us better understand and ultimately change habits and behaviors that can lead to better weight management. 🔍 p. 1

- Truth - If many changes need to be made or deep psychological trauma has been experienced, professional help from a dietitian, social worker or psychologist may be necessary to overcome some behaviors.

Final decision: Thumbs up 👍

How to improve this diet: Additional calories may be needed for very active individuals. Be sure to monitor the number of calories consumed necessary to reach individual goals.

Potato Hack Diet (aka Potato Diet)

Premise of the Diet: Potatoes contain proteinase inhibitor 2 that may help decrease hunger.

Claims of the Diet: Lose up to 1 pound a day, strengthen the immune system, improve gut health, and acquire necessary nutrients during weight loss.

Diet Description: For 3-5 days, eat 2-5 pounds of plain potatoes daily.

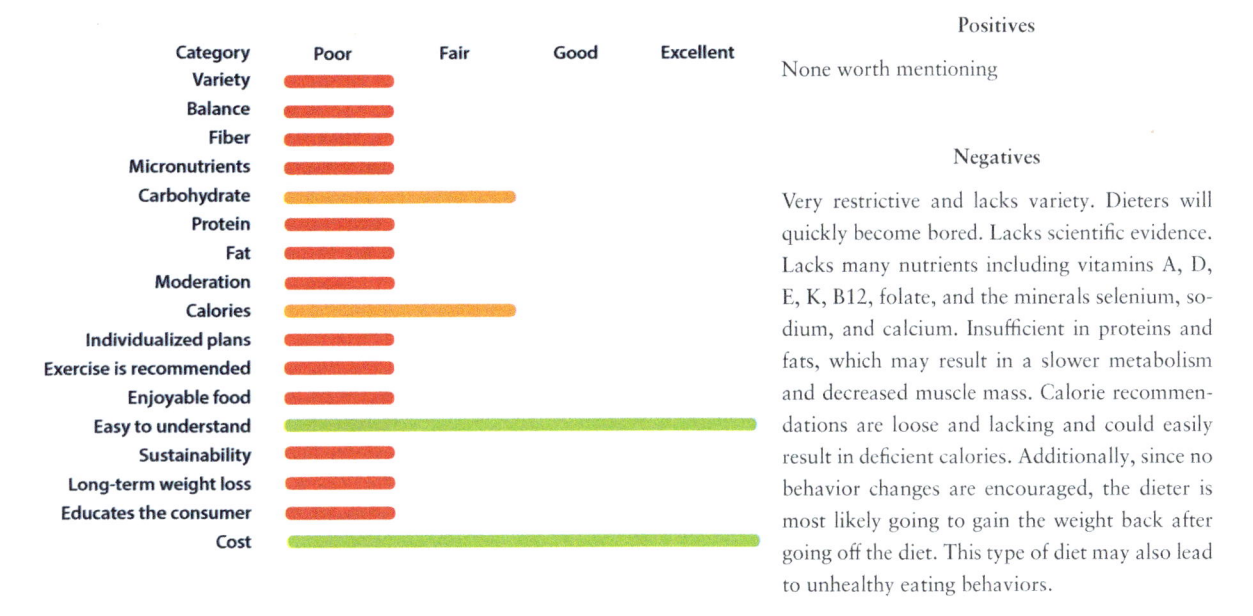

Category	Poor	Fair	Good	Excellent
Variety	▬			
Balance	▬			
Fiber	▬			
Micronutrients	▬			
Carbohydrate		▬▬▬		
Protein	▬			
Fat	▬			
Moderation	▬			
Calories		▬▬		
Individualized plans	▬			
Exercise is recommended	▬			
Enjoyable food	▬			
Easy to understand				▬▬▬▬▬
Sustainability	▬			
Long-term weight loss	▬			
Educates the consumer	▬			
Cost				▬▬▬▬▬

Positives
None worth mentioning

Negatives
Very restrictive and lacks variety. Dieters will quickly become bored. Lacks scientific evidence. Lacks many nutrients including vitamins A, D, E, K, B12, folate, and the minerals selenium, sodium, and calcium. Insufficient in proteins and fats, which may result in a slower metabolism and decreased muscle mass. Calorie recommendations are loose and lacking and could easily result in deficient calories. Additionally, since no behavior changes are encouraged, the dieter is most likely going to gain the weight back after going off the diet. This type of diet may also lead to unhealthy eating behaviors.

The hook/catch or brilliant selling point: So simple and calls to people who love potatoes.

Truths/Myths

- *Myth* - Potatoes are the "best diet pill ever invented."

- *Truth* - Diets need to provide adequate nutrients for growth, repair and maintenance of the body. Too many nutrients are missing for this diet to be healthy or sustainable.

- *Truth* - Dieters will get bored quickly with this repetitive, monotonous intake. 🔍 p. 29

Final decision: Thumbs down 👎

How to improve this diet: Can't be improved

The Pritikin Principle
(aka The Pritikin Principle: The Calorie Density Solution)

Premise of the Diet: The basic idea is to choose foods that are "nutrient-dense" and plant-based.

Claims of the Diet: This diet outlines principles for losing weight and maintaining a healthy fitness level.

Diet Description: The Pritikin Principle provides many charts listing the caloric density of foods. Recommends eating foods that have a lot of fiber and water, such as vegetables, fruits, beans, and natural, unprocessed grains. The dieter calculates the "average caloric density of meals," then keeps that average number in goal range.

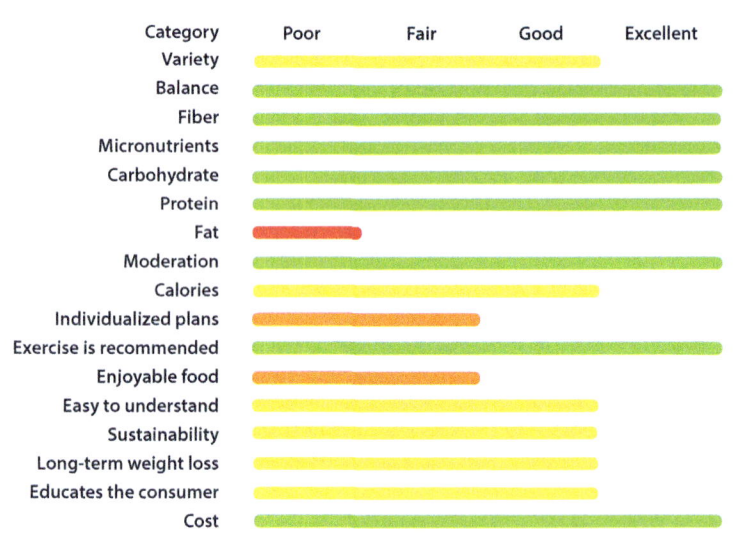

Category	Poor	Fair	Good	Excellent
Variety			███	
Balance				███
Fiber				███
Micronutrients				███
Carbohydrate				███
Protein				███
Fat	██			
Moderation				███
Calories			███	
Individualized plans		██		
Exercise is recommended				███
Enjoyable food		██		
Easy to understand			███	
Sustainability			███	
Long-term weight loss			███	
Educates the consumer			███	
Cost				███

Positives

Includes menu plans, recipes, and exercise routines. Follows many of the key recommendations from the DIETARY GUIDELINES FOR AMERICANS 2015-2020, including: a variety of vegetables from all of the subgroups: dark green, red and orange, legumes (beans and peas), starchy, fruits, whole grains, fat-free or low-fat dairy, including milk, yogurt, cheese, and/or fortified soy beverages, seeds, and soy products, less than 10% of calories per day from saturated fats, less than 10% of calories per day from added sugars, and less than 2,300 milligrams (mg) per day of sodium. Recommends 45 minutes of moderate exercise daily.

Negatives

For some, the very low-fat content may make the plan difficult to follow.

The hook/catch or brilliant selling point: Appeared on the "60 Minutes" program in 1977 and soon became the most popular diet of the 1970s.

Truths/Myths

- **Myth** - None worth noting.

- **Truth** - Weight will be lost on the Pritikin diet when strictly followed.

- **Truth** - It is nutritionally-rich/nutrient-dense.

- **Truth** - Usually, a very low-fat diet leaves people feeling hungry. In other words, fat makes us feel full. Being hungry usually causes people to eat. However, the foods/plans provided in Pritikin are high in fiber, which can cause fullness and satisfaction.

- **Truth** - The Pritikin Plan recommends fewer than 10% of calories from fats. This is lower than the (AMDR) for fat intake, which is between 20 to 35% of total dietary calories. 🔍 p. 55

Final decision: Thumbs up 👍

How to improve this diet: Increase healthy fats to individual satisfaction within AMDR.

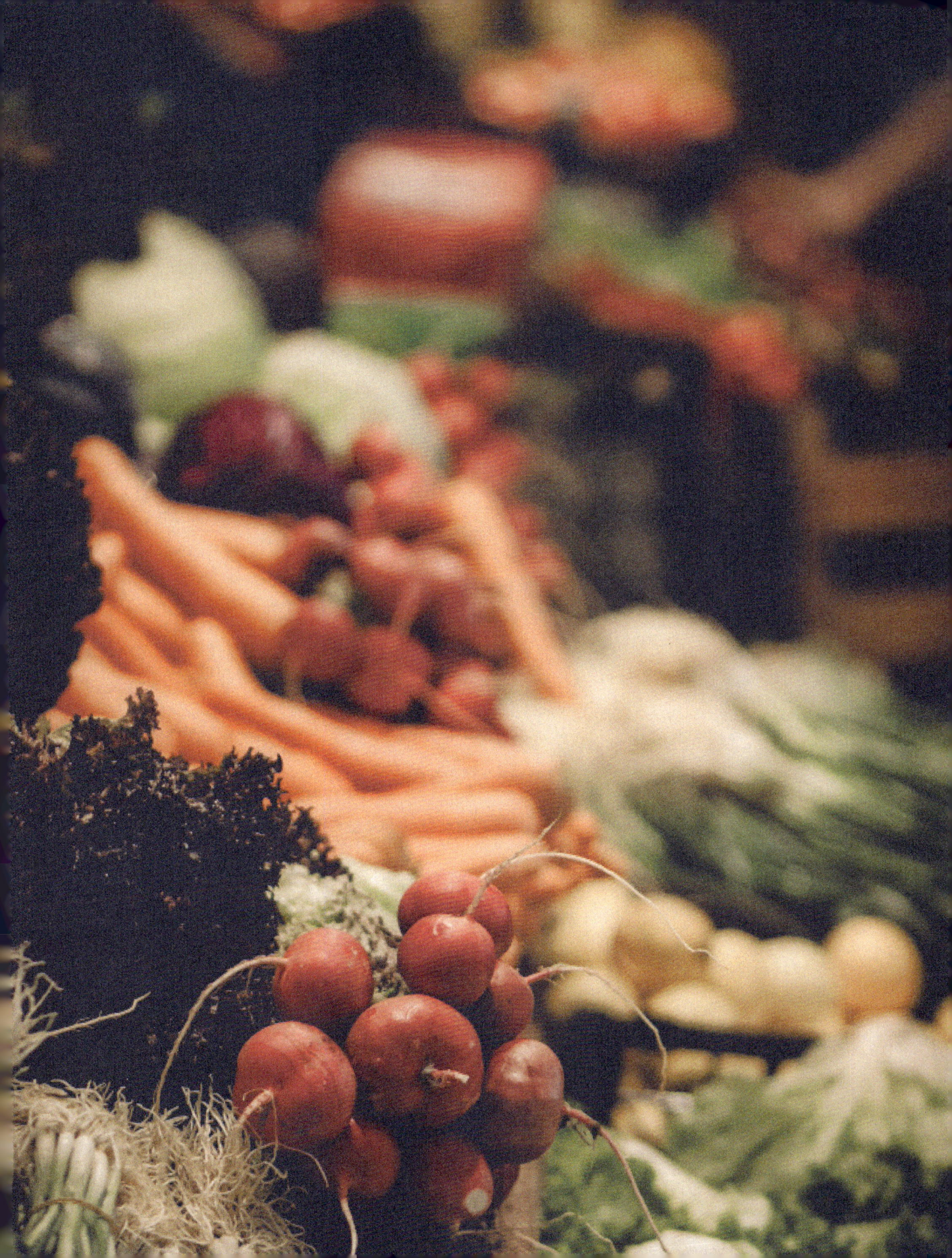

Protein Power Diet

Premise of the Diet: A low-carb diet (< 20% of total calories or less than 100 grams of carbs per day).

Claims of the Diet: This is a revolutionary and deliciously satisfying plan that has helped thousands lose weight and achieve life-saving health benefits.

Diet Description: Similar in many ways to the Atkins program, except in the way caloric values are determined. Atkins does not limit calories. It only limits carbohydrates, while the Protein Power Diet directly links caloric intake to protein requirements. Reduce carbohydrate intake until the body switches to ketosis (using fat for fuel). Slowly reintroduce low-glycemic carbs back into the diet, until carbohydrates consumption is slightly more than protein consumption. More specifically, Phase 1 should be implemented by individuals 20% over their healthy body weight. They are required to reduce carbohydrates to a maximum of 30 grams per day. Phase 2 is for those individuals who are less than 20% over their ideal body weight. It is recommended that those individuals reduce their carbohydrate intake to 55 grams per day.

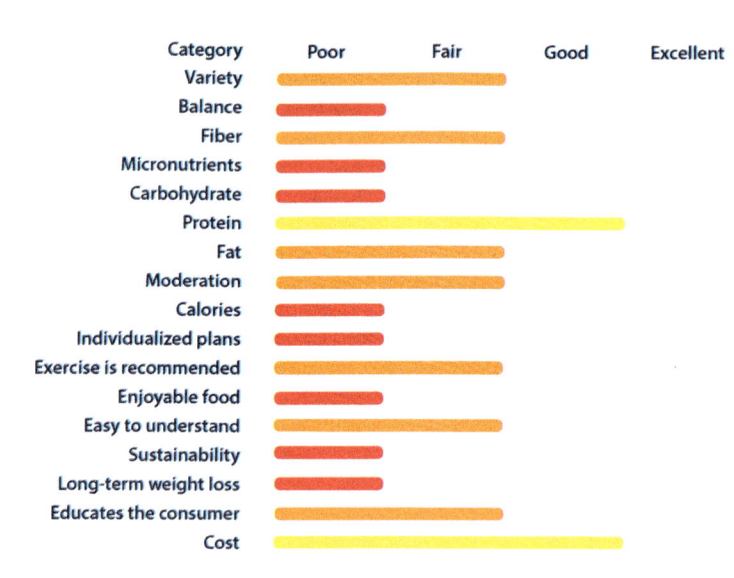

Category	Poor	Fair	Good	Excellent
Variety		██		
Balance	█			
Fiber		██		
Micronutrients	█			
Carbohydrate	█			
Protein				████
Fat		██		
Moderation		██		
Calories	█			
Individualized plans	█			
Exercise is recommended		██		
Enjoyable food	█			
Easy to understand		█▌		
Sustainability	█			
Long-term weight loss	█			
Educates the consumer		█▌		
Cost				████

Positives

Provides explanations, encouragement, and practical suggestions for eating out. Allows numerous vegetables. Suggests resistance training, such as weight-lifting, to help burn stored fat. Recommends 25 grams of fiber daily.

Negatives

Too much protein can raise uric acid levels, which can cause gout and can exacerbate problems for those with kidney problems. It is easy to consume too much fat on this diet if careful attention is not focused on choices. Women of childbearing age need folate, which is added to many grain products. Thus, this diet is concerning for women of child-bearing age. Pre-pregnancy weight loss is best done with a balanced diet. While weight training is healthy, so are cardiovascular exercises, which are not adequately recommended. A daily supplement is needed to cover the nutritional gaps that emerge from eliminating various food groups.

The hook/catch or brilliant selling point: Protein is good! Right?

Truths/Myths

- **Myth** - Carbs and weight loss are closely related.

- **Truth** - Actually, calories and weight loss are closely related.

- **Myth** - Limiting carbohydrates (sugar) means the body will burn fat, including body fat, for fuel. 🔍 p. 21, 73

- **Truth** - Limiting calories (regardless of their source) means the body may have to tap into body fat for fuel. Eating calories that provide carbs, proteins, and fats in recommended amounts and in sufficient amounts to meet BMR while exercising is the best way to burn body fat.

- **Myth** - There are no dangers associated with this style of eating.

- **Truth** - This type of diet should only be conducted under the close supervision of a physician. Attempting to try this diet without a physician's supervision can be dangerous. 🔍 p. 78

Final decision: Thumbs down 👎

How to improve this diet: Add adequate carbohydrates in the form of complex carbohydrates. Carbohydrates should be at least 45-65% of all calories consumed. Continue to eat a variety of fruits, vegetables and lean meats, and consume no more than 35% of calories from fat sources.

Raw Food Diet

Premise of the Diet: Three quarters of the diet involves unprocessed, whole, plant-based (preferably organic) foods.

Claims of the Diet: Eating mostly raw foods is healthier and provides more energy, better digestion, clearer skin, and a lower risk of developing heart disease than eating cooked foods.

Diet Description: Food needs to be prepared a special way. The only heating allowed is with a dehydrator, using temperatures that do not exceed 116 Fahrenheit. Dehydrators blow hot air through food. Grain and bean seeds are eaten soaked and sprouted. Nuts can also be soaked. Fruits and vegetables may be juiced or used in smoothies.

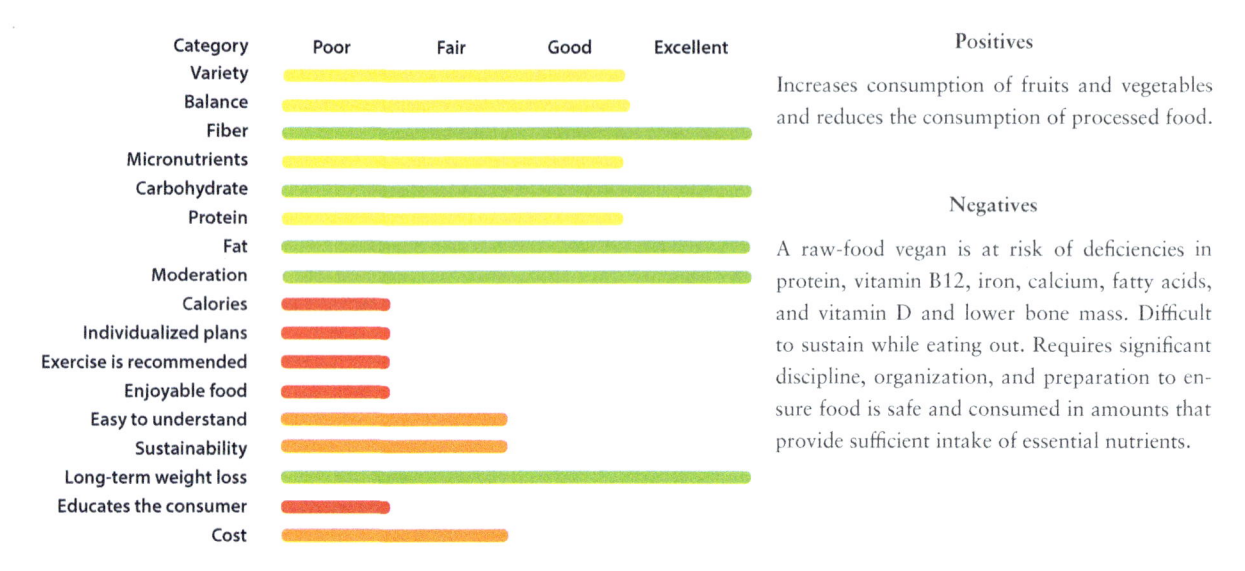

Category	Rating
Variety	Fair
Balance	Fair
Fiber	Excellent
Micronutrients	Fair
Carbohydrate	Excellent
Protein	Fair
Fat	Excellent
Moderation	Excellent
Calories	Poor
Individualized plans	Poor
Exercise is recommended	Poor
Enjoyable food	Poor
Easy to understand	Fair
Sustainability	Fair
Long-term weight loss	Excellent
Educates the consumer	Poor
Cost	Fair

Positives

Increases consumption of fruits and vegetables and reduces the consumption of processed food.

Negatives

A raw-food vegan is at risk of deficiencies in protein, vitamin B12, iron, calcium, fatty acids, and vitamin D and lower bone mass. Difficult to sustain while eating out. Requires significant discipline, organization, and preparation to ensure food is safe and consumed in amounts that provide sufficient intake of essential nutrients.

The hook/catch or brilliant selling point: Let's get back to nature. The more natural the better.

Truths/Myths

- Myth - A raw-food diet is better able to prevent and fight diseases, especially chronic diseases, because raw and living foods contain essential enzymes. Heating food destroys these enzymes. Enzymes are the life force of a food, allowing human bodies to fully digest foods without having to rely on human digestive enzymes. Cooked foods take longer to digest and clog up the digestive system and arteries with partially digested foods.

- Truth - Scientific research has not confirmed this.

- Truth - Some water-soluble vitamins, particularly B and C, are reduced or destroyed by cooking, so eating food raw ensures a better supply of these.

- Truth - Studies have indicated a plant-based diet (but not necessarily raw) can lead to weight loss and reduce the risk of chronic disease, including cardiovascular disease, cancer, obesity, and type 2 diabetes.

- Truth - Some vegetables may be more beneficial when cooked. For example, cooking tomatoes makes the antioxidant lycopene available.

- Truth - Cooking kills some toxins, bacteria, and harmful compounds in food. The following foods should not be eaten raw:

  - Alfalfa sprouts contain canavanine, which has a lupus-inducing potential.

  - Apricot kernels contain amygdalin, an extract derived from apricot pits and other plants. It can be broken down by human intestine enzymes to produce cyanide, a known poison.

  - Buckwheat contains fagopyrins in the greens and if eaten raw in large quantities can trigger photosensitivity and other skin problems in people with fair skin.

  - Cassava is a root vegetable (a tuber crop). It is the underground part of the cassava shrub. It is critical to peel cassava and never eat it raw because it contains dangerous levels of cyanide unless cooked thoroughly.

  - Kidney beans contain phytohaemagglutinins, or lectins. Thus, some raw kidney beans and kidney bean sprouts may be toxic when eaten raw. When consumed raw, they interfere with digestion in the small intestine. Lectins resist digestion, bind to surface receptors, and cause changes in the metabolism of the epithelial cells. These changes include cell hypertrophy (cell expansion) and hyperplasia (cell overproduction), which can result in increased sensitivity to bacterial infection and reduced nutrient absorption. Legume species with the highest amounts of lectin include *Phaseolus vulgaris*, aka the kidney bean; *Phaseolus coccineus*, aka the scarlet runner bean; and *Phaseolus acuifolius*, aka the tepary bean. As such, these should not be eaten raw. A safer alternative, like legume species with little to no lectin activity, include *Cicer arietinum*, aka the chickpea; *Vigna unguiculata*, aka cow peas (black-eyed peas, field peas, or Southern peas); *Vicia faba*, aka fava bean; *Lens culinaris*, aka lentil; *Vigna radiate*, aka mung bean; *Pisum sativum*, aka peas; *Cajanus cajan*, aka the pigeon pea; and *Glycine max*, aka the soybean. Beans with high amounts of lectins can be rendered safe by long soaking and heat treatment prior to consumption.

  - Meat can pass on dangerous bacteria, parasites, and viruses. Cooking to the right temperature kills harmful germs.

  - Milk, when not pasteurized, can contain *Mycobacteria bovis (M. bovis)*, which can cause non-pulmonary tuberculosis and can affect the lungs, lymph nodes, and other parts of the body. The most common way people are infected with *M. bovis* is by eating or drinking contaminated, unpasteurized dairy products. The heating and cooling process of pasteurization destroys disease-causing organisms in milk products.

  - Pea seeds of the Lathyrus type can cause neurological weakness of the lower limbs, tremors, muscular weakness, and paraplegia.

  - Parsnips contain furanocoumarins chemicals produced by plants as a defense mechanism against predators. Furanocoumarins can be toxic.

  - Raw eggs can contain salmonella bacteria, which can cause serious illness and death. Cooking eggs kills the bacteria.

Final decision: Thumbs down 👎

How to improve this diet: Continue to eat an adequate amount of fruits and vegetables, but cook all the above foods that are dangerous if eaten raw.

Rice Diet Solution (aka Rice Diet)

Premise of the Diet: A physical, emotional, and spiritual program that will improve life.

Claims of the Diet: Lose weight by "cleansing and detoxifying" and reducing calories, sodium, fat, sugar, and protein without feeling hungry.

Diet Description: Three phases. The first phase permits 800 calories daily, then the calorie level gradually increases to 1,200 daily. Servings of starch, nonfat dairy, fruits, and vegetables are consumed daily. Plan is low-fat, including low- or no-fat dairy, while all the protein is very lean.

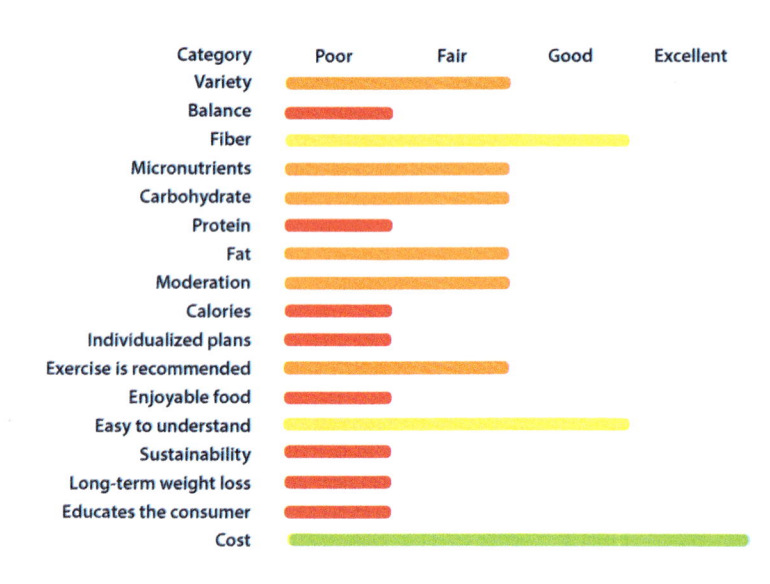

Category	Poor	Fair	Good	Excellent
Variety		▇		
Balance	▇			
Fiber			▇	
Micronutrients		▇		
Carbohydrate		▇		
Protein	▇			
Fat		▇		
Moderation		▇		
Calories	▇			
Individualized plans	▇			
Exercise is recommended		▇		
Enjoyable food	▇			
Easy to understand			▇	
Sustainability	▇			
Long-term weight loss	▇			
Educates the consumer	▇			
Cost				▇

Positives

Recommends exercise, keeping a food journal, and meditation to manage stress. Includes fresh fruits and vegetables, whole grains, low-salt beans, and lean protein. The abundant amount of high-fiber foods can reduce hunger and help fill up.

Negatives

Doesn't provide enough calcium and vitamin D. Insufficient protein is provided. Rather inflexible, low in calories and restrictive, thus challenging to stay on, especially at social events and while eating out. The low amount of protein may lead to loss of muscle mass and hinder feelings of fullness. The rules and limited food choices may take away some of the pleasure of eating. p. 29

The hook/catch or brilliant selling point: Non-offensive and not intimidating

Truths/Myths

- Myth - Will detoxify the body. p. 13

- Truth - There is no evidence that diets that claim to detoxify the body actually remove toxins.

Final decision: Thumbs down

How to improve this diet: Can't be improved.

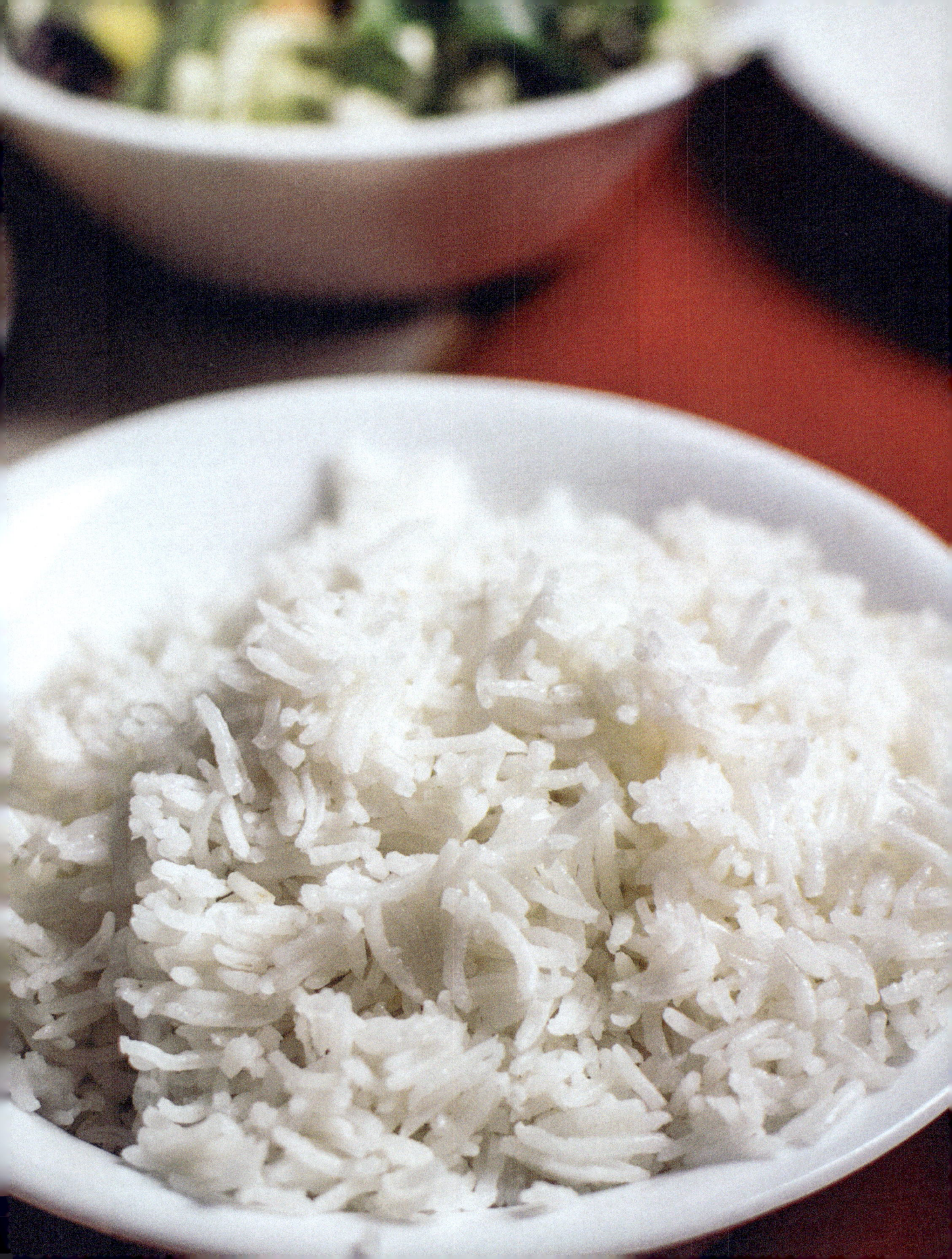

Senza (Ketogenic and Fasting Diet)

Premise of the Diet: Keto and fasting go hand in hand. Discover just how good you'll feel when you maximize the benefits of both.

Claims of the Diet: Keto isn't the only way to recover your health, but in our experience, it is the most measurable one.

Diet Description: Senza is an app dedicated to keto dieting. It verifies net carbs with time-based logging, provides a directory of keto-friendly meal ideas, and offers digital health coaching. Senza also provides shopping lists and meal plans that include products they sell, such as spices that cost $10 for 1.5 oz, keto cacao powder 8 oz for $13, 3.9 oz of salt for $8, 11 oz of keto granola cereal for $12, and fat fuel coffee for $2.75 a cup. Meal planning assistance can be requested on the Order page in exchange for points. Points are earned by using the app to log, share, and monitor progress.

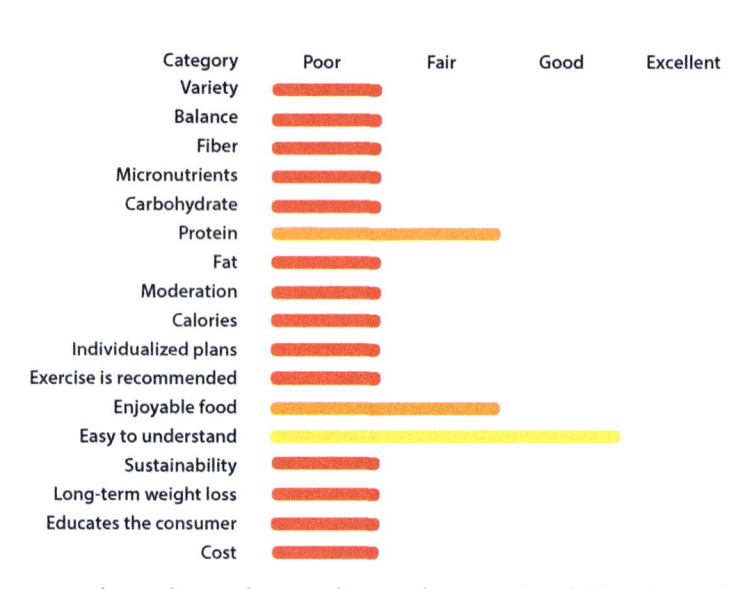

Category	Poor	Fair	Good	Excellent
Variety	■			
Balance	■			
Fiber	■			
Micronutrients	■			
Carbohydrate	■			
Protein		■		
Fat	■			
Moderation	■			
Calories	■			
Individualized plans	■			
Exercise is recommended	■			
Enjoyable food		■		
Easy to understand			■	
Sustainability	■			
Long-term weight loss	■			
Educates the consumer	■			
Cost	■			

Positives

While this diet might not provide health benefits for an otherwise healthy person, under close doctor supervision, it may be beneficial for diabetics because reducing carbohydrate consumption reduces the need for insulin to be secreted, which can improve insulin sensitivity. May feel fuller for a longer period of time. Some healthy unsaturated fats are allowed on the keto diet—like nuts (almonds, walnuts), seeds, avocados, tofu, and olive oil.

Negatives

Keeping the body in a state of ketosis requires strict adherence. Cheating or sneaking just a few carbohydrates is enough to disrupt the state of ketosis. Ketosis is a slower process of producing energy, thus no bursts of energy after a meal are experienced. There is no calorie restriction. Carbohydrates, which are restricted on this diet, are a large source of daily fiber. Weight loss may be short-lived because the diet is difficult to stick with long term, so the likelihood of returning to old eating habits is great. Many experience "keto flu" their first week on the diet, which leaves them feeling fatigue, brain fog, nausea, headaches, and muscle cramps. Protein sources come from both lean protein foods and foods high in saturated fat.

The hook/catch or brilliant selling point: Everything is provided to follow the keto diet.

Truths/Myths

- **Myth** - The big food system which everyone is familiar with is unhealthy and all wrong. The Senza system believes the only solution is to start over with a small-scale system built around real foods.

- **Truth** - The Senza system states that its system is built around "real foods" yet sells mostly highly processed products.

- **Myth** - The only solution to the big food system everyone is familiar with is to start over with a small-scale system built around the current understanding of nutrition science, which includes the 43 essential nutrients humans need to thrive. These nutrients come from about 100 basic foods, not from mass-produced mono-crop products.

- **Truth** - The current understanding of nutrition science is that we don't know what we don't even know yet. In addition to the macro- and micronutrients, science has discovered thousands of phytochemicals found in real foods that are beneficial to health.

• Myth - We are building the foundation for a decentralized food system—one that will restore human health and foster authentic social connections, one community at a time.

• Truth - Their food system is centralized in the Senza company, and prepackaged keto-friendly foods do not foster authentic social connections, but rather isolation.

• Myth - Because there is solid evidence showing a ketogenic diet is beneficial in reducing seizures in children, these neuroprotective effects must be beneficial for other brain disorders like Parkinson's, Alzheimer's, multiple sclerosis, and autism.

• Truth - While there is strong evidence showing a ketogenic diet reduces seizures in children, sometimes as effectively as medication, there is little to no human research that supports recommending ketosis to treat these other conditions. In fact, because it is not easy to get an adult body into deep ketosis, which is necessary to have an impact on epilepsy, health care providers in general do not attempt or recommend this approach except in the case of diabetes. In the case of diabetes, close monitoring of patients for potential problems and to ensure they are actually staying in ketosis is required. Because the truth is, staying in true, deep ketosis is especially challenging for adults. That is why the medical diet is used to treat children and infants with epilepsy because it's easier. In many instances dieters trying this diet for weight loss oftentimes are not even in ketosis. If they are in ketosis, they are not in deep ketosis, which has problems of its own.

• Myth - It is a weight-loss wonder. 🔍 p. 85

• Truth - Keto is actually a medical diet that comes with serious risks when not under a doctor's supervision. It is not the type of diet with which to leisurely experiment. It is used to help reduce seizures in children with epilepsy. In a manner of speaking, only short-term results have been studied. We still need long-term studies as we do not know much about the long-term effects, possibly because this approach to nutrition is difficult to stick with long term. If this diet can't be sustained for a long time, it is also important to remember that "yo-yo dieting" leads to rapid weight-loss fluctuation and is associated with increased mortality.

• Truth - Weight loss is the primary reason my patients use the ketogenic diet.

• Myth - Burning ketones instead of other fuels is the ideal way to lose weight.

• Truth - In order to get the body to burn ketones, we must deprive ourselves of carbohydrates, consuming fewer than 20–50 grams per day. It typically takes a few days to reach a state of ketosis, during which time a "keto flu" may be experienced. Eating too much protein can also interfere with ketosis. But eating too little protein can cause the body to strip its own lean tissue, which is not helpful for people trying to lose weight.

• Myth - Keto diets are great for athletes and body builders. 🔍 p. 48

• Truth - Since this diet requires such a high percentage of calories coming from fat (75%–90%) and such a low percentage from carbohydrates (less than 5%), very little room is left for protein, which is essential for maintaining muscle mass. Moreover, decades of research indicate that carbohydrates are the body's preferred source of fuel, which is essential for physically active individuals.

• Myth - So many people are on this diet that it must be safe and effective.

• Truth - Many people are on this diet, but that does not mean it is safe or effective long term. This diet is seen and heard about everywhere, and nearly all of us have heard anecdotal reports of lots of weight loss. We do not yet have enough information to know the long-term effects. What we do know is eating any restrictive diet is difficult to sustain. Once "off" the diet, most will return to their normal way of eating, and the weight lost will likely be regained. 🔍 p. 13

• Myth - The keto diet is safe, healthy, and nutritionally balanced. 🔍 p. 39

• Truth - Whole grain and unrefined carbohydrates lower the risk of stroke, dementia, and certain cancers. This diet removes those protective foods. Not eating a wide variety of vegetables, fruits, and grains puts us at risk for deficiencies in several micronutrients, including selenium, magnesium, phosphorus, and vitamins B and C. Because so much fat is consumed and needs to be metabolized, the diet could make existing liver conditions worse. The low intake of carbohydrates can cause confusion, irritability, and mood swings. Constipation may result due to consuming low amounts of fibrous foods like grains and legumes.

• Truth - Due to the high saturated-fat content, the American Heart Association cautions against this diet, indicating it can be hard on the heart, kidneys, and bones. 🔍 p. 56

• Truth - Due to the lack of carbohydrates, the body mobilizes its stored carbohydrates in the form of glycogen from the liver and muscle tissues. In this process water is lost, thus, much of the rapid weight loss in the beginning is water weight. 🔍 p. 15

• Truth - For the most part, not all types of this diet have been studied. Overall, only the standard and high-protein types have been examined to any degree.

• Truth - A ketogenic diet has been shown to improve blood sugar levels in people with type-2 diabetes, at least in the short term.

• Truth - There is no long-term research analyzing this diet's effects over time on diabetes and high cholesterol.

• Truth - Some have expressed the following concern: Once someone has reached his or her goal weight and gotten a taste preference for foods with no carbs in them, it might be hard to keep calorie levels high enough to maintain that lower weight because of being satisfied with fewer calories than was once needed before excess fat has been burned off.

Final decision: Thumbs down 👎

How to improve this diet: Eat a balanced, unprocessed diet with adequate quantities of colorful fruits and vegetables, lean meats, fish, whole grains, nuts, seeds, olive oil, and lots of water.

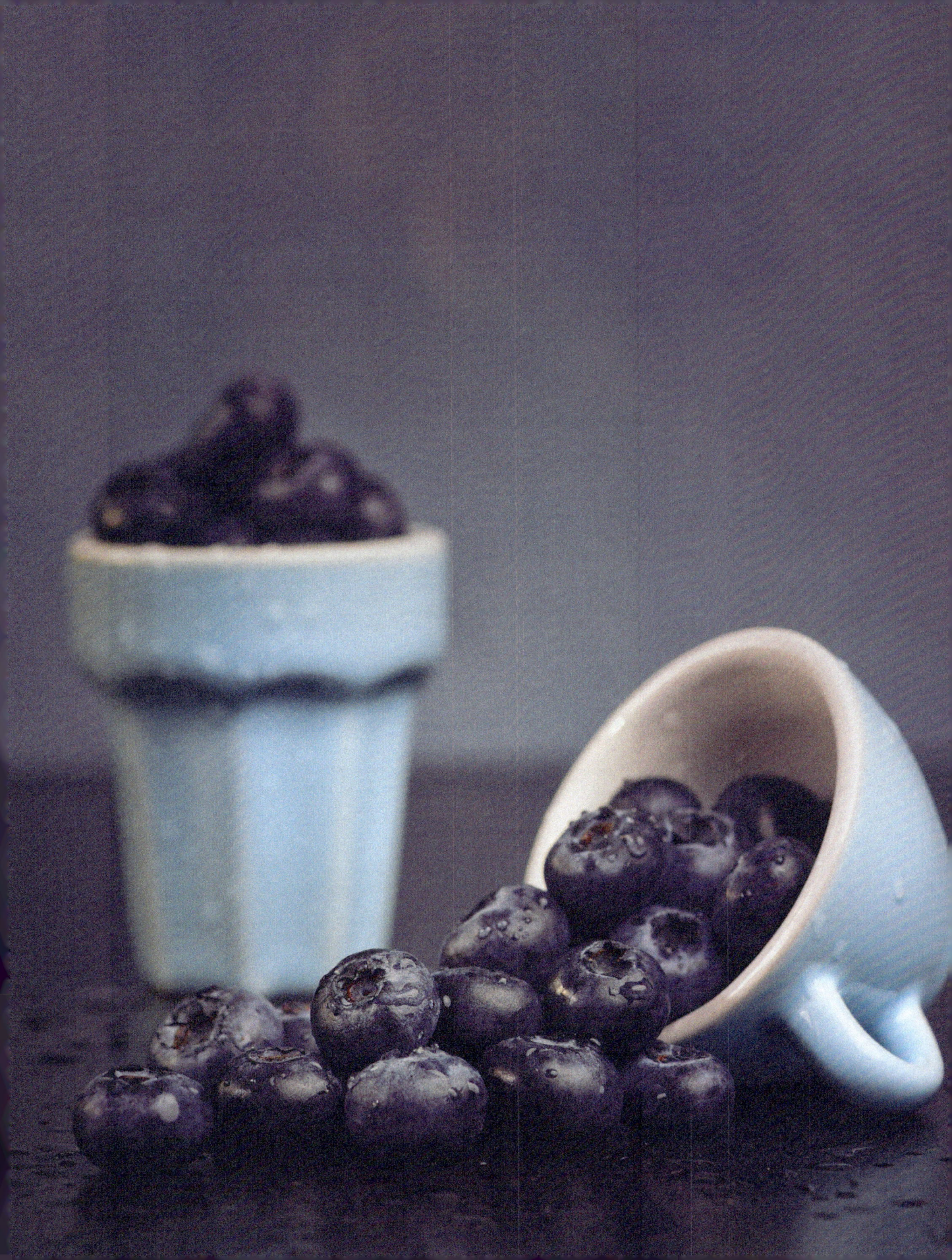

Seventeen Day Food Diet

Premise of the Diet: Changing calorie count and food combinations every 17 days for four cycles keeps the metabolism in a fat-burning state because causing the metabolism to stay "confused" will allow for weight loss and avoidance of plateaus.

Claims of the Diet: Will rev up a fat-burning metabolism; lose up to 10–12 pounds in 17 days and build healthy new habits.

Diet Description: This diet is divided into four cycles, starting with the "Accelerate Cycle," which is a restrictive 1,200 calorie, lean protein, healthy fat, minimal starch, antioxidant and probiotic rich plan that then proceeds to the "Activate," "Achieve," and "Arrive Cycles." The first three cycles each last 17 days, with new foods being introduced with each cycle. The "Arrive Cycle" is meant to be followed for life. The diet does not prescribe a certain number of calories for each cycle. Instead, calories are progressively increased by introducing more calorie-rich options with each cycle. Processed foods, salty foods, fried foods, and sugar are not allowed, and fruit can only be eaten before 2 pm. Progression through the diet eventually allows an occasional drink, 100-calorie snack, or a cheat meal.

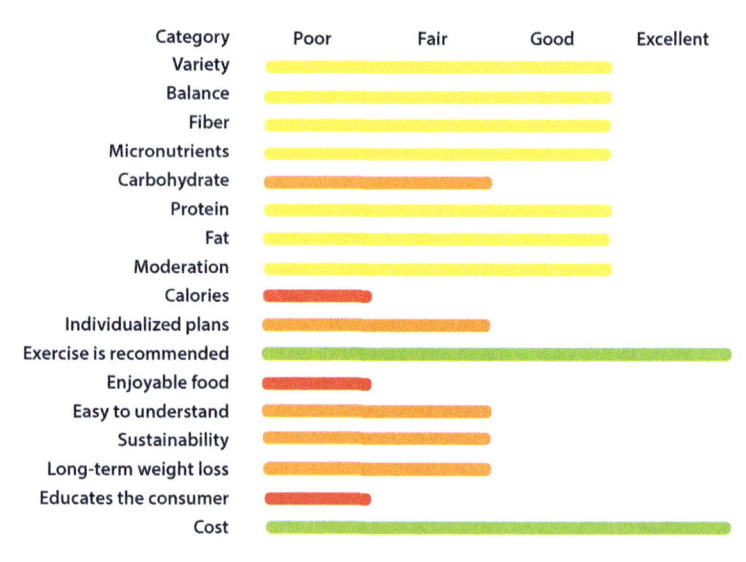

Category	Rating
Variety	Fair/Good
Balance	Fair/Good
Fiber	Fair/Good
Micronutrients	Fair/Good
Carbohydrate	Poor/Fair
Protein	Fair/Good
Fat	Fair/Good
Moderation	Fair/Good
Calories	Poor
Individualized plans	Poor/Fair
Exercise is recommended	Excellent
Enjoyable food	Poor
Easy to understand	Poor/Fair
Sustainability	Poor/Fair
Long-term weight loss	Poor/Fair
Educates the consumer	Poor
Cost	Excellent

Positives

Provides recipes that can be used to accommodate individual preferences. Recommends low-salt foods and probiotic-rich dairy products. Recommends whole foods and regular exercise. Exercise recommendations start off slow and gradually increase and include both weightlifting and cardio. A maintenance phase and a rather strong support network are available to help reinforce long-term success.

Negatives

May provide too much protein for some. A 1200-calorie diet is too low for most and may result in a drop in metabolic rate and nutrient deficiencies if foods are not carefully selected. Numerous claims associated with this diet are not supported by quality research. Because the first two cycles of the diet are lower in calories and carbohydrates, they may negatively impact exercise ability. One edition of the diet recommends costly supplements. Since favorite meals can be eaten three times per week during the last cycle, it may be easy to overeat, thus preventing weight loss.

The hook/catch or brilliant selling point: The magical number is 17.

Truths/Myths

- Myth - Changing calorie count and food combinations every 17 days for four cycles keeps the metabolism in a fat-burning state.

- Truth - Research does not support this claim.

- Myth - Carbohydrates eaten later in the day are harder to burn.

- Truth - Research does not support this claim.

- Myth - The 17 Day Diet can help more with weight loss because it is more effective than conventional, calorie-restricted, whole-foods diets.

- *Truth* - Research does not support this claim.

- *Truth* - Evidence for the role of both prebiotics and probiotics in weight management is emerging. In the meantime, their aid in general wellness is realized. Dysbiosis, or dysbacteriosis, is a term for microbial imbalance on or inside the body. This refers to human microbiota, such as skin flora, gut flora, or vaginal flora. Higher levels of the bacteria Prevotella in the human gut are correlated with increased risk of type 2 diabetes and high blood glucose levels. The gut bacteria Akkermansia, on the other hand, may help stabilize blood sugar levels in those with type 2 diabetes. Akkermansia has also been linked to reduced GI inflammation, reduced appetite and obesity, and potentially less risk of diabetes.

- *Truth* - Consumption of vegetables and fruits helps to normalize gut bacteria to healthy levels. 🔍 p. 40

Final decision: Thumbs down 👎

How to improve this diet: No need to follow all the numerous rules. While this diet provides a good framework to help with weight loss, the most restrictive phase should be avoided. While the diet can aid weight loss by restricting calories and food groups, it makes a number of questionable claims and rules that are not supported by research, making dieting more complicated than it needs to be.

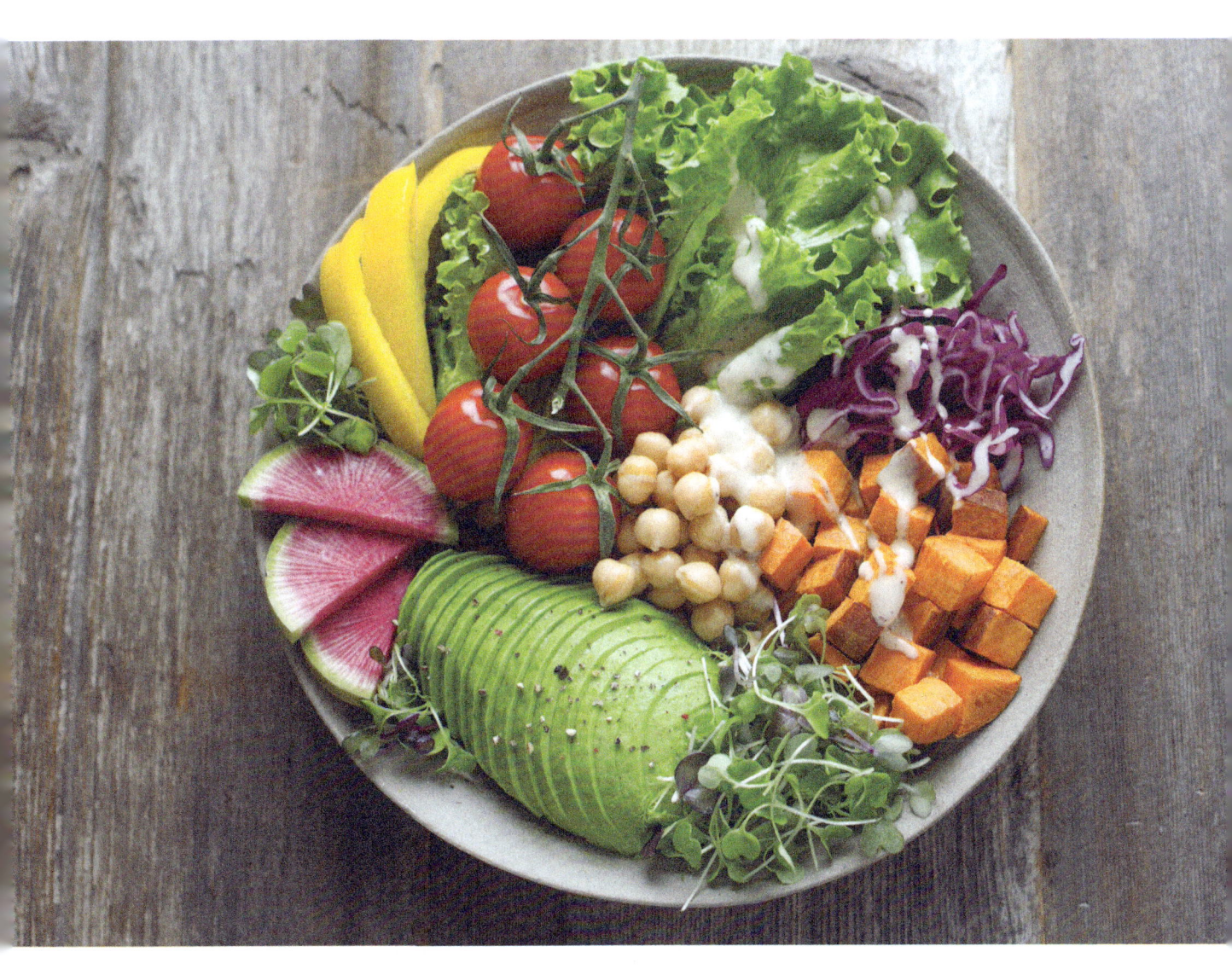

Shangri-La Diet

Premise of the Diet: The body has a "set point," a weight level that it seeks to maintain. The key to weight loss is controlling or altering the body's perception of what weight it wants to maintain. Different foods can increase or decrease the body's desired "set point."

Claims of the Diet: This diet puts people at peace with food. Promises freedom from hunger and cravings through teaching the body to desire less food.

Diet Description: Take 1-3 tablespoons of extra light olive oil and/or 1-2 tablespoons of sugar water twice daily, between meals.

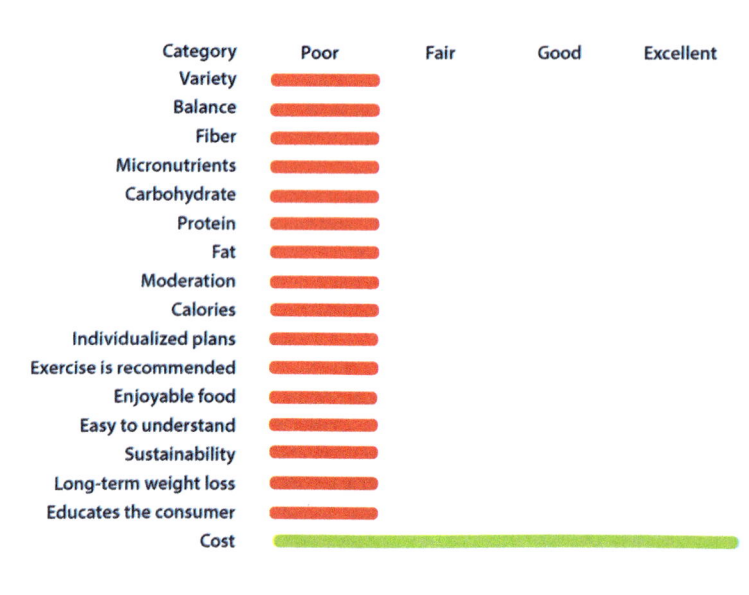

Category	Poor	Fair	Good	Excellent
Variety	■			
Balance	■			
Fiber	■			
Micronutrients	■			
Carbohydrate	■			
Protein	■			
Fat	■			
Moderation	■			
Calories	■			
Individualized plans	■			
Exercise is recommended	■			
Enjoyable food	■			
Easy to understand	■			
Sustainability	■			
Long-term weight loss	■			
Educates the consumer	■			
Cost				■

Positives

All foods are allowed. No food is off-limits. All that is required is adding a small amount of extra light olive oil or sugar water daily. It is "almost as easy as taking a pill, and 100 times safer and less expensive."

Negatives

Recommends holding your nose or stopping it up in some way to avoid smelling the aroma of tasty foods, which will then make them less flavorful. It does not require any real lifestyle changes. Does not discuss or provide portion control guidelines. Adding sugar water or olive oil to a daily routine of unhealthy calorie-dense food won't help with weight loss or improve health. It is a big assumption and a leap of faith to believe that people will desire less food or that this could be sustained when surrounded by flavorful foods.

The hook/catch or brilliant selling point: Conjures up images of Shangri-La, which is often associated with peace and tranquility

Truths/Myths

- **Myth** - Over time, our bodies learn to associate flavorful foods with calories. This leads to overindulging in our favorite foods and results in uncontrollable weight gain.

- **Truth** - There is no scientific evidence to support this. Furthermore, if the body were, in fact, to associate flavor with calories and it didn't want to gain weight, wouldn't it guide us away from foods with which we might overindulge?

- **Myth** - Since olive oil and sugar water have calories but little taste, the body can be taught to stop associating flavor with calories. Eventually the body will signal that it wants less food. 🔍 p. 1

- **Truth** - It is debatable if olive oil and sugar are void of taste. For survival purposes, it makes more sense that the body would not discontinue signaling that it wants food.

- **Myth** - The key to weight loss is predetermining, in advance, the weight your body wants to maintain. In other words, thoughts and desires from the brain can override gene expression.

• Myth - Unfamiliar foods means the body will not have a past association with which to connect. Unfamiliar foods help lower the set point.

• Truth - Eating bland foods, such as bread without butter or plain soup or adding an "off" flavor to a familiar food most likely will result in less pleasure in the new flavor combination, thus resulting in it being less eaten. It also means less satisfaction and possibly less satiation, both of which translate into less likelihood of remaining on the diet.

Final decision: Thumbs down

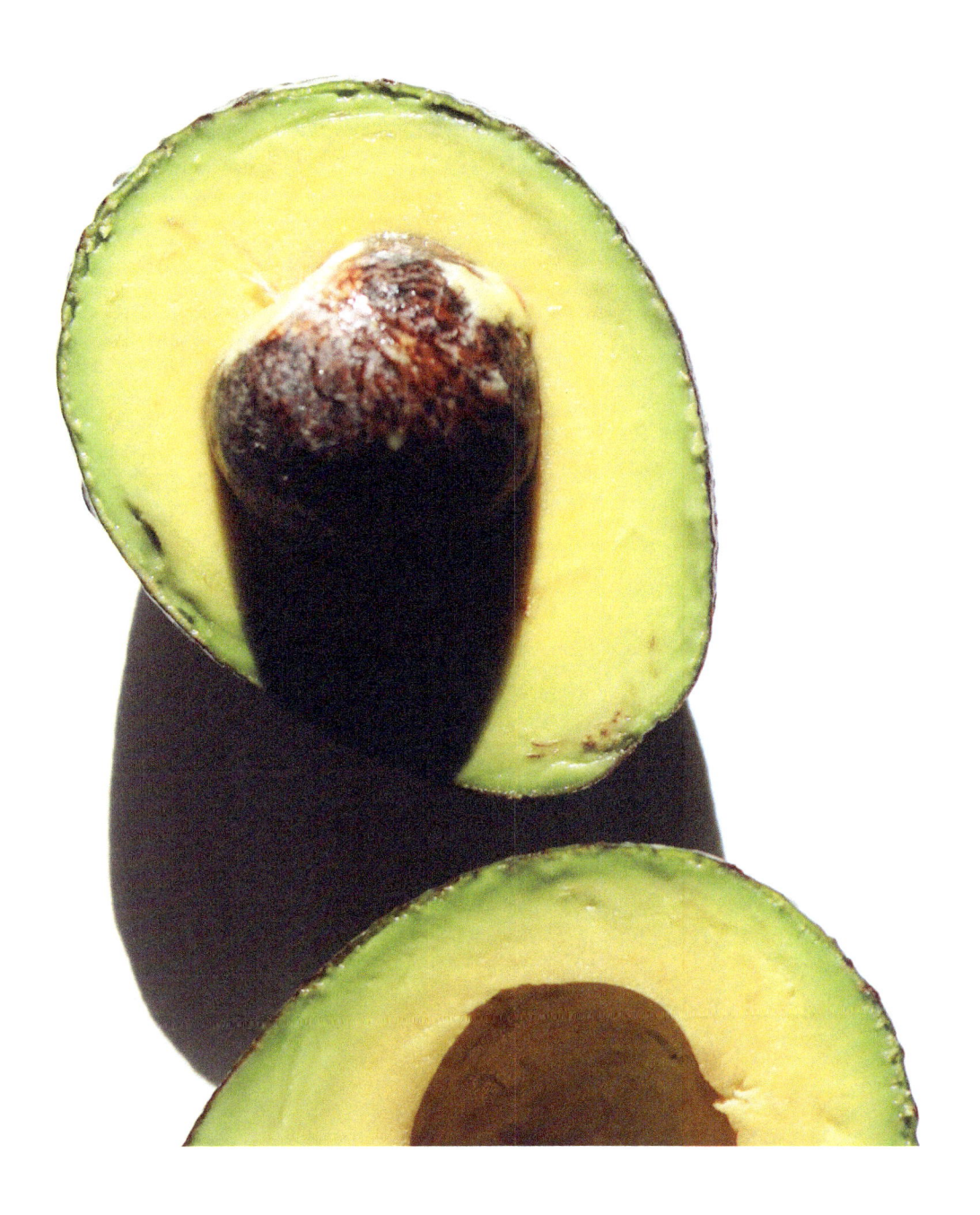

How to improve this diet: Can't be improved.

Skinny Bastard Diet:

A Kick-in-the-Ass for Real Men Who Want to Stop Being Fat and Start Getting Buff

Premise of the Diet: This is a vegan diet for men who want to lose weight and be the envy of the board room or locker room.

Claims of the Diet: Will transform men into lean and clean-eating loving machines.

Diet Description: Meat, dairy, simple carbohydrates, and sugar are replaced with fruits, vegetables, nuts, seeds, legumes, and grains. Lists of specific foods and brands are provided.

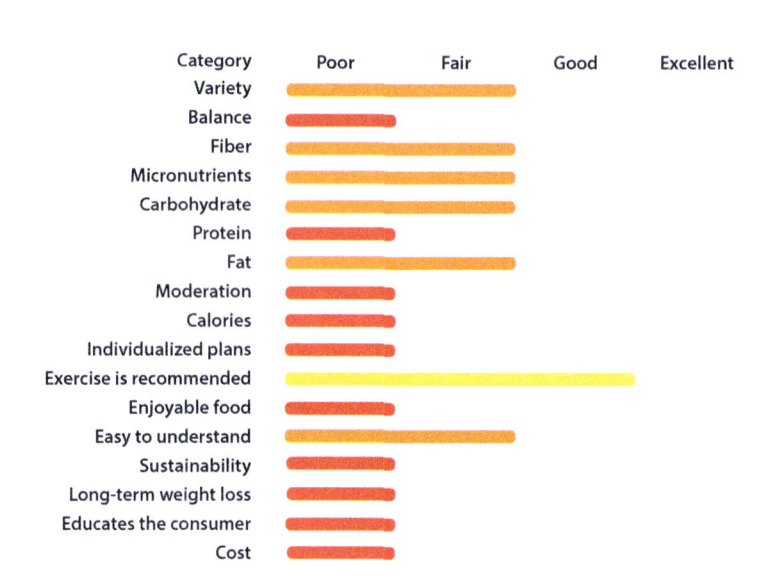

Category	Poor	Fair	Good	Excellent
Variety		██		
Balance	█			
Fiber		██		
Micronutrients		██		
Carbohydrate		██		
Protein	█			
Fat		██		
Moderation	█			
Calories	█			
Individualized plans	█			
Exercise is recommended			███	
Enjoyable food	█			
Easy to understand		██		
Sustainability	█			
Long-term weight loss	█			
Educates the consumer	█			
Cost	█			

Positives

Does not recommend fast food or processed food. Recommends high-fiber foods like fruits, vegetables, soy products, and whole grains. Encourages regular exercise.

Negatives

Blunt with harsh language. Cuts out all meat, dairy, eggs, and fish. Discourages snacking. Recommends not eating until famished. High risk of deficiency in calcium, vitamin D, iron, and B12. Provides little guidance on portion sizes. Recommends organic foods, which are more expensive than non-organic choices. Requires a high level of motivation and a strong desire to eat a vegan diet and thus, remain on this diet. May feel deprived, angry, overwhelmed, and frustrated. Dining out could be difficult.

The hook/catch or brilliant selling point: Men, too, can be hated for being skinny and fit.

Truths/Myths

- **Myth** - Skinny automatically means healthy.

- **Truth** - Skinny does not necessarily mean healthy. Many cancer patients are skinny.

- **Myth** - Feelings of deprivation, anger, and frustration are necessary when dieting.

- **Truth** - This buys into the "no pain no gain" concept, leading the dieter to the common misconception that the "dieting" process needs to be miserable. In fact, the more misery felt, the better the "diet" is going. This thinking can lead to an unhealthy relationship with food.

- **Myth** - Fasting is necessary to jump-start weight loss.

- **Truth** - This is not true. In fact, not eating can decrease the metabolic rate, which slows weight loss as the body begins to conserve energy.

Final decision: Thumbs down 👎

How to improve this diet: Can't be improved.

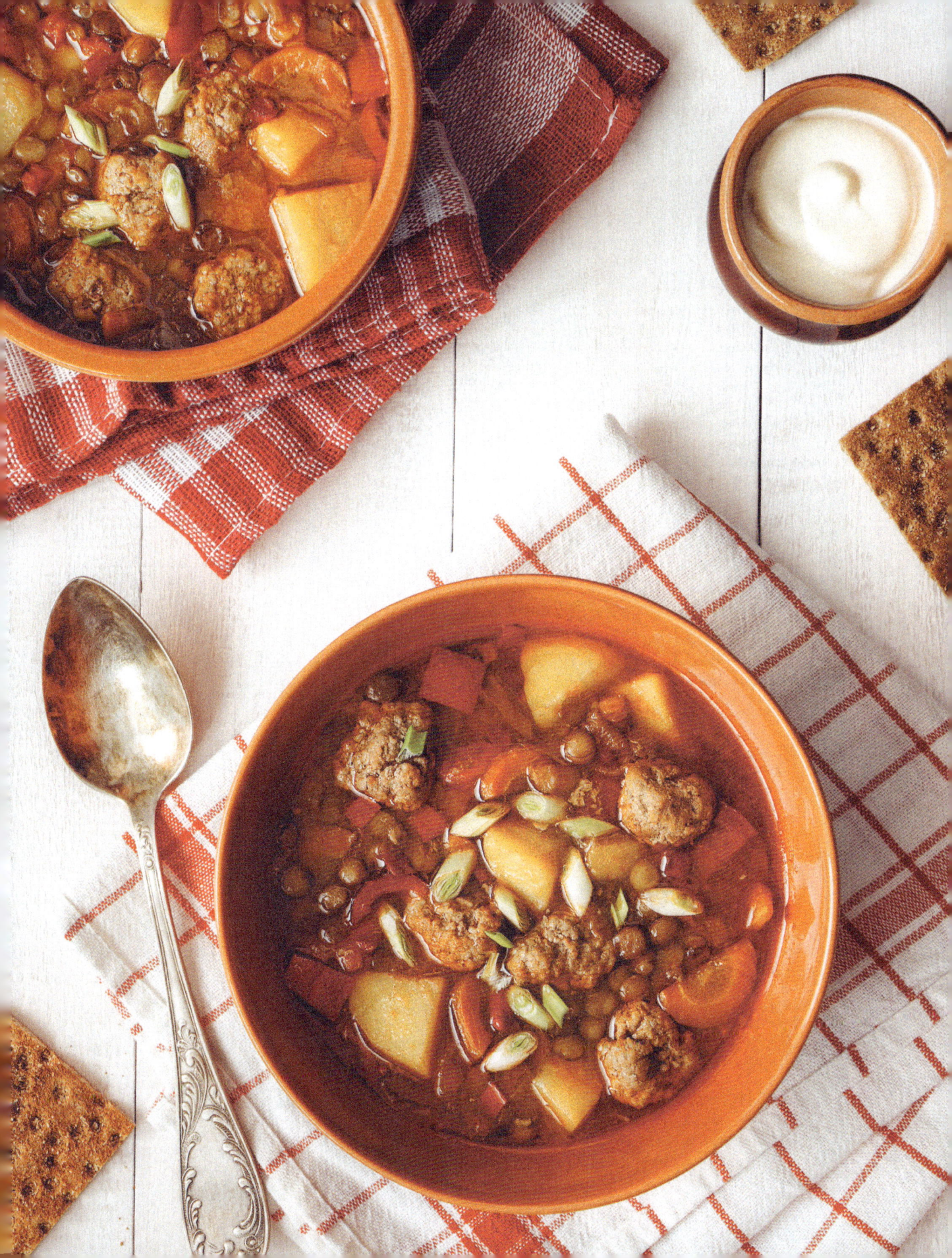

Skinny Vegan Diet (aka Skinny Bitch Diet)

Premise of the Diet: Goes back to the popular high-school girl mentality of "Do what I do, and you, too, can be popular."

Claims of the Diet: Promotes health, happiness, energy, and a skinny body.

Diet Description: Eat as much fruit, vegetables, legumes, nuts, seeds, and whole grains as you want, but only when you get famished.

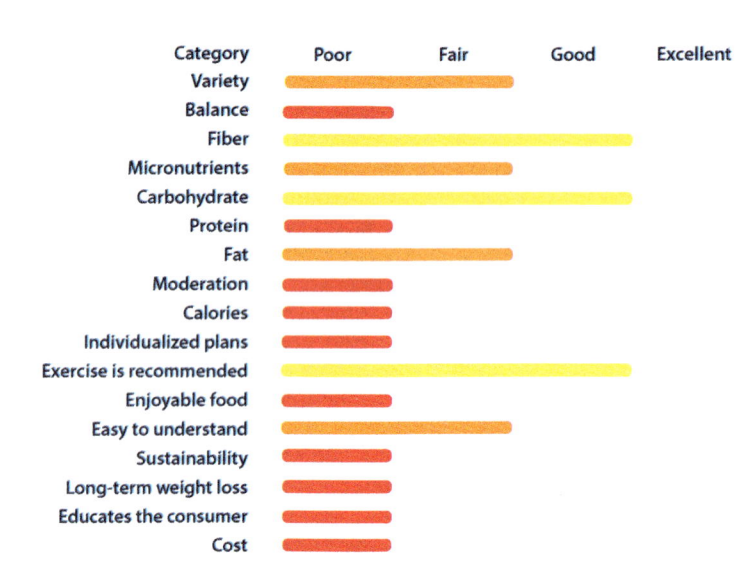

Category	Poor	Fair	Good	Excellent
Variety	██			
Balance	█			
Fiber			██	
Micronutrients	██			
Carbohydrate			██	
Protein	█			
Fat	█			
Moderation	█			
Calories	█			
Individualized plans	█			
Exercise is recommended			██	
Enjoyable food	█			
Easy to understand	██			
Sustainability	█			
Long-term weight loss	█			
Educates the consumer	█			
Cost	█			

Positives

Does not recommend fast food or processed food. Recommends high-fiber foods like fruits, vegetables, soy products, and whole grains. Encourages regular exercise.

Negatives

Cuts out all meat, dairy, eggs, and fish. Discourages snacking. Recommends not eating until famished. High risk of deficiency in calcium, vitamin D, iron, and B12. Provides little guidance on portion sizes. Recommends organic foods, which are more expensive than non-organic choices. Requires a high level of motivation and a strong desire to eat vegan to remain on this diet. May feel deprived, angry, overwhelmed, and frustrated. Dining out could be difficult.

The hook/catch or brilliant selling point: Uses the strong platform of a high-profile former modeling agent, former model. The authors of the book *Skinny Bitch* invite followers into their clique.

Truths/Myths

- Myth - Skinny automatically means healthy.

- Truth - Skinny does not necessarily mean healthy. Many cancer patients and those suffering with anorexia nervosa are skinny. Healthy weights do not always coincide with the images portrayed in the media. A healthy weight is defined as a weight that minimizes health risks. Having a body mass index under 18.5 is considered underweight and can accompany a higher risk of anemia, osteoporosis and bone fractures, heart irregularities, depression, anxiety and amenorrhea in women. 🔍 p. 78, 18

- Myth - Feelings of deprivity, anger and frustration are necessary when dieting.

- Truth - This buys into the "no pain no gain" concept, leading the dieter to the common misconception that the "dieting" process needs to be miserable. In fact, the more misery felt, the better the "diet" is going. This thinking can lead to an unhealthy relationship with food.

- Myth - Fasting is necessary to jump-start weight loss. 🔍 p. 67

- Truth - This is not true. In fact, not eating can decrease the metabolic rate, which slows weight loss as the body begins to conserve energy.

Final decision: Thumbs down

How to improve this diet: Can't be improved.

Slim Fast Diet

Premise of the Diet: Meal-replacement shakes and food products are designed to promote weight loss.

Claims of the Diet: Keeps metabolism burning and wards off hunger while 1–2 pounds are lost each week.

Diet Description: Eat two meal replacements and three 100-calorie snacks every day. Make one 500-calorie meal where at least half the plate is vegetables, one quarter protein, and about one quarter starch. The diet provides approximately 1,200 calories per day for women and 1,600 calories per day for men. Shakes come in regular, low-sugar, and high-protein varieties.

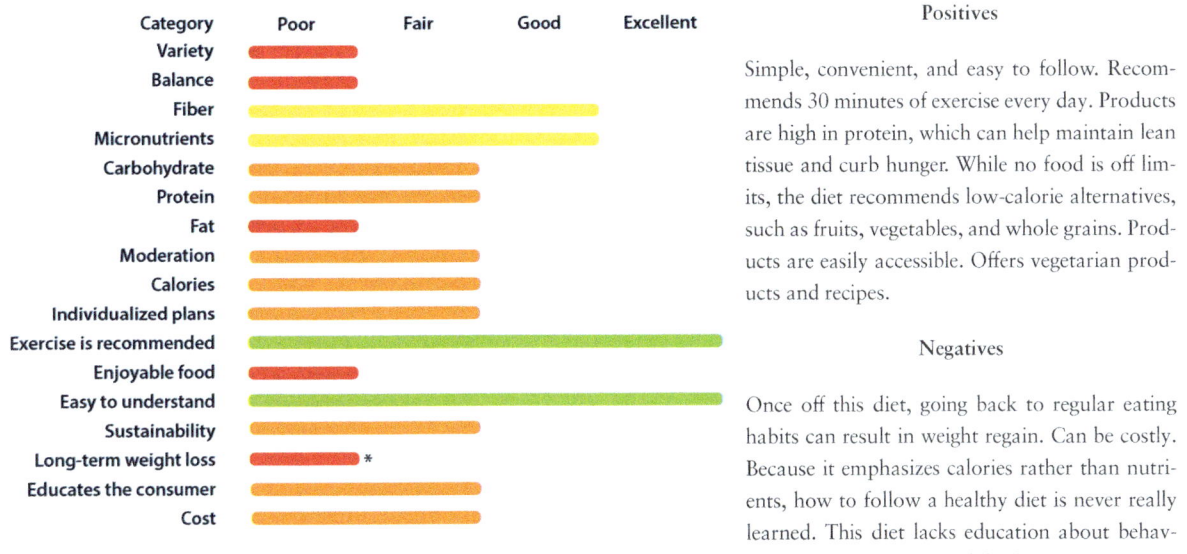

Category	Poor	Fair	Good	Excellent
Variety	■			
Balance	■			
Fiber			■	
Micronutrients			■	
Carbohydrate		■		
Protein		■		
Fat	■			
Moderation		■		
Calories		■		
Individualized plans		■		
Exercise is recommended				■
Enjoyable food	■			
Easy to understand				■
Sustainability		■		
Long-term weight loss	■*			
Educates the consumer		■		
Cost		■		

Positives

Simple, convenient, and easy to follow. Recommends 30 minutes of exercise every day. Products are high in protein, which can help maintain lean tissue and curb hunger. While no food is off limits, the diet recommends low-calorie alternatives, such as fruits, vegetables, and whole grains. Products are easily accessible. Offers vegetarian products and recipes.

Negatives

Once off this diet, going back to regular eating habits can result in weight regain. Can be costly. Because it emphasizes calories rather than nutrients, how to follow a healthy diet is never really learned. This diet lacks education about behavioral modifications and the development of other healthy habits such as portion control, which are needed for long-term success. Dieting without changing behaviors is only effective short-term. Recommended foods are primarily processed foods. Does not provide a structured transition or maintenance plan. Does not meet the USDA's definition of a healthy meal plan.

*Most research indicates weight loss is sustained for about a year.

The hook/catch or brilliant selling point: Simple, no need to learn anything.

Truths/Myths

- Myth - This is a healthy method to lose weight.

- Truth - Because diets that promote eating processed prepackaged foods like bars and shakes instead of real foods aren't sustainable or nutritious, they are not healthy and won't result in long-lasting and satisfying results.

Final decision: Thumbs down

How to improve this diet: Instead of eating two meal replacements and three 100-calorie prepackaged snacks every day along with one "real" 500-calorie meal, go ahead and eat "real" meals that follow the same calorie level but that are fresh, satisfying, full of variety, and meet the US Dietary Guidelines.

Sonoma Diet

Premise of the Diet: Focus on 10 power foods and portion control to lose weight.

Claims of the Diet: Through learning how to satisfy cravings with healthy foods, a trimmer waist and better health will be achieved in 10 days without feelings of deprivation.

Diet Description: Three "waves" to the diet:

The first wave lasts 10 days. Numerous foods are banned, including sugar, artificial sweeteners, anything sweet, processed foods and refined grains. It is designed to promote quick weight loss. The second wave adds some fruit, vegetables, sugar-free treats, and up to 6 ounces of wine. This is the main wave, or phase, until the desired weight is achieved. The third wave begins once the goal is reached. It makes the Sonoma Diet the new lifestyle.

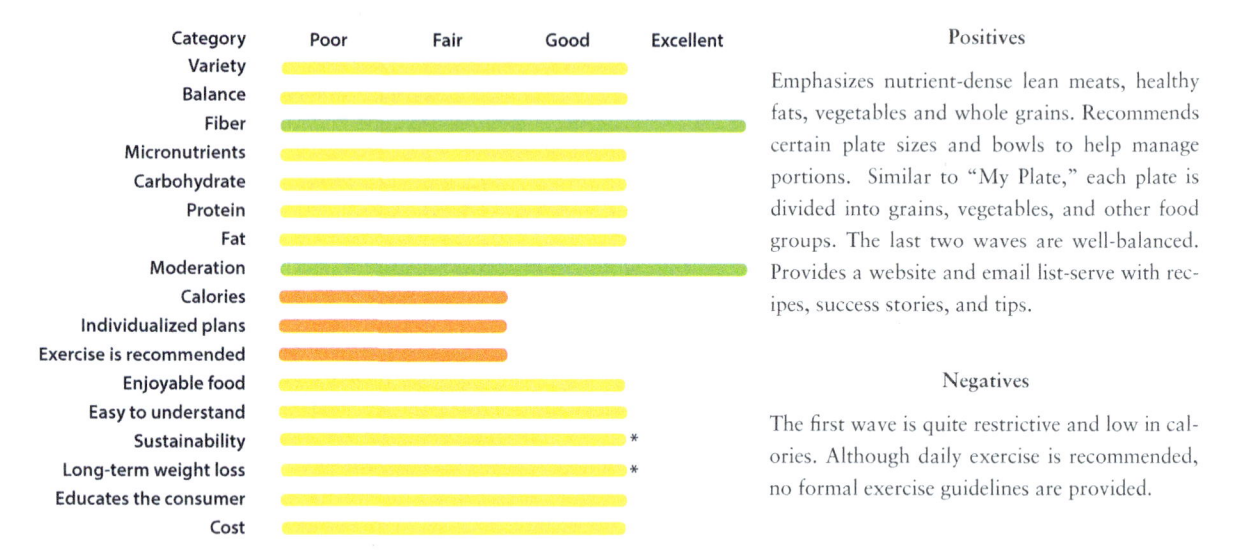

Category	Poor	Fair	Good	Excellent
Variety			Good	
Balance			Good	
Fiber				Excellent
Micronutrients			Good	
Carbohydrate			Good	
Protein			Good	
Fat			Good	
Moderation				Excellent
Calories		Fair		
Individualized plans		Fair		
Exercise is recommended		Fair		
Enjoyable food			Good	
Easy to understand			Good	
Sustainability			Good*	
Long-term weight loss			Good*	
Educates the consumer			Good	
Cost			Good	

Positives

Emphasizes nutrient-dense lean meats, healthy fats, vegetables and whole grains. Recommends certain plate sizes and bowls to help manage portions. Similar to "My Plate," each plate is divided into grains, vegetables, and other food groups. The last two waves are well-balanced. Provides a website and email list-serve with recipes, success stories, and tips.

Negatives

The first wave is quite restrictive and low in calories. Although daily exercise is recommended, no formal exercise guidelines are provided.

* The restrictive nature of the first wave may decrease the diet's sustainability and potential for long-term weight loss.

The hook/catch or brilliant selling point: Eat power foods to power through and maintain weight loss.

Truths/Myths

- **Myth** - The restrictions recommended in wave 1 are important to jump-start a diet.

- **Truth** - There is no scientific evidence to support that restricting nutritious foods, such as fruit and potatoes, is necessary for weight loss. Moreover, there is no scientific proof indicating elimination of sweets and fruit will reduce cravings for those foods.

- **Myth** - It is important to begin a diet with a strict, restrictive plan.

- **Truth** - Potential weight gain may result after the very restrictive first wave, due to decreased metabolic rate and physiological responses to severe restriction. 🔍 p. 78

- **Myth** - It is important to consume "power foods."

- **Truth** - This is confusing food advice. Some of the so-called "power foods" are actually restricted in wave 1. Variety is important.

Final decision: Thumbs down 👎

How to improve this diet: Skip the first wave and begin with Wave 2.

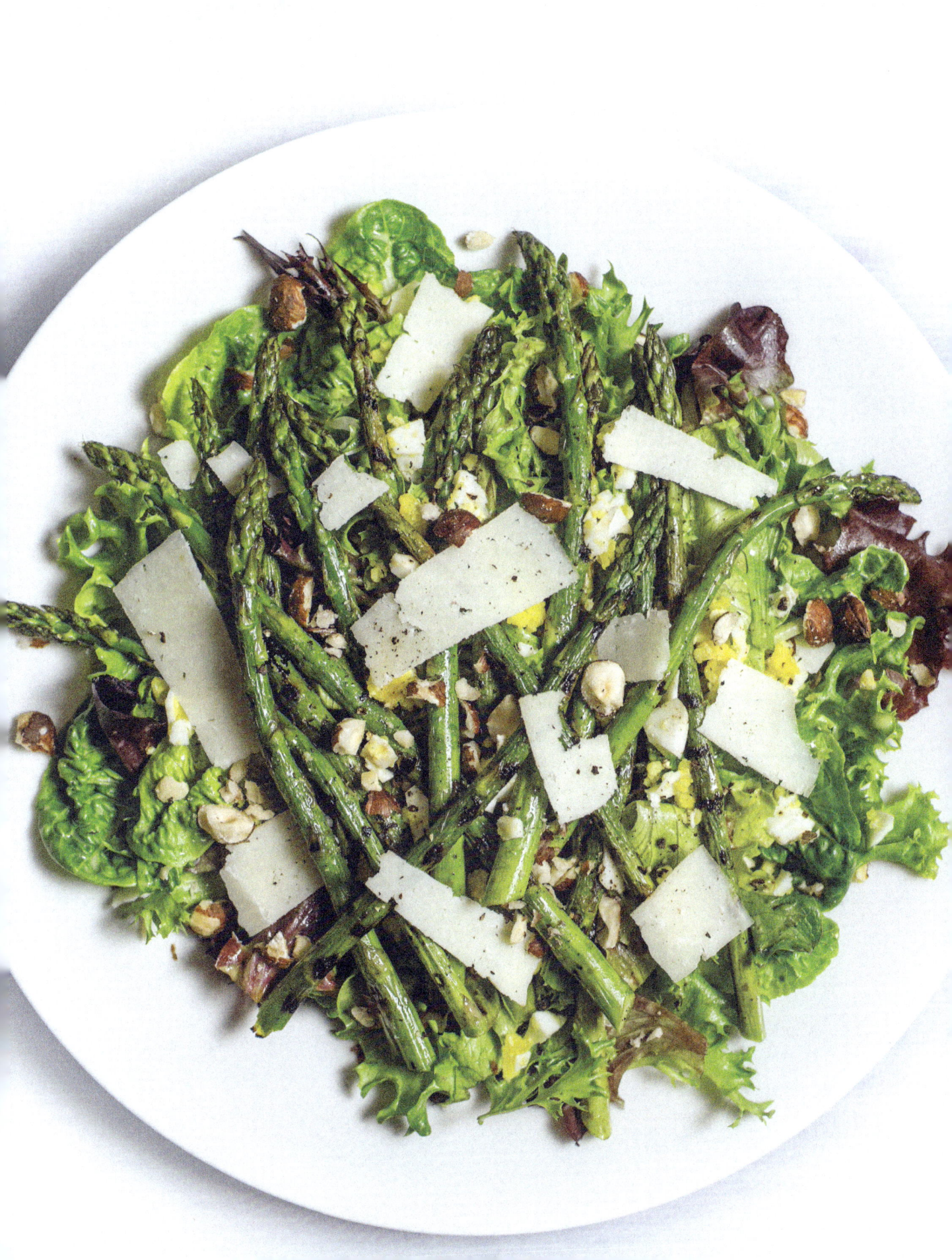

South Beach Diet
(aka The South Beach Diet Supercharged)

Premise of the Diet: A cardiologist-created, lower-carb diet that emphasizes lean meats, unsaturated fats, and low-glycemic-index carbohydrates.

Claims of the Diet: Lose 8–13 pounds during phase 1 and 1–2 pounds per week during phase 2.

Diet Description: Three different phases.

Phase 1 is the strictest phase. Fruit, grains, and other higher-carb foods are limited in an attempt to decrease blood sugar and insulin levels, stabilize hunger, and reduce cravings. Can expect to lose 8–13 pounds during this phase. Requires three meals of lean protein, non-starchy vegetables, healthy fats and legumes, and two mandatory snacks daily. Fruit, fruit juices, starchy foods, dairy products, and alcohol are off-limits. This phase lasts 2 weeks.

Phase 2 begins on day 15 and is to be maintained until the goal weight is achieved. An average of 1–2 pounds will be lost per week. In addition to the foods allowed in phase one, limited portions of fruit and "good carbs," such as whole grains and certain types of alcohol, are also allowed.

Phase 3 begins once the target weight is achieved. In this stage, treats are allowed. No foods are off limits.

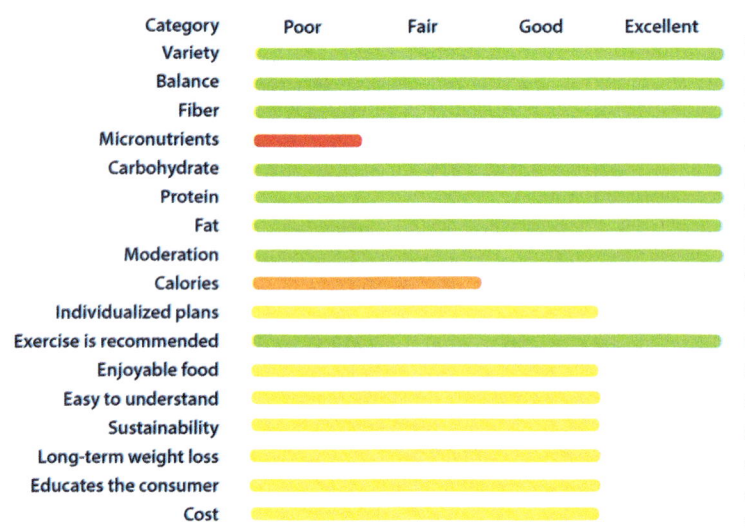

Category	Poor	Fair	Good	Excellent
Variety				●
Balance				●
Fiber				●
Micronutrients	●			
Carbohydrate				●
Protein				●
Fat				●
Moderation				●
Calories		●		
Individualized plans			●	
Exercise is recommended				●
Enjoyable food			●	
Easy to understand			●	
Sustainability			●	
Long-term weight loss			●	
Educates the consumer			●	
Cost			●	

Positives

Rich in low-glycemic-index carbohydrates, lean proteins, and unsaturated fats. In The South Beach Diet Supercharged version, regular exercise is recommended and a three-phase fitness program is suggested. Online tools, including tracking weight, recipes, customizing meal plans, guides for dining-out, and support are available. Relies on proven methods and suggestions for weight loss such as eating whole grains, healthy fats, lean protein, low-fat dairy, and high-fiber foods. Embraces the behavioral changes necessary for long-term success. Is reasonably customizable to fit individual schedules and preferences. Plenty of protein is provided, which can help reduce hunger and promote feelings of fullness.

Negatives

In phase 3, 28 percent of daily calories may come from carbohydrates. This is not within the recommended range. Severely restricting carbohydrates may result in ketosis.

The hook/catch or brilliant selling point: Created by a cardiologist and named for a glamorous area of Miami.

Truths/Myths

- **Myth** - It is healthy to lose 8-13 pounds in 2 weeks. 🔍 p. 13

- **Truth** - Since fruit, grains, and other higher-carb foods are limited, especially in the first phase, glycogen stores will quickly be depleted. Water will be lost alongside the loss of glycogen. Thus, much of the weight loss in the first two weeks of this diet will not be much fat loss. Instead, the weight loss will be glycogen and water loss. 🔍 p. 67

Final decision: Thumbs down 👎

How to improve this diet: Increase whole grain, low-glycemic carbohydrates to within the AMDR. Skip the first phase and begin with phase 2.

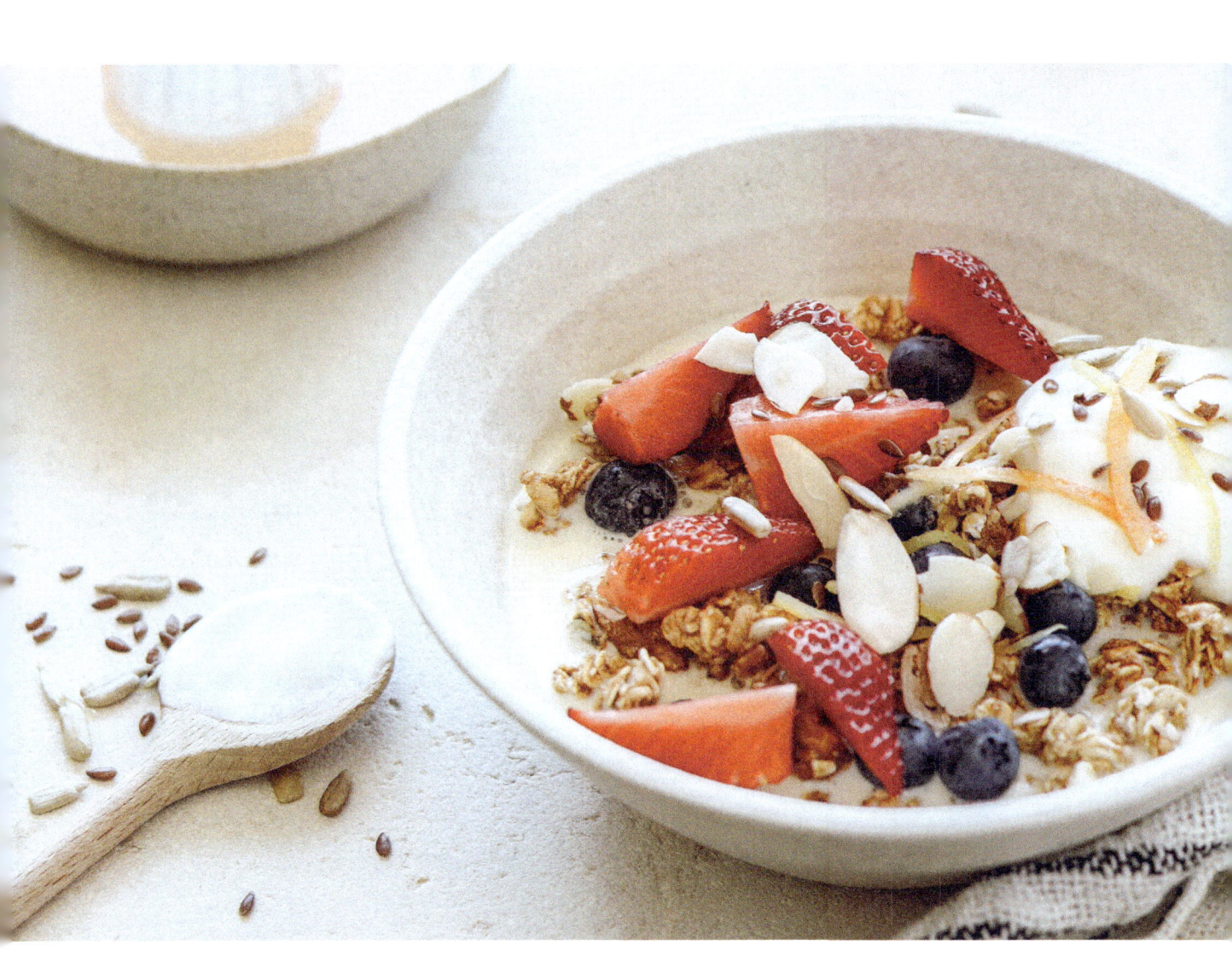

Special K Diet (aka The Special K Challenge)

Premise of the Diet: Eating Special K cereal instead of two meals for 2 weeks will assist in losing weight.

Claims of the Diet: Lose up to 6 pounds, or drop a pants size, in 2 weeks.

Diet Description: Replace two meals each with one bowl of Special K cereal (with skim milk) for 2 weeks. Eat a regular evening meal.

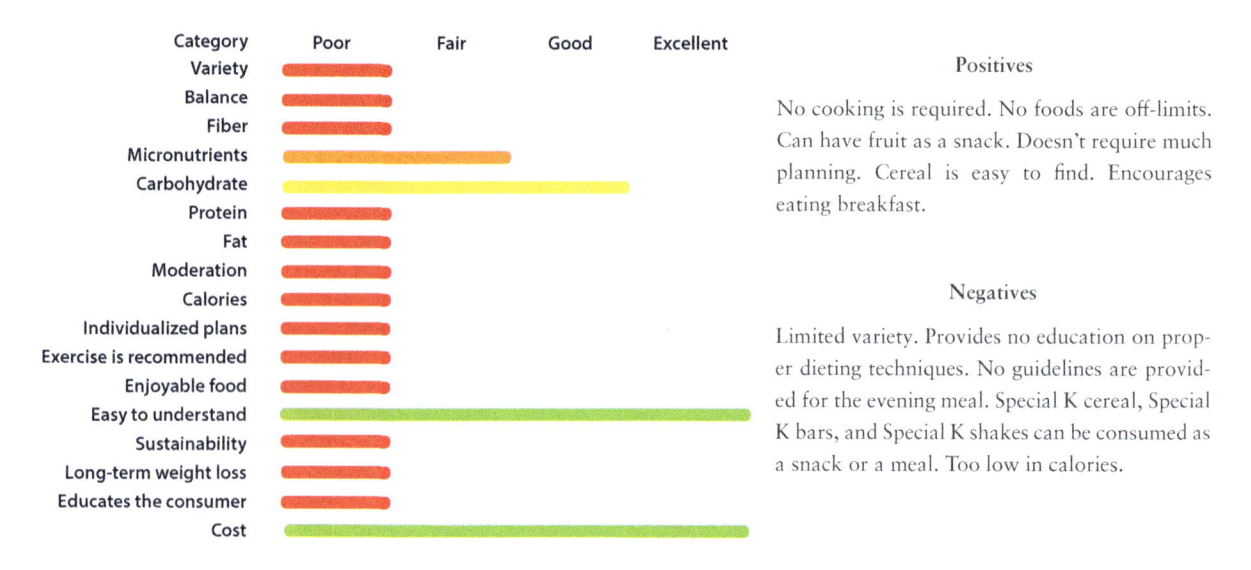

Category	Poor	Fair	Good	Excellent
Variety	■			
Balance	■			
Fiber	■			
Micronutrients		■		
Carbohydrate			■	
Protein	■			
Fat	■			
Moderation	■			
Calories	■			
Individualized plans	■			
Exercise is recommended	■			
Enjoyable food	■			
Easy to understand				■
Sustainability	■			
Long-term weight loss	■			
Educates the consumer	■			
Cost				■

Positives

No cooking is required. No foods are off-limits. Can have fruit as a snack. Doesn't require much planning. Cereal is easy to find. Encourages eating breakfast.

Negatives

Limited variety. Provides no education on proper dieting techniques. No guidelines are provided for the evening meal. Special K cereal, Special K bars, and Special K shakes can be consumed as a snack or a meal. Too low in calories.

The hook/catch or brilliant selling point: So easy to use! With this prepackaged, convenient cereal as meal replacements, anyone can lose weight.

Truths/Myths

- **Myths** - Eating Special K cereal is a better alternative than consuming two well-balanced, portion-controlled meals to lose weight.

- **Truths** - Will quickly become bored with this diet. It is not sustainable, which increases the risk that weight lost will be regained once off the diet. 🔍 p. 13

Final decision: Thumbs down 👎

How to improve this diet: Substitute 2 well-balanced, portion-controlled meals in place of the 2 meals consisting of cereal.

Spectrum Diet

Premise of the Diet: Since the program is really about lowering disease risk, it is not only about food consumption, but a guide to wellness. There are three components: nutrition, stress management, and exercise. People assess their life and determine where they are on the spectrum. Significant emphasis is placed on exercise, meditation, and lowering stress.

Claims of the Diet: This diet works for anyone, but targets those with or at risk for heart disease.

Diet Description: Foods are put into 5 categories and each category is ranked from the healthiest "Group 1" to the least healthy "Group 5." To lose weight and gain health, eat foods from the healthy end of the spectrum. Takes a gradual approach to making healthier lifestyle choices using a step-wise approach.

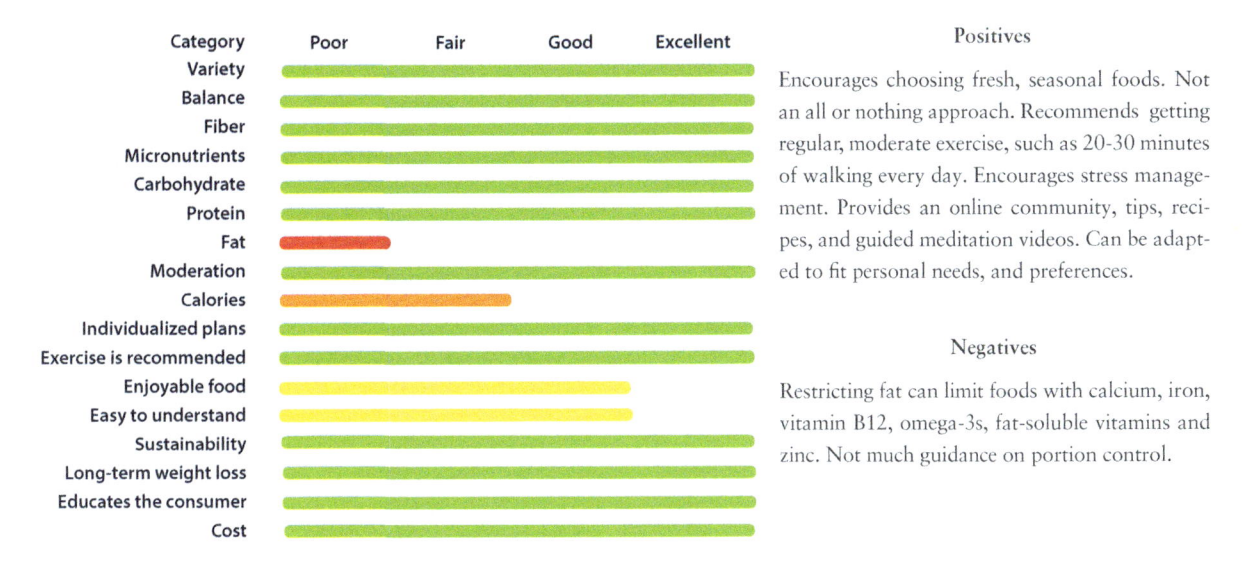

Category	Poor	Fair	Good	Excellent
Variety				✓
Balance				✓
Fiber				✓
Micronutrients				✓
Carbohydrate				✓
Protein				✓
Fat	✓			
Moderation				✓
Calories		✓		
Individualized plans				✓
Exercise is recommended				✓
Enjoyable food			✓	
Easy to understand			✓	
Sustainability				✓
Long-term weight loss				✓
Educates the consumer				✓
Cost				✓

Positives

Encourages choosing fresh, seasonal foods. Not an all or nothing approach. Recommends getting regular, moderate exercise, such as 20-30 minutes of walking every day. Encourages stress management. Provides an online community, tips, recipes, and guided meditation videos. Can be adapted to fit personal needs, and preferences.

Negatives

Restricting fat can limit foods with calcium, iron, vitamin B12, omega-3s, fat-soluble vitamins and zinc. Not much guidance on portion control.

The hook/catch or brilliant selling point: It is about freedom, flexibility and choice.

Truths/Myths: None worth noting.

Final decision: Thumbs up. 👍

How to improve this diet: Be sure to understand portion sizes and complementary proteins, since many animal protein sources are in groups 4 and 5. Monitor nutrients for deficiencies. Need a good mix of groups 1 and 2, or deficiencies become a concern. Be sure to consume adequate fat. 🔍 p. 23, 47, 29

Step Diet

Premise of the Diet: A collection of suggestions to permanently change eating and exercise patterns.

Claims of the Diet: Results in slow and steady 1-2 pounds weekly weight loss.

Diet Description: Walk 10,000 steps every day and cut portions eaten by a quarter. Eat a healthy diet that satisfies hunger. Use a pedometer or Fitbit to assess usual number of daily steps, then continually add steps until the goal of 10,000 daily steps is reached.

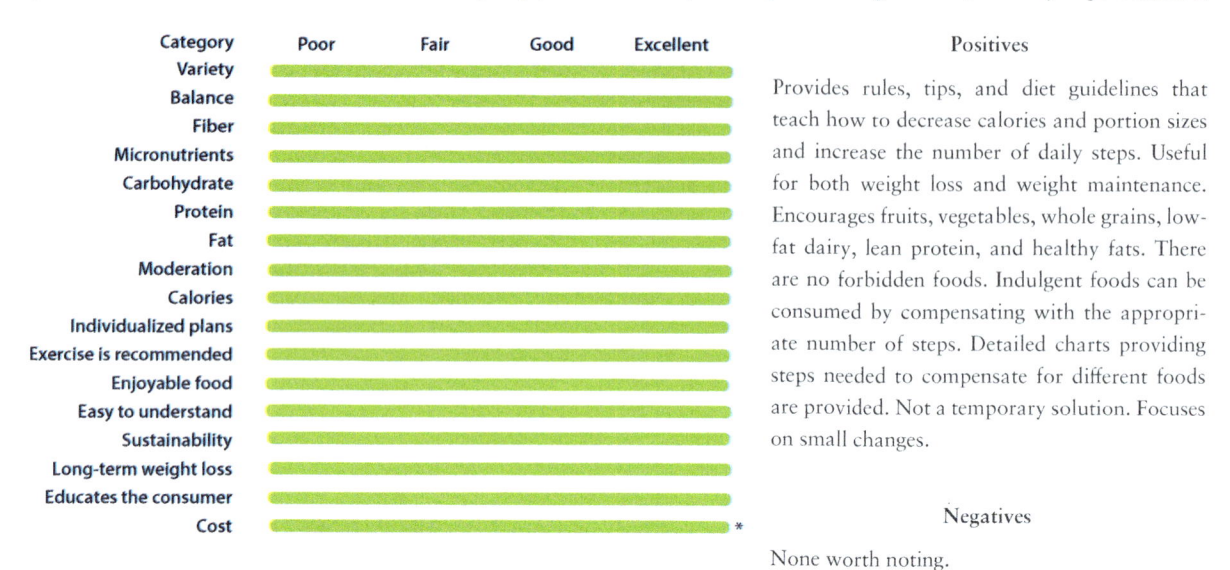

Category	Poor	Fair	Good	Excellent
Variety				●●●
Balance				●●●
Fiber				●●●
Micronutrients				●●●
Carbohydrate				●●●
Protein				●●●
Fat				●●●
Moderation				●●●
Calories				●●●
Individualized plans				●●●
Exercise is recommended				●●●
Enjoyable food				●●●
Easy to understand				●●●
Sustainability				●●●
Long-term weight loss				●●●
Educates the consumer				●●●
Cost				●●●*

Positives

Provides rules, tips, and diet guidelines that teach how to decrease calories and portion sizes and increase the number of daily steps. Useful for both weight loss and weight maintenance. Encourages fruits, vegetables, whole grains, low-fat dairy, lean protein, and healthy fats. There are no forbidden foods. Indulgent foods can be consumed by compensating with the appropriate number of steps. Detailed charts providing steps needed to compensate for different foods are provided. Not a temporary solution. Focuses on small changes.

Negatives

None worth noting.

*Cost is low if using a pedometer ($5-$10) rather than a FitBit ($70+)

The hook/catch or brilliant selling point: Fitbits are a big craze… everyone is counting steps.

Truths/Myths

- Myth - None worth noting

- Truth - Small, permanent lifestyle changes promoting healthy energy balance is key to long-term weight control. 🔍 p. 105

Final decision: Thumbs up 👍

How to improve this diet: Nothing worth noting.

Sugar Busters

Premise of the Diet: Emphasizes low glycemic index (GI) foods.

Claims of the Diet: Will lower cholesterol, help achieve optimal wellness, increase energy, and treat diabetes.

Diet Description: Cuts out refined carbohydrates and added sugars while encouraging select fruits, vegetables, whole grains, lean proteins, and healthy fats. High-carb foods like pasta, pastries, and white flour are replaced with low-glycemic, fiber-rich foods like legumes and whole grains. The distribution of calories is carbohydrates about 40%, fats and protein each 30%.

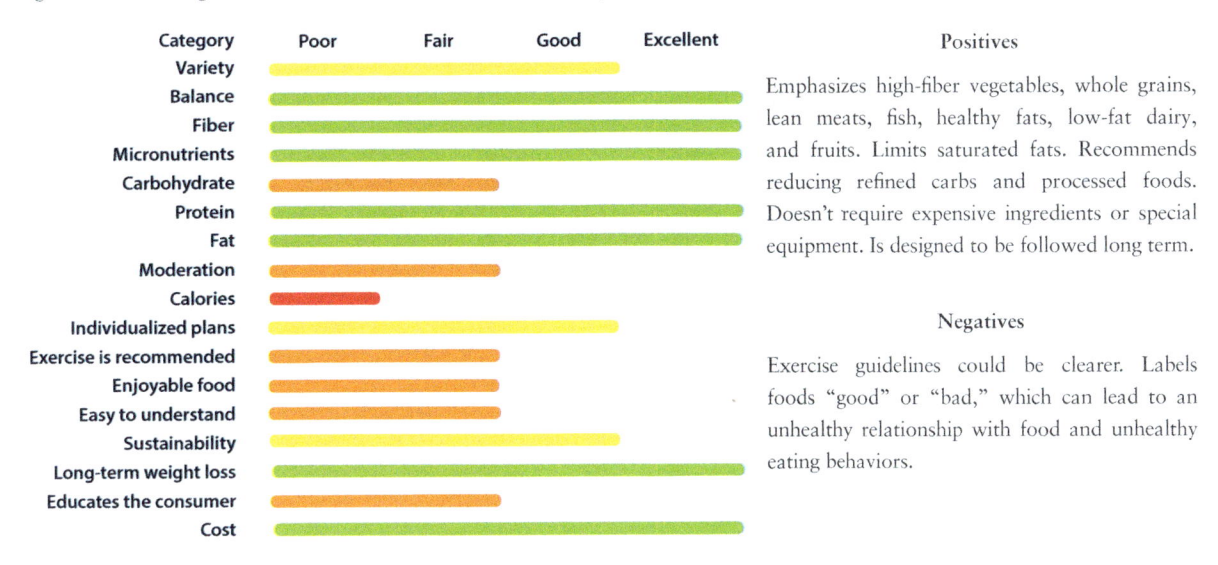

Category	Poor	Fair	Good	Excellent
Variety			Good	
Balance				Excellent
Fiber				Excellent
Micronutrients				Excellent
Carbohydrate		Fair		
Protein				Excellent
Fat				Excellent
Moderation		Fair		
Calories	Poor			
Individualized plans			Good	
Exercise is recommended		Fair		
Enjoyable food		Fair		
Easy to understand		Fair		
Sustainability			Good	
Long-term weight loss				Excellent
Educates the consumer		Fair		
Cost				Excellent

Positives

Emphasizes high-fiber vegetables, whole grains, lean meats, fish, healthy fats, low-fat dairy, and fruits. Limits saturated fats. Recommends reducing refined carbs and processed foods. Doesn't require expensive ingredients or special equipment. Is designed to be followed long term.

Negatives

Exercise guidelines could be clearer. Labels foods "good" or "bad," which can lead to an unhealthy relationship with food and unhealthy eating behaviors.

The hook/catch or brilliant selling point: Lose weight by getting rid of toxic sugar.

Truths/Myths

- Myth - Sugar is "toxic" and causes weight gain by increasing insulin levels. 🔍 p. 39

- Truth - Sugar is not toxic. We have lots of sugar in our bodies and it doesn't kill us. However, when we eat simple sugars, glucose and fructose (sucrose), they are digested and absorbed quickly and can result in an insulin spike. Sugars in complex form require more digestion. Weight gain is mainly from increased consumption of calories. 🔍 p. 73

- Myth - Eliminating insulin will result in weight loss.

- Truth - The above statement is too simple. We need insulin in our body to get glucose into muscles and liver to be stored as glycogen and used during times of fasting or fight/flight. A correlation between excess body fat and insulin resistance has been shown. Insulin resistance is when the pancreas releases a sufficient amount of insulin, but its signal has a reduced effect on the target tissues, muscle, adipose and liver. In essence, the body can't store the fuel consumed and, as a result, sugar levels remain elevated in the blood which results in more insulin to be secreted, a catch-22.

Final decision: Thumbs up 👍

How to improve this diet: Although this is a good template for eating healthy, loosening the restrictions of natural foods (even though they may be higher in natural sugars) may increase sustainability. Increase consumption of healthy complex carbohydrates so that at least 45% of all daily calories come from carbohydrates.

Thin for Life Diet

Premise of the Diet: Do what people who have been able to lose weight and keep it off have done.

Claims of the Diet: You will get secrets & recipes from people who have lost weight & kept it off

Diet Description: A 6-week plan which focuses on making one change to one food group each week. Eat three meals and one snack daily. A number of food items are not allowed, such as fried foods, baked goods, and processed foods. 10 keys for losing and maintaining weight are provided.

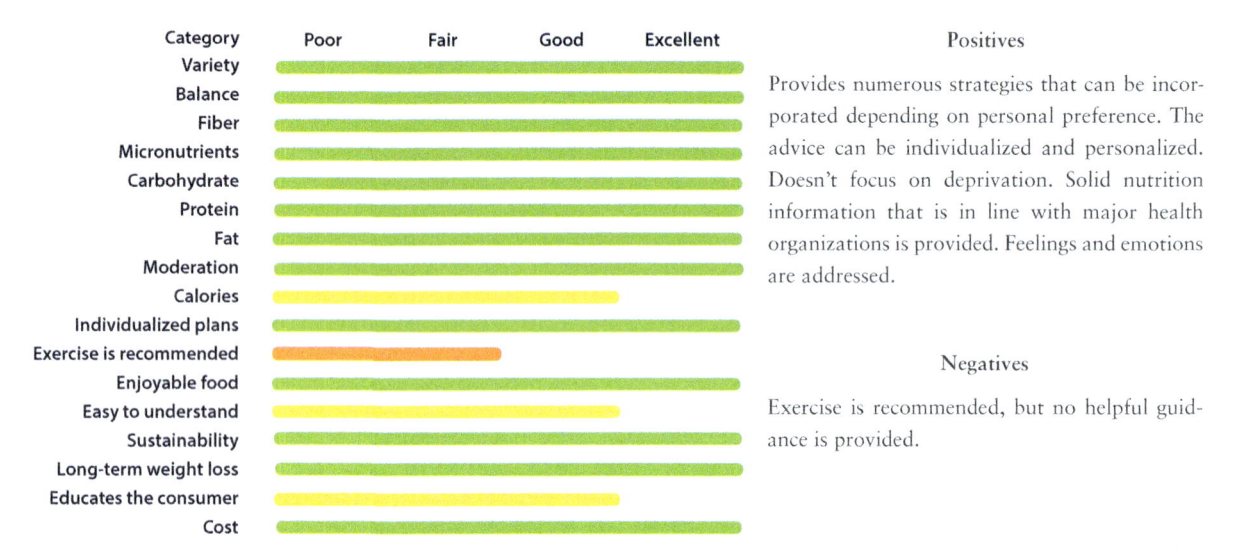

Category	Poor	Fair	Good	Excellent
Variety				■
Balance				■
Fiber				■
Micronutrients				■
Carbohydrate				■
Protein				■
Fat				■
Moderation				■
Calories			■	
Individualized plans				■
Exercise is recommended		■		
Enjoyable food				■
Easy to understand			■	
Sustainability				■
Long-term weight loss				■
Educates the consumer			■	
Cost				■

Positives

Provides numerous strategies that can be incorporated depending on personal preference. The advice can be individualized and personalized. Doesn't focus on deprivation. Solid nutrition information that is in line with major health organizations is provided. Feelings and emotions are addressed.

Negatives

Exercise is recommended, but no helpful guidance is provided.

The hook/catch or brilliant selling point: Learn from the experts – people who have lost weight and kept it off.

Truths/Myths

- Myth - None worth noting

- Truth - It can be helpful to hear from others what techniques and tips helped them to lose weight. It is also important to keep in mind that people are unique and there will be individual differences in the weight loss process.

Final decision: Thumbs up 👍

How to improve this diet: Consume fewer calories than are expended.

This Is Why You're Fat Diet

Premise of the Diet: "Being fat isn't your fault; staying fat is."

Claims of the Diet: You will become "hot and healthy" without feeling deprived. Replacing sugar, white flour, caffeine, artificial sweeteners, processed foods, fatty meats, and alcohol with healthy foods will correct body chemistry, satisfy hunger, and reduce cravings.

Diet Description: For two weeks, in addition to lemon water and herbal tea, add foods like eggs, oatmeal, vegetables, and whey protein shakes to put the body into "fat burn" mode. Starting the third week, there is continual consumption of 1,500-1,800 calories of unprocessed healthy foods, including lean protein, two cups of vegetables, two pieces of fruit, two servings of whole grains, and small amounts of plant-based fats.

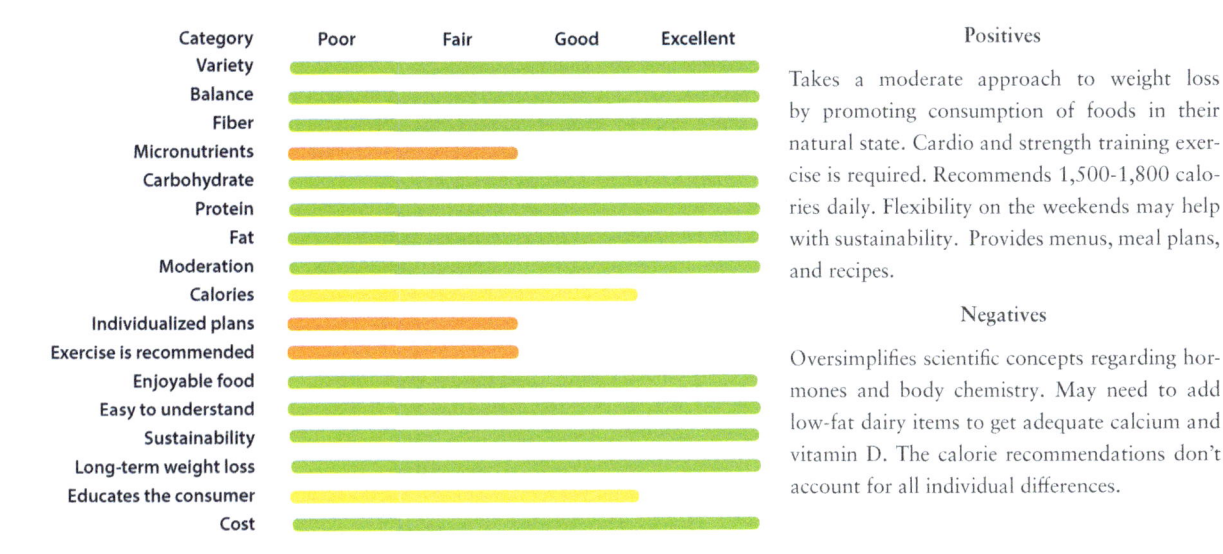

Category	Poor	Fair	Good	Excellent
Variety				██
Balance				██
Fiber				██
Micronutrients		██		
Carbohydrate				██
Protein				██
Fat				██
Moderation				██
Calories			██	
Individualized plans		██		
Exercise is recommended		██		
Enjoyable food				██
Easy to understand				██
Sustainability				██
Long-term weight loss				██
Educates the consumer			██	
Cost				██

Positives

Takes a moderate approach to weight loss by promoting consumption of foods in their natural state. Cardio and strength training exercise is required. Recommends 1,500-1,800 calories daily. Flexibility on the weekends may help with sustainability. Provides menus, meal plans, and recipes.

Negatives

Oversimplifies scientific concepts regarding hormones and body chemistry. May need to add low-fat dairy items to get adequate calcium and vitamin D. The calorie recommendations don't account for all individual differences.

The hook/catch or brilliant selling point: Catchy title by TV personality.

Truths/Myths

- **Myth** - People get fat because the wrong foods eaten alter body chemistry and toxify the body.

- **Truth** - The main reasons many people get fat is due to a slowing metabolism that accompanies aging, along with eating too many calories than expended. 🔍 p. 65, 21

Final decision: Thumbs up 👍

How to improve this diet: May need to add low-fat dairy items to get adequate calcium and vitamin D. 🔍 p. 29

Three Day Diet
(aka The Military Diet, Navy Diet, Army Diet, and Ice Cream Diet)

Premise of the Diet: Combines food in such a way as to increase metabolism and burn fat.

Claims of the Diet: Lose up to 10 pounds in 3 days.

Diet Description: A 3-day set menu is followed by 4 days off, and the weekly cycle is repeated until goal weight is reached. Sauces and dressings are not allowed, but vanilla ice cream can be consumed every day. Although there are no rules for the remaining 4 days of the diet, limiting portion sizes and keeping the total calorie amount under 1,500 daily is recommended.

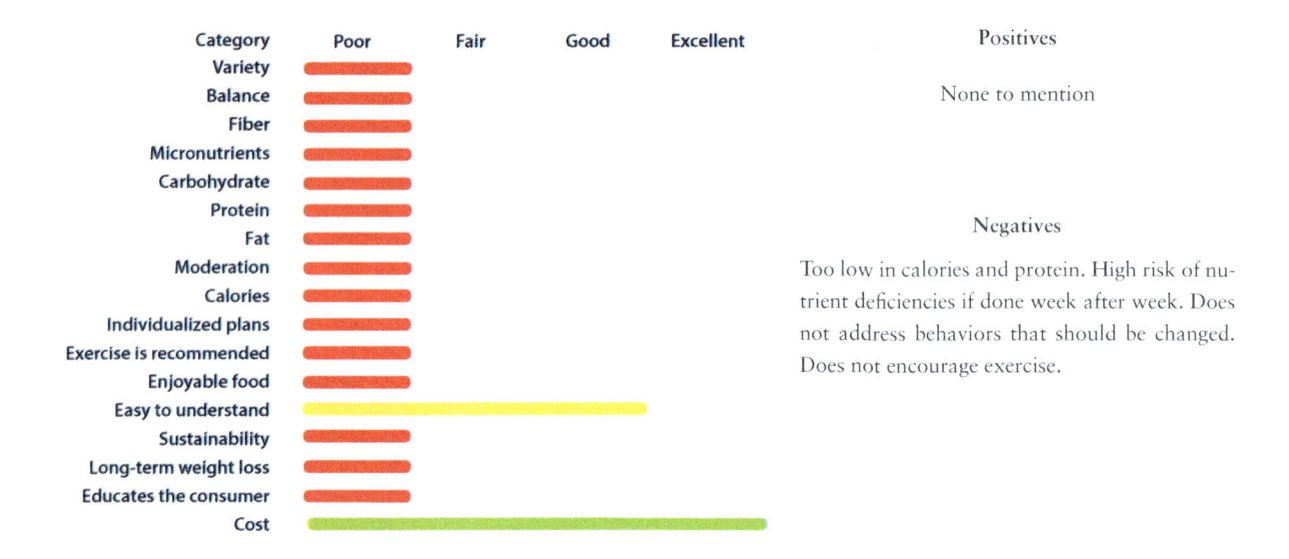

Category	Poor	Fair	Good	Excellent
Variety	■			
Balance	■			
Fiber	■			
Micronutrients	■			
Carbohydrate	■			
Protein	■			
Fat	■			
Moderation	■			
Calories	■			
Individualized plans	■			
Exercise is recommended	■			
Enjoyable food	■			
Easy to understand			■	
Sustainability	■			
Long-term weight loss	■			
Educates the consumer	■			
Cost				■

Positives

None to mention

Negatives

Too low in calories and protein. High risk of nutrient deficiencies if done week after week. Does not address behaviors that should be changed. Does not encourage exercise.

The hook/catch or brilliant selling point: Lose a lot of weight fast.

Truths/Myths

- Myth - Is chemically and enzyme balanced. 🔍 p. 13

- Truth - There are no standard definitions for these terms in order to know what is "in balance" or "out of balance."

- Truth - Not affiliated with any military or governmental institutions.

- Myth - It is possible to lose 10 pounds of fat in 3 days.

- Truth - If the scale drops by 10 pounds in 3 days, some combination of lean tissue, glycogen and water have been lost. 🔍 p. 15

Final decision: Thumbs down 👎

How to improve this diet: Can't be improved.

Three Hour Diet

Premise of the Diet: Eating consistently will keep the metabolism up, which helps burn fat throughout the day.

Claims of the Diet: Eating every three hours helps keeps the metabolism high and helps lose belly fat. Will lose belly fat and will decrease the stress hormone cortisol.

Diet Description: Eat small portions of food every 3 hours throughout the day. Stop eating at least 3 hours before going to sleep. Consume around 1,450 calories per day.

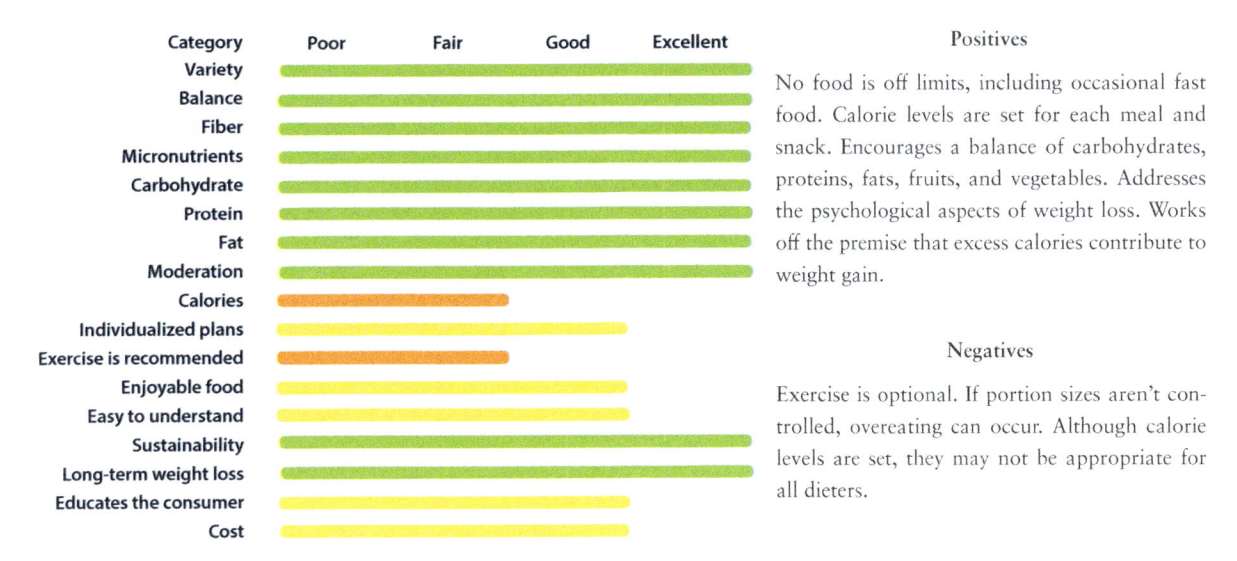

Category	Poor	Fair	Good	Excellent
Variety				■
Balance				■
Fiber				■
Micronutrients				■
Carbohydrate				■
Protein				■
Fat				■
Moderation				■
Calories		■		
Individualized plans		■		
Exercise is recommended		■		
Enjoyable food			■	
Easy to understand			■	
Sustainability				■
Long-term weight loss				■
Educates the consumer			■	
Cost			■	

Positives

No food is off limits, including occasional fast food. Calorie levels are set for each meal and snack. Encourages a balance of carbohydrates, proteins, fats, fruits, and vegetables. Addresses the psychological aspects of weight loss. Works off the premise that excess calories contribute to weight gain.

Negatives

Exercise is optional. If portion sizes aren't controlled, overeating can occur. Although calorie levels are set, they may not be appropriate for all dieters.

The hook/catch or brilliant selling point: Snack to lose weight

Truths/Myths

- *Myth* - Not eating for more than 3 hours puts the body into "starvation mode," which means fat is more likely to be stored and muscle more likely to be broken down for fuel which can also slow the metabolism. 🔍 p. 71

- *Truth* - While many experts are not in agreement that small portions eaten regularly translate into weight loss, eating every three hours may prevent a dieter from binging due to becoming famished.

Final decision: Thumbs up 👍

How to improve this diet: Include some type of physical activity.

The Trinity Diet

Premise of the Diet: To show how the trinity of macronutrients can mirror the concept of the Triune God. In this context, protein symbolizes God the Father, carbohydrates symbolize Jesus the bread of life, and fats symbolize the Holy Spirit. The diet focuses on providing an adequate balance of the nutrients needed by the body to optimize its ongoing detoxification process. To reach and maintain ideal weight, it is important to identify the causes of weight gain and make fundamental lifestyle changes.

Claims of the Diet: Moving away from prescription drugs, toxic foods, and negative thoughts can heal. Through a properly executed Trinity Diet program, a male will burn an average of 11 calories per pound of body weight and a female 10 calories per pound of body weight each day. The maximum amount of fat loss possible in a week is 4–6 pounds.

Diet Description: A number of steps and suggestions for making the transition to the Trinity Diet are provided. These include things like: Make meals a positive family experience, only buy foods you want eaten by the family, pray before each meal for the Lord to strengthen your body for His service, take responsibility for the way your family eats by planning ahead, try healthy alternatives so you do not feel deprived, don't skip meals, and avoid soft drinks, caffeine, packaged and processed foods, and dairy products, sugar, and simple carbohydrates.

A major part of the diet involves herbs and phytonutrients for cardiovascular and circulation support; detoxification and digestive support; stress, mood, and energy support; blood sugar support; female menopause support and male reproductive support; and depression, anxiety, and nervous tension support.

The diet identifies three different cycles that the body goes through in a 24-hour period—Detoxification, Assimilation, and Restoration—and the dieter eats according to these cycles.

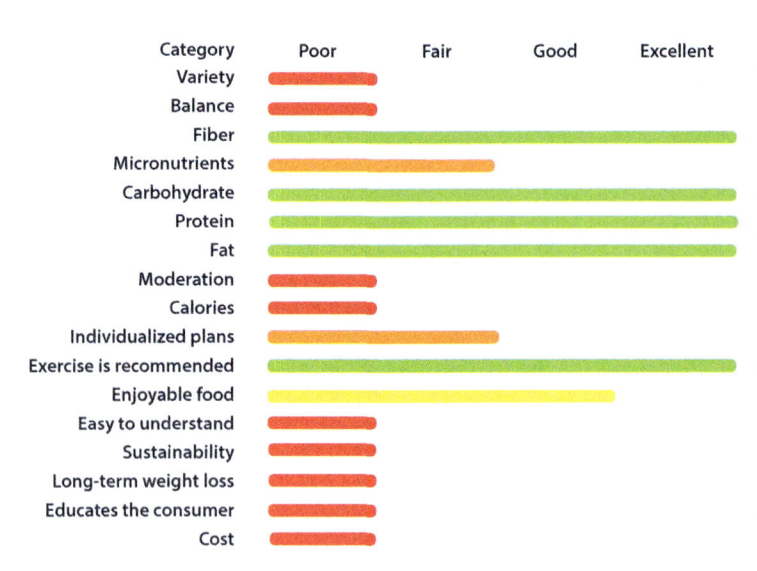

Category	Rating
Variety	Poor
Balance	Poor
Fiber	Excellent
Micronutrients	Fair
Carbohydrate	Excellent
Protein	Excellent
Fat	Excellent
Moderation	Poor
Calories	Poor
Individualized plans	Fair
Exercise is recommended	Excellent
Enjoyable food	Good
Easy to understand	Poor
Sustainability	Poor
Long-term weight loss	Poor
Educates the consumer	Poor
Cost	Poor

Positives

Includes aerobic, strength, and flexibility training. Promotes many positive and accepted healthy eating practices such as minimizing soft drinks, making meals a positive family experience, and planning ahead. Provides recipes. Recommends eating every 3–4 hours.

Negatives

Heavily recommends supplements. Eliminates a number of foods such as dairy (including all cheeses), all gluten-containing products, oranges, coffee, caffeine, peanuts, and all canned and creamed vegetables. Offers unproven reasons for many of the recommendations and suggestions. Requires dieters to determine their "lean body mass," which is a great idea but isn't possible for all dieters. Elimination of medication in lieu of natural plant hormone-supportive nutrients is recommended.

The hook/catch or brilliant selling point: Familiar terminology that is enticing to Christians.

Truths/Myths

- Myth - The most active period for the body to cleanse is between 4 am and 12 pm; when we consume excess calories late in the day, the body lacks the energy to digest food into smaller, usable molecules; in a 24-hour period the body goes through three different cycles.

- Truth - No credible scientific evidence exists to indicate that the body cleanses best between 4 am and 12 pm, nor to reliably say that the body lacks energy to digest food at certain times of the day. No credible scientific evidence exists to suggest that in a 24-hour period, everyone's body goes through three cycles.

- Myth - Rejecting the entire medication approach and embracing the natural remedies available through God's abundant creation sets you free to be healed. Your body will often heal faster without the interference of pharmaceuticals.

- Truth - God heals who He chooses to heal. There is no guarantee that following the Trinity Diet will lead to healing.

- Myth - Supplementation of quality nutrients such as those recommended are a vital part of making the Trinity Diet work more effectively at the cellular level. 🔍 p. 99

- Truth - Environments may influence the function of molecules. Thus, if the molecule is removed from its source or the chemical is extracted from the chemical matrix of the plant, there is no guarantee that it functions as it did in its original source.

- Myth - All herbal drugs are safe and free from side effects.

- Truth - A number of phytotherapeutic preparations have been studied and are fairly widely accepted including:

    - Preparations derived from the leaves of Ginkgo biloba—this is used to treat specific cognitive disorders and certain other disorders of the central nervous system.

    - Aerial parts of St. John's wort (Hypericum perforatum) to treat mild to moderate depression.

    - Aerial parts and roots of Echinacea angustifolia are used to treat and prevent the common cold and other respiratory conditions.

    - Parts of African devil's body/claw are used to fight inflammation and relieve arthritis pain.

- Truth - Drug interactions exist, and long-term interactions with prescription drugs have not been systematically studied with rigor, so caution must be exercised.

- Truth - Although the human body involves complex chemistry, biology, and physiology, in an age of choice, empowerment, convenience, and questioning authority, phytotherapy is appealing for those wishing to self-medicate. 🔍 p. 8

- Truth - Our bodies are temples of the Holy Spirit, precious gifts from our Father in Heaven.

- Truth - In order to detoxify itself, the body removes toxic waste via the feces, urine, carbon dioxide, and sweat, while organs such as the liver, kidney, lungs, and gallbladder also remove wastes from the body. 🔍 p. 89

Final decision: Thumbs down 👎

How to improve this diet: Do not invest in the purchase of the supplements but instead eat a variety of unprocessed foods in moderation. Include low-fat dairy products; avoid gluten if a gluten sensitivity is present. Approach with caution.

Ultrametabolism Diet

Premise of the Diet: Diet can reprogram genes.

Claims of the Diet: Lose 6 to 11 pounds during weeks 2-4.

Diet Description: An 8-week program.

Week 1: Eliminate processed food, sugars, alcohol, and caffeine.

Weeks 2 to 4: Cut out wheat, dairy, and eggs.

Weeks 5 to 8: Choose healthy fats, high-fiber starches, plant proteins, and lean meat. At this point, fewer than three glasses of wine per week and one cup of coffee a day can be incorporated. Requires calcium, magnesium with vitamin D, and omega-3 fatty acid supplements.

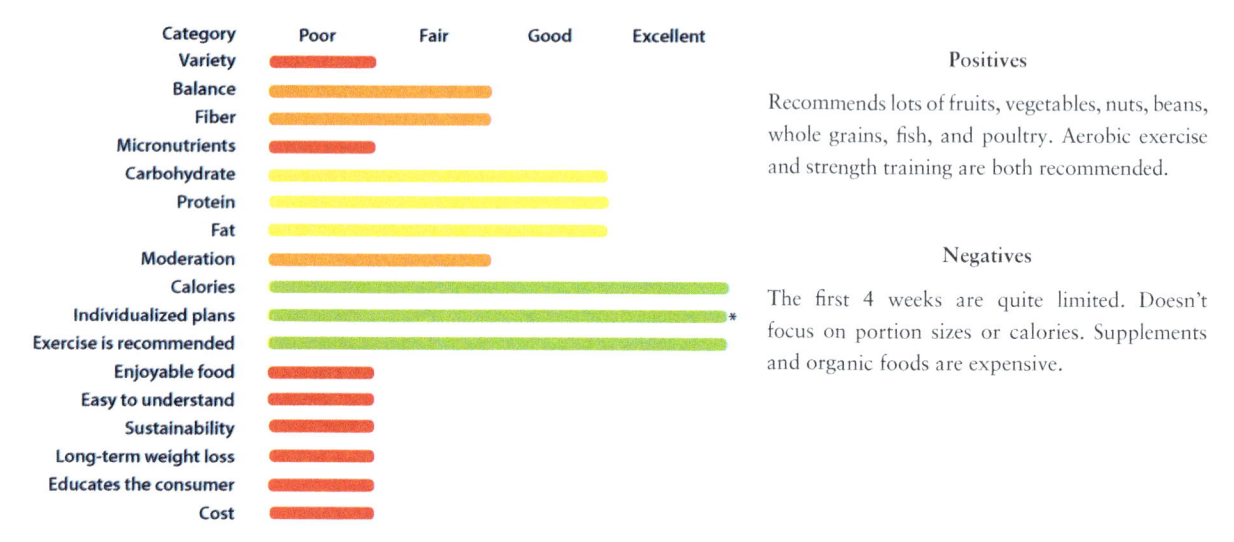

Category	Rating
Variety	Poor
Balance	Fair
Fiber	Fair
Micronutrients	Poor
Carbohydrate	Good
Protein	Good
Fat	Good
Moderation	Fair
Calories	Excellent
Individualized plans	Excellent*
Exercise is recommended	Excellent
Enjoyable food	Poor
Easy to understand	Poor
Sustainability	Poor
Long-term weight loss	Poor
Educates the consumer	Poor
Cost	Poor

Positives

Recommends lots of fruits, vegetables, nuts, beans, whole grains, fish, and poultry. Aerobic exercise and strength training are both recommended.

Negatives

The first 4 weeks are quite limited. Doesn't focus on portion sizes or calories. Supplements and organic foods are expensive.

*Based on the quizzes a person must take prior to starting the diet, this scored excellently. Unfortunately, it is not necessarily individualized in ways that have a scientific basis.

The hook/catch or brilliant selling point: The magic bullet has been found – it's the perfect individualized diet!

While a balance of proteins, carbs, and fats is recommended, clarity is needed on amounts because one size does not meet the needs for everyone and without portion sizes, weight loss cannot be guaranteed.

Truths/Myths

- Myth - We know enough about the human genome to make specific diet recommendations for each of the specific genes.

- Truth - We still have much to learn about the interaction between different foods and different genes. To date, the traditional Mediterranean diet's influence on genes has been studied more than any other diet. The Mediterranean diet seems to exert beneficial effects on risk factors for stroke, improved lipid profile, and even emotional eating.

- Truth - While nutrigenomics is a real emerging field, it is still young. We cannot yet say with confidence if certain food/gene combinations speed up metabolism or help with weight loss. The idea behind this diet is very complex. The complexity of relationships between foods, nutrients and genes is great and the field is still in the infancy stage. Exactly how food and genes interact isn't clear yet.

Final decision: Thumbs down

How to improve this diet: Consume a diet high in whole grains, fresh fruit, vegetables, healthy fats and lean meats that corresponds to required caloric needs. Exercisenomics indicates regular exercise is important.

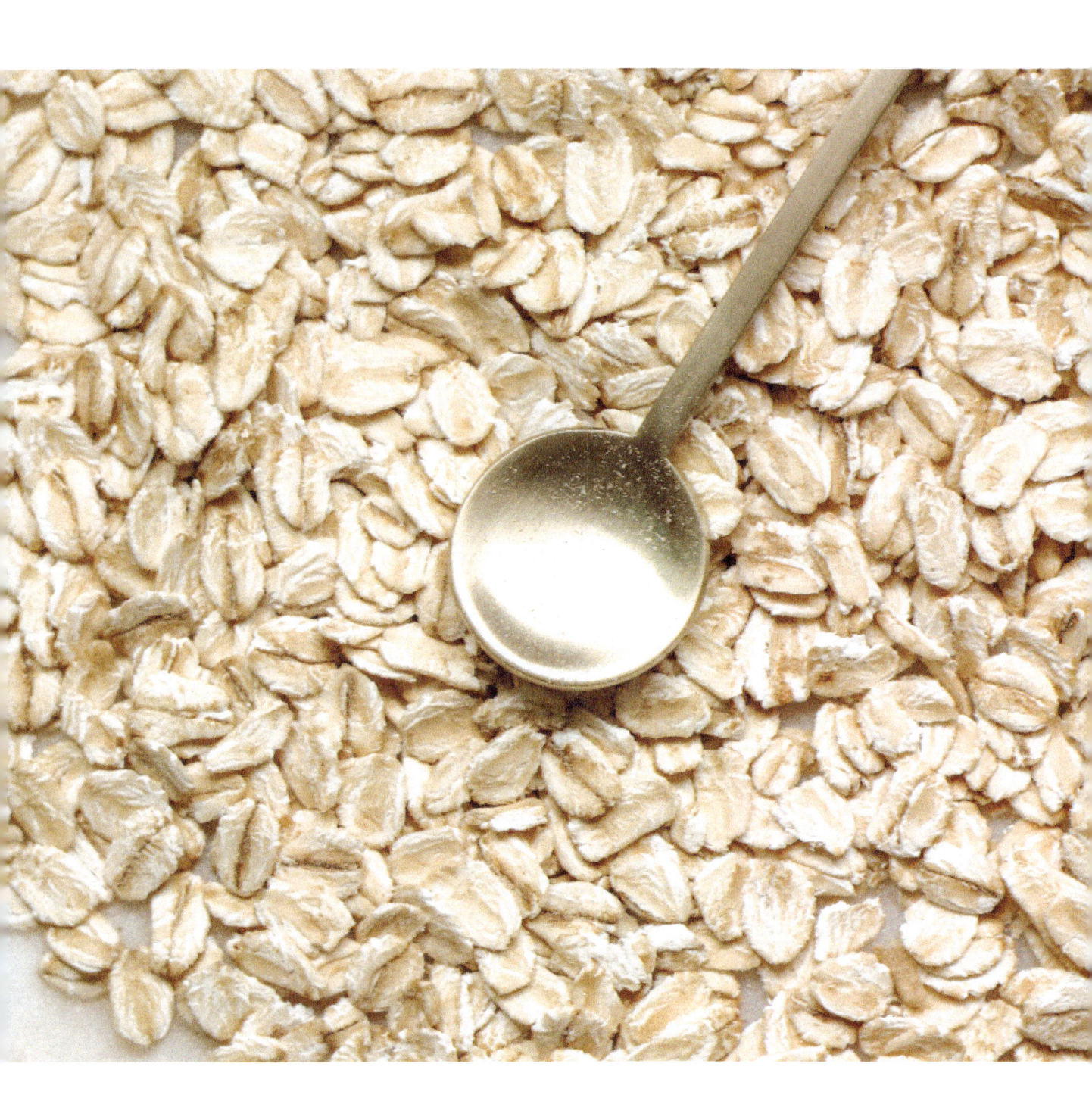

Volumetrics (aka The Ultimate Volumetrics Diet)

Premise of the Diet: By filling up on low-calorie foods, there is a decrease in caloric intake, which encourages weight loss.

Claims of the Diet: Promises weight loss of 1 to 2 pounds weekly while on the plan.

Diet Description: Consume foods that are low-calorie and high-volume with a lot of water and fiber to increase the sense of fullness. No food is banned if it is consumed within the recommended calorie intake. Foods are divided into 4 categories. 1 includes "free" or "anytime" fruits, non-starchy vegetables, and broth-based soups. 2 includes sensible portions of whole grains, lean proteins, legumes, and low-fat dairy. 3 includes small portions of foods such as breads, desserts, fat-free baked snacks, cheeses, and higher-fat meats. 4 allows scant portions of fried foods, candy, cookies, nuts, and fats. The plan divides food into three meals, two snacks, and a dessert each day.

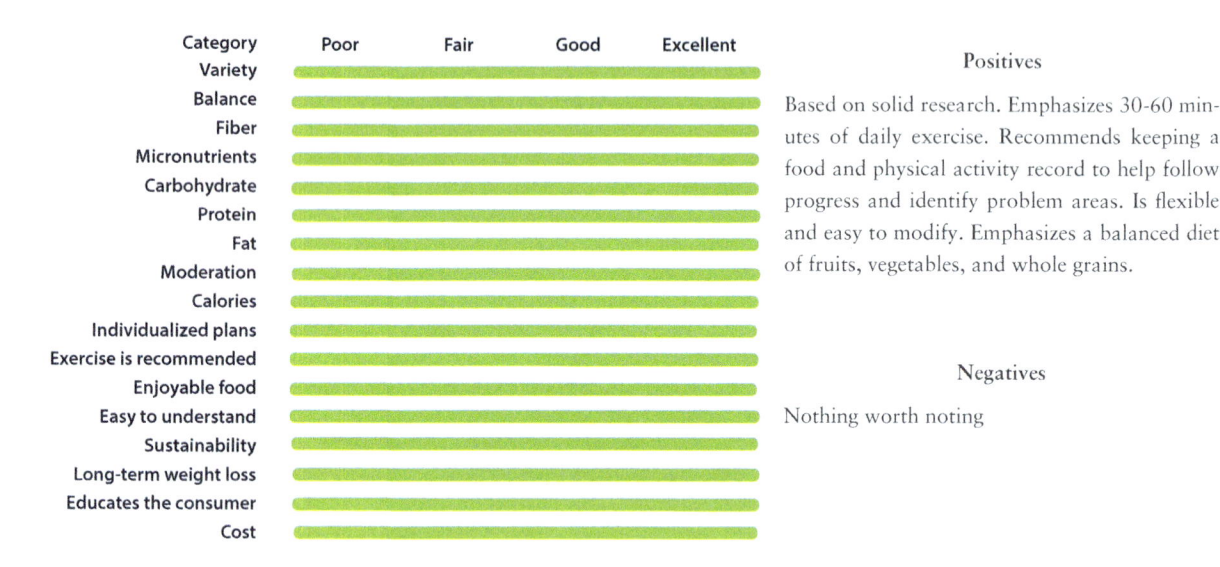

Category	Poor	Fair	Good	Excellent
Variety				████
Balance				████
Fiber				████
Micronutrients				████
Carbohydrate				████
Protein				████
Fat				████
Moderation				████
Calories				████
Individualized plans				████
Exercise is recommended				████
Enjoyable food				████
Easy to understand				████
Sustainability				████
Long-term weight loss				████
Educates the consumer				████
Cost				████

Positives

Based on solid research. Emphasizes 30-60 minutes of daily exercise. Recommends keeping a food and physical activity record to help follow progress and identify problem areas. Is flexible and easy to modify. Emphasizes a balanced diet of fruits, vegetables, and whole grains.

Negatives

Nothing worth noting

The hook/catch or brilliant selling point: Achieve long-term weight loss. Focuses on feeling full.

Truths/Myths

- Truth - No claims made that need to be explained.
- Myth - No false claims made

Final decision: Thumbs up 👍

How to improve this diet: No recommendations

Warrior Diet

Premise of the Diet: Eat in the manner of ancient warriors, who fasted for 20 hours then ate large amounts of food for 4 hours in the evening.

Claims of the Diet: Helps dieters get slim, healthy bodies.

Diet Description: Overall, the diet promotes a fast throughout the day, except for a 4-hour window of time in which the dieter "overeats." It is a strict intermittent fasting plan that is divided into phases.

The first phase takes one week, with the goal of detoxing by consuming clear broth, water, tea, coffee, vegetables and vegetable juice, olive oil and vinegar, eggs, and raw fruits. These are allowed during the 20-hour fast. During the 4-hour eating window, nutrient-dense foods such as vegetables, legumes, rice, quinoa, and unprocessed barley products are allowed.

The second phase also lasts for one week and in addition to the foods allowed in phase one, high-fat foods such as 4-6 ounces of lean meat and poultry, low-fat dairy, and nuts are allowed, but no starches or grains.

The third phase lasts for a week and alternates between high-carbohydrates (rice, oats, quinoa, corn, peas, potatoes, sweet potatoes, butternut squash, pumpkin, pasta, and bread) and high-protein days. This 3-week cycle is then repeated.

Category	Rating
Variety	Fair
Balance	Poor
Fiber	Fair
Micronutrients	Poor
Carbohydrate	Fair*
Protein	Fair*
Fat	Poor
Moderation	Fair
Calories	Poor
Individualized plans	Poor
Exercise is recommended	Fair
Enjoyable food	Poor
Easy to understand	Fair
Sustainability	Poor
Long-term weight loss	Poor
Educates the consumer	Poor
Cost	Fair

Positives

Minimizes fried foods and highly-processed foods. Preliminary short-term studies on intermittent fasting indicate a possible decrease in cholesterol and blood sugar levels.

Negatives

Lacks long-term scientific evidence. Based on the author's personal experience. Because food groups are limited or missing, multivitamins are required. May lead to binge-eating. Fatigue, stress and hormonal disruption may accompany this diet, due to the long periods of time without food. The diet is difficult to follow, due to its restrictiveness. May lead to binging on unhealthy foods. Long periods without fuel can limit exercise, which is essential to health and weight loss. Milk or milk products are not promoted, which can lead to nutrient deficiencies. p. 71, 29

*Depends on which day is being examined.

The hook/catch or brilliant selling point: The word "Warrior" is invigorating, strong and victorious. Very enticing!

Truths/Myths

- Myth - Eating this way will make the dieter a lean, mean fighting machine.

- Truth - This approach is very restrictive. It takes nutrient-dense foods and makes them difficult to incorporate into a healthy, sustainable lifestyle.

Final decision: Thumbs down

How to improve this diet: Can't be improved without major revision and restructuring.

Weigh Down Diet

Premise of the Diet: One can improve their relationship with food by strengthening their relationship with God. Reach out to God instead of food when the soul is in need. Helps the dieter recognize the difference between emotional eating and physical hunger.

Claims of the Diet: Gives new hope to millions who have failed on conventional diets.

Diet Description: Addresses how much is eaten more than avoiding or including certain foods. Mindful eating should be instituted by listening to body signals, which will indicate when to stop eating. To begin to understand the sensation of hunger, don't eat anything until your stomach begins growling. Proceed by eating a favorite food, even if it contains salt, sugar, or fat. Eating regular food, rather than diet food, is recommended. Experiment first by cutting your normal portion in half. Recommends eating slowly, paying attention to flavors, textures and fullness level, attempting to stop before feeling stuffed.

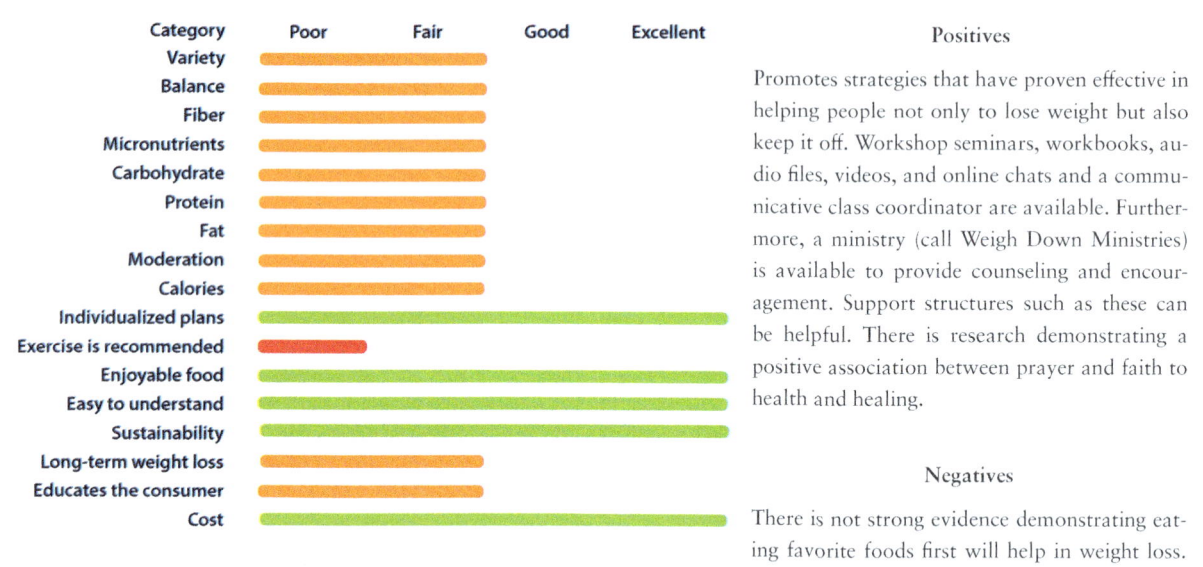

Category	Poor	Fair	Good	Excellent
Variety		█		
Balance		█		
Fiber		█		
Micronutrients		█		
Carbohydrate		█		
Protein		█		
Fat		█		
Moderation		█		
Calories		█		
Individualized plans				█
Exercise is recommended	█			
Enjoyable food				█
Easy to understand				█
Sustainability				█
Long-term weight loss		█		
Educates the consumer		█		
Cost				█

Positives

Promotes strategies that have proven effective in helping people not only to lose weight but also keep it off. Workshop seminars, workbooks, audio files, videos, and online chats and a communicative class coordinator are available. Furthermore, a ministry (call Weigh Down Ministries) is available to provide counseling and encouragement. Support structures such as these can be helpful. There is research demonstrating a positive association between prayer and faith to health and healing.

Negatives

There is not strong evidence demonstrating eating favorite foods first will help in weight loss. For many, their favorite foods may not be the most nutritious. Self-control will need to be displayed in order to not overeat on these foods. Since the goal of any diet should be to stay on it long-term, in this case, it is up to the dieter to be sure foods are nutrient dense and meals are balanced and full of variety.

The hook/catch or brilliant selling point: Developed by the pioneer of faith-based weight loss.

Truths/Myths

- Myth - This approach will help everyone trying to lose weight and achieve health. 🔍 p. 9

- Truth - People who always seem to be hungry, who feel they have no control over their binges, who find their desire for food irresistible when feeling sad, depressed, lost or lonely, may very well lose weight and benefit from incorporating these strategies.

Final decision: Thumbs down 👎

How to improve this diet: Incorporate the strategies recommended by this diet that have been proven effective in helping people not only to lose weight but also to keep it off. While these approaches alone may help certain people lose weight, food selections should be nutrient-dense and full of variety and balance. Keep in mind that healthy eating involves many areas. This diet addresses the emotional aspect of dieting well.

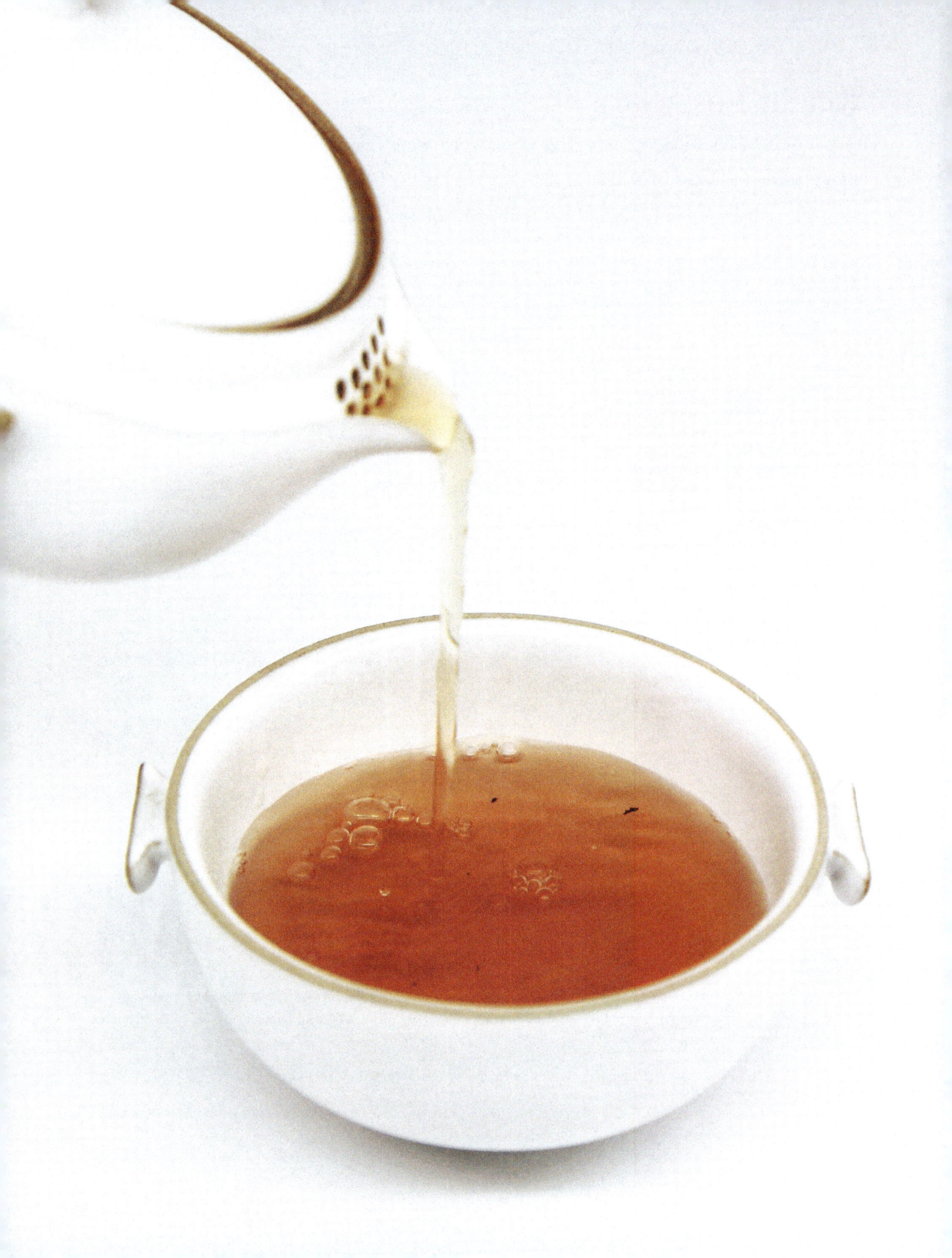

Weight Loss Cure Diet

Premise of the Diet: A strict organic diet with a secret protocol to help with weight loss.

Claims of the Diet: Will maximize fat-burning.

Diet Description: This three-phase diet is a strict organic diet that includes herbal supplements, along with practices such as hormone shots of human chorionic gonadotropin (hCG) and colon cleansings, or colonics. The first phase requires consuming only organic foods and engaging in internal cleansings, such as colonics. The second phase then adds daily human chorionic gonadotropin (hCG) injections. During the third phase, you will focus again on eating according to the specific recommendations of the diet and continuing with activities that allegedly cleanse your body and various organs, such as your liver.

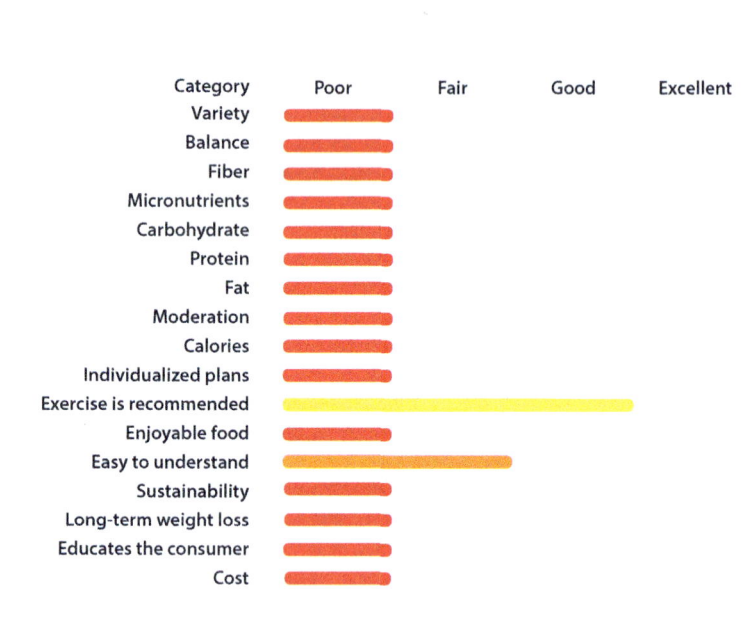

Category	Poor	Fair	Good	Excellent
Variety	Poor			
Balance	Poor			
Fiber	Poor			
Micronutrients	Poor			
Carbohydrate	Poor			
Protein	Poor			
Fat	Poor			
Moderation	Poor			
Calories	Poor			
Individualized plans	Poor			
Exercise is recommended			Good	
Enjoyable food	Poor			
Easy to understand		Fair		
Sustainability	Poor			
Long-term weight loss	Poor			
Educates the consumer	Poor			
Cost	Poor			

Positives

Focuses on fruits and vegetables. Exercise recommendations exceed the national guidelines. Recommends reducing sugars and sweets. Minimizes refined foods high in white flour and sugar.

Negatives

Recommends the unapproved use of hCG shots, and unnecessary colon cleansings. Emphasizes coconut oil, which is about 90% saturated fat. The required foods and protocols are expensive. The restrictive nature of the food recommendations makes sustainability difficult and nutritional deficiencies are likely. In phase 2, people consume 500 calories a day. Discusses legal loopholes for getting hCG, which is often promoted for weight loss, despite not being proven for weight loss. Filled with erroneous and questionable information. 🔍 p. 108

The hook/catch or brilliant selling point: Sounds farfetched, so it must work wonders.

Truths/Myths

- Myth - The author claims this approach to weight loss is known by diet experts but is being kept from the public.

- Truth - This diet is based on the work of British physician, Simeons, who in the 1950s declared hCG shots were helpful for weight loss. His work has been discredited in the Journal of the American Medical Association.

- Truth - The author does not have a medical background and has had encounters with the Federal Trade Commission (FTC) which resulted in him being banned for life from the infomercial industry.

- Truth - Governmental court decisions established advertised claims made by this diet did not contain much truth and as a result in 2009, a federal judge ordered consumers be repaid millions of dollars. FTC sent hundreds of thousands of refund checks to people who bought the book The Weight Loss Cure.

- Myth - hCG, which is usually found in the urine of pregnant women, helps with weight loss.

- Truth - hCG is approved by FDA as a prescription drug for the treatment of female infertility. It is not approved for weight loss.

- Truth - Any weight loss achieved while being on the hCG diet is due to a low calorie intake alone. hCG does not boost metabolism or help with weight loss.

- Truth - No credible studies support the claims of this diet.

Final decision: Thumbs down

How to improve this diet: Can't be improved.

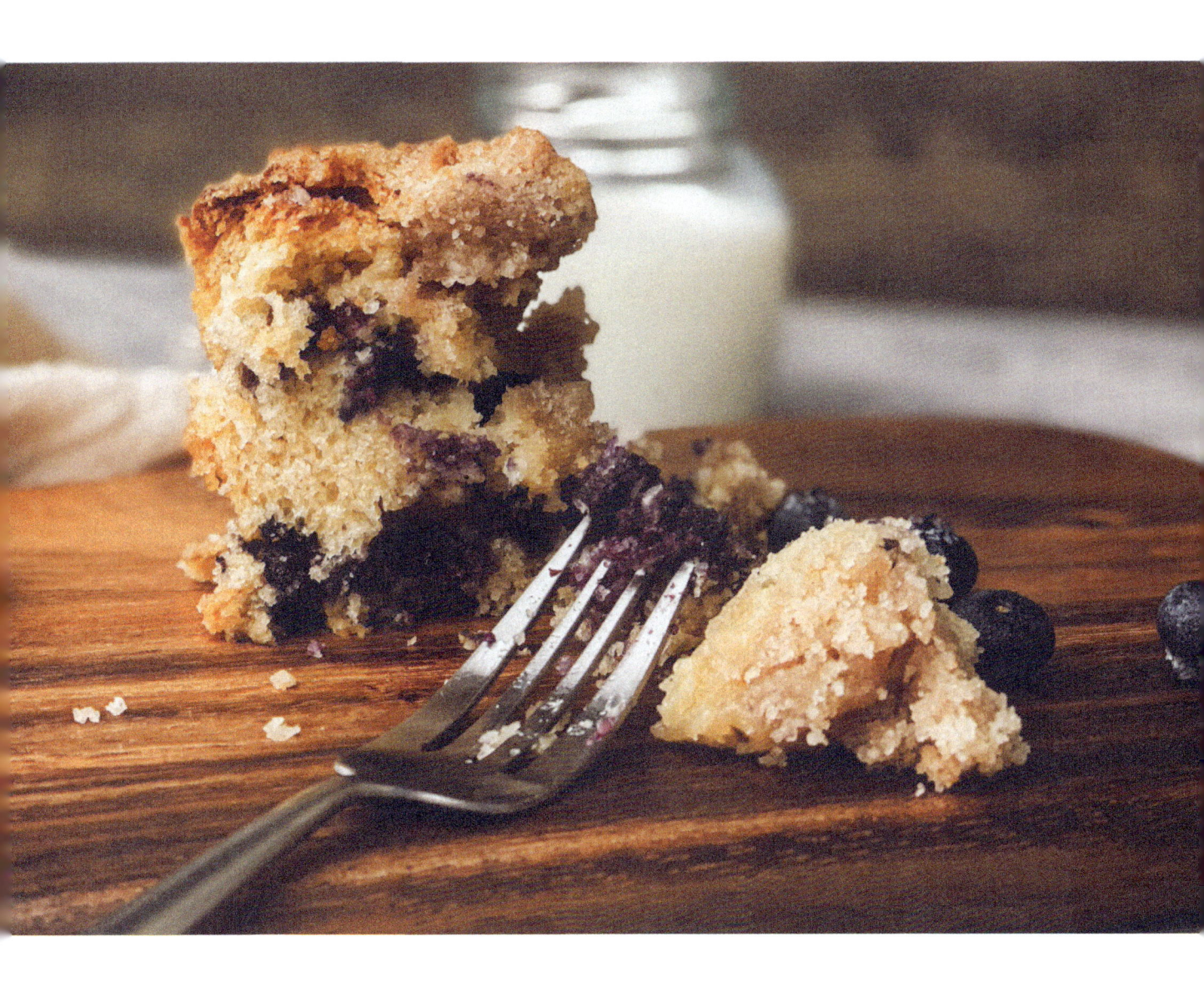

WW (Weight Watchers, Wellness that Works)

Premise of the Diet: Lifestyle modification that includes better decisions that prioritize healthy foods.

Claims of the Diet: Expect to lose .5 to 2 pounds per week.

Diet Description: This program, which was started in 1963, has gone through several changes over the years. Initially, it used an exchange system where foods were counted based on their food group. In the 1990s, it presented a points-based system where values were assigned to foods and drinks based on their fiber, fat, and calorie contents. Then in 2015 the program came out with the SmartPoints system. SmartPoints take into account calorie, fat, protein, and sugar contents. In 2017 the program adjusted again to become more flexible and user-friendly and is now called WW Freestyle. The main difference is the inclusion of more than 200 foods that do not have to be weighed, measured, or tracked because they contribute zero points. Zero-point foods include eggs, skinless chicken, plain Greek yogurt, many fish, and unsweetened plain yogurt. In an attempt to encourage dieters to make healthier food choices instead of basing decisions solely on how many points they are allotted, in the newest system a number of foods higher in protein contribute a lower point value.

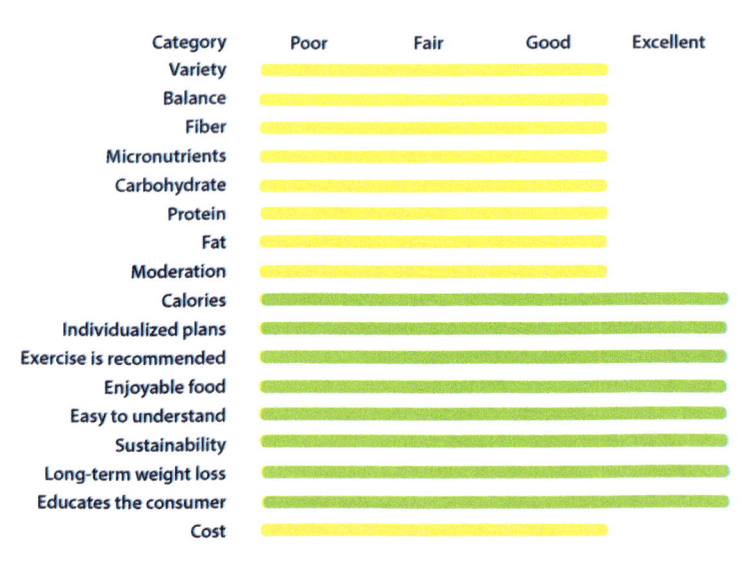

Category	Poor	Fair	Good	Excellent
Variety			■	
Balance			■	
Fiber			■	
Micronutrients			■	
Carbohydrate			■	
Protein			■	
Fat			■	
Moderation			■	
Calories				■
Individualized plans				■
Exercise is recommended				■
Enjoyable food				■
Easy to understand				■
Sustainability				■
Long-term weight loss				■
Educates the consumer				■
Cost			■	

Positives

Provides a slow, steady weight loss through dietary and lifestyle changes. Has a support network that includes a 24/7 online chat, apps, in-person group meetings or one-on-one support, a personal coach, and access to an online database of foods and recipes. No foods are off limits. Allows users to indulge within reason. Encourages physical activity by assigning FitPoints that can be logged into an app. Provides fitness videos and workout routines. Prepackaged foods are also available. Emphasizes portion control. Randomized controlled trials support the effectiveness of this program.

Negatives

It can be time-consuming to daily keep track of the foods eaten. May be expensive for some people. Because theoretically unhealthy food can make up all allotted SmartPoints, this program may be too lenient for those who struggle with self-control.

The hook/catch or brilliant selling point: Has longevity as a diet program.

Truths/Myths: None worth noting.

Final decision: Thumbs up 👍

How to improve this diet: No suggestions other than be sure to follow the MyPlate recommendations when making food choices.

Werewolf Diet
aka The Moon Diet, The Lunar Diet

Premise of the Diet: Based on lunar phases.

Claims of the Diet: Can lose 6 pounds in 24–26 hours. Cleanses the body of toxins.

Diet Description: The idea behind this diet is that since the human body is made up of mostly water, and the moon influences the tides of the ocean, the moon must also then influence the water in human bodies. When the moon is full or at a new phase, there is a strong 24-hour gravitational pull that will influence how much water weight one can gain or lose. Dieters have the choice of two plans, the basic Moon Diet plan or the extended version. The basic version is a 24-hour day of fasting during either a new or full moon. It includes only drinking water, detox teas, and juice. The extended version starts with fasting at these same times but then follows specific eating plans for the various phases of the moon: full moon, waning moon, new moon, and waxing moon.

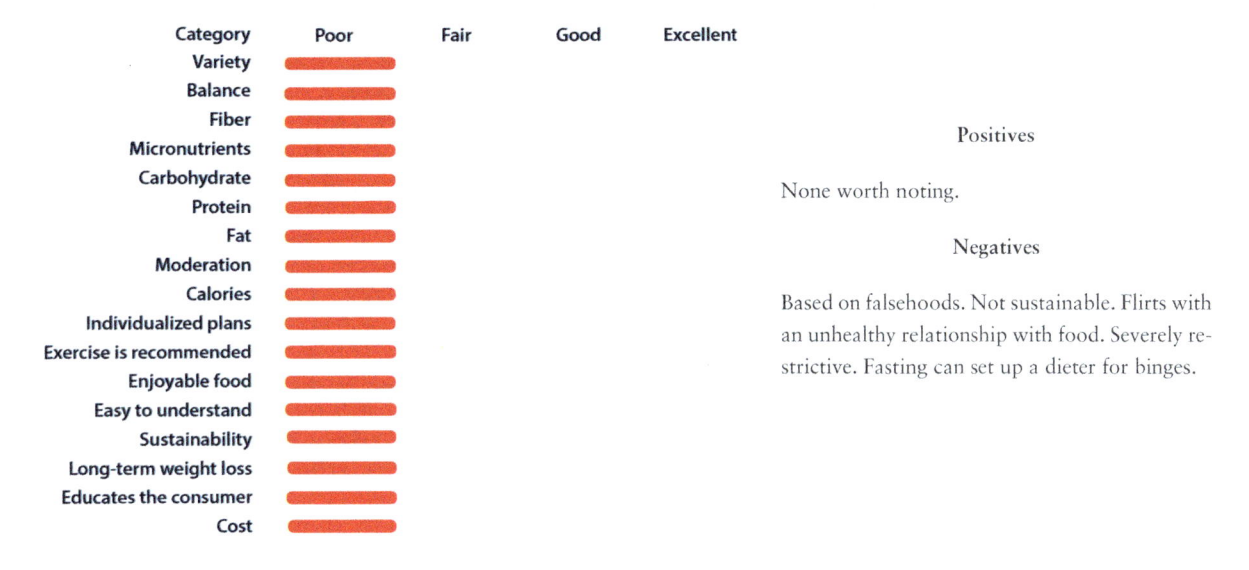

Category	Poor	Fair	Good	Excellent
Variety	●			
Balance	●			
Fiber	●			
Micronutrients	●			
Carbohydrate	●			
Protein	●			
Fat	●			
Moderation	●			
Calories	●			
Individualized plans	●			
Exercise is recommended	●			
Enjoyable food	●			
Easy to understand	●			
Sustainability	●			
Long-term weight loss	●			
Educates the consumer	●			
Cost	●			

Positives

None worth noting.

Negatives

Based on falsehoods. Not sustainable. Flirts with an unhealthy relationship with food. Severely restrictive. Fasting can set up a dieter for binges.

The hook/catch or brilliant selling point: Popularized by various celebrities.

Truths/Myths

- Myth - The phases of the moon can affect weight loss.

- Truth - No credible scientific evidence supports this claim.

- Myth - Can lose 6 pounds in 24–26 hours.

- Truth - Restriction of any calories can lead to weight loss. But this type of loss will not be fat loss. Weight will be regained as soon as the dieter goes "off" the diet.

Final decision: Thumbs down

How to improve this diet: No way to improve this diet.

What Color Is Your Diet?

Premise of the Diet: Health can be achieved and weight can be lost by eating a wide range of fruits and vegetables.

Claims of the Diet: Will supercharge health while promoting losing weight.

Diet Description: Eating one serving (1/2 cup cooked or 1 cup raw) daily from each of the following seven color categories:

1. Red foods rich in lycopene (tomatoes, pink grapefruit, watermelon)
2. Red/purple foods rich in anthocyanin (grapes, berries, prunes, red apples)
3. Orange foods rich in both alpha- and beta-carotene (carrots, mangoes, apricots, cantaloupe)
4. Orange/yellow foods rich in carotenoids and vitamin C (oranges, tangerines, peaches, nectarines, papaya)
5. Yellow/green foods rich in lutein and zeaxanthin (bell peppers, spinach, kale, collard greens, corn)
6. Green foods rich in sulforaphane, isothiocyanate, and indoles (broccoli, kale, bok choy)
7. White/green flavonoid-rich foods (garlic, onion, celery, pears, chives)

The diet includes lean protein, lower-fat dairy, healthy fats, and a focus on whole grains, fiber, and spices.

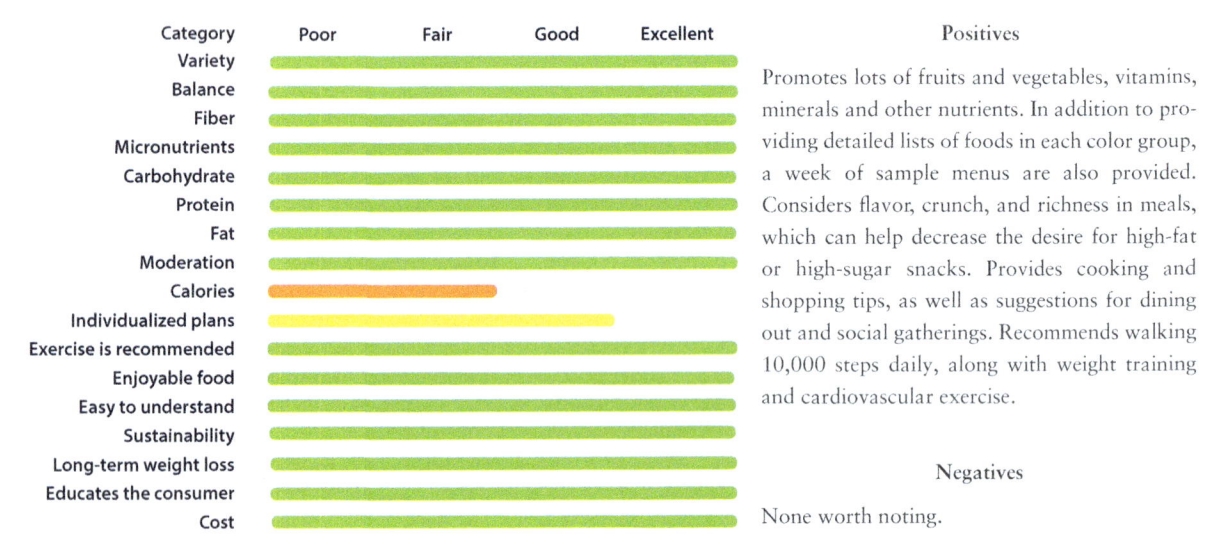

Category	Poor	Fair	Good	Excellent
Variety				✓
Balance				✓
Fiber				✓
Micronutrients				✓
Carbohydrate				✓
Protein				✓
Fat				✓
Moderation				✓
Calories		✓		
Individualized plans			✓	
Exercise is recommended				✓
Enjoyable food				✓
Easy to understand				✓
Sustainability				✓
Long-term weight loss				✓
Educates the consumer				✓
Cost				✓

Positives

Promotes lots of fruits and vegetables, vitamins, minerals and other nutrients. In addition to providing detailed lists of foods in each color group, a week of sample menus are also provided. Considers flavor, crunch, and richness in meals, which can help decrease the desire for high-fat or high-sugar snacks. Provides cooking and shopping tips, as well as suggestions for dining out and social gatherings. Recommends walking 10,000 steps daily, along with weight training and cardiovascular exercise.

Negatives

None worth noting.

The hook/catch or brilliant selling point: Sounds fun.

Truths/Myths: None worth noting

Final decision: Thumbs up 👍

How to improve this diet: Introducing too much fiber and whole grains too quickly or all at once can negatively affect the digestive system. Gradually introduce new foods and slowly increase quantities so as to not shock the system.

Wheat Belly Diet

Premise of the Diet: A gluten-free lifestyle.

Claims of the Diet: Giving up wheat helps with weight loss and increases energy.

Diet Description: Eliminate all foods made with wheat, barley, rye, oats, rice, potatoes, legumes, cornstarch, rice starch, potato starch, tapioca starch, high-fructose corn syrup, sucrose, salt, sugary foods, soda, fruit juice, and dried fruit. Avoid trans fats, fried foods, and cured meats on this plan. Focuses on replacing all grain-based carbohydrates with natural gluten-free whole foods, like protein, healthy fats, and vegetables, with a limited variety of fruits.

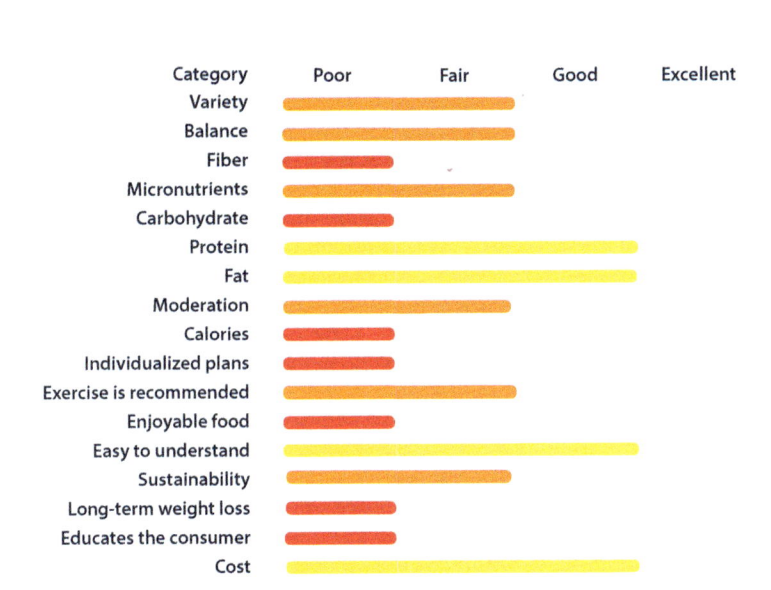

Category	Rating
Variety	Fair
Balance	Fair
Fiber	Poor
Micronutrients	Fair
Carbohydrate	Poor
Protein	Excellent
Fat	Excellent
Moderation	Fair
Calories	Poor
Individualized plans	Poor
Exercise is recommended	Fair
Enjoyable food	Poor
Easy to understand	Excellent
Sustainability	Fair
Long-term weight loss	Poor
Educates the consumer	Poor
Cost	Excellent

Positives

Minimizes consumption of highly-processed foods.

Negatives

While regular exercise is encouraged, it doesn't offer specific recommendations. Does not monitor calories and macronutrient proportions. It eliminates foods that are good sources of fiber and provide carbohydrates, such as potatoes, rice, quinoa, and legumes. These are staples in a healthy gluten-free diet. It also eliminates cornstarch, tapioca starch, potato starch, and rice starch which, in a gluten-free diet, are allowed occasionally in "sometimes" foods like birthday cake. This would be a very bland diet and therefore likely unsustainable, even for someone who is sensitive to gluten.

The hook/catch or brilliant selling point: The culprit has been found and we can eliminate it.

Truths/Myths

- **Myth** - All forms of wheat and grains are detrimental to health because they have been hybridized over the years. 🔍 p. 39

- **Truth** - Many farm-grown foods have been modified over the years to increase nutrient content.

- **Myth** - This diet is a good approach for weight loss.

- **Truth** - Regarding weight loss, portion sizes matter and guidelines for overall healthful eating or calorie control are lacking with this diet. Any weight loss will most likely not be from eliminating gluten. There is no scientific evidence suggesting foods without gluten cause more weight loss than other foods. However, eliminating items like soda, fried foods, and foods with added sugar can help with weight loss. 🔍 p. 22

- **Myth** - Consuming wheat can lead to insulin resistance, which makes the body store extra fat.

- **Truth** - This is not scientifically proven.

Final decision: Thumbs down 👎

How to improve this diet: Can't be improved.

Whole 30 Diet

Premise of the Diet: Does not focus solely on weight loss. Instead of restricting calories, various food categories are restricted.

Claims of the Diet: Removes groups of foods that harm health. Over 95% of participants have lost weight and improved their body composition. People experience more energy, sharper mental focus, better sleep, clearer skin, improved mood and increased athletic performance.

Diet Description: The goal is to "reset" the body, which then allows someone to slowly add foods back into their diet while checking for adverse reactions. Potentially harmful food groups include dairy, sugar, grains, and legumes. This is a temporary diet designed to last 30 days.

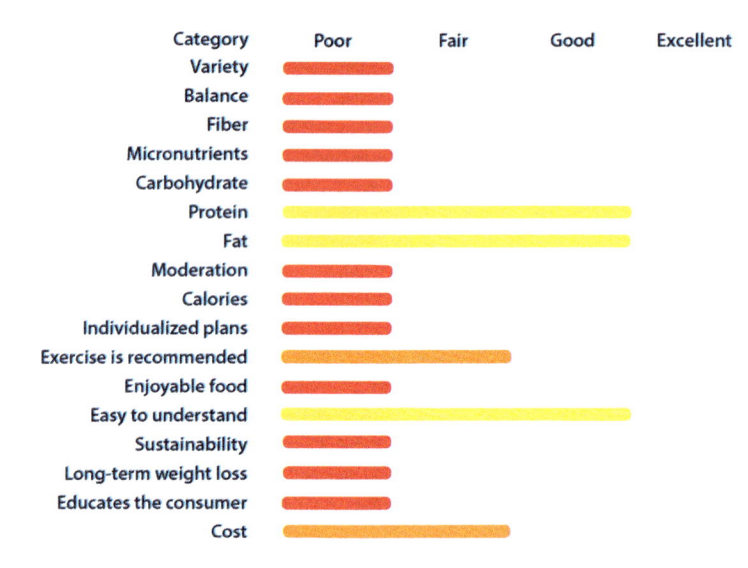

Category	Poor	Fair	Good	Excellent
Variety	■			
Balance	■			
Fiber	■			
Micronutrients	■			
Carbohydrate	■			
Protein				■
Fat				■
Moderation	■			
Calories	■			
Individualized plans	■			
Exercise is recommended		■		
Enjoyable food	■			
Easy to understand				■
Sustainability	■			
Long-term weight loss	■			
Educates the consumer	■			
Cost		■		

Positives

Recommends eating whole foods. Eliminates refined grains and sugars. No calorie counting or measuring is required. Encourages label reading.

Negatives

There are no cheat days during these 30 days. If the rules are broken at any time, returning to day 1 and starting again is a must. Is very restrictive and takes a lot of self-discipline. Because entire food groups are eliminated, it may take more time than usual to plan and prepare meals for an entire month. Even though this is a temporary diet and a plan must be in place to transition to a balanced, healthful diet that can be long term, little assistance is provided to guide this long-term transition. No exercise is recommended. Constipation and a disruption of healthy gut flora could be a problem. Many nutrient-dense foods are eliminated, which increases the risk of nutrient deficiencies, including fiber, phytochemicals, folate, vitamin E, iron, magnesium, B vitamins, calcium, potassium, and vitamin D. A number of the foods eliminated have been linked to a lower risk of heart disease, some cancers, and diabetes. This is a costly diet, as it recommends organic, wild-caught or pasture-raised meats, and oils and drinks that are much more expensive than many people would normally consume.

The hook/catch or brilliant selling point: Promotes the idea we can add or eliminate foods and be in control of our health.

Truths/Myths

- Myth - Cutting out said food groups for 30 consecutive days will allow the body to heal from the underlying issues (inflammation, gut-disruption, psychological harm, and hormone imbalance.) In essence, the diet hits a reset button. 🔍 p. 29

- Truth - Other than allergies or intolerances, there is no science-based nutrition reason to cut out the food groups this diet requires.

Final decision: Thumbs down 👎

How to improve this diet: Focus on foods that can be eaten, rather than the foods which are off-limits. With the exception of allergy or intolerance, there is no reason to cut out so many food groups.

You on a Diet (aka Dr. Oz's Ultimate Diet)

Premise of the Diet: Learning how to change our environment helps us achieve our waistline goals.

Claims of the Diet: Will take up to 2 inches off the waist in 2 weeks.

Diet Description: Foods are eliminated (actually thrown out of the house) if they don't follow the "Rule of 5s," which means foods with sugars, syrups, white flours, saturated fats, or trans fats as one of the first five ingredients on the label. New foods introduced emphasize fiber and lean protein. This diet starts with a strict and repetitive 2-week introduction that recommends the same healthy foods for breakfast and lunch. The idea is that limiting food choices will help with weight loss. More variety is offered for the evening meal. Thirty minutes of daily walking and additional stretching is recommended. A guide to strength training is also provided. Throughout the program, waistline measurements are taken to track progress.

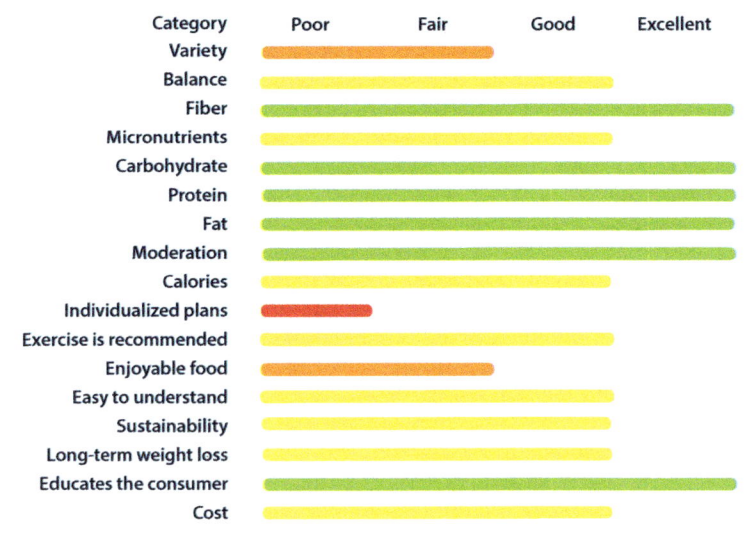

Category	Poor	Fair	Good	Excellent
Variety		■		
Balance			■	
Fiber				■
Micronutrients			■	
Carbohydrate				■
Protein				■
Fat				■
Moderation				■
Calories				■
Individualized plans	■			
Exercise is recommended			■	
Enjoyable food		■		
Easy to understand			■	
Sustainability			■	
Long-term weight loss			■	
Educates the consumer				■
Cost			■	

Positives

Emphasizes whole grains, fruits, vegetables, and healthy fats. Recommends exercise. Recommends tracking progress, which can be rewarding. Attempts to educate consumers. Does not take a "quick fix" approach. Recommends finding a "weight-loss buddy" for support. Follows the nutritional guidelines of the American Heart Association and the American Diabetes Association. Provides helpful tips on how to stick with the diet for a lifetime.

Negatives

Although variety in food choices increases as the diet progresses, the limited list of acceptable foods could frustrate some people, especially in the beginning. Research does not support the notion that having fewer choices causes less eating. Eating out may be difficult while trying to follow the "Rule of 5s." Does not take individual differences into account and does not adequately address emotional eating. This diet reduces calories by about 100 calories per day, which will produce a slow, steady weight loss; however, it would be such a slow weight loss that dieters may become frustrated with the lack of progress.

The hook/catch or brilliant selling point: Celebrity endorsement.

Truths/Myths

- **Myth** - Having fewer choices causes less eating.

- **Truth** - While this may be true in an environment with little food, in an environment of plenty it has not been established as fact. 🔍 p. 7

Final decision: Thumbs down

How to improve this diet: While some dieters like routine, others do not. Sufficient variety needs to exist for each individual dieter. Emotional eaters may need additional support to make this work. Work in reasonable "cheat meals" for eating out or social gatherings.

Zero Belly Diet

Premise of the Diet: Turns off fat genes.

Claims of the Diet: Will attack fat cells on a genetic level to help eliminate visceral fat around organs.

Diet Description: Focuses on nine power foods which are to be consumed in three meals and one to two snacks daily. Includes lots of smoothies made from plant-based protein powder to help reduce hunger. Provides two different eating schedules. One schedule accounts for daytime exercise and the other for nighttime exercise.

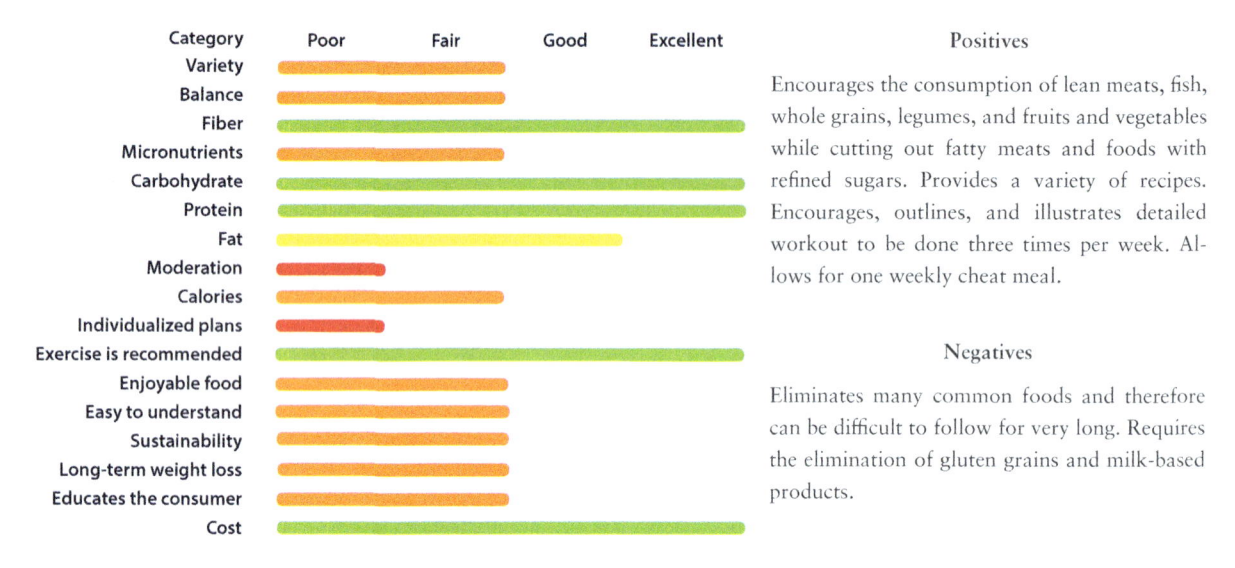

Category	Rating
Variety	Fair
Balance	Fair
Fiber	Excellent
Micronutrients	Fair
Carbohydrate	Excellent
Protein	Excellent
Fat	Good
Moderation	Poor
Calories	Fair
Individualized plans	Poor
Exercise is recommended	Excellent
Enjoyable food	Fair
Easy to understand	Fair
Sustainability	Fair
Long-term weight loss	Fair
Educates the consumer	Fair
Cost	Excellent

Positives

Encourages the consumption of lean meats, fish, whole grains, legumes, and fruits and vegetables while cutting out fatty meats and foods with refined sugars. Provides a variety of recipes. Encourages, outlines, and illustrates detailed workout to be done three times per week. Allows for one weekly cheat meal.

Negatives

Eliminates many common foods and therefore can be difficult to follow for very long. Requires the elimination of gluten grains and milk-based products.

The hook/catch or brilliant selling point: We love the idea of zero fat on our bellies!

Truths/Myths

- **Myth** - Uses foods that are high in specific nutrients (like choline and folate) to "turn off fat genes."

- **Truth** - The human genome is vast and complex. Much research is being done in this area, but not enough is yet known to make specific recommendations like this.

- **Myth** - Specifically targets belly fat. p. 61

- **Truth** - We cannot dictate where we lose body fat. We cannot spot-reduce through exercise or diet. We can only tone areas of the body through exercise. p. 24

Final decision: Thumbs down

How to improve this diet: Be sure to consume adequate dairy products to ensure getting adequate calcium and vitamin D. If you are not sensitive to gluten, there is no need to cut it from the diet.

Zone Diet

Premise of the Diet: Reduces inflammation in the body.

Claims of the Diet: Optimizes hormones and escorts the body into "the Zone" where inflammation is controlled, energy is boosted, and excess body fat is lost without feeling hunger and fatigue.

Diet Description: Designed to be followed for a lifetime, the diet requires 40% of all calories to come from low glycemic index carbohydrates, 30% from low-fat protein sources, and 30% of calories from mostly monounsaturated fats. The goal is to design a Zone-friendly plate, by first dividing the plate into thirds where 1/3 is lean protein about the size and thickness of the palm of your hand. Two-thirds of the plate should be low-glycemic carbohydrates which, in essence, translate into legumes and non-starchy vegetables. Then one serving of monounsaturated fat. There are two approaches to this diet. The easiest is the hand-eye method where the eyes estimate portion sizes while the hand serves the portion. Five fingers remind us to eat five times a day and never go without food for five hours. The second method uses Zone food blocks. Zone food blocks work to personalize the Zone Diet by calculating how many grams of protein, carbs and fat should be consumed daily based on weight, height, waist, and hip measurements. The average male needs 14 Zone blocks per day, while the average female needs about 11 Zone blocks per day. Breakfast, lunch, and dinner generally contain three to five Zone blocks, while a snack provides one Zone block. Each Zone block is made up of a protein block which contains 7 grams of protein, a Carb block which contains 9 grams of carbohydrates and a Fat block which contains 3 grams of fat (1.5 grams of fat if it is an animal source.)

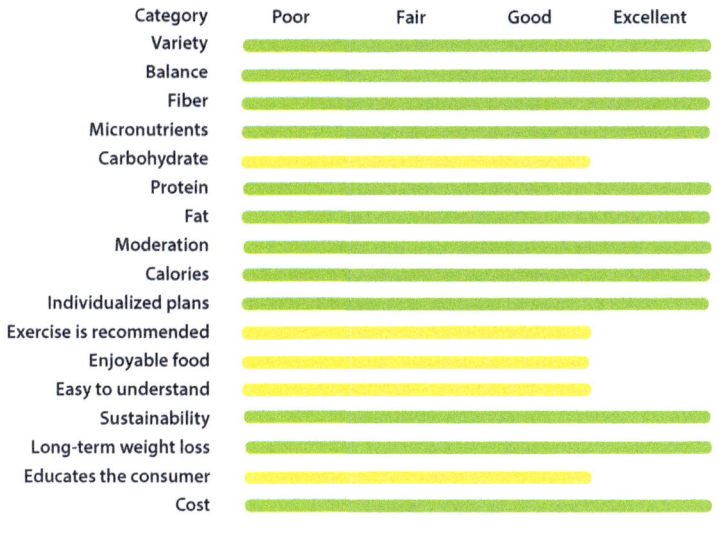

Category	Poor	Fair	Good	Excellent
Variety				✓
Balance				✓
Fiber				✓
Micronutrients				✓
Carbohydrate			✓	
Protein				✓
Fat				✓
Moderation				✓
Calories				✓
Individualized plans				✓
Exercise is recommended			✓	
Enjoyable food			✓	
Easy to understand			✓	
Sustainability				✓
Long-term weight loss				✓
Educates the consumer			✓	
Cost				✓

Positives

Is flexible and provides guidance for eating out. Provides appropriate proportions of macronutrients spread throughout the day that fall within the ranges recommended by the Institute of Medicine. While processed foods with added sugar are not recommended, it does not strictly eliminate any food choices. Whereas primarily designed to lower inflammation, it can aid in fat loss because it controls calories consumed per day. Moderate, consistent exercise is recommended. Recommends realistic, healthy weight loss. Website offers helpful tools including a food journal, grocery guide, tips for dining-out, and healthy recipes.

Negatives

Evidence supporting the Zone Diet's 40% carb, 30% protein, and 30% fat ratio as the optimal ratio for fat loss is lacking. While this diet recommends choices similar to the Mediterranean diet, which is widely accepted as one of the healthiest dietary approaches, this diet makes claims such as it will help one perform better and think faster, which are not sufficiently proven.

The hook/catch or brilliant selling point: Excess body fat is lost without feeling hunger and fatigue substantiated.

Truths/Myths

- **Myth** - Recommended supplements are necessary for weight loss. 🔍 p. 99

- **Truth** - Polyphenol supplements are molecules in plants that have antioxidant properties. Some research shows they decrease iron absorption. Eating plenty of plant foods should be sufficient to achieve health benefits.

Final decision: Thumbs up 👍

How to improve this diet: None with noting.

Blanket Template

Name(s) of the Diet:

Premise of the Diet:

Claims of the Diet:

Diet Description:

Category	Poor	Fair	Good	Excellent
Variety				
Balance				
Fiber				
Micronutrients				
Carbohydrate				
Protein				
Fat				
Moderation				
Calories				
Individualized plans				
Exercise is recommended				
Enjoyable food				
Easy to understand				
Sustainability				
Long-term weight loss				
Educates the consumer				
Cost				

Positives

Negatives

The hook/catch or brilliant selling point:

Truths/Myths:

- Myth -

- Truth -

Final decision: Thumbs down

How to improve this diet:

References for Rating the Diets

Alkaline Diet

1. Blackburn KB. Alkaline diet: what cancer patients should know. MD Anderson. https://www.mdanderson.org/cancerwise/alkaline-diet--what-cancer-patients-should-know.h00-159223356.html. Published April 2018. Accessed July 2, 2020.

2. de Santo NG, Capasso G, Malnic G, Anastasio P, Spitali L, D'Angelo A. Effect of an acute oral protein load on renal acidification in healthy humans and in patients with chronic renal failure. J Am Soc Nephrol. 1997;8(5):784-792.

3. Fenton TR, Lyon AW, Eliasziw M, Tough SC, Hanley DA. Phosphate decreases urine calcium and increases calcium balance: a meta-analysis of the osteoporosis acid-ash diet hypothesis. Nutr J. 2009;8:41. doi:10.1186/1475-2891-8-41.

4. Fenton TR, Lyon AW, Eliasziw M, Tough SC, Hanley DA. Meta-analysis of the effect of the acid-ash hypothesis of osteoporosis on calcium balance. J Bone Miner Res. 2009;24(11):1835-1840. doi:10.1359/JBMR.090515.

5. Fenton TR, Tough SC, Lyon AW, Eliasziw M, Hanley DA. Causal assessment of dietary acid load and bone disease: a systematic review & meta-analysis applying Hill's epidemiologic criteria for causality. Nutr J. 2011;10:41. doi:10.1186/1475-2891-10-41.

6. Koeppen BM. The kidney and acid-base regulation. Adv Physiol Educ. 2009;33(4):275-281. doi:10.1152/advan.00054.2009.

7. Robey IF. Examining the relationship between diet-induced acidosis and cancer. Nutr Metab (Lond). 2012;9(1):72. doi:10.1186/1743-7075-9-72.

Biggest Loser Diet

1. Amidor T. Diet 101: The Biggest Loser Diet. Food Network. https://www.foodnetwork.com/healthyeats/diets/2010/03/diet-101-the-biggest-loser-diet. Published March 2017. Accessed June 2, 2020.

2. Health. Diet Review: The Biggest Loser. Health. https://www.health.com/weight-loss/diet-review-the-biggest-loser. Published October 2010. Accessed June 12, 2020.

3. U.S. News. Biggest Loser Diet. https://health.usnews.com/best-diet/biggest-loser-diet. Accessed June 12, 2020.

DASH Diet

1. Schwingshackl, L. Bogensberger, B. Hoffmann, G. Diet quality as assessed by the healthy eating index, alternate healthy eating index, dietary approaches to stop hypertension score, and health outcomes: An updated systematic review and meta-analysis of cohort studies. J of Nutr and Dietetics. https://jandonline.org/article/S2212-2672(17)31260-1/fulltext. Published October 27, 2017. Accessed July 28,2020. doi:https://doi.org/10.1016/j.jand.2017.08.02

Fast Away Fat Loss

1. Langer A. Faster way to fat loss- welcome to diet confusion. Abby Langer Nutrition. 2020. Accessed November 1, 2021. https://abbylangernutrition.com/faster-way-to-fat-loss-welcome-to-diet-con-fusion/.

F-Factor Diet

1. Oh R. Uppaluri KR. Low carbohydrate diet. StatPearls. Treasure Island, FL: StatPearls; 2020. https://www.ncbi.nlm.nih.gov/books/NBK537084/. Accessed June 12, 2020.

Gene Smart Diet

1. Fito M, Konstantinidou V. Nutritional genomics and the Mediterranean diet's effects on human cardiovascular health. Nutrients. 2016;8(4):218. doi:10.3390/nu8040218.

2. McAllister EJ, Dhurandhar NV, Keith SW et al. Ten putative contributors to the obesity epidemic. Crit Rev Food Sci Nutr 2009; 49(10): 868–913.

3. Tam V, Turcotte M, Meyre D. Established and emerging strategies to crack the genetic code of obesity. *Obesity Reviews*. 2019;212-240. doi: 10.1111/obr.12770.

4. U.S. National Library of Medicine. SLC19A3 gene: solute carrier family 19 member 3. U.S. National Library of Medicine. https://ghr.nlm.nih.gov/gene/SLC19A3#conditions. Published June 2020. Accessed July 5, 2020.

Genotype Diet

1. McAllister EJ, Dhurandhar NV, Keith SW et al. Ten putative contributors to the obesity epidemic. Crit Rev Food Sci Nutr 2009; 49(10): 868–913.

2. Tam V, Turcotte M, Meyre D. Established and emerging strategies to crack the genetic code of obesity. *Obesity Reviews*. 2019;212-240. doi: 10.1111/obr.12770.

3. U.S. National Library of Medicine. What did the Human Genome Project accomplish? U.S. National Library of Medicine. https://ghr.nlm.nih.gov/primer/hgp/accomplishments. Published May 2020. Accessed May 14, 2020.

hCG Diet

1. Bosch B, Venter I, Stewart RI, Bertram SR. Human Chorionic Gonadotrophin and weight loss. A double-blinded, placebo-controlled trial. S Afr Med J. 1990;77(4):185-189.

2. Kennedy L, Salinas R. Does the "HCG diet" provide additional weight loss compared with a low-calorie diet alone? Evidence-Based Practice. 2020 https://journals.lww.com/ebp/Citation/9000/Does_the__HCG_diet__provide_additional_weight_loss.99310.aspx. Accessed July 31. 2020. doi: 10.1097/EBP.0000000000000815

3. Stein MR, Julis RE, Peck CC, Hinshaw W, Sawicki JE, Deller JJ. Ineffectiveness of Human Chorionic Gonadotropin in weight reduction: a double-blind stuy. Am J Clin Nutr. 1976;29(9):940-948. doi:10.1093/ajcn/29.9.940.

4. U.S. Food & Drug Administration. HCG diet products are illegal. U.S. Food & Drug Administration. https://www.fda.gov/consumers/consumer-updates/hcg-diet-products-are-illegal. Updated September 2013. Accessed June 12, 2020.

Instinct Diet

1. Deckersbach T, Das SK, Urban LE, et al. Pilot randomized trial demonstrating reversal of obesity-related abnormalities in reward system responsivity to food cues with a behavioral intervention. Nutr Diabetes. 2014;4:e129. doi:10.1038/nutrd.2014.26.

Intermittent Fasting Diet Plan

1. Betts JA, Chowdhury EA, Gonzalez JT, Richardson JD, Tsintzas K, Thompson D. Is breakfast the most important meal of the day? Proceedings of the Nutrition Society. 2016, 75, 464–474 doi:10.1017/S0029665116000318

2. Carlson O, Martin B, Stote KS, Golden E, Maudsley S, Najjar SS, Ferrucci L, Ingram DK, Longo DL, Rumpler WV, Baer, DJ, Egan J, Mattson MP. Impact of reduced meal frequency without calorie restriction on glucose regulation in healthy, normal weight middle-aged men and women. Metabolism. 2007 Dec; 56(12):1729–34.

3. Cioffi I, Evangelistra A, Ponzo V, Ciccone G, Soldati L, Santarpia L, Contaldo F, Pasanisi F, Ghigo E, Bo S. Intermittent versus continuous energy restriction on weight loss and cardiometabolic outcomes: a systematic review and meta-analysis of randomized controlled trials. J Transl Med 2018;16:371-386. doi:10.1186/s12967-018-1748-4

4. De Cabo R, Mattson MP. Effects of intermittent fasting on health, aging, and disease. N Engl J Med. 2019; 381:26:2541-51.

5. Harvie M, Howell A. Potential benefits and harms of intermittent energy restriction and intermittent fasting amongst obese, overweight and normal weight subjects – A narrative review of human and animal evidence. Behav. Sci. 2017;7:4. doi:10.3390/bs7010004

6. Keys A. The residues of malnutrition and starvation. Science. 1950;112:371-373.

7. Most, J, Redman, LM. Impact of calorie restriction on energy metabolism in humans. Experimental Gerontology. 2020; Volume 133, May 2020, 110875 https://doi.org/10.1016/j.exger.2020.110875 -- https://www.sciencedirect.com/science/article/abs/pii/S0531556519308642

8. Patterson RE, Sears DD. Metabolic effects of intermittent fasting. Ann Rev Nutr. 2017;37:371-393. doi:10.1146/annurev-nutr-071816-064634.

9. Schnitker M, Mattman P, Bliss T. A clinical study of malnutrition in Japanese prisoners of war. Ann Intern Med. 1951;35:69-96.

Keto Diet Hypnosis

1. Mott T, Roberts J. Obesity and hypnosis: A review of literature. *American Journal of Clinical Hypnosis*. 2011;22(1):3-7. https://doi.org/10.1080/00029157.1979.10403994.

Keto Fast Diet

1. Pons V, Riera J, Capo X, et al. Calorie restriction regime enhances physical performance of trained athletes. J Int Soc Sports Nutr. 2018;15:12. doi:10.1186/s12970-018-0214-2.

Ketogenic Diet

1. Dudgeon WD, Kelley EP, Scheett TP. In a single-blind, matched group design: branched-chain amino acid supplementation and resistance training maintains lean body mass during a caloric restricted diet. J Int Soc Sports Nutr. 2016;13(1).

2. Fogelholm M. Effects of bodyweight reduction on sports performance. Sports Med. 1994;18(4):249–267. doi: 10.2165/00007256-199418040-00004.

3. Mettler S, Mitchell N, Tipton KD. Increased protein intake reduces lean body mass loss during weight loss in athletes. Med Sci Sports Exerc. 2010;42(2):326–337. doi: 10.1249/MSS.0b013e3181b2ef8e.

4. Nelms M, Sucher K, Lacey K, Roth SL. Nutrition Therapy & Pathophysiology. 2nd ed. Belmont, CA: Cengage; 2011.

5. Paoli A, Grimaldi K, Toniolo L, Canato M, Bianco A, Fratter A. Nutrition and acne: therapeutic potential of ketogenic diets. Skin Pharmacol Physiol. 2012;25:111–1174

The Makers Diet

1. Bissette A. The five most poisonous substances: from polonium to mercury. The Conversation. https://theconversation.com/the-five-most-poisonous-substances-from-polonium-to-mercury-29619. Published July 2014. Accessed May 13, 2020.

2. Soloway RAG. Do fillings cause mercury poisoning? Dental amalgams and mercury. National Capital Poison Center. https://www.poison.org/articles/2010-dec/do-fillings-cause-mercury-poisoning. Accessed May 13, 2020.

3. Toxicology Data Network. ChemIDplus. U.S. National Library of Medicine. https://chem.nlm.nih.gov/chemidplus/jsp/chemidheavy/help.jsp. Accessed May 13, 2020.

4. World Health Organization. Mercury and health. World Health Organization. https://www.who.int/news-room/fact-sheets/detail/mercury-and-health. Published March 2017. Accessed May 13, 2020.

New Atkins for a New You

1. Feinman RD, Pogozelski WK, Astrup A, et al. Dietary carbohydrate restriction as the first approach in diabetes management: critical review and evidence base. Nutrition. 2015;31:1-13. doi:10.1016/j.nut.2014.06.011

2. Nelms M, Sucher K, Lacey K, Roth SL. Nutrition Therapy & Pathophysiology. 2nd ed. Belmont, CA: Cengage; 2011.

Noom

Robinson-Walker D. Noom diet review: pros, cons and how it works. Forbes Health. 2021. Accessed November 1, 2021. https://www.forbes.com/health/body/noom-diet-review/.

The Obesity Code

1. Betts JA, Chowdhury EA, Gonzalez JT, Richardson JD, Tsintzas K, Thompson D. Is breakfast the most important meal of the day? Proc Nutr Soc. 2016;75(4):464-474. doi:10.1017/S0029665116000318.

2. Longo VD, Mattson MP. Fasting: molecular mechanisms and clinical applications. Cell Metab. 2014;19(2):181-192. doi:10.1016/j.cmet.2013.12.008.

3. Rigaud D, Hassid J, Meulemans A, Poupard AT, Boulier A. A paradoxical increase in resting energy expenditure in malnourished patients near death: the king penguin syndrome. Am J Clin Nutr. 2000;72(2):355-360. doi:10.1093/ajcn/72.2.355.

4. Zauner C, Schneeweiss, Kranz A. Resting energy expenditure in short-term starvation is increased as a result of an increase in serum norepinephrine. Am J Clin Nutr. 2000;71(6):1511-1515. doi:10.1093/ajcn/71.6.1511.

Raw Food Diet

1. Alcocer-Varela J, Iglesias J, Llorente L, Alarcon-Segovia D. Effects of L-canavanine on T cells may explain the induction of systemic lupus erythematosus by alfalfa. Arthritis Rheum. 1985;28(1):52-57. doi:10.1002/art.1780280109.

2. Brazier Y. The raw food diet: should I try it? Medical News Today. https://www.medicalnewstoday.com/articles/7381#what-can-i-eat. Published April 2020. Accessed May 13, 2020.

3. Division of Tuberculosis Elimination. Mycobacterium bovis (bovine tuberculosis) in humans. Centers for Disease Control and Prevention. https://www.cdc.gov/tb/publications/factsheets/general/mbovis.htm. Reviewed September 2012. Accessed May 13, 2020.

4. Hill GD. Plant Antinutritional Factors and Characteristics. In: Caballero B, Finglas P, Toldra F, ed. Encyclopedia of Food Sciences and Nutrition. 2nd ed. Cambridge, MA: Academic Publishing; 2003:4578-4587.

5. Memorial Sloan Kettering Cancer Center. Amygdalin. Memorial Sloan Kettering Cancer Center. https://www.mskcc.org/cancer-care/integrative-medicine/herbs/amygdalin. Updated February 2019. Accessed May 13, 2020.

6. National Resources Conservation Service. Phaseolus vulgaris L. kidney bean. https://plants.usda.gov/core/profile?symbol=PHVU. Accessed May 13, 2020.

Sugar Busters

1. Baskin DG, Porte D, Schwartz MW. Insulin signaling in the central nervous system: a critical role in metabolic homeostasis and disease from C. elegans to humans. Diabetes. 2005;54:1264-1276.

2. Blazquez E, Velazquez E, Hurtado-Carneiro V, Ruiz-Albusac JM. Insulin in the brain: its pathophysiological implications for states related with central insulin resistance, type 2 diabetes and Alzheimer's disease. Front Endocrinol (Lausanne). 2014;5:161. doi:10.3389/fendo.2014.00161.

3. Craft S. Insulin resistance and Alzheimer's disease pathogenesis: potential mechanisms and implications for treatment. Curr Alzheimer Res. 2007;4(2):147-152. doi: 10.2174/156720507780362137.

4. Craft S. Insulin resistance syndrome and Alzheimer disease: pathophysiologic mechanisms and therapeutic implications. Alzheimer Dis Assoc Discord. 2006;20(4):298-301.

5. Flint A, Gregersen NT, Gluud LL, et al. Associations between postprandial insulin and blood glucose responses, appetite sensations and energy intake in normal weight and overweight individuals: a meta-analysis of test meal studies. Br J Nutr. 2007;98:17-25. doi: 10.1017/S000711450768297X.

6. Neth BJ, Craft S. Insulin resistance and Alzheimer's disease: bioenergetic linkages. Front Aging Neurosci. 2017;9:345. doi: 10.3389/fnagi.2017.00345.

7. Neumann KF, Rojo L, Navarrete LP, Farias G, Reyes P, Maccioni RB. Insulin resistance and Alzheimer's disease: molecular links & clinical implications. Curr Alzheimer Res. 2008;5:000-000. doi: 10.2174/1567205087859019.

8. Park S. Hong SM, Sung SR, Junk HK. Long-term effects of central leptin and resistin on body weight, insulin resistance, and b-cell function and mass by the modulation of hypothalamic leptin and insulin signaling. Endocrinol. 2008;149(2):445-454. doi: 10.1210/en.2007-0754.

9. Porte D. Central regulation of energy homeostasis: the key role of insulin. Diabetes. 2006;55(2):S155-S160. doi: 10.2337/db06-S019.

10. Sharma MD, Garber AJ, Farmer JA. Role of insulin signaling in maintaining energy homeostasis. Endocr Pract. 2008;14(3):373-380.

11. Willett G. Sweet talk: the insulin connection. Institute for Natural Resources. February 2013-K.

Trinity Diet

1. Calixto J. Efficacy, safety, quality control, marketing and regulatory guidelines for herbal medicines (phytotherapeutic agents). 2000;33(2). https://doi.org/10.1590/S0100-879X2000000200004.

2. Niemeyer K, Bell I, Koithan M. Traditional knowledge of western herbal medicine and complex systems science. *J Herb Med*. 2013;3(3):112-119. doi:10.1016/j.hermed.2013.03.001.

3. Wilt T, Ishani A, Rutks I, et al. Phototherapy for benign photostatic hyperplasia. *Public Health Nutrition*. 2007;3(4):459-472. https://doi.org/10.1017/S1368980000000549.

Weight Down Diet

1. DeHaven MJ, Hunter IB, Wilder L, Walton JW, Berry J. Health programs in faith-based organizations: are they effective? Am J Public Health. 2004;94(6):1030-1036.

2. Kim KH, Linnan L, Campbell MK, Brooks C, Koenig HG, Wiesen C. The WORD (Wholeness, Oneness, Righteousness, Deliverance): a faith-based weight-loss program utilizing a community-based participatory research approach. Health Educ Behav. 2008;35(5):634-650. doi:10.1177/1090198106291985.

Weight Loss Cure Diet

1. Fair L. One true to take from the Trudeau story. Federal Trade Commission. https://www.ftc.gov/news-events/blogs/business-blog/2016/07/one-truth-take-trudeau-story. Published July 2016. Accessed May 12, 2020.

2. Greenway FL, Bray GA. Human chorionic gonadotropin (HCG) in the treatment of obesity: a critical assessment of the Simeons method. West J Med. 1977;127(6):461-463.

Werewolf Diet

1. UVA Health. The moon diet plan. MoonConnection.com. 2021. https://www.moonconnection.com/moon-diet.phtml.

Zone Diet

1. Mennen LI, Walker R, Bennetau-Pelissero C, Scalbert A. Risks and safety of polyphenol consumption. Am J Clin Nutr. 2005;81(1S):326S-329S. doi:10.1093/ajcn/81.1.326S.

2. Pandey KB, Rizvi SI. Plant polyphenols as dietary antioxidants in human health and disease. Oxid Med Cell Longev. 2009;2(5):270-278. doi:10.4161/oxim.2.5.9498.

Printed by Amazon Italia Logistica S.r.l.
Torrazza Piemonte (TO), Italy